Diatrizoate
Diazepam
Diazoxide
Diethylstilbestrol
Digitoxin
Diphenhydramine
Diphenylhydantoin
Doxepin
Erythromycin
Ethacrynic acid
Ethambutol
Ethanol
Ethosuximide
Fluorocytosine
Fluphenazine
Furosemide
Gentamicin
Glutethimide
Gold
Griseofulvin
Guanidine
Haloperidol
Heparin
Hydralazine
Hydrochlorothiazide
Hydroxychloroquine
Ibuprofen
Idoxuridine
Imipramine
Indomethacin
Insecticides
Iodides
Iopanoic acid
Isoniazid
Isoproterenol
Isotretinoin
Levodopa
Lincomycin
Marijuana
Measles vaccine
Mefenamic acid
Mephenytoin
Meprobamate
Mercury
Methapyrilene
Methicillin
Methimazole
Methyldopa
Methylthiouracil
Methysergide
Mumps vaccine
Nalidixic acid
Neomycin
Nitrofurantoin
Novobiocin
Orphenadrine
Oxacillin
Oxazepam
Oxyphenbutazone
Oxytetracycline
Paramethadione
Penicillamine
Penicillin
Pentamidine isethionate
Pentazocine
Pentobarbital
Phenacemide
Phenacetin
Phenformin
Phenindione
Phenobarbital
Phenylbutazone
Poliomyelitis vaccine
Polythiazide
Potassium

Practolol
Prednisone
Primidone
Probenecid
Procainamide
Procarbazine
Prochlorperazine
Propoxyphene
Propranolol
Propylthiouracil
Protriptyline
Pyrimethamine
Quinacrine
Quinidine
Quinine
Reserpine
Rifampin
Ristocetin
Rubella vaccine
Salicylamide
Salicylazosulfapyridine
Smallpox vaccine
Solvents
Spironolactone
Stibophen
Streptomycin
Sulfadiazine
Sulfadoxine
Sulfamerazine
Sulfamethazine
Sulfamethizole
Sulfamethoxazole
Sulfamethoxydiazine
Sulfamethoxypyridazine
Sulfanilamide
Sulfapyridine
Sulfathiazole
Sulfisoxazole
Tamoxifen
Tetracycline
Thallium
Thioridazine
Tolazamide
Tolbutamide
Toluene
Triamcinolone
Trifluoperazine
Trimeprazine
Trimethoprim
Trimethoprim-sulfamethoxazole
Typhoid-paratyphoid vaccine
Vitamin A
Vitamin K
Xylene

Thrombocytosis
Azathioprine
Benzene
Cefazolin
Cephalothin
Epinephrine
Ethanol
Fluoride
Penicillamine
Sulfamethoxypyridazine

Thrombotic Thrombocytopenic Purpura (TTP)
Contraceptive agents, oral
Hydralazine
Influenza vaccine
Methyldopa
Penicillin
Pertussis vaccine
Tetanus antitoxin

Typhoid-paratyphoid vaccine

Immunologically Mediated Thrombocytopenia
Analgesics
  Acetaminophen
  Antipyrine
  Aspirin
  Oxyphenbutazone
  Phenylbutazone
  Sodium salicylate
Antibacterials
  Ampicillin
  Cephalothin
  Lincomycin
  Novobiocin
  Oxytetracycline
  Para-aminosalicylate
  Penicillin
  Pentamidine
  Rifampicin
  Streptomycin
  Sulfonamides
Cinchona alkaloids
  Quinidine
  Quinine
Sedatives, hypnotics
  Allylisopropylacetylurea
  Allylisopropylbarbiturate
  Butabarbitone
  Carbamazepine
  Centalun
  Clonazepam
  Diphenylhydantoin
  Ethyl-allyl-acetylurea
  Ethylchlorvinyl
  Ethyl-phenylhydantoin
  Meprobamate
  Paramethadione
  Primidone
Sulfonamide derivatives
  Acetazolamide
  Chlorpropamide
  Chlorthalidone
  Clopamide
  Diazoxide
  Furosemide
  Glymidine
  Tolbutamide
Miscellaneous
  Alpha-methyldopa
  Antazoline
  Arsenical antiluetics
  Chloroquine
  Chlorothiazide
  Chlorpheniramine
  Copper sulfate
  Desimipramine
  Digitoxin
  Disulfiram
  Gold salts
  Hydrochlorothiazide
  Iopanoic acid
  Isoniazid (INH)
  Mercurial diuretics
  Nitrofurantoin
  Nitroglycerin
  Penicillamine
  Pertussis vaccine
  Prochlorperazine
  Propylthiouracil
  Spironolactone
  Stibophen
  Tetanus toxoid
  Thiouracil

(Adapted from Swanson M, Cook R: Drugs, Chemicals, Blood Dyscrasias. Hamilton, IL, Drug Intelligence Publishers, 1977. Kindly provided by Jerry L. Bauman, Pharm.D.)

Hemostasis and Thrombosis in the Clinical Laboratory

J. B. Lippincott Company

Philadelphia   London   Mexico City   New York   St. Louis   São Paulo   Sydney

Hemostasis and Thrombosis

IN THE CLINICAL LABORATORY

Edited by

Donna M. Corriveau, M.A., M.T.(A.S.C.P.), C.L.Sp.(H.)

Adjunct Assistant Professor,
Medical Technology Program,
Sangamon State University,
Springfield, Illinois

George A. Fritsma, M.S., M.T.(A.S.C.P.)

Associate Professor and Associate Head,
Department of Medical Laboratory Sciences,
University of Illinois at Chicago,
Chicago, Illinois

With 6 contributors

Acquisitions Editor: Lisa A. Biello
Sponsoring Editor: Delois Patterson
Manuscript Editor: Lee Henderson
Indexer: Angela Holt
Design Coordinator: Michelle Gerdes
Production Manager: Carol A. Florence
Production Coordinator: Barney Fernandes
Compositor: Progressive Typographers, Inc.
Printer/Binder: R. R. Donnelley & Sons Company

Library of Congress Cataloging-in-Publication Data

Hemostasis and thrombosis in the clinical laboratory.

Includes bibliographies and index.
1. Blood—Coagulation, Disorders of.   2. Thrombosis.
3. Blood—Coagulation.   4. Hemostasis.   I. Corriveau,
Donna M.   II. Fritsma, George A.   [DNLM: 1. Hemostasis.
2. Hemostatic Technics.   3. Technology, Medical.
4. Thrombosis.   WH 310 H4894]
RC647.C55H455   1988   616.1'57   87-3837
ISBN 0-397-50769-0

The authors and publishers have exerted every effort to ensure
that drug selection and dosage set forth in this text are in accord
with current recommendations and practice at the time of
publication. However, in view of ongoing research, changes in
government regulations, and the constant flow of information
relating to drug therapy and drug reactions, the reader is urged to
check the package insert for each drug for any change in
indications and dosage and for added warnings and precautions.
This is particularly important when the recommended agent is a
new or infrequently employed drug.

In Memoriam

Ruth M. French
1920 – 1987

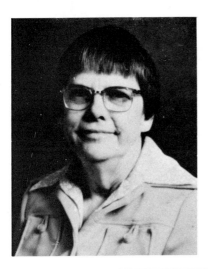

Ruth M. French was a Certified Medical Technologist who had been the first Head of the Department of Medical Laboratory Sciences of the University of Illinois at Chicago (1966 – 1972) and Associate Dean for Academic Affairs for the College of Associated Health Professions (1972 – 1984). She was Associate Dean, Emerita, from 1984 until her death. She was active in the National Accrediting Agency for Clinical Laboratory Sciences from 1974 to 1987 and held numerous positions of leadership in the American Society for Medical Technology and the American Society of Allied Health Professions. She was a noted author, and in addition to several book chapters, wrote *Guide to Diagnostic Procedures,* now in its fifth edition, and *Dynamics of Health Care,* in its third edition. Over her life, Ms. French received numerous honors.

Ruth French was a noted authority and consultant in allied health education. She founded the Department of Medical Laboratory Sciences of the University of Illinois at Chicago and was instrumental in the founding of the University's College of Associated Health Professions. She was particularly respected for her foresight, gifted self-expression of innovative ideas, and ability to support and promote the growth of her colleagues. Through thoughtful suggestions and open support, Ruth French encouraged the advancement of countless developing professionals. Her ability to elicit the best from those who respected her contributed immeasurably to an attitude of excellence in the allied health professions. The editors owe a great deal of their personal growth to the concern and encouragement of Ruth French, and we therefore dedicate this textbook in her memory.

In Memoriam

Andrew E. Weiss
1930–1987

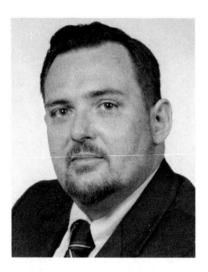

The editors regret to report the untimely death of Andrew E. Weiss, M.D., November 12, 1987. Dr. Weiss was a pediatric hematologist who founded and directed the Regional Comprehensive Hemophilia Center of Central and Northern Illinois. He was a nationally recognized expert in coagulation whose life was never limited by hemophilia. He wrote from a personal perspective that illuminates his chapters in this text. His wisdom, enthusiasm, and friendship are missed by the editors, his colleagues, and his friends.

Contributors

Larry D. Brace, Ph.D., M.T.(A.S.C.P.)S.H.
Associate Professor,
Department of Medical Laboratory Sciences,
University of Illinois at Chicago,
Chicago, Illinois

Donna M. Corriveau, M.A., M.T.(A.S.C.P.), C.L.Sp.(H.)
Adjunct Assistant Professor,
Medical Technology Program,
Sangamon State University,
Springfield, Illinois

Gerald L. Davis, M.T.(A.S.C.P.), C.L.S.(N.C.A.), Ph.D.
Director, Medical Laboratory Science,
Northeastern University,
Boston, Massachusetts

Barrett W. Dick, M.D.
Clinical Professor of Pathology,
Southern Illinois School of Medicine;
Pathologist,
Director of Hematology Laboratory,
Department of Laboratory Medicine,

Memorial Medical Center,
Springfield, Illinois

George A. Fritsma, M.S., M.T.(A.S.C.P.)
Associate Professor and Associate Head,
Department of Medical Laboratory Sciences,
University of Illinois at Chicago,
Chicago, Illinois

Harlene Stapf Palkuti, B.S., M.T.(A.S.C.P.)
Hemostasis Consultant,
Sunnyvale, California

Jeanine M. Walenga, Ph.D., M.T.(A.S.C.P.), C.L.S.(N.C.A.)
Supervisor and Research Associate,
Hemostasis Research Laboratories,
Department of Pathology,
Loyola University Medical Center,
Maywood, Illinois

Andrew E. Weiss, M.D.
Associate Professor and Head,
Pediatric Hematology–Oncology,
University of Illinois College of Medicine at Peoria,
Peoria, Illinois

Forewords

Medical science is at a very exciting age. New technologies allow the body to be studied in greater detail than ever in both the research and clinical laboratories. Recent developments in monoclonal biochemistry and, subsequently, in immunoassay testing have found practical applications in many other laboratories, including microbiology, chemistry, and hematology. Computerization of clinical laboratory instruments has increased the precision, sensitivity, and specificity of tests, resulting in more rapid diagnoses and faster, better-targeted treatment. Furthermore, cooperation between medical laboratories and health care specialists is greater than ever. These technological advances and improvements in health care teamwork promise exciting new developments in testing methodologies, leading to a better understanding of how the body functions.

Blood dynamics — hemostasis — has fascinated mankind for ages. Even today it remains intriguing because of its complexity. For example, a delicate balance exists between the mechanisms of clot formation and clot lysis: What happens when this balance is upset? Platelets detect and repair vessel damage: How do they accomplish this? What initiates a clot, and what prevents it from growing too large? These are some of the questions that are answered in *Hemostasis and Thrombosis in the Clinical Laboratory*.

The authors begin with a brief historical perspective of coagulation, providing a colorful backdrop against which hemostasis unfolds. The reader meets the Crown Prince Alexis and his mysterious disease and discovers that Plato and Aristotle were among the first to observe fibrin formation. Coagulation tests such as the prothrombin time and the activated partial thromboplastin time are introduced, along with the scientists who developed them and originated terms such as *hemophilia*. Hence, the reader experiences the science of hemostasis at its birth. The text steps lightly into the realm of pathology and histology, with more emphasis on physiology and biochemistry. One particularly intricate chapter, Chapter 8, provides a challenging discussion of platelet biochemistry.

An exceptional characteristic of this text is the inclusion of case studies preceding each chapter. Most cases present clinical and laboratory manifestations of a specific bleeding disorder and raise questions concerning coagulation testing and diagnosis. The cases are interesting and provide good examples of the practical application of coagulation testing. Other helpful features include illustrations and tables that are organized to facilitate study, a glossary, and thorough discussion of complex concepts.

From the perspective of a recent graduate, this text is excellent not only for the student first encountering hemostasis, but also for the more advanced student.

Jeanne M. Manganello, M.T.(A.S.C.P.), C.L.S.(N.C.A.)
Staff Technologist
University of Illinois Hospital
Chicago, Illinois

The field of hemostasis and blood coagulation is experiencing significant growth and change as its importance in the diagnosis and management of clinical disorders is rapidly becoming appreciated.

Until recently, the primary concern of the hemostasis laboratory was to diagnose simple bleeding problems and assess anticoagulant therapy. Now it is essential to identify patients at risk for thrombosis or to differentiate among a variety of potential bleeding disorders to better manage the patient as new techniques become available.

The hemostasis laboratory now determines the level and function of plasma procoagulant proteins and their activators and inhibitors, as well as evaluates platelet and endothelial cell functions.

These advances have been made possible by incorporating protein biochemistry, immunology, molecular biology, and other disciplines into the field.

The changes that have occurred have had a profound effect on the technology in the laboratory. Progress has been made from water bath, stopwatch, tilt-tube clotting tests to automated, multipurpose, optical instruments. Spectrophotometers, electrophoresis chambers, and chromatographic equipment are becoming prominent. Technologists are faced with a tremendous task of reeducation to remain current and proficient.

This important new text provides the reader with a clear, concise guide to the laboratory management of disorders of hemostasis.

The contributors to *Hemostasis and Thrombosis in the Clinical Laboratory* are well qualified and active in laboratory practice and in education. The various chapters offer views and ideas based on current practice in different locations, representing state-of-the-art technology blended into a cohesive, timely publication.

Gordon E. Ens, M.T.(A.S.C.P.)
Laboratory Director
Colorado Coagulation Consultants;
Editor
Clinical Hemostasis Review
Denver, Colorado

Preface

Hemostasis and Thrombosis in the Clinical Laboratory is a comprehensive learning guide for the student of medical technology, the medical student, and the pathology resident. It is also designed to be a shelf reference for the clinical laboratory that performs routine and special coagulation procedures. All of the important areas of hemostasis are presented, including vascular integrity, the platelet's role, coagulation, and fibrinolysis. Normal physiology of each of these systems is stressed, as are the control mechanisms.

The organization of the book reflects the editors' intent to provide a text that begins with the basics and proceeds to intermediate, then advanced principles of hemostasis. The language is both active and direct, with ample illustrations to aid the learner in understanding hemostasis. The physiological aspects of hemostasis are combined with the complex biochemical reactions to give the reader a complete picture.

Laboratory techniques are described in detail, reflecting the standard progression of principle, materials, protocol, expected results, and clinical application. Each technique is keyed to its particular role in the hemostatic mechanism and the pathophysiologic problems that affect test results. Separate chapters are devoted to the commonly described disorders of hemostasis, including congenital and acquired coagulation and platelet defects, platelet number problems, hypercoagulation, vascular disease, and fibrinolysis.

Each chapter begins with a case study, illustrating the clinical application for that chapter. The overall chapter organization proceeds from simple to complex, beginning with historic perspectives and common laboratory practice, then proceeding to a discussion of more complex biochemical mechanisms, such as internal cellular messengers and advanced instrumental techniques of immunoassay and chromogenic substrates. The book concludes with a look toward the future of testing in hemostasis.

Donna M. Corriveau, M.A., M.T.(A.S.C.P.), C.L.Sp.(H.)

George A. Fritsma, M.S., M.T.(A.S.C.P.)

Acknowledgments

It is our privilege to acknowledge those whose support, materials, skills, encouragement, and patience have made this textbook possible. Jeanne Manganello, Elmer Koneman, Larry Brace, Jean Corriveau, and Mary Anne Loafman skillfully reviewed manuscript drafts, providing many helpful suggestions. Leon LeBeau, Owen Rugg, Rich Doering, Tom Gunter, and Marcin Hiolski provided expert assistance with the preparation of the artwork and photomicrographs. Jerry Bauman, Andrew Weiss, and Judy Sutherland were generous with a variety of source materials. President Durwood Long and Vice-President of Academic Affairs Michael Ayers, of Sangamon State University, supported the artwork by kindly granting use of the institution's resources. Andrew Maturen, head of the Department of Medical Laboratory Sciences at the University of Illinois at Chicago, generously provided the time and materials for manuscript preparation, while Lorean Schroeder, Carrie O'Rourke, and Monica Rassoul assisted with word processing. Several colleagues relieved the editors of administrative and scholastic duties during this time: Christopher Anderson, Mary Anne Loafman, Barbara Glinski, David Reid, Lauralyn Lebeck, Scott Duratinsky, Larry Brace, Andrew Maturen, Bev Fiorella, Larry Schoeff, and Joanne Bradna. Finally, the book would never have been completed without the encouragement and patience of our families. Special thanks to Gregory, Jean-Paul, Teri Jo, and Robert Georges, and most of all to our spouses, Paula and Jean.

Contents

Hemostasis and Thrombosis in the Clinical Laboratory

Major Elements of Hemostasis

Donna M. Corriveau

Hemostasis is the mechanism by which the body controls bleeding after injury. Originally, this term meant only the formation of a clot, an insoluble barrier to blood loss. Today, the definition of hemostasis includes the chemical responses of the blood vessels, platelet activation, and the biochemical reactions that lead to clot formation and dissolution.

This chapter will begin with a case study and history of hemostasis up to the 1960s. A basic overview of the subject will follow, presenting the concepts of the 1980s. Biochemical experiments, electron microscopy, and immunologic techniques — all inventions of the 20th century — are now being applied extensively to the study of hemostasis to reveal its physiological complexity.

The historical perspective is presented as an aid in developing a preliminary understanding of and appreciation for the research efforts that led to our current level of knowledge, although the concepts currently held acceptable are sometimes quite different from the hypotheses of the past. For instance, hemophilia was once thought to be a singular bleeding disorder. We now know that there are several biochemical defects that can each lead to bleeding problems. The finding of these specific biochemical defects has altered the theory of blood clotting. There are valuable lessons that can be learned from history, and the history of hemostasis is no exception. Several excellent textbooks give a more detailed historical account for the interested reader.[8a,37,41]

CASE STUDY   In Spala, Poland, in September 1912, Crown Prince Alexis, age 8, of Russia experienced extreme pain following a jostling carriage ride. The pain, located in the left leg and lower abdomen, was of such severity that the young tsarevich was immobilized.

History and Physical Examination

Alexis was the son of Tsar Nicholas II and Tsarina Alexandra. He was examined by the physician to the royal family, Dr. Eugene Botkin, and several other eminent physicians of Russia. They examined the young prince repeatedly in an attempt to alleviate the problem, yet hemorrhaging, the cause of the pain, continued. The mother and physicians reported several previous episodes of joint and abdominal pain following various normal childhood activities like climbing trees or playing games.

Records indicate that young Alexis was diagnosed with femoral neuropathy secondary to retroperitoneal bleeding.[56] The left hip was flexed outward. Femoral nerve involvement was indicated by the external rotation of the hip and the thigh drawn up to the chest. There was a large hematoma over the medial thigh and groin. The child was in agony, semiconscious, groaning, and delirious.

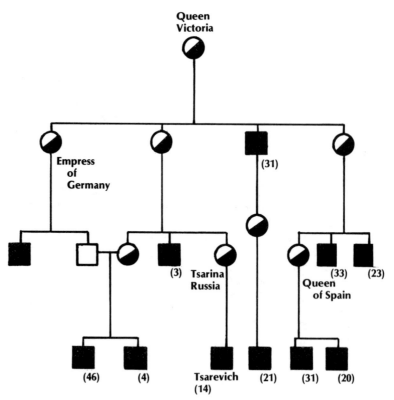

FIG. 1-1. Pedigree of classic hemophilia in the royal families of Europe. Affected males are shown by darkened boxes and carrier females by half-darkened circles. Numbers below the boxes indicate the year of death.

The physicians agreed that the child was suffering from hemophilia, a bleeding disorder, but they were unsuccessful in treating the problem. The Tsarina had other family members, including her brother, her uncle, three cousins, and five nephews, with similar conditions. Several had died. Later records showed documentation of hemorrhagic disorders in several lines of the royal families of Europe (Fig. 1-1). The disease appeared to be caused by a sex-linked recessive gene, with a hereditary pattern in which the women were carriers and the men were symptomatic. Apparently the Tsarina was a carrier.

Course

The boy's symptoms continued for 2 weeks while physicians continued their prodding examinations. Meanwhile, the mother, desperate for her son's life, sought the help of a Siberian peasant priest by the name of Grigori Rasputin (Fig. 1-2). Rasputin belonged to a deviate religious sect and was believed to have many mysterious powers. It was his reputation as a healer that attracted the Tsarina to seek his expertise. His words to the Tsarina were, "God has seen your tears and heard your prayers. Do not grieve. The

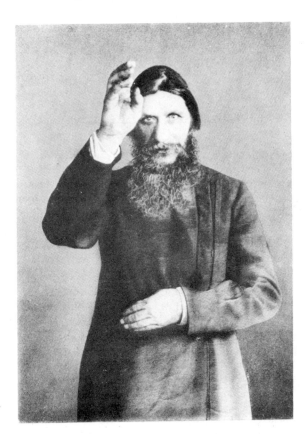

FIG. 1-2. Grigori Efimovich Rasputin. (Culver Pictures)

Little One will not die. Do not allow the doctors to bother him too much."[56] Two days later the bleeding stopped, and the boy was again free from pain. Rasputin was credited with the cure of this particular case in spite of not examining Alexis. Once the physicians stopped the constant probing, a clot was able to form without being dislodged.

Rasputin gained influence over the Tsar and Tsarina by his ability to stop other bleeding episodes in Alexis. Some say these events may have influenced the course of Russian history. Alexis died at the age of 14, the same year that his entire family was executed (July 16–17, 1918).

This case study exemplifies an interesting event of the past, connecting history with hemostasis. For years scientists puzzled over how Rasputin was able to stop the bleeding in the tsarevich. Did he really possess strange, demonic powers? In the above case, common sense was the reason for his success, but later accounts of his treatments attribute his powers to hypnosis. It is interesting to note that scientists are again beginning to appreciate the use of hypnosis in treating hemophiliacs.[26]

We can learn from those before us who have paved the way in hemostasis research. Many dedicated investigators have contributed to our current understanding through their successful discoveries and through their failures. Sometimes, what is not proven is also vital information about a problem. It is not possible to name all of the scientists or their research in this chapter. Selected significant contributions will be highlighted. By no means should this imply that those not mentioned were insignificant or unimportant. Many enhanced the development of our understanding of the processes of hemostasis to be what it is today.

HISTORY

Hemophilia is the oldest recognized bleeding disorder; references to it date back to the Babylonian Talmud in Tractate Yevamouth 64b.[2,43] In this treatise by Yevamouth, it was recognized in the second century that a bleeding condition existed if, after two male children were circumcised, they died. The famous talmudist and physician Moses Maimonides writes in the Mishneh Torah about hemophilia:

> If a woman had her first son circumcised and he died as a result of the circumcision which enfeebled his strength and she similarly had her second circumcised — whether the latter child was from her first husband or from her second husband — the third son may not be circumcised at the proper time. Rather one postpones the operation for him until he grows up and his strength is established.[32]

This disorder was not called hemophilia (love of hemorrhage) until 1828 with the publication of a thesis by Dr. Friedrich Hopff.[8] Dr. Hopff credits his teacher, Schönlein, with origination of the term.[27,46] Clinical descriptions of hemophilia date back to 1803, when Otto wrote of several bleeder families.[36] Others have also described elaborate pedigrees of famous hemophilic families from Tenna and Wald, Switzerland; Ipswich, Massachusetts; and Württemberg and Kirchheim, Germany; and in the royal families of Europe.[10,16,17,22,52] The entire historical account of hemophilia can be found in *Handbook of Hemophilia*, edited by Brinkhous and Hemker.[8]

Fibrin Formation

The first to note that fibers formed when blood cooled were Plato and Aristotle.[39] Malpighi, however, has been credited as the first major contributor to our understanding of fibrin clot formation. In the mid – 17th century, he washed cells from a blood clot, studying the morphology of the remaining fibers and cells under the microscope.[33]

In 1780 William Hewson demonstrated that these fibers came from plasma, documenting Petit's earlier observation that clots form to stop bleeding.[25,38] Collecting blood in basins, he experimented with the clotting of whole blood, observing that the clotting time was shortened in patients with inflammatory diseases and infinitely prolonged in a woman after delivery.[24] Fibrinogen (later designated Factor I), the precursor plasma protein to fibrin, was described in 1845 by the Scottish physiologist Andrew Buchanan.[9] Others then began to look for a mechanism or factor that would cause the fibrin to form. The existence of this factor that we now call thrombin was debated until the present century.

Thrombin Formation

Alexander Schmidt has been called "the father of blood coagulation" because he realized that thrombin could not circulate in blood but must be in an inactive, precursor form.[45] This precursor, called prothrombin by Pekelharing in 1891 and later designated Factor II, was not purified until 1960 by Walter Seegers.[48]

Assembling the work of others, Morawitz wrote his classic theory of blood coagulation in 1905 (Fig. 1-3).[35] Clotting, or *coagulation,* as it was then called, appeared to require two steps: (1) the conversion of prothrombin to thrombin by tissue thromboplastin (later designated Factor III) and (2) the conversion of fibrinogen to fibrin by thrombin. Calcium (later designated Factor IV) was thought necessary for only step one.

Morawitz's theory was upheld until the 1930s, at which time other plasma clotting factors like Factor VII (1948) were discovered as a result of new methods to measure thrombin generation. With these new tests it was possible to detect diseases associated with certain factor deficiencies. Morawitz's theory, however, provided the foundation for these later discoveries.

The discovery of additional coagulation factors led to the distinction between the extrinsic and the intrinsic pathways of coagulation. Similar to Schmidt's hypothesis, a theory of Thackrah in 1819 described the extrinsic path as initiated by tissue injury and thromboplastin release.[51] This was confirmed by de Bainville several years later when he infused brain tissue into the vessels of animals and observed total occlusion of those vessels by a clot.[14]

The theories of Morawitz and Schmidt delayed acceptance of the intrinsic pathway theory of coagulation, which held that contact with a foreign surface activated coagulation. At the time scientists believed that only one theory could be true and that the extrinsic path had been proven; therefore, the other theory must be false. It took the discovery of additional biochemical factors involved in coagulation to prove that both

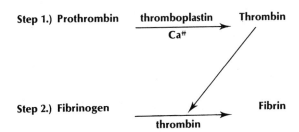

FIG. 1-3. The first theory of blood coagulation.

theories were right. It is now realized that these two pathways of proteins converge and interact in several ways to form thrombin, which eventually leads to fibrin formation. The intrinsic system of coagulation, involving Factor VIII (discovered in 1937 and originally named antihemophilic globulin [AHG]) and other plasma proteins, was found to be more complicated because more coagulation proteins were involved.

As plasma clotting factors were discovered, others worked on tests to measure their activity. Warner, Brinkhous, and Smith at the University of Iowa in 1936 devised a two-step method to measure prothrombin.[54] At the same time Armand Quick invented the still-used one-stage prothrombin time.[40] He had difficulty getting his work published until 1959. Later, investigators discovered discrepancies between the results of the two methods. When stored blood and blood from persons with bleeding disorders were tested, normal results were obtained under certain conditions but not all the time. Although the factors had not been given their formal nomenclature at that time, it is now known that Factor IX was present in the stored blood, but Factor VIII was not. The deficient factor in the patient sample was present in the stored sample for some patients, but not all of them. This finding differentiated hemophiliacs into type A (Factor VIII deficiency) and type B (Factor IX deficiency).[3] Factor IX deficiency was reported in the December 1952 issue of the British Medical Journal as Christmas Disease. A rather interesting letter to the editor followed this issue:

> hastening through its pages to discover what seasonable though morbid experiences had been enjoyed by no less than seven distinguished haematologists, we were similarly disappointed to find that this festal title was merely a ferial eponym for an all-the-year-round disease, derived from the name of its victims.[12]

Factors X, XI, XII, and XIII, Fletcher factor, and Fitzgerald factor were discovered in 1956, 1953, 1955, 1944, 1965, and 1975, respectively. In 1962 an international committee on nomenclature met in Rome to establish the use of Roman numerals in designating the factors. Elucidation of these factors allowed researchers to further understand the intrinsic pathway of coagulation, in which they were found. Initiation of coagulation without tissue thromboplastin was clarified, and various hemophilias could be separated by their specific factor deficiency. Macfarlane, in 1964, proposed the term *cascade* to describe his hypothesis for factor activation.[31] Davie and Ratnoff described a similar coagulation scheme as the waterfall cascade. Both proposed that the factors were enzymes that must be activated in order to activate the next protein in the sequence.

In the meantime, Seegers' group had conceived of another theory centered on the prothrombin molecule. That hypothesis involves a variety of subunits of prothrombin designated *autoprothrombins* (see Autoprothrombins).[47] All of these are dependent on vitamin K for production. The simplicity of Seegers' theory is appealing, but the cascade reaction (in a modified form) is now the generally accepted model.

Vitamin K

The story of vitamin K is another dramatic one in the history of hemostasis. The discovery of a "Koagulations-Vitamin" by Henrik Dam led to his being awarded a Nobel Prize in physiology in 1943 for his work on chicks fed a diet of ether-extracted grain.[13] Following this diet, the chicks developed bleeding tendencies. His co–Nobel Prize winner, Edward Doisy, is credited with the isolation of the naphthoquinone structure for the vitamin K family and its presence in green leafy plants. Later work led to the

AUTOPROTHROMBINS*

Prethrombin: a subunit of prothrombin from which thrombin is generated. It is the substrate for the reaction.
Autoprothrombin Ip: a procoagulant from prothrombin when calcium and platelet factor 3 (PF$_3$) are present
Autoprothrombin Ic: an equivalent of Factor X that results from activation of prothrombin by autoprothrombin C
Autoprothrombin II: an equivalent of Factor VIII or platelet factor 1, or perhaps Factor IX. It is generated from prothrombin by thrombin in the absence of calcium.
Autoprothrombin III: an intermediate between prothrombin and autoprothrombin C
Autoprothrombin C: the enzyme that actually splits thrombin from the prothrombin molecule

* Autoprothrombins are derivatives of the prothrombin molecule, which is the center of Seegers' concept of coagulation.
(Data from Owen CA, Bowie EJ, Thompson JH: The Diagnosis of Bleeding Disorders, 2nd ed, pp 51–52. Boston, Little, Brown & Co, 1975)

actual discovery of vitamin K's role in the production of certain coagulation proteins and its relationship with liver disease.[55]

In the 1930s a farmer noted hemorrhagic disease in his herd of cattle following dehorning or castration. He requested Paul Link, a biochemist at the University of Wisconsin, to investigate the problem. A similar incident in 1921 in Canada suggested that the culprit was spoiled sweet clover ingested by the cattle. In spoiling, biochemical changes occurred in the clover. Link extracted from this spoiled feed a chemical, bishydroxycoumarin—dicumarol. In connection with Quick, he learned that the prothrombin time of the cows' blood was prolonged, showing that the production of prothrombin was decreased in those cattle that ate the spoiled clover.[29] They concluded that somehow dicumarol was an antagonist to vitamin K, producing hypoprothombinemia and bleeding. Warfarin, a derivative of dicumarol, received its name from the Wisconsin Agricultural Research Foundation (WARF), where the research took place. Warfarin is still used today as a rat poison and anticoagulant. The use of dicumarol derivatives marked the advent of anticoagulant therapy for thromboembolic disease.

Platelets

Independent of one another, Donne,[15] Gerber,[18] Addison,[1] and Simon[49,53] first described the platelet in 1842. Donne concluded that platelets were derived from the fatty particles in the chyle. The other hypotheses suggested that platelets were precipitates from plasma or fragments of the endothelium. Hayem, in 1878, confirmed that the platelet was a unique element of the blood.[23] He also showed that it changed shape in conjunction with fibrin formation. He postulated that the platelet exchanged coagulant substances with the plasma.

In 1882, Bizzozero wrote his classic paper describing "viscous metamorphosis" of platelets.[4] In it he stated, "Platelets become granular within the lumen of an injured vessel; and this change produces a substance which activates the coagulation system to form fibrin."

A bridge was crossed in 1906 when Wright confirmed Bizzozero's theory of the origin of the platelet from the bone marrow megakaryocyte.[60]

In 1896 Hayem recognized the importance of platelets in clot retraction and the ability of the clot to shrink. Studying a patient with a clinical bleeding problem characterized by the inability of the clot to retract even in the presence of normal platelet numbers, Glanzmann theorized that some internal platelet constituent was necessary for clot retraction.[19] How that contractile protein, called thrombosthenin or actomyosin, worked was unclear. The disorder was named Glanzmann's thrombasthenia, and it was the first recorded qualitative platelet disorder.

With the introduction of the electron microscope in the 1940s, scientists could view the platelet and its functions at the molecular level.[59] In 1947 both Quick and Brinkhous independently described platelet factors that contributed to thrombin formation.[7] In 1951 Harrington discovered an antiplatelet antibody that destroyed not only platelets but those cytoplasmic portions of megakaryocytes from which platelets are derived.[21]

In 1956 Braunsteiner and Pakesch showed that in thrombopathy (the old term for a platelet abnormality), the platelet was unable to provide a substance called platelet factor 3 for coagulation.[6] The same year, Born noted that adenosine triphosphate (ATP, a source of energy) was consumed in platelet transformation.[5] These discoveries were vital to the study of platelet function. The key roles of ATP and PF_3, coupled with advancements in research techniques (histochemical, biochemical, and immunologic), opened the door for further platelet investigations. From the 1950s to the present, there has been an abundance of research on the platelet and its central role in hemostasis.[20,34,50]

Fibrinolysis

At the end of the 18th century, John Hunter observed that blood from people who died of accidents, seizures, electrical injury, or lightning strikes, or who died in anger, did not clot.[28] In 1937 Macfarlane confirmed that observation with further research suggesting that an activator of plasminogen (the precursor to the protein that aids in clot breakdown) was in those tissues.[30] When the tissues were damaged, this activator was released, starting the process of clot dissolution. In essence, it made the blood fluid when normally the blood would clot following death. The ability of plasma to allow blood to clot when necessary, yet also to dissolve that clot, is a remarkable process. No doubt future research in thrombosis and fibrinolysis will enhance our understanding of the mechanisms causing coronary heart disease and thromboembolic disorders.

OVERVIEW OF HEMOSTASIS

Hemostasis is the mechanism by which the body prevents loss of blood from the vascular system. It is a complex system, involving cells and biochemicals, that maintains a state of fluidity in normal circulation but forms a barrier when trauma or pathologic conditions cause vessel damage. In most cases the hemostatic mechanism repairs minute vascular changes without noticeable signs or symptoms. However, in certain instances, with trauma resulting from laceration, abrasion, or bruise, the mechanism is called upon to participate extensively in a process of clot formation. When there is major damage like this, platelets, vessels, and certain plasma proteins react to form a thrombus. The wound is closed, and other biochemicals are released to aid in initiating healing and tissue growth.

Hemorrhage, the loss of blood from the vascular system, triggers the hemostatic mechanism. In congenital hemophilias part of the mechanism is missing or does not function properly. In persons with hemophilia, hemorrhage may proceed unchecked, resulting in disability and pain. Some acquired hemostatic disorders, caused by systemic disease or the presence of toxins, lead to a total loss of control of the hemostatic mechanism resulting in shock or even death.

Other hereditary and acquired defects and deficiencies result in the tendency to form clots or thrombi inappropriately. These are associated with stroke, heart disease, and deep vein thrombosis, resulting in death, paralysis, or damage to tissues.

Normal hemostasis, then, is a complex system of many checks and balances that allows our body to maintain the fluidity of the blood with minimal bleeding, while clotting only at the site of trauma (Fig. 1-4). Simply stated, hemostasis can be divided into two stages: primary and secondary.

Primary hemostasis is the direct closure of a damaged blood vessel by vessel constriction or platelet adhesion of individual platelets sticking to the vessel wall. This happens immediately after trauma and is often sufficient to stop the bleeding. The role of the platelet and vasculature in primary hemostasis is a simple one of ongoing vascular repair. However, many times a more complex clot is required than the fragile clot of primary hemostasis.

In *secondary hemostasis* a tougher clot composed of fibrin and platelets is formed. It requires the enzymatic reactions of the coagulation proteins to produce the fibrin along with the platelet factors to establish a firmer, more stabilized fibrin clot (hemostatic plug).

The clot gradually dissolves, and tissue repair takes place normally. Clot dissolution is called fibrinolysis, a process that involves certain proteolytic enzymes to degrade the fibrin in the clot. Fibrinolysis completes the process of hemostasis.

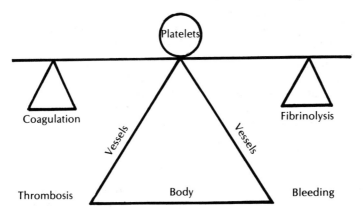

FIG. 1-4. The balance of hemostasis. The vasculature (vessels), coagulation and fibrinolytic proteins, and platelets all work together to aid in thrombus formation when needed at a certain point. The platelet is the center of thrombogenesis. A swing of the balance to the right (*i.e.,* too much fibrinolysis or too little coagulation) can result in bleeding, whereas a swing to the left (*i.e.,* too much coagulation or lowered fibrinolytic factors) can result in pathologic thrombosis.

In summary, primary and secondary hemostasis involves three important elements: blood vessels, platelets, and coagulation and fibrinolytic proteins. The interaction of these three components maintains our ability to avoid bleeding to death from trauma. When there is a defect due to a deficiency in one component, a hemorrhagic diathesis (tendency to bleed) may occur. However, there are parts of each component that, when deficient, could result in a tendency to thrombose. The study of hemostasis is a complicated one that involves many interrelated components that are not separable. One should study each part individually but then attempt to put all concepts together. The hemostatic mechanism is a dynamic one with many overlapping sequences and systems.

The Role of Blood Vessels

Blood vessels conduct the blood supply to and from all parts of the body. The vasculature is a closed system that maintains blood in a fluid state unless a rupture occurs. Thick-walled arteries conduct blood away from the heart, and thinner-walled veins direct blood back to the heart. Large *elastic arteries* near the heart branch into intermediate *muscular arteries* that distribute the blood throughout the body. Muscular arteries branch into *arterioles* that in turn branch into *capillaries,* the thinnest of the vessels, composed of a single layer of endothelium. Capillaries converge into *post-capillary venules* that, together with the capillaries, form an exchange bed for nutrients and wastes. Polymorphonuclear neutrophils, monocytes, and lymphocytes can also pass from the blood to the intracellular spaces through the gaps and fenestrations in the thin capillary walls. Venules combine to form *intermediate veins* that further converge to form *large veins*. Almost every artery has its corresponding vein. Figure 1-5 schematically illustrates the circulatory system. Following is a discussion of the normal histologic and physiologic features of the vasculature and how each plays a role in hemostasis.[42]

Histology of the Blood Vessels
The walls of arteries and veins have three layers in cross section. From innermost to outermost, these are the *tunica intima,* the *tunica media,* and the *tunica adventitia.* The layers are made up of the following tissue components:

- Tunica intima: a single endothelial cell layer, the basal lamina (basement membrane) associated with the endothelium and composed of collagenous fibers, subendothelial connective tissue with smooth muscle cell fibers, and an internal elastic lamina composed of elastic connective tissue
- Tunica media: smooth muscle cells and elastic tissue embedded in loose connective tissue
- Tunica adventitia: external elastic lamina at the border of the media and adventitia, loose connective tissue with collagen fibers, fibroblasts

The histologic composition of the blood vessel layers varies with the size of the vessel and whether it is an artery or vein. The structure of each type of vessel reflects its function.

ELASTIC ARTERIES. The elastic arteries (*i.e.,* the aorta, subclavian arteries, and carotid arteries) are those arteries closest to the heart. They are structured to respond to the mechanical pressures of a pumping heart, dissipating the heart pulse and pressure. Elastic arteries can expand and return to their normal size, due to the elastic compo-

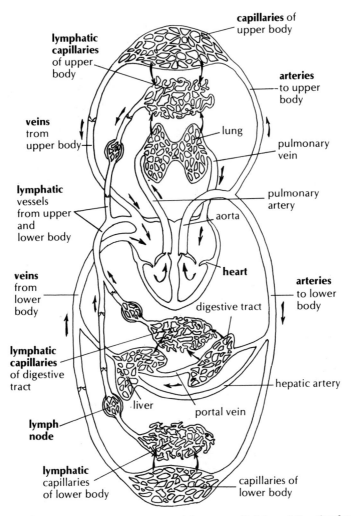

FIG. 1-5. Schematic representation of the arterial–venous division of the circulatory system. Arrows indicate the flow of blood.

nent; but they do not contract, because there is little muscle cell content. The intima of the elastic artery is thicker than in any other artery or vein. It includes endothelium, basal lamina or membrane, and collagenous connective tissue with a few elastic fibers. The internal elastic lamina is indistinct, since it is mixed with the elastic tissue of the tunica media. The media is the thickest of the three layers. It is composed primarily of elastic tissue interspersed with a few smooth muscle cells. The adventitia is composed of collagenous fibers in loose connective tissue, along with capillaries, arterioles, and venules (the vasa vasorum). The external elastic lamina is indistinct; it is mixed with the elastic tissues of the media. Figure 1-6 illustrates these components of the elastic artery in cross section.

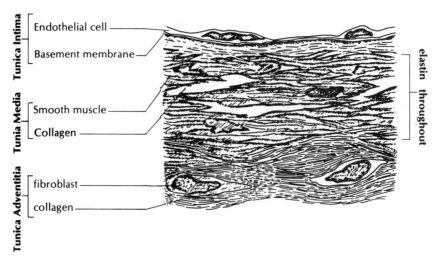

FIG. 1-6. Cross section of an elastic artery showing the histologic features in each layer. (Modified from Harker LA: Hemostasis Manual, 2nd ed, p 2. Philadelphia, FA Davis, 1976)

LARGE VEINS. The large veins correspond to the elastic arteries. The intima of these vessels is composed of endothelium surrounded by loose connective tissue. The media is narrow, containing some smooth muscle and elastic fibers in a loose connective tissue matrix. The adventitia is dense and contains elastic connective tissue with collagenous fibers.

MUSCULAR ARTERIES. Muscular or intermediate arteries distribute blood to the tissues. The intima is thinner than in elastic arteries but features a prominent internal elastic lamina that has a wavy outline in histologic preparation. Smooth muscle predominates in the media, with a few elastic or collagen fibers also present. The media is the thickest of the three layers in a muscular artery. There is a visible external elastic lamina surrounded by an adventitia of loose connective tissue with small vessels and nerves.

Muscular arteries are able to expand and contract. Impulses from the autonomic nervous system control the degree of vasoconstriction or vasodilation and regulate the supply of blood distributed to the tissues. Injury to a muscular artery results in vasoconstriction, a reaction that minimizes the loss of blood from the site of damage. Vasodilation occurs in response to an increased need for blood, oxygen, or other nutrients to a site.

INTERMEDIATE VEINS. Intermediate veins resemble muscular arteries in cross section (Fig. 1-7). The two vessels can be distinguished by the minimal muscle cell component and increased loose connective tissue of the media of the vein versus the large component of muscle in the media of the artery. The vein lacks an elastic lamina, and the lumen has an irregular outline. Nerve endings of the autonomic nervous system are also found in the intermediate vein.

See Table 1-1 for a histologic comparison of all sizes of veins and arteries.

ARTERIOLES. Arterioles are much smaller in cross section than muscular arteries. The intima is composed of only endothelium, while the media is made up of one or two layers of smooth muscle (Fig. 1-8). When two layers are present, they are arranged in planes perpendicular to each other. The adventitia is indistinguishable from the surrounding tissue. Arterioles provide a "reduction valve" mechanism that protects the capillary bed from the high blood pressure found in the larger arteries. High pressure is required to deliver blood through the arteries to the tissues, but capillaries are unable to withstand such pressure. The degree of pressure in the arterioles, and thus in the capillaries, is regulated by muscle tone, activity of the autonomic nervous system, and the presence of certain vasoactive chemicals like serotonin, epinephrine, and norepinephrine. Arterioles control the distribution of blood to various capillary beds by vasoconstriction and vasodilation. They are the prime regulators of blood pressure.

CAPILLARIES. Capillaries are composed of a single, contiguous endothelial cell layer with a lumen that is large enough for only a single red blood cell to pass (see Fig. 1-8). The thin walls, the presence of fenestrae (or windows) throughout the endothelial cells, and the gaps between endothelial cells all promote the passage of nutrients and wastes in the direction necessary. Leukocytes can pass from the capillary lumen to the surrounding tissue fluid through the gaps, but red cells do not normally escape the circulatory system.

VENULES. Venules are composed histologically of endothelium surrounded by an adventitia of loose connective tissue (Fig. 1-9). There is no visible tunica media. Blood enters the venule via the capillary under low pressure; thus the walls of the venule are

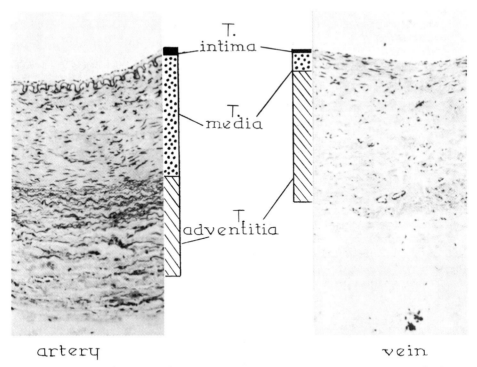

artery   vein

FIG. 1-7. *(Left)* Medium-power photomicrograph of a cross section of the wall of a distribution or muscular artery. *(Right)* Photomicrograph, taken at the same magnification, of a cross section of the wall of its companion vein. (Ham A: Histology, 7th ed. Philadelphia, JB Lippincott, 1974)

TABLE 1-1
Summary of the Important Aspects of Hemostasis for Each Major Type of Vessel*

Vessel Type	Composition			Type of Bleeding	Requirement to Stop Bleeding	Hemostatic Response
	Tunica Intima	*Tunica Media*	*Tunica Adventitia*			
Artery						
Elastic	++	++++	++	Hemarthrosis, hemorrhage	Pressure, surgery, tourniquet	V, C, P
Muscular	+	++++	+	Hemarthrosis, hemorrhage	Pressure, surgery, tourniquet	V, C, P
Arteriole	+	++++	+	Hemarthrosis, hemorrhage	Pressure, surgery, tourniquet	V, C, P
Vein						
Large	+	+	++++	Hematoma	Rare	V, C, P
Medium	+	++	+++	Hematoma	Rare	V, C, P
Small (venule)				Hematoma	Rare	V, C, P
Capillary				Petechiae		P

* The histologic components of the vasculature (tunica intima, tunica media, and tunica adventitia) are graded for each vessel type. As can be seen, the main component of the arteries is the tunica media, which is rated 4+, whereas the tunica intima and adventitia are rated 1+ and 2+ to indicate that the amount of those layers is less in the artery. The veins in relation to the arteries have a much thicker tunica adventitia, except for the small venule. It consists of an endothelium with basal lamina and pericytes. The capillary consists of a single endothelial cell wall. Each vessel type responds to trauma through one of the hemostatic mechanisms: vasculature or vasoconstriction (V), coagulation (C), or platelets (P).

quite thin, while the lumen is large. Blood flows in a laminar fashion, more rapidly through the center and slowing near the margins to allow for easy interaction of platelets, plasma proteins, and the vessel wall.

Pericytes, unspecialized cells that probably differentiate into various vessel-related cell types, are found in the adventitia of the arteriole and venule adjacent to the endothelium of the capillary.

Seventy percent of the total blood supply is located in the veins. Collagen-rich valves in the muscular veins enable the blood to overcome the forces of gravity and return the blood to the heart. Muscle tone in the veins is weak and is under the control of the autonomic nervous system. Venous smooth muscle operates in conjunction with surrounding skeletal muscle to aid in that return.

The Function of Vessels in Hemostasis

Physical and biochemical properties of blood vessels help to maintain normal circulation. The physical properties include vasoconstriction, vasodilation, and changes in

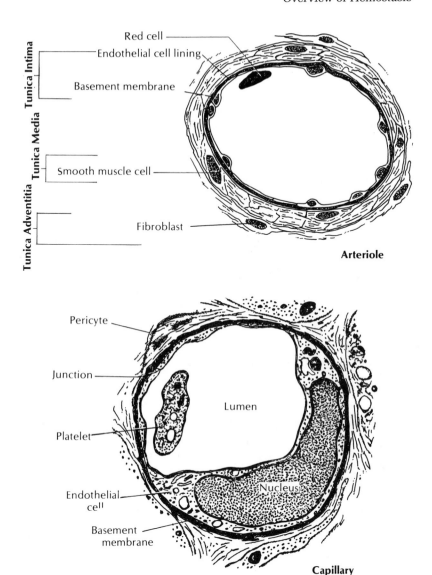

FIG. 1-8. Comparison of capillary and arteriole structure viewed through the vessel lumen.

vessel permeability. All of these actions are controlled by the smooth muscle tissue of the tunica media. Biochemical properties are associated with the intima and include the secretions of endothelial cells and subendothelial smooth muscle tissue.

ANTITHROMBOTIC FACTORS. Certain physical characteristics of the blood vessel function to maintain blood in the fluid state. These are said to be *antithrombotic*. The most important physical property is the ability of the vessel to maintain a normal blood flow rate. Blood in motion does not have the opportunity to activate platelets and the coagulation mechanism. Blood that is slowed or that encounters turbulence is prone to

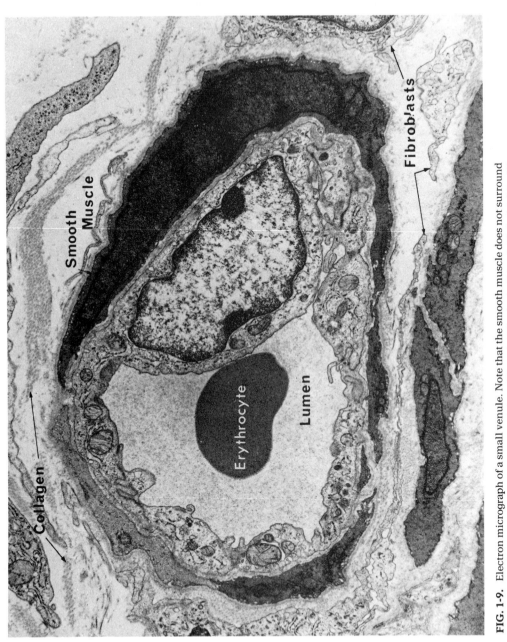

FIG. 1-9. Electron micrograph of a small venule. Note that the smooth muscle does not surround the lumen of the venule as it does in arterioles. (Ham A: Histology, 7th ed. Philadelphia, JB Lippincott, 1974)

thrombosis. Endothelial cells form a smooth, contiguous surface that promotes blood flow, reduces turbulence, and provides no site for platelet activation. Blood flow is regulated by vasoconstriction and vasodilation.[61]

Endothelial cells secrete certain antithrombotic biochemicals. *Prostacyclin (PGI_2)* is a powerful local hormone that inhibits platelet activation and induces vasodilation. Certain enzymes metabolize adenine nucleotides (adenosine diphosphate [ADP] and ATP [adenosine triphosphate]) to release the adenine nucleoside adenosine, a vasodilator that regulates blood flow. *Thrombomodulin* is a large molecule produced by the endothelium that enhances the anticoagulant property of *protein C,* an important plasma regulator of coagulation. (See Chap. 2 for a complete discussion of regulators of coagulation and fibrinolysis.) *Protease nexin* is an enzyme that inactivates thrombin by binding covalently at its active site. The protease – thrombin complex is internalized and degraded by the endothelial cell. Deficiencies in any of these secretions can result in thromboembolic disorders.

Heparan sulfate, a structural glycosaminoglycan on the endothelial cell surface, accelerates the activity of antithrombin III, a plasma anticoagulant. The action of heparan sulfate is much like that of heparin, a circulating anticoagulant and antithrombotic agent. Endothelial cells also secrete small concentrations of a heparinlike substance to the subendothelial smooth muscle tissue.[11] The function of this heparin is unknown.

FACTORS PROMOTING THROMBUS FORMATION. Although normal blood vessels inhibit thrombogenesis (the growth of a thrombus), injured vessels promote coagulation, or thrombus formation. Vasoconstriction is the physical reaction to trauma, as described previously. The reaction consists of an early, neurogenic component and a sustained, myogenic component. The neurogenic response lasts 10 to 30 seconds and depends on an intact nerve supply. The second lasts up to an hour and is not clearly understood.[44] Platelet secretions of the prostaglandin *thromboxane A_2* and *serotonin* contribute to vasoconstriction.

Two biochemical elements of the tunica intima promote thrombogenesis. *Tissue thromboplastin,* a complex biochemical mixture, is released from vascular tissue, as it is from any injured tissue, and promotes coagulation through the extrinsic system. Collagen, a component of the basement membrane, is exposed upon injury to provide a surface that induces activation of the contact factors of the intrinsic path of coagulation (Factor XII, Factor XI, prekallikrein, and Fitzgerald factor) and platelets. Activated platelets enhance the intrinsic coagulation pathway by providing a reaction surface and several procoagulants to the system. Figure 1-10 summarizes the response of the vessel to trauma and damage.

FACTORS OF FIBRINOLYSIS AND REPAIR. The endothelium provides *tissue plasminogen activator (tPA).* tPA catalyzes the conversion of circulating plasminogen to plasmin. Plasmin is the enzyme most active in fibrinolysis. As clot formation begins, tPA is released, providing the mechanism for clot dissolution.

Vascular repair follows lysis of the clot. Normally, endothelial cells grow independent of external influences as long as there is an intact subendothelium. With vascular damage, the subendothelium is exposed. Mitogenesis of the fibroblasts and smooth muscle cells of the subendothelium depends in part on *platelet-derived growth factor,* a secretion of platelets. This results in proliferation and repair of those cells.

Vascular Damage and Diseases

Vascular damage results from accidental or mechanical rupture of the vessel due to trauma or from loss of vessel tone, contractibility, or wall integrity due to disease.

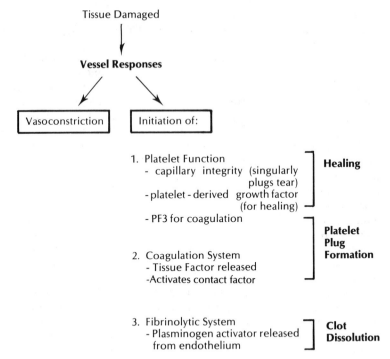

FIG. 1-10. Summary of the blood vessel response to damage or trauma.

Infection, inflammation, and other conditions can aggravate and damage the vasculature.

Stress, surgery, and hormones from both the adrenals and pituitary glands influence capillary integrity. Capillary integrity is the vessel's ability to withstand normal blood pressure and trauma. Loss of capillary integrity or resistance results in the formation of petechiae (seen as pinpoint red dots on the skin surface). Formation of petechiae results from red blood cells escaping from the capillary bed and infiltrating the tissue. It is important to remember that petechiae are seen only in vascular or platelet problems. They are not a common finding in coagulation or fibrinolytic defects.

Other clinical features of vascular disorders are purpura or ecchymoses. These are commonly associated with petechiae. *Purpura* is the general term that describes a variety of hemorrhagic lesions in which the bleeding is confined to the skin, mucous membranes, or serosal surfaces. Ecchymoses are a type of purpura in which the superficial bleeding extends over a large area, but not into deep tissue. Purpura range in size from very small pinpoint lesions to diffuse erythemas. Examples of petechiae and ecchymoses of several vascular disorders can be seen in Figures 1-11 through 1-14.

Small ecchymoses and a few petechiae are normal in some women and children. The reason for their occurrence is unknown.

Vascular disorders are classified as either acquired or hereditary.[57] Wintrobe classifies bleeding disorders by cause: (1) an autoimmune phenomenon, (2) infection, (3) structural problems, and (4) a miscellaneous category that includes skin diseases, proteinemias, and syndromes with sensitization to one's own red cells or DNA (see

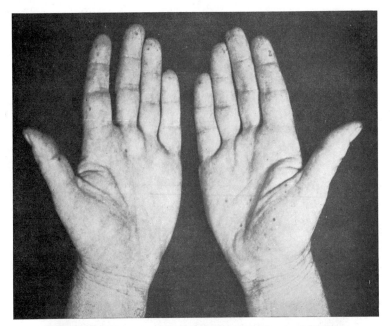

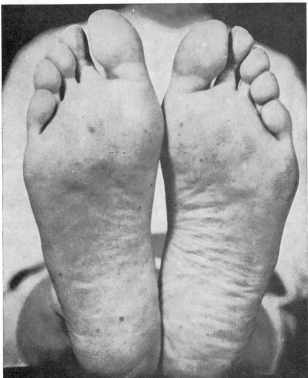

FIG. 1-11. Hands and feet of a 55-year-old man with hereditary hemorrhagic telangiectasia. Bleeding began at the age of 4, and the patient later developed cirrhosis of the liver. (Wintrobe MM: Hematology, 8th ed, p 1081. Philadelphia, Lea & Febiger, 1981)

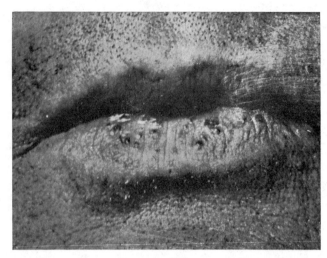

FIG. 1-12. Characteristic lesions on the lips of a patient with hereditary hemorrhagic telangiectasia. (Wintrobe MM: Hematology, 8th ed, p 1080. Philadelphia, Lea & Febiger, 1981)

Classification of Bleeding Disorders on p 22).[58] Most vascular disorders are secondary to another disease or acquired, while only hereditary hemorrhagic telangiectasia and hereditary collagen disorders are inherited.

The bleeding time is increased in patients suffering from vascular problems and all other coagulation tests, including the platelet count and platelet function, are normal. These latter two tests should always be performed to differentiate a vascular disorder from a platelet problem. Laboratory testing specific for vascular disorders is not available, biopsy is not helpful, and therapy is usually not effective, except as support in severe hemorrhage.

The defective mechanism of bleeding in many vascular conditions is not known. Bleeding ranges from mild to severe, with lesions most commonly located on the legs and buttocks.

Senile purpura is a benign problem seen in elderly patients. Dark blue ecchymoses are found on the forearms of these patients due to a loss of elasticity of the skin and vasculature. Vasculitis, an inflammation of the small vessels from allergies, drug reactions, or autoimmune processes, is probably due to the deposition of complement and immune complexes on the small vessel wall. Activation of the complement initiates the inflammatory response that affects the skin as well as internal organs (see Fig. 1-14).

Patients with *infections* can develop petechiae. These lesions are probably due to an inflammatory response similar to the autoimmune process described above. Figure 1-13 illustrates the extensive purpuric lesions that occurred in a case of scarlet fever. Immune complexes have been detected in some cases of endocarditis.

Hereditary telangiectasia is an autosomal-dominant disorder in which small lesions (1 mm – 3 mm) are found on the skin of the face, especially the mouth and nose (see Figs. 1-11 and 1-12). Internal organs like the liver and spleen can be enlarged. The lesions are dilations of capillaries and venules that accumulate over time. Patients usually do not have severe bleeding until later in life, when transfusion may be necessary.

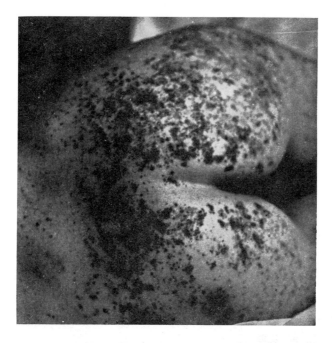

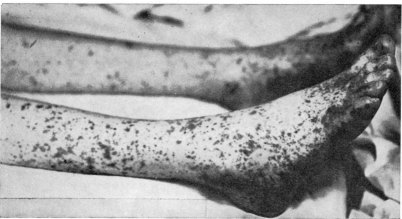

FIG. 1-13. Purpuric lesions in a patient with scarlet fever. There was no thrombocytopenia. (Fox MJ, Enzer N: A consideration of the phenomenon of purpura following scarlet fever. Am J Med Sci 196:321, 1938)

Ehlers-Danlos syndrome is also inherited as an autosomal-dominant disorder. In this condition the joints are hyperextensible, and skin is hyperplastic, as seen in the "rubberman" of the circus. There is a defect in the body's supportive tissues of skin, bone, and vasculature. Patients with Ehlers-Danlos syndrome tend to bruise easily and form hematomas of the skin. Bleeding from the gums, postpartum bleeding, and gastrointestinal bleeding are common.

CLASSIFICATION OF BLEEDING DISORDERS

AUTOIMMUNE VASCULAR PURPURAS

Allergic purpura (Henoch-Schönlein)
Drug-induced vascular purpura (iodides, belladona, atropine, quinine, procaine, penicillin, aspirin, merbaphen, chloral hydrate, sulfonamides, coumarins, and others)
Purpura fulminans

INFECTIONS

Bacterial (meningococcemia, septicemia, typhoid fever, diphtheria, tuberculosis, endocarditis, leptospirosis)
Viral (measles, smallpox, influenza, and others)
Rickettsial (Rocky Mountain spotted fever, typhus)

STRUCTURAL ABNORMALITIES

Hereditary telangiectasia
Hereditary connective tissue disorders (Ehlers-Danlos syndrome, osteogenesis imperfecta, pseudoxanthoma elasticum)
Acquired connective tissue disorders (scurvy, corticosteroid therapy, Cushing's disease, senile purpura)

MISCELLANEOUS

Autoerythrocyte sensitization (psychogenic purpura, Gardner-Diamond syndrome, DNA hypersensitivity)
Paraproteinemias (Waldenström's macroglobulinemia, cryoglobulemic purpura)
Purpura simplex
Purpura associated with certain skin diseases
Others (Kaposi's sarcoma, snake envenomation, amyloidosis, hemochromatosis)

(Modified from Wintrobe MM: Clinical Hematology, 8th ed, p 1073. Philadelphia, Lea & Febiger, 1981)

Vitamin C is a necessary chemical for maintenance and formation of basement membranes. *A deficiency of ascorbic acid, or scurvy,* results in the formation of petechiae, bleeding from gums, bone pain, and even intramuscular hemorrhage in severe cases.

The Role of Platelets

The platelet, a refractile cell 2 μm to 4 μm in diameter, is a disc-shaped searcher of hemostatic trouble in the peripheral bloodstream. The cytoplasm of the platelet stains light blue in Wright's stain. There are numerous and evenly distributed red-purple cytoplasmic granules. See Figures 1-15 and 1-16 to study the features as viewed under light microscopy.

Platelets are cytoplasmic fragments of megakaryocytes, cells that are 35 μm to 150 μm in diameter and are found in the bone marrow and lung. Megakaryocytes have multilobulated nuclei that stain purple with Wright's stain, as seen in Figures 1-16 and 1-17. Platelets are formed by a process called demarcation, a simultaneous fragmenta-

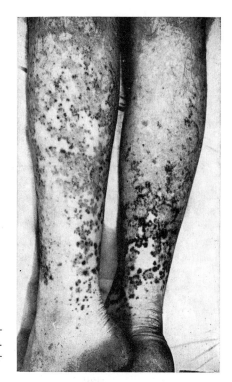

FIG. 1-14. The ecchymoses and erythematous lesions associated with Henoch-Schönlein purpura. (Wintrobe MM: Hematology, 8th ed, p 1076. Philadelphia, Lea & Febiger, 1981). (Reduced to 81%)

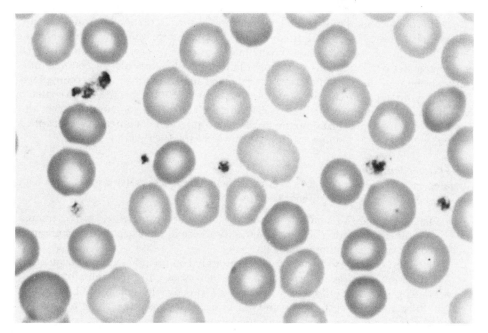

FIG. 1-15. Photomicrograph of circulating platelets at 100× magnification. (Reduced to 81%)

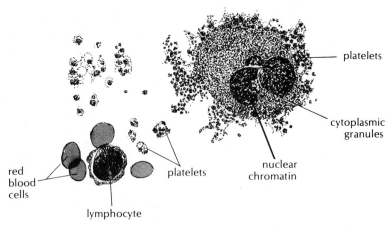

FIG. 1-16. Platelets and megakaryocyte *(right)* with red cells and a lymphocyte for comparison of size. Not a depiction of peripheral blood or bone marrow.

tion of the entire cytoplasm of the megakaryocyte. Approximately 50 platelets per nuclear lobe are formed, or about 35,000 per microliter of peripheral blood per day, replacing old or nonfunctional platelets that are removed from the circulation. The life span of the platelet is 9.5 to 10.5 days, with macrophages in the spleen, liver, and bone marrow removing the aged platelet. Younger platelets are larger (4 μm to 6 μm in diameter), less dense, and physiologically more active than older platelets.

Normal whole blood contains approximately 150 to 400 platelets per microliter. Two thirds of peripheral blood platelets are found in the circulation, and one third are sequestered in the spleen. Splenic platelets are in dynamic equilibrium with circulating platelets and are exchanged freely. Direct platelet counting is performed manually on a hemocytometer or by automated instrumentation. Platelets may also be counted indirectly through the use of a stained peripheral blood smear. In the indirect count, platelets and erythrocytes are counted simultaneously under 1000X magnification so that a ratio of platelets to erythrocytes can be determined. The ratio is then multiplied by the erythrocyte count to give an approximate platelet count. Platelet kinetics are described in detail in Chapter 7. Platelet counting techniques are described in Chapter 9.

Platelet Function

As stated earlier, the platelet plays a central role in the process of hemostasis. There are several separate yet interdependent functions:

- Platelets adhere to small defects of the vascular intima when minor trauma results in sloughing of endothelial cells or formation of gaps between margins of the adjacent endothelial cells.
- Platelets aggregate to form hemostatic plugs in conjunction with the coagulation mechanism to repair large ruptures of the vessel wall from trauma.
- Platelets provide a phospholipid surface and procoagulants such as fibrinogen in the generation of thrombin and fibrin for the hemostatic platelet plug.
- Platelets secrete an array of substances to promote aggregation, coagulation, vasoconstriction, and vascular repair.

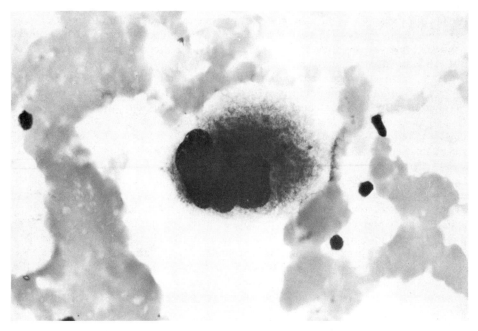

FIG. 1-17. Photomicrograph of a megakaryocyte at 100✕ in the process of demarcation. Note the platelets being released. (Reduced to 81%)

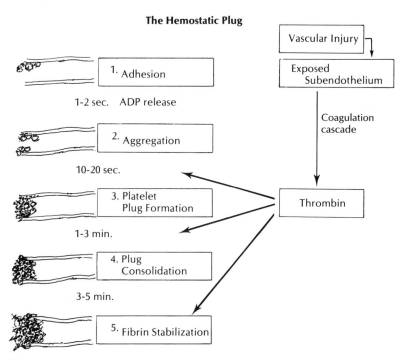

FIG. 1-18. Hemostatic platelet plug formation.

Platelets accomplish these functions by participating in adhesion, aggregation, and secretion. While each of these functions can be individually measured by clinical testing, all three are involved in the formation of the hemostatic platelet plug. Figure 1-18 demonstrates the initiation and growth of the plug over 3 to 5 minutes.

Platelet adhesion occurs after minor trauma that causes disruption of the endothelium, exposing collagen microfibrils of the subendothelium. Adhesion depends on the presence of von Willebrand factor and the platelet surface receptor glycoprotein Ib (see Chap. 8 for an explanation of the surface receptors on platelets). On attachment of the platelet to the ruptured vessel wall, the platelet swells, releases ADP and ATP, and causes adjacent platelets to change shape. Thromboxane A_2 is also released to aid in vasoconstriction.

Platelet aggregation is the adhesion of platelets to one another. *In vitro* studies employing platelet aggregometry reveal that aggregation proceeds in stages. (See Chap. 9 for a complete explanation of aggregometry methods.) Although it is impossible to actually study a platelet's activity in the human body, the simulation studies of aggregometry are thought to parallel the platelet functioning *in vivo*. The first stage, *primary aggregation,* includes shape change of the platelet and formation of small aggregates. Platelet shape change in this stage is also called reorganization, which involves the formation of pseudopods and centralization of organelles. Primary aggregation is reversible. *Secondary aggregation* follows primary aggregation after a brief period. In secondary aggregation, platelet energy is spent on formation of large aggregates that remain clumped for an extended period, resulting in an irreversible reaction. Platelets secrete organelle materials in sequence during primary and secondary aggregation. The first secretions come from the dense bodies — granules that contain ADP, ATP, ionic calcium, and serotonin. ADP and ionic calcium from the dense bodies recruit additional platelets to the site, building secondary aggregation. Serotonin is a potent vasodilator, but the role of ATP is not clear. The second group of secretions of group 1 and 2 are often termed *release I* and *release II*. A series of proteolytic enzymes are also secreted from platelet lysosomes after platelet release II. The effects of these substances are not clear at this time.

Summary

Primary aggregation, secondary aggregation, release I, and release II are phenomena that have been measured by *in vitro* testing but are ill-defined *in vivo*. Platelets first

---

FIG. 1-19. Summary of platelet responses and requirements. *(Step 1)* When subendothelial collagen is exposed through traumatic removal of endothelium, adhesion is instantaneous. Von Willebrand factor bridges the gap between the platelet and the collagen by neutralizing the inhibitory effects of negatively charged chemicals on both. The platelet does not become activated and does not secrete its contents. *(Step 2)* If the trauma is extensive, a hemostatic platelet plug is necessary. In the early stages, platelets aggregate. Cohesion requires fibrinogen and the specific receptor site glycoprotein IIbIIIa. Contraction of microfilaments is begun with centralization of organelles. Biochemical requirements for platelet aggregation include agonists, the receptor site, fibrinogen, aerobic energy from the mitochondria, free calcium, thrombosthenin, and the prostacyclin product thromboxane A_2, which potentiates platelet activation. *(Step 3)* As the platelet plug forms, the contents of the platelet are secreted: ADP, ATP, serotonin, and calcium from the dense bodies, procoagulants such as PF_4 and β-thromboglobulin from the alpha granules, and acid hydrolases from the lysosomes. *vWF,* von Willebrand factor; *PLT,* platelet; *GP,* glycoprotein.

FUNCTION	MORPHOLOGY	BIOCHEMICAL REQUIREMENTS

Step I: Adhesion

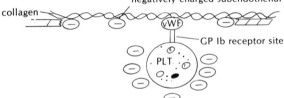

1. Von Willebrand factor

2. Glycoprotein Ib receptor to neutralize negative charges of platelet and collagen

Step II: Primary Aggregation

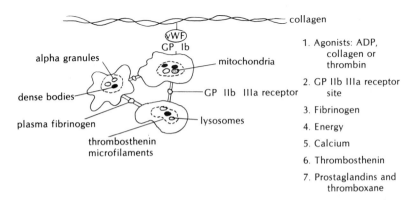

1. Agonists: ADP, collagen or thrombin

2. GP IIb IIIa receptor site

3. Fibrinogen

4. Energy

5. Calcium

6. Thrombosthenin

7. Prostaglandins and thromboxane

Step III: Secondary Aggregation

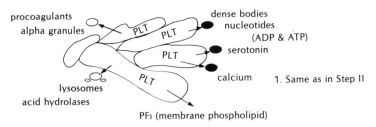

1. Same as in Step II

Step IV: Clot Retraction

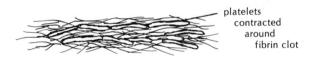

platelets contracted around fibrin clot

adhere to the subendothelial collagen, undergo shape change within 1 to 2 seconds, secrete ADP to attract other platelets, and form loose platelet aggregates. Secretion of platelet procoagulants enhances intrinsic fibrin formation that is also initiated directly by the exposed collagen. Platelet surface membrane phospholipid provides the main site for fibrin to form and thrombogenesis to occur. The original platelet aggregates are stabilized in a firm fibrin mesh. The combination of platelet aggregates, erythrocytes,

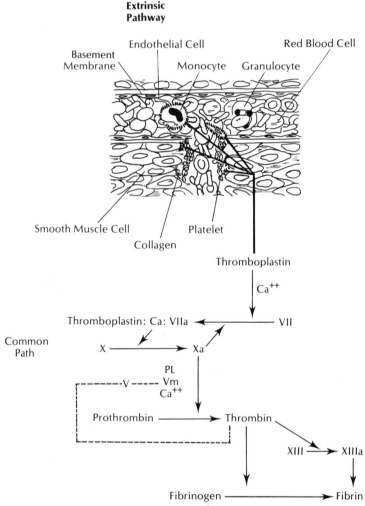

FIG. 1-20. The extrinsic pathway of the coagulation system and the vessel wall response. Upon vessel wall injury, thromboplastin, the inducer of the extrinsic pathway, is exposed on the surface of disrupted or stimulated endothelial cells and smooth muscle cells. Monocytes also possess thromboplastin in their membranes, and the thromboplastin becomes available on the surface after stimulation. *PL*, phospholipid; *Vm*, Factor V modified; Ca^{++}, calcium. (Osterud B: Activation of pathways of the coagulation system in normal hemostasis. Scand J Haematol 32:337–345, 1984)

Intrinsic Pathway

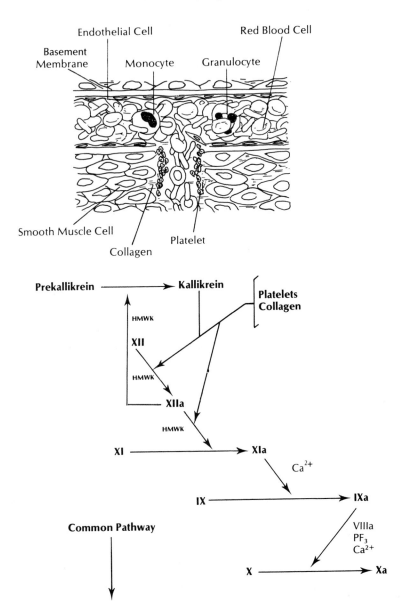

FIG. 1-21. The intrinsic pathway of the coagulation system and the vessel wall. Platelets are activated and adhere to collagen upon vessel wall injury. They aggregate together with preformed kallikrein to activate Factors XII and XI. The activation of Factor XI may occur even in the absence of Factor XII. Factor XI$_a$, in turn, activates Factor IX, which feeds into the common pathway of coagulation with the activation of Factor X. *HWWK*, high-molecular weight kininogen. (Osterud B: Activation of pathways of the coagulation system in normal hemostasis. Scand J Haematol 32:337–345, 1984)

and fibrin is termed the *hemostatic platelet plug.* The plug may seal off the entire lumen of a vessel or seal only the damaged area. Platelets in the center of the plug lose individual structure and become a consolidated mass by the surrounding fibrin. Platelets on the periphery of the plug retain their internal structures. Actomyosin (thrombosthenin) within the peripheral platelets slowly contracts to diminish the size and volume of the plug. The ability of platelets to contract the plug is energy dependent, proceeding only when magnesium is present. This platelet phenomenon is also referred to as clot retraction. Figure 1-19 provides an overview of the morphologic and biochemical events of hemostatic platelet plug formation.

The Role of Coagulation and Fibrinolysis

Coagulation, or fibrin formation, is a complex series of enzymatic reactions that involve coagulation proteins. Extrinsic coagulation, as seen in Figure 1-20, starts when tissue thromboplastin (Factor III) is released from damaged cells or tissue. Intrinsic coagulation (as seen in Fig. 1-21) is a slower mechanism that is initiated by exposure of collagen to Hageman factor (Factor XII) from the plasma and activation of platelets. Extrinsic coagulation requires the presence of Factor VII, while intrinsic coagulation requires Factors XII, XI, IX, and VIII and high-molecular-weight kinogen and prekallikrein. Both pathways require phospholipid and calcium from the platelets and join together in the activation of Factor X at a point called the "common pathway." Factors necessary for function of the common pathway to produce fibrin include Factor V, prothrombin, fibrinogen, phospholipid, and calcium. Finally, the fibrin plug is stabilized by Factor XIII. The pathways involve each protein activating the next protein in the pathway, thus creating a dynamic reaction that builds up fibrin formation in the hemostatic platelet plug.

   A separate series of biochemicals, nearly as complex as those involved in coagulation, provide for ultimate removal of the thrombus formed (Fig. 1-22). The process of clot dissolution is known as *fibrinolysis.* Plasminogen, the plasma-borne precursor of

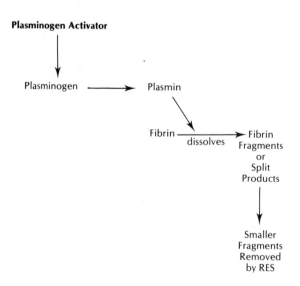

FIG. 1-22. Fibrinolytic proteins and the pathway of fibrinolysis.

the proteolytic enzyme plasmin, attaches to the fibrin formed and is laid down in the clot. Damage to a vessel wall releases tPA, which catalyzes the conversion of plasminogen to plasmin. Plasmin breaks down the clot proteolytically, causing it to disappear. The fibrin fragments of the broken-up thrombus are removed by the reticuloendothelial system.

REFERENCES

1. Addison W: On the colorless corpuscles and on the molecules and cytoblasts in the blood. London Med Gaz (NS) 30:144, 1842
2. Alfasi on Tractate Yevamouth 64b: Babylonian Talmud. edition of Otzar Hasefarim. New York, 1957
3. Biggs RD, Macfarlene RG et al: Christmas disease: A condition previously mistaken for hemophilia. Br Med J 2:1378, 1952
4. Bizzozero J: Über eine neuen Formbestand there des blutes und desen Rolle bei der Thrombose und der Blutgerinnerung. Virchows Arch Pathol Anat 90:261, 1882
5. Born GR: The breakdown of adenosine triphosphate in platelets during clotting. J Physiol 133:61, 1956
6. Braunsteiner H, Pakesch F: Thrombocytasthenia and thrombocytopathia—old names and new diseases. Blood 11:965, 1956
7. Brinkhous KM: Clotting defect in hemophilia: Deficiency in a plasma factor required for platelet utilization. Proc Soc Exp Biol Med 66:117, 1947
8. Brinkhous KM: A short history of hemophilia with some comments on the word hemophilia. In Brinkhous KM, Hemker HC: Handbook of Hemophilia, a, pp 3–5; b, pp 3–19. New York, Elsevier, 1975
9. Buchanan A: On coagulation of the blood and other fibriniferous liquids. Lond Med Gaz (NS) 1:617, 1845. Reprinted in J Physiol 2:158–168, 1879–1880
10. Chelius MJ: Beobachtungen einer Blut Familie Heidelberger. Klin Ann 3:344, 1827
11. Cochran DL, Castellot JJ, Karnovsky MJ: Effect of heparin on vascular smooth muscle cells. II. Specific protein synthesis. J Cell Physiol 124:29–36, 1985
12. Collins DH: Correspondence: Discussion of Christmas disease. Br Med J 1:97, 1953
13. Dam H: Cholesterinstoffwechsel in Huhnereiern und Huhnchen. Biochem Z 215:475–492, 1929
14. de Bainville HM: Injection de matiere cerebrale dans les veins. Gaz Med Paris (S2) 2:524, 1834
15. Donne AD: L'origine des globules der san, de leur mode de formation et de leur fin. CK Acad Sci 14:366, 1842
16. Elsaesser JA: Geschichte eine Familie von Blutern in Württemberg. J Pract Heilkd 58:89, 1824
17. Fischer M: Die bluterkrankheit in europaischen furstenhauser. Forsch Fortschr 12:425, 1936
18. Gerber F: Elements of General and Minute Anatomy of Man and Mammals. London, G. Gulliver, 1842
19. Glanzmann E: Hereditare hamorrhagische thrombasthenie: Ein beitrag zur pathologie der blutpattchen. Jahrb Kinderheilkd 88:113, 1918
20. Grette K: The mechanism of thrombin catalyzed hemostatic reactions in platelets. Acta Physiol Scand (Suppl) 195:1–93, 1962
21. Harrington WJ, Minnick V, Hollingswirth JW et al: Demonstration of a thrombocytopenic factor in the blood of patients with thrombocytopenic purpura. J Lab Clin Med 38:1, 1951
22. Hay J: Account of a remarkable haemorrhagic disposition existing in many individuals of the same family. N Engl J Med Surg 2:221, 1813
23. Hayem G: Recherches sur l'evolution des hematies dans le sang de l'homme et des vertebres. Arch Physiol Norm Pathol 5:692, 1878

24. Hewson W: Experimental Inquiries Into the Properties of Blood, With Remarks on its Morbid Appearances, 3rd ed. London, J. Johnson, 1780
25. Hewson W: The Works of William Hewson. Gulliver FRS (ed): London, The Sydenham Society, 1846
26. Heyden MJ: Rasputin provides clue for modern treatment. Dent Angles (United States) 10:11, September 1969
27. Hopff F: Ueber die Haemophilie oder die erbliche Anlage zu todtlichen Blutungen. Thesis, Wurzburg, Germany, 1828
28. Hunter J: A Treatise on the Blood, Inflammation, and Gun-Shot Wounds, 3rd ed. London, Sherwood, Gilbert and Piper, 1828
29. Link KP: The discovery of dicumarol and its sequels. Circulation 19:97–107, 1959
30. Macfarlane RG: Fibrinolysis after operation. Lancet i:10–12, 1937
31. Macfarlane RG: An enzyme cascade in the blood clotting mechanism and its function as a biochemical amplifier. Nature 202:498, 1964
32. Maimonides M: Laws of Circumcision, Book of Adoration (Sefer Ahavah). In Code of Maimonides (Mishneh Torah), Chap 1, Paragraph 18. Jerusalem, Pardes, 1957
33. Malpighi M: DePolypo Cordis. Forester JM (trans): Uppsala, Almqvist & Wiksels, 1956
34. Marcus AJ, Zucker MB: The Physiology of Blood Platelets. New York, Grune & Stratton, 1965
35. Morawitz P: Die Chemie der Blutgerinnuns. Ergeb Physiol 4:307–422, 1905
36. Otto JC: An account of an hemorrhagic disposition existing in certain families. Med Respository 6:1–4, 1803
37. Owen CA, Bowle EJ, Thompson JH: Introduction and historical perspective. In The Diagnosis of Bleeding Disorders, 2nd ed. Boston, Little, Brown & Co, 1975
38. Petit JE: Dissertation sur la maniere d'arreter le sang dans les hemorrhagies: Avec la description d'une machine on bandage propre à procurer la consolidation des vaisseaux, apres l'amputation des membres, par le seule compression. Mem Acad R Sci (Amsterdam edition) 1:122, 1731
39. Plato: Timaeus. In Jewett B (ed): The Dialogues of Plato, 3rd ed, Vol 3, pp 339–543. New York, Macmillan, 1892
40. Quick AJ: The development and use of the prothrombin tests. Circulation 19:92–96, 1959
41. Ratnoff OD: The Evolution of Knowledge About Hemostasis. In Ratnoff O, Forbes CD: Disorders of Hemostasis, pp 1–20. New York, Grune & Stratton, 1984
42. Reith JE, Ross MH: Histology: A Text and Atlas. Philadelphia, JB Lippincott, 1985
43. Rosner F: Hemophilia in the Talmud and rabbinic writings. Ann Intern Med 70(4):833–837, 1969
44. Saito H: Normal hemostatic mechanisms in disorders of hemostasis. In Ratnoff OD, Forbes CD (eds): Disorders of Hemostasis, p 24. New York, Grune & Stratton, 1984
45. Schmidt A: Zur Blutlehre. Leipzig, Vogel, 1892
46. Schönlein JL: Haemorrhaphilie (erbliche Anlage zu Blutungen) in Allgemeine und specielle Pathologie und Therapie. In Nach JL: Schönleins Vorlesungen niedergeschrieben und herausgegeben von einem seiner Zuhorer, 2nd ed, Vol. 2, pp 88–90. Whurzburg, Germany, Etlinger, 1832
47. Seegers WH, Johnson SA: Conversion of prothrombin to auto prothrombin II (platelet cofactor II) and its relation to the blood clotting mechanism. Am J Physiol 184:259, 1956
48. Seegers WH: Prothrombin, pp 111–113. Cambridge, Harvard University Press, 1962
49. Simon JF: Physiologische und pathologische antropochemie mit Berucksichtigung der eigentlichen Zoochemie. Handbuch der angewandten medizinischen chemie nach dem neuesten Standpunkte der wissenschaft und nach zahlreichen eigenen untersuchungen. Theil II. Berlin, A. Förstner, 1842
50. Stuart JJ: Inherited defects of platelet function. Semin Hematol 12(3), July 1975
51. Thackrah CT: An Inquiry Into the Nature and Properties of the Blood. London, Cox and Sons, 1819
52. Thormann F: Haemotocele bei einem Jungling aus einer Beuter-Familie Schweiz. Natur und Heilk 2:340, 1837

53. Tocantins LM: Historical notes on blood platelets. Blood 3:1073, 1948
54. Warner ED, Brinkhous KM, Smith HP: A quantitative study on blood clotting: Prothrombin fluctuations under experimental conditions. Am J Physiol 114:667–675, 1936
55. Warner ED, Brinkhous KM, Smith HD: Bleeding tendency of obstructive jaundice: Prothrombin deficiency and dietary factors. Proc Soc Exp Biol Med 37:628–630, 1938
56. Willbanks W: Femoral neurapathy due to retroperitoneal bleeding. Am J Surg 145:196, 1983
57. Williams WJ: Disorders of hemostasis—classification. In Williams WJ, Beutler E, Erslev AJ, Lichtman MA (eds): Hematology, 3rd ed, pp 1288–1289. New York, McGraw-Hill, 1983
58. Wintrobe MM: Clinical Hematology, 8th ed, p 1073. Philadelphia, Lea & Febiger, 1981
59. Wolper C, Ruska H: Strukturuntersuchangen zur Blutgerrinung. Klin Wochenschr 18:1077, 1939
60. Wright JH: The origin and nature of the blood platelet. Boston Med Surg J 154:643, 1906
61. Yaffe E: Vascular function in hemostasis. In Williams WJ, Beutler E, Erslev AJ, Lichtman MA (eds): Hematology, 3rd ed, pp 1277–1281. New York, McGraw-Hill, 1983

Plasma Proteins: Factors of the Hemostatic Mechanism

2

Donna M. Corriveau

CASE STUDY A 3-year-old girl was brought to her family physician for suture of a severe laceration to the left foot that resulted from stepping on a piece of broken bottle while swimming. Following successful closing of the wound, she was sent home. Two weeks later, the physician removed the stitches and observed poor wound healing and severe dehiscence, or gaping of the wound. There was no prior history of bleeding problems. Laboratory results showed

Prothrombin time (PT): prolonged
Thrombin time (TT): prolonged
Fibrinogen: 300 mg/dl (Normal = 200–400 mg/dl)
Reptilase time: prolonged more than the TT
Thromboelastograph: decreased tensile strength
Urea solubility test: abnormal

The physician puzzled about the prolonged TT, which indicated a problem with fibrin formation, although the fibrinogen concentration was normal. The patient was not on heparin. The technologist observed and reported that in each test the clot was small and friable or fragile with excessive red cell fallout. The thromboelastograph confirmed that the clot formed had a defective tensile strength, meaning that the clot was not able to withstand normal stress without breaking. The fibrinogen level was normal, but the form of fibrinogen was not. Although the screening test for Factor XIII (urea solubility) was abnormal, the prolonged PT and TT indicated a problem in the coagulation phase of hemostasis. If Factor XIII were deficient, as found in patients with poor wound healing and oozing from wounds, these tests would be normal, with an abnormal urea solubility test. A defect in fibrinolysis also produces a prolonged TT and PT, but decreased amounts of fibrinogen are expected. Heparin therapy produces a prolongation of the PT, activated partial thromboplastin time (APTT), and TT, but the Reptilase test and the fibrin concentration are normal. In this case the abnormality in coagulation is the fibrinogen molecule itself, as detected by the thromboelastograph test and gross clot observation.

This patient has dysfibrinogenemia, a hereditary condition in which there is an amino acid substitution in the fibrinogen molecule, thus forming an abnormal fibrinogen. It is inherited as an autosomal-dominant trait.

These forms of fibrinogen do not perform like normal fibrinogen. They lack the ability to release fibrinopeptides or cause a delay in the polymerization or stabilization of the fibrin to be formed. The result is the friable clot observed by the technologist. A simple procedure of gross clot observation provides vital information for diagnosis of the patient. Dysfibrinogenemias may be classified by immunoelectrophoresis. To date, more than 80 types of abnormal fibrinogens, all named after their city of origin (*e.g.*, fibrinogens Amsterdam, Baltimore, Detroit, Metz, Zurich, St. Louis, Iowa City, and others) have been described. Upon electrophoresis of the plasma from this patient, two populations of fibrinogen molecules were found. These were determined to be a normal gamma chain and an abnormal gamma chain. This finding, along with the clinical data, narrowed the qualitative defect to Paris I, an abnormal fibrinogen molecule that inhibits the crosslinking of the normal alpha and beta chains by Factor XIII$_a$.[15] Patients with this type of dysfibrinogenemia are usually asymptomatic except for poor wound healing.

The patient received cryoprecipitates to aid wound healing. Recovery was uneventful.

The plasma proteins involved in hemostasis include *procoagulants* for coagulation and factors of fibrinolysis and the control mechanism. All of the factors of hemostasis except calcium, thromboplastin, and platelet factor 3 (PF$_3$), a phospholipid, are proteins that circulate in the plasma. Calcium, a factor in coagulation, does circulate in the plasma. Thromboplastin and phospholipid provide surfaces on which the coagulation reactions occur. Most of the biochemical factors of coagulation, fibrinolysis, and control are glycoproteins.

All of the proteins are synthesized in the liver, except the macromolecular-weight portion of the Factor VIII molecule (VIII : vWF [von Willebrand factor]), which is produced in endothelium and megakaryocytes. Factors II, VII, IX, and X, protein C, and protein S are dependent on vitamin K for proper production.

The procoagulant factors of coagulation, the fibrinolytic proteins, and the proteins of the control mechanism are substrates, cofactors, or enzymes that are precursors of serine proteases or transglutaminases. Procoagulants, the precursor coagulation proteins, are proenzymes that, when activated, activate the next precursor in a waterfall or cascade sequence of events that leads to fibrin formation. Figure 2-1 illustrates this cascade phenomenon of the enzymatic proteins involved in coagulation. Fibrinolytic proteins function to activate plasminogen, the circulating zymogen or enzyme precur-

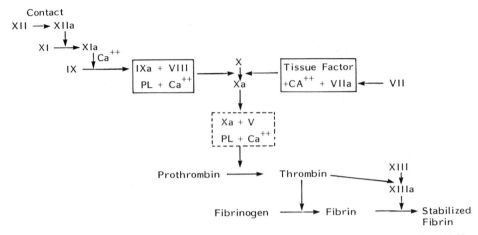

FIG. 2-1. Overview of the coagulation cascade. The boxed factors indicate a complex. Ca^{++}, calcium; *PL*, platelet phospholipid. (Courtesy of George Fritsma)

sor of plasmin. Other proteins of the control mechanism (antithrombin III, protein C, and antiplasmin) neutralize procoagulants and fibrinolytic substances.

The enzymes, cofactors, and substrates of the two systems interact in two types of allosteric reactions, each designed to expose serine-rich active enzyme sites. The first type of allosteric change is a conformational one, a physical change that occurs in the presence of a cofactor(s) converting the zymogen to an active enzyme. The molecule may be turned, twisted, or bent during a conformational change, but it is not cleaved. This enzyme in turn activates the next proenzyme in the sequence. The second type of activation, hydrolytic cleavage of the precursor protein, requires a phospholipid surface, the zymogen, a possible cofactor(s), and a serine protease that hydrolyzes the zymogen at a specific peptide bond. This cleavage exposes the active serine residue, thus creating another serine protease enzyme. Early reactions in the coagulation mechanism are usually conformational changes, whereas later reactions are of the cleavage type, occurring on the surface of aggregated platelets. This produces a dynamic hemostatic system in which the initial stimulus can be both amplified and modulated.[29] Cascade mechanisms like coagulation are common in nature, providing a means for amplification of a reaction to a minute stimulus, while simultaneously maintaining control.

This chapter will describe the coagulation and fibrinolytic mechanisms in detail, showing how the properties of each factor relate to its function.

INTERNATIONAL NOMENCLATURE

The international system for naming the procoagulants uses roman numerals plus the subscripts $_a$ to denote activation, $_m$ for modification, and $_f$ for fragmentation.[36] Table 2-1 summarizes the classification, providing the common names as well. The synonyms were the original names for the factors, named after the bearer of the deficiency or the discoverer.

TABLE 2-1
International Nomenclature for Coagulation Proteins

Factor	Synonym(s)
I	Fibrinogen
II	Prothrombin, prethrombin
III	Tissue thromboplastin, tissue factor
IV	Calcium
V	Proaccelerin, labile factor, accelerator globulin
VI	Not assigned
VII	Proconvertin, stable factor, serum prothrombin conversion accelerator (SPCA), autoprothrombin I
VIII	Antihemophilic factor (AHF), antihemophilic globulin (AHG), platelet cofactor I
IX	Plasma thromboplastin component (PTC), Christmas factor, antihemophilic factor B, autoprothrombin II, platelet cofactor II
X	Stuart-Prower factor, Stuart factor, autoprothrombin III
XI	Plasma thromboplastin antecedent (PTA), antihemophilic factor C
XII	Hageman factor
XIII	Fibrin-stabilizing factor, fibrinase, Laki-Lorand factor
Prekallikrein	Fletcher factor
HMWK	High-molecular-weight kininogen, Fitzgerald factor, Flaujeac factor

The terms for Factors III and IV, tissue thromboplastin and calcium, respectively, are the currently used names. Factor VI, once called accelerin, has since been determined to be a modified form of Factor V. The number VI has been unassigned since that finding. The factors were assigned numbers in the order of their discovery, not based on their location in the coagulation scheme.

Upon activation by thrombin, Factors V and VIII become cofactors. Many experts prefer to call activated V and VIII V_m and VIII_m rather than V_a and VIII_a. This is to demonstrate that activation does not imply an enzyme formation but a modification of the protein.

Factor II_a, activated prothrombin, is called thrombin. When fibrinogen (Factor I) is cleaved, the product is called fibrin. The designation I_a is never used to refer to fibrin.

Prekallikrein and high-molecular-weight kininogen have never been assigned roman numerals because they are more closely linked to the kinin system and the inflammatory response. Their participation in the coagulation mechanism is, however, firmly established. Based on the family name in which prekallikrein and HMWK deficiencies were first detected, prekallikrein is also known as Fletcher factor and HMWK is called Fitzgerald factor.

The fibrinolytic precursor protein is called plasminogen, while the activated form is plasmin. Tissue plasminogen activator, a glycoprotein released from the damaged tissues, activates plasminogen to do its duties as part of the fibrinolytic system. Thus, the name of this activator of fibrinolysis describes its function in the fibrinolytic system. Other proteins of the control mechanism also have descriptive titles (*e.g.*, antithrombin, antiplasmin, etc.).

GROUPS OF COAGULATION FACTORS

The coagulation proteins can arbitrarily be divided into a fibrinogen group, the members of which are sensitive to thrombin; a prothrombin group, the proteins of which are dependent on vitamin K for production; and a contact group. The list below provides the general properties and physical characteristics of each group, which can be useful in understanding their functions in coagulation testing and aiding in specific factor identification.

Fibrinogen group (I, V, VIII, XIII)
  Present in plasma
  Absent in serum, except XIII
  Not adsorbed by barium sulfate or other salts
  Consumed during coagulation
  Destroyed by plasmin
  Present in platelet alpha granules
  Acute-phase reactants
  High molecular weights (>250,000)
  Heat labile (I, V, VIII)
  Storage labile (V, VIII)
  Unaffected by oral anticoagulants
Prothrombin group (II, VII, IX, X, protein C, protein S)
  Not consumed during coagulation, except II
  Adsorbed by barium sulfate and aluminum hydroxide
  Present in serum and stored plasma, except II
  Vitamin K dependent for production
  Affected by oral anticoagulants
  Low molecular weights (55,000–70,000)
  Storage stable
  Heat labile, except II
Contact group (XI, XII, Fletcher factor, Fitzgerald factor)
  Medium molecular weights (80,000–200,000)
  Fairly stable
  Partially consumed in coagulation
  Absorbed by kaolin, but only partially adsorbed by aluminum hydroxide or barium sulfate

The fibrinogen group (I, V, VIII, and XIII) is characterized by its *lability* and consumption during coagulation. The term *lability* refers to the changeability or lack of stability of these proteins under certain physical conditions such as a temperature increase or storage. Factor V, for instance, will deteriorate rapidly at room temperature and disappear from refrigerated, citrated blood bank units at the rate of approximately 6% per day. Factor VIII can survive longer in blood stored at 4°C but still deteriorates moderately or rapidly at 15% to 20% per week. The survival of V and VIII in oxalated blood is shorter. The stability of the factors does not correlate with their half-lives *in vivo*. All of the proteins of this group have high molecular weights (greater than 250,000 daltons) and are not adsorbed by salts like barium sulfate. The enzyme thrombin activates or modifies these factors. Small amounts of thrombin enhance the coagulant activities of Factors V and VIII, while large amounts of thrombin destroy the factors. They are substrates for plasmin, the fibrinolytic enzyme.

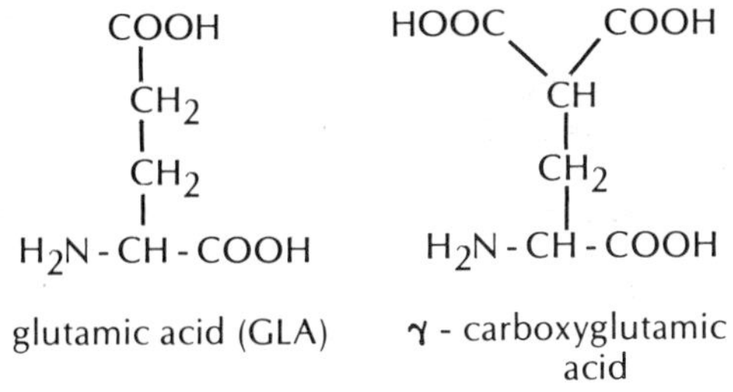

$$COOH$$
$$|$$
$$CH_2$$
$$|$$
$$CH_2$$
$$|$$
$$H_2N - CH - COOH$$

glutamic acid (GLA)

$$HOOC \diagdown \diagup COOH$$
$$CH$$
$$|$$
$$CH_2$$
$$|$$
$$H_2N - CH - COOH$$

γ - carboxyglutamic acid

FIG. 2-2. Vitamin K–dependent prefactors carry several glutamic acid moieties near the amino terminus that are converted to carboxyglutamic acid by a vitamin K–dependent reaction.

The prothrombin group (II, VII, IX, X, and proteins S and C) have low molecular weights of 55,000 to 70,000 daltons. Although protein S and protein C are procoagulant inhibitors, they are included here because of their biochemical similarities and requirement for vitamin K for adequate production. The glycoproteins of the prothrombin group all have a region near the N-terminal end that is rich in glutamic acid. In the liver, vitamin K participates in the carboxylation reaction affecting the gamma carbon of glutamic acid, yielding the modified amino acid γ-carboxyglutamic acid. This amino acid region is responsible for the binding of calcium that is characteristic of the prothrombin group. Figure 2-2 shows the biochemical configuration of this unique amino acid sequence found on all vitamin K–dependent factors. Calcium binding is necessary for any molecule to complex with a phospholipid molecule. Chapter 6 discusses all the aspects, normal and pathologic, of the hydroxyquinone–epoxyquinone cycle in the formation of the vitamin K–dependent factors. These factors, except prothrombin, are not consumed during coagulation and are *adsorbed* by the salts of barium sulfate and aluminum hydroxide. They are heat and storage stable. Oral anticoagulants interfere with production of the vitamin K–dependent factors. Upon initiation of anticoagulant therapy, these factors will disappear in order of their half-lives, with Factor VII first, then IX and X, and finally prothrombin.

The contact family of coagulation proteins (XII, XI, Fletcher, and Fitzgerald) have medium molecular weights of 80,000 to 200,000 daltons and are relatively stable. They are involved in the activation of the coagulation and fibrinolytic processes.

BIOCHEMISTRY OF HEMOSTATIC PROTEINS

Table 2-2 provides the biologic half-life and concentration for all of the factors involved in the hemostatic mechanism. Table 2-3 summarizes the important biochemical features of each factor of the coagulation, fibrinolytic, and control mechanisms. The factors are presented in order of their function.

Fibrinogen

Fibrinogen is a *glycoprotein* that migrates between the beta and gamma globulin regions on electrophoresis. Its dimer structure consists of three pairs of polypeptide chains, alpha, beta, and gamma, linked by disulfide bonds.[8,13] The molecule is designated $A\alpha_2$, $B\beta_2$, γ_2 (Fig. 2-3). The concentration of fibrinogen is the highest of all the procoagulant proteins. It is heat labile and storage stable. At 56°C, fibrinogen precipitates irreversibly. At 4°C, cryofibrinogen precipitates out as a fraction, although this

TABLE 2-2
Plasma Factor Concentrations and Biologic Half-Lives

Factor	Concentration (mg/dl)	Half-Life
I	300–400	90 hr.
II	20	60 hr.
III	0	
IV	4–5	
V	0.5–1	12–36 hr.
VII	0.2	6–8 hr.
VIII	1–2	12 hr.
IX	0.3–0.4	12 hr.
X	0.6–0.8	48–72 hr.
XI	0.4	48–84 hr.
XII	3	48–52 hr.
XIII	2.5	3–5 days
Fletcher	5	35 hr.
Fitzgerald	2.5	6.5 days
Plasminogen	10–15	0.8–2.2 days
Protein C	0.4	5–7 hr.
Protein S (free form)	1.5	
α_2-Macroglobulin	150–350	
α_2-Plasmin inhibitor	5–7	2.6 days
α_1-Antitrypsin	200–400	
Antithrombin III	18–35	68 hr.
C1 inactivator	15–35	

reaction is reversible upon warming. As an *acute-phase reactant,* fibrinogen concentration increases with a variety of stimuli. The body's response to inflammation is the main cause of a rise in fibrinogen levels. Fibrinogen has been reported within platelet granules and adsorbed to the platelet surface. See Chapters 7 and 8 for a full discussion concerning platelet fibrinogen. Platelet fibrinogen is different from plasma fibrinogen in that it is not as sensitive to the enzyme thrombin.[35]

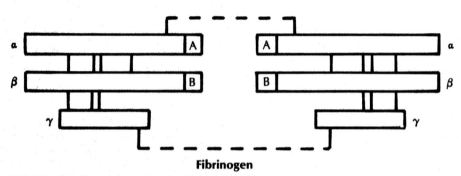

Fibrinogen

FIG. 2-3.   The fibrinogen molecule. (Courtesy of George Fritsma)

TABLE 2-3
Classification, Function, and Biochemistry of Hemostatic Factors of the Coagulation, Fibrinolytic, and Control Mechanisms

Factor	Molecular Weight/(No. Chains)	Active Form
EXTRINSIC SYSTEM		
Factor III	45,000/(1)	Cofactor
Factor VII	55,000/(1)	Serine protease
INTRINSIC SYSTEM		
Factor XII	80,000/(1)	Serine protease
Prekallikrein	85,000/(1)	Serine protease
HMWK	120,000/(1)	Cofactor
Factor XI	160,000/(2, dimer)	Serine protease
Factor IX	57,100/(1)	Serine protease
Factor VIII	1–2 million (6–10, multimer)	Cofactor
COMMON PATH		
Factor X	59,000/(2)	Serine protease
Platelet Factor 3		Cofactor
Factor V	330,000/(1)	Cofactor
Prothrombin(II)	75,500/(1)	Serine protease: Thrombin
Fibrinogen	340,000/(6)	Fibrin clot
Factor XIII	300,000/(4)	Transglutaminase
FIBRINOLYSIS		
Plasminogen	90,000/(1)	Serine protease: Plasmin
CONTROL MECHANISM		
α_2-Macroglobulin	820,000/(multimer)	Serine protease
α_2-Antiplasmin	65,000	Serine protease
Antithrombin III	65,000/(1)	Serine protease
C1 inactivator	104,000	Serine protease
Protein C	62,000/(2)	Serine protease
Protein S		Cofactor

Fibrinogen is converted to a fibrin gel through the action of thrombin, which catalyzes the removal of polar peptides. These peptides, fibrinopeptides A and B (indicated by small boxed areas toward the center of the α and β branches, as seen on Fig. 2-3) constitute approximately 3% of the total fibrinogen molecule. Following fibrin formation and polymerization of fibrin monomer, Factor XIII$_a$ catalyzes the formation of peptide bonds by crosslinking the γ and α chains. This stabilizes the fibrin clot.

Plasmin first attacks the α chains of the molecule in the degradation of the fibrin clot.[9]

Unlike thrombin, which catalyzes the hydrolysis of both the α and β fibrinogen chains with release of fibrinopeptides A and B, certain snake venoms hydrolyze only the α chain, releasing only fibrinopeptide A. Many of these venoms are used as reagents in specific tests like the Reptilase test, which uses the venom of *Bothrops atrox*. Another venom, ancrod, comes from *Bothrops jararaca*, the Malayan pit viper. These venoms

TABLE 2-4
Partial Listing of Some Abnormal Fibrinogens

		Defect in			
		Release of			
Dysfibrinogen	Symptoms	*Fibrino-peptide A*	*Fibrino-peptide B*	*Polymerization*	*Fibrin Stabilization*
Detroit	B	X			
Baltimore	B, T	X		X	X
Paris I	A			X	X
Oklahoma	U				X
Bethesda I	B	X	X		
Giessen II	B			X	
New York	T	?	?		
St. Louis	A			X	
Zurich I	A	X			
Metz	B	X			

B, bleeding; *T*, thrombosis; *A*, asymptomatic; *U*, uncertain; *X*, defect or problem

bypass the effects of heparin and antithrombin III, acting on fibrinogen. In addition, they result in the formation of a friable fibrin clot, one that crumbles or is easily broken.

Dysfibrinogens are structurally abnormal or qualitatively defective fibrinogen molecules. These forms of fibrinogen result in the formation of a soft, friable clot. Table 2-4 is a partial list of dysfibrinogens, along with classification by defects of polymerization, fibrinopeptide release, or fibrin crosslinking when known. The first listing that was developed recorded more than 30 abnormal fibrinogens; now there are more than 80.[5,15] Dysfibrinogens are named after their city of origin and are differentiated by immunoelectrophoresis.

Prothrombin

Prothrombin is a single-chain glycoprotein that migrates with the α_2-globulins.[32] Near the free amino acid terminal end are several γ-carboxyglutamic acids that bind phospholipid, calcium, and inorganic salts such as barium sulfate. The formation of the unique carboxylated portion is altered when vitamin K is absent or is suppressed by oral anticoagulants (coumarin). Inactive forms of prothrombin are then produced. These forms of prothrombin, along with other inactive forms of the vitamin K–dependent factors, are called PIVKAs—proteins induced by vitamin K antagonists.

Normal prothrombin is heat and storage stable; however, it is almost entirely consumed in serum.[23] Only a small amount remains in serum.[24]

Thrombin is activated prothrombin. This reaction requires the proteolytic enzyme Factor X_a and three mediators: platelet phospholipid, calcium, and a cofactor, Factor V_a. The thrombin produced is a strong proteolytic enzyme or serine protease that initiates irreversible hemostatic plug formation. Thrombin is also a trypsinlike enzyme, in that it can act on a variety of substrates, not one specifically. In trace amounts thrombin also enhances the efficiency of Factors V and VIII. It converts fibrinogen to fibrin, as stated earlier, and activates Factor XIII and the fibrinolytic system. Thrombin, in high concentrations, inhibits Factors V and VIII.

Tissue Thromboplastin

Tissue factor (high-molecular-weight lipoprotein) is found in all tissues, although the brain, liver, and placenta have the highest concentrations. Tissue factor is a complex of two components, a phospholipid and a protein. Both are required for full activity of the molecule. Tissue factor is necessary for activation of Factor VII in the extrinsic pathway of coagulation. Upon heating, the protein portion of the factor is denatured, thus decreasing its activity.[39]

Factor V

Factor V is a single-chain glycoprotein that migrates with the albumin fraction on electrophoresis. It is the most heat labile of all the factors and is unstable in plasma, especially when the specimen is collected in a chelating anticoagulant. Factor V deteriorates rapidly at room temperature. Purified, Factor V becomes stable. Platelet Factor V has a slightly different structure from that of normal circulating factor V, but the procoagulant activity of the two is the same (see Chap. 7).[18]

Factor V is activated by thrombin, which can increase Factor V's activity 300-fold. As a cofactor, V_a (V_m) is bound to prothrombin, enhancing the activation of prothrombin. It is thought that this reaction involves a conformational change of the prothrombin molecule, allowing cleavage to be more efficiently accomplished by Factor X_a.[6]

Factor VII

The vitamin K–dependent Factor VII is also a single-chain glycoprotein that migrates on electrophoresis between the α and β globulins. It is the coagulation protein present in the lowest concentration in the plasma. Factor VII is heat labile and storage stable. Refrigerated at 4°C, it remains stable for 2 weeks or more.

Without tissue thromboplastin, Factor VII cannot be activated to VII_a, the serine protease that cleaves Factor X to produce X_a. In a reverse reaction, X_a can attack Factor VII in the presence of phospholipid to enhance Factor VII activity. It has been reported that X_a hydrolyzes VII to yield a two-chain form of VII that has 85 times the procoagulant activity.[28,30a] Yet large amounts of X_a can inactivate Factor VII, limiting X_a's own activation.

It is now documented that Factor VII_a also activates Factor IX through an alternate pathway. This reaction is also dependent on thromboplastin as the cofactor.[26]

If the plasma has been exposed to glass or other surfaces, Factor XII_a, Factor IX_a, and kallikrein can indirectly activate Factor VII.[1]

Factor VIII

Factor VIII is a large multimeric molecule that can be concentrated as *cryoprecipitate.* This commercial preparation of the factor contains two portions of the molecule (VIII:C and VIII:vWF). Factor VIII migrates with the α_2-globulins and is heat and storage labile.

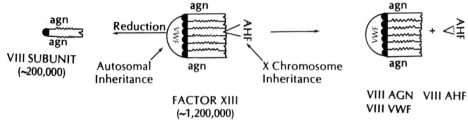

FIG. 2-4.   The Factor VIII complex and its substructures. The multimeric Factor VIII is composed of multiple subunits. VIIIAGN in this figure refers to VIIIR : Ag, the part that possesses antigenic properties. Von Willebrand factor (vWF) is part of the high-molecular-weight portion of the Factor VIII complex that is necessary for platelet adhesion. Another name for this part is VIIIR : Co (ristocetin cofactor), referring to the reagent required to test platelet function by aggregation studies. The small, low-molecular-weight portion of the Factor VIII molecule is antihemophilic globulin (AHG) or antihemophilic factor (AHF). It is now called VIII : C because it possesses the procoagulant activity of the factor. (Modified from Hoyer LW: Von Willebrand's disease. Prog Hemost Thomb 3:231, 1976)

Upon treatment with a high salt concentration of NaCl or $CaCl_2$, the protein complex dissociates into a low-molecular-weight (LMW) portion and a high-molecular-weight (HMW) portion (Fig. 2-4).[14] The LMW component is produced by sex-linked genes and is also called the procoagulant portion (VIII:C). Decreased Factor VIII:C activity causes hemophilia A. The site of production of Factor VIII:C remains unclear. The HMW portion of the molecule is controlled by autosomal inheritance. It contains both Factor VIIIR : Ag and von Willebrand factor (VIII : vWF) activity and is synthesized by the endothelium and megakaryocytes (Fig. 2-5).[37,38] A decrease in concentration in

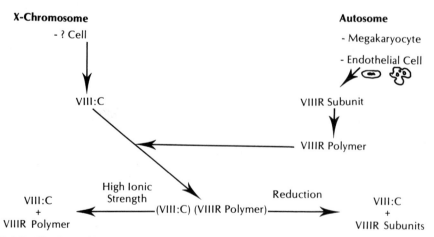

FIG. 2-5.   The Factor VIII complex. This diagram shows the two main parts, their genetic control, and the effects of ionic strength and reduction. (VIIIR is now referred to as vWF.) (Modified from Hoyer LW: The factor VIII complex: Structure and function. Blood 58:1, 1981)

either of these factors plus VIII : C results in von Willebrand disease. Chapter 5 differentiates hemophilia A from von Willebrand disease and provides a full description of the Factor VIII molecule as it relates to these disorders. The entire molecular structure of Factor VIII is still being investigated.

Factor VIII$_a$ is a cofactor to Factor X activation. In response to thrombin, it can be enhanced with small amounts of thrombin but inhibited by large amounts. Factor VIII is sensitive to degradation by plasmin and is also inactivated by protein C.

Below is the nomenclature for Factor VIII as proposed by the International Committee on Thrombosis and Haemostasis. The terminology reflects different methods of testing applied to determine physical and functional abilities of the two parts of the Factor VIII molecule. There is currently some evidence that the HMW portion may indeed have several subparts that are seen as different activities of that part of the molecule.

VIII/vWF. The Factor VIII molecule, composed of VIII : C and vWF portions that are noncovalently bound and circulate in the plasma

VIIIR : RCo. Ristocetin cofactor activity is the Factor VIII – related activity required for the aggregation of human platelets with ristocetin.

VIII : vWF. The von Willebrand factor activity as determined by bleeding time

VIIIR : Ag. Factor VIII – related antigen as measured by immunologic techniques of laurel rocket or immunoradiometric assay

VIII : C. Factor VIII procoagulant activity as measured by the modified APTT, a factor-specific assay

VIIIC : Ag. The antigen reflecting the procoagulant portion of the molecule as measured by immunologic monoclonal antibody technique

Factor IX

Factor IX is a single-chain glycoprotein that migrates with the β globulins. It is a vitamin K – dependent protein that is heat labile and storage stable at 4°C for several weeks. Upon activation, it is converted to a two-chain molecule linked by disulfide bonds. Factor IX level is also controlled by sex-linked inheritance, with a deficiency resulting in hemophilia B.

Factor IX is activated by XI$_a$, a reaction that cleaves the Factor IX molecule at two sites. This provides a highly negatively charged enzyme that can aid in the activation of Factor X. An enzyme from Russell's viper venom can also activate Factor IX.[2]

Factor X

The glycoprotein Factor X consists of two chains, a light chain and a heavy chain, connected by disulfide bonds. The molecule migrates between the α and prealbumin bands on electrophoresis. As a vitamin K – dependent protein, it is relatively heat stable and can be stored at 4°C for weeks to several months.

Factor X is activated by Factor VII$_a$ in the extrinsic system and by a IX$_a$ – calcium – phospholipid complex in the intrinsic system. Activation of Factor X is the first step of the common pathway. Factor X can also be activated by Russell's viper venom and dilute trypsin.[12]

Factor XI

Factor XI consists of two similar polypeptide chains. This protein is somewhat heat labile, and its concentration increases upon storage. It is a glycoprotein that migrates with the β or γ globulins. It circulates in the plasma with HMWK.

Factor XI is activated by both trypsin and Factor XII$_a$ through limited proteolysis. Factor XI, in turn, activates Factor IX as part of the contact activation system.[31]

Factor XII

Factor XII is the earliest enzyme of the intrinsic pathway of coagulation to become activated. It is heat labile after 30 minutes at 60°C. It is stable stored at 4°C for up to 3 months. As a single-chain glycoprotein, it migrates with the β globulins. It can be activated by exposure to negatively charged surfaces such as glass, ellagic acid, collagen, celite, homocysteine, fatty acids, endotoxin, and others.[11]

Once activated, Factor XII$_a$ activates prekallikrein to convert it to kallikrein and activates Factor XI, with the aid of HMWK, initiating the kinin and coagulation systems.

Factor XIII

Factor XIII is a member of the enzyme group called transglutaminases. XIII consists of two pairs of nonidentical polypeptide chains. It is heat labile and storage stable. It migrates in the α_2-globulin region. Factor XIII is trapped in the fibrin clot as it is formed and is activated by thrombin. Factor XIII$_a$, an enzyme, is essential in forming the covalent bonds between adjacent fibrin monomers. This crosslinking of fibrin, the final step in fibrin formation, produces a stable fibrin clot that can withstand dissolution in 5M urea. Evidence also points to Factor XIII's involvement in strengthening the attachment of fibrin to platelets and fibroblasts with the substance *fibronectin*.[21]

Persons deficient in Factor XIII tend to form *keloids*, resulting from the overproduction of collagen within a scar.

Fletcher Factor

Also called prekallikrein, Fletcher factor has been isolated in two forms of equal molecular weight and function. Prekallikrein circulates in the plasma complexed to HMWK. It migrates as a fast γ-globulin.

Factor XII$_a$ hydrolyzes a peptide bond of prekallikrein to convert it to kallikrein. Kallikrein then attacks prekallikrein to activate plasminogen and the fibrinolytic system.

Fitzgerald Factor

Fitzgerald factor, or HMWK, is thought to be produced by the liver. As a single-chain glycoprotein involved in contact activation, it has no proteolytic action. It circulates complexed with prekallikrein and Factor XI.[20]

Kallikrein acts on HMWK to release bradykinin and several other components. Only the light chain of one of the small subunits has procoagulant activity.

Other Factors

Phospholipid and calcium are essential accelerators of blood coagulation. They mediate the conversion of X to X_a and prothrombin to thrombin. Phospholipid is found within tissue. Platelets are a source of both. In addition, free calcium circulates at concentrations of 8.4 mEq to 10.2 mEq/liter in plasma. Ionized calcium is an important cofactor in other coagulation reactions. Hypocalcemia could never cause bleeding problems, however, for the level decrease that causes tetany is less than that needed to cause bleeding.

Fibrinolytic Proteins

Plasminogen

The zymogen plasminogen circulates as a single-chain glycoprotein that is produced in the liver. It is found in plasma and other body fluids. Plasminogen is present in barium sulfate– or aluminum hydroxide–adsorbed plasma, but not in serum. It migrates on plasma electrophoresis in the β-globulin region. When a clot is formed, plasminogen becomes bound to fibrin and incorporated into the clot. Nearby endothelial cells and smooth muscle cells release tissue plasminogen activator (tPA), which converts plasminogen to active plasmin. Plasmin digests fibrin and is the essential component of fibrinolysis. Free plasmin is indiscriminate in its action, digesting fibrinogen, Factor V, fibrin, and Factor VIII. Free plasmin activity is pathologic and is mediated by such activators as urokinase, streptokinase, Factor XII_a, or kallikrein.

Tissue Plasminogen Activator

Tissue activators are located in most tissues. They are single- or double-chain serine proteases that have a high affinity for fibrin. Derived from the endothelium and secreted into the plasma at the site of destruction, tPA cleaves plasminogen at its arginine–valine site. All extrinsic activators share common functional and structural properties, except urokinase, the activator synthesized by renal cells and secreted into the urine. Urokinase has diminished ability to bind to fibrin and activate plasminogen; however, it is responsible for dissolution of clots in the collecting system of the kidney.[10]

Control Mechanisms: Physiologic Anticoagulants

Naturally occurring anticoagulants are inhibitors of both the coagulation and fibrinolytic systems that keep the body's hemostatic mechanism in check.

Antithrombin III (ATIII), called the heparin cofactor, is produced in the liver as a single polypeptide chain. Heparin is the essential accelerator for ATIII's complexing with thrombin. ATIII is the main inactivator of thrombin but also inhibits Factors XII_a, X_a, and IX_a, kallikrein, and plasmin.

Protein C is a vitamin K–dependent glycoprotein dimer with disulfide-linked chains of unequal length. The light chain carries several γ-carboxyglutamic acids near its free amino-terminal end. The modified glutamic acid moieties form the site that binds ionic calcium. A serine-rich active site is found on the heavy chain.

Protein C, also termed *autoprothrombin II* by Seegers, becomes activated (C_a) in the presence of thrombin. Activation is enhanced by attachment to the endothelium and binding to thrombomodulin. Thrombin ceases to function as protein C is activated.

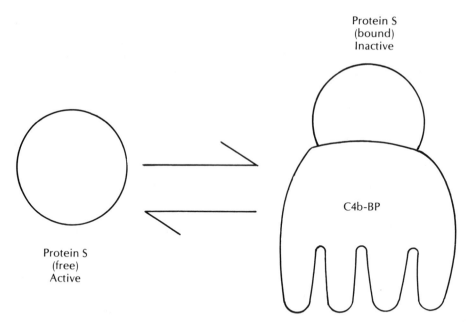

Protein S
(bound)
Inactive

C4b-BP

Protein S
(free)
Active

FIG. 2-6. Two pools of protein S exist in plasma. Only free protein S serves as a cofactor for the anticoagulant effects of activated protein C. The majority of protein S–deficient patients have the protein S–C4b-binding protein complex but little or no free protein S.

Factor V and Factor VIII : C are the most important substrates for protein C, degrading them and providing a feedback mechanism to limit clot formation.[3,4]

Protein S, another vitamin K–dependent protein, is a necessary cofactor for protein C. It exists in two pools, one free and the other bound to a component of complement (C4b). The free pool is the active form (Fig. 2-6).[3]

The most important inhibitor of plasmin is α_2-*antiplasmin.* This is a circulating glycoprotein that migrates to the α_2-globulin position in plasma electrophoresis. α_2-Antiplasmin forms a covalent complex with plasmin, thus inactivating that proteolytic enzyme. It continues with complex formation of Factors VIII and IX to activate Factor X.

α_2-*Macroglobulin* is a large glycoprotein that consists of several subunits. It inhibits kallikrein, thrombin, and plasmin but is not as potent as ATIII.

α_1-*Antitrypsin* has a molecular weight of 50,000 daltons and migrates to the α_1 position on electrophoresis. It inhibits Factor XI_a and plasmin.

C' inactivator inhibits plasmin, kallikrein, Factor XII_a, and Factor XI_a.

THE COAGULATION MECHANISM

The Coagulation Cascade

Thrombus formation requires a complex series of enzymatic reactions called the coagulation cascade. The cascade is a humoral amplification mechanism in which several plasma glycoproteins, termed *procoagulants,* are activated to serine protease enzymes or enzyme cofactors. Each procoagulant and activated enzyme factor in the cascade has been purified and studied biochemically. Although the majority of the coagulation factors behave as enzymes that act on a given substrate, several are cofactors involved in complex formation, thus enhancing the reaction. Thromboplastin, ionic calcium, and phospholipid are additional participants in complex formation, also enhancing the reactions.

The cascade theory arbitrarily divides the reaction into three pathways: intrinsic, extrinsic, and common. The intrinsic pathway begins with contact activation, involving Factors XII and XI, prekallikrein, and HMWK. It continues with complex formation of Factors VIII and IX to activate Factor X. The extrinsic pathway begins with trauma to tissue, causing release of tissue thromboplastin and activation of Factor VII. The pathways converge at the common pathway in activating Factor X.

Factors V and X_a form another complex that converts prothrombin to thrombin, the crucial enzyme in the system that acts on fibrinogen, converting it to fibrin. Figure 2-7 illustrates the currently accepted version of the cascade hypothesis. Each part of the scheme will be discussed in this section: contact activation, intrinsic pathway, extrinsic pathway, common pathway/thrombin generation, and fibrin formation. Alternate pathways are also shown in Figure 2-7 and will be discussed.

Contact Activation

In vivo activation of the coagulation system is initiated by contact with a negatively charged surface, such as collagen or basement membrane exposed when endothelium is damaged. Some alternate, pathologic activators are serum, urate crystals, fatty acids, or endotoxin. The pathologic activators are implicated in conditions of hypercoagulability or disseminated intravascular coagulation. Glass, kaolin (clay), Celite (diatomaceous earth), ellagic acid, and dextran sulfate are some exogenous substances with repetitive negative charges that can activate the contact factors *in vitro*.[19]

The four contact factors (XII, XI, prekallikrein, and HMWK) do not require the presence of calcium for their reactions, and they are all readily adsorbed onto negatively charged surfaces. This adsorption onto the surface allows for close interaction among the factors, enhancing factor XII_a activation of Factor XI. Prekallikrein and HMWK are necessary in the reaction to provide optimal results. *In vitro* studies indicate that the contact phase also activates fibrinolysis and the inflammatory systems of kinin and complement.

The exact events that lead to activation of Factor XII *in vivo* are unclear. One theory is that a conformational change occurs as Factor XII is adsorbed onto the surface. This exposes a serine-rich site that is the active portion of the molecule.[25] Another theory postulates that bound Factor XII is activated by increased enzymatic attack by kallikrein. Unactivated Factor XII has slight enzymatic activity that might contribute to initiation of the coagulation cascade.[33]

Factor XII_a, in the presence of HMWK, activates prekallikrein to generate kallikrein and activates Factor XI to XI_a. Kallikrein and Factor XI_a then reciprocally activate Factor XII in a feedback system that amplifies the reaction (Fig. 2-8). Studies have shown that a single deficiency of prekallikrein, Factor XII, or Factor XI does not totally inhibit contact activation, although it is greatly slowed. Patients with a deficiency of a contact factor have been known to show no signs of clinical bleeding. Factor XII can also autoactivate, thus bypassing the need for prekallikrein and HMWK. The autoactivation of XII still requires a negatively charged surface, but it proceeds much more slowly than normal activation.

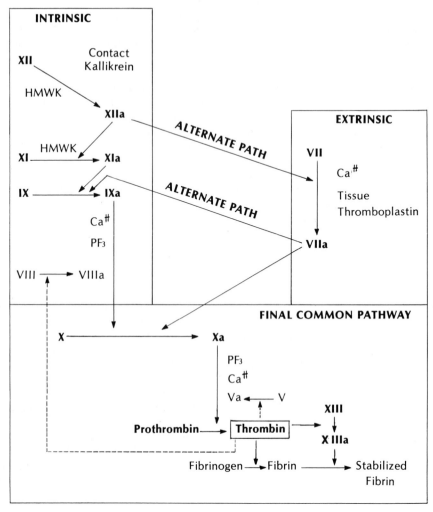

FIG. 2-7. The coagulation cascade. The dotted lines indicate thrombin's feedback action to modify Factors V and VIII.

A second feature of contact activation is autodigestion and kallikrein hydrolysis of Factor XII. These two processes result in the formation of Factor XII fragments (XII$_f$) that are effective in activating prekallikrein and plasminogen proactivator (see Fig. 2-8). The products of these activation reactions (plasminogen activators and kallikrein) activate the fibrinolytic and kinin systems, respectively. Kallikrein acts on HMWK to produce bradykinin, a small polypeptide. Bradykinin is of physiological importance because it increases vascular permeability, dilates small vessels, and contracts smooth muscle, causing pain. Plasminogen proactivator is a complex of kallikrein and Factor XII$_a$. Together they convert plasminogen to plasmin, initiating fibrinolysis.

Contact activation is complete with activation of Factor IX.

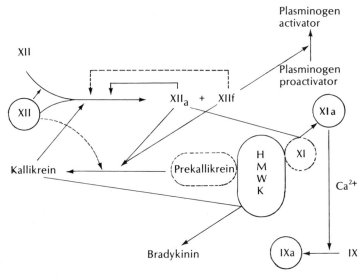

FIG. 2-8. Contact activation. (Courtesy of Larry Brace)

Intrinsic Pathway of Factor X Activation

The intrinsic pathway of coagulation (see Fig. 2-7) technically begins with contact activation of Factor XII to produce XII_a, the enzyme that acts on XI to form XI_a. Factor XI_a, in turn, is the enzyme that cleaves the substrate, Factor IX. This reaction requires calcium. The product of the reaction, Factor IX_a, is a potent serine protease that complexes with Factor VIII, phospholipid, and calcium to convert Factor X to X_a.

Factor VIII requires modification by thrombin in order to function as a cofactor (VIII_a or VIII_m). The phospholipid supplied by platelets provides a surface for the multimolecular complex. This complex formation accelerates the reaction several thousand times over an uncomplexed IX_a *in vitro*.

Extrinsic Pathway of Factor X Activation

The extrinsic pathway, shorter and less complex than the intrinsic pathway, is initiated by tissue thromboplastin (tissue factor) in the presence of calcium. Tissue thromboplastin is a lipoprotein component of all cell membranes that becomes exposed following trauma and activates Factor VII. Activation of Factor VII is a function of its ability to bind to thromboplastin. The phospholipid portion of tissue factor binds to the γ-carboxyglutamic acid on the free amino acid terminus of Factor VII. Thromboplastin then forms a complex with Factor VII_a and calcium to convert Factor X to X_a, the first step of the common pathway.

Alternate Pathways

In the past decade, two alternate pathways or reactions linking the intrinsic and extrinsic paths have been demonstrated (see Fig. 2-7).[26,27] Factor VII_a – tissue thromboplastin–calcium complex activates Factor IX *in vitro*. Also, Factor XII_a activates Factor VII in a cleavage reaction, different from the conformational change of VII by complex formation. The XII_a reaction creates a two-chain form of VII_a that has increased activity on Factor X. The latter reactions implicate Factor XII_a in activation of both the intrinsic and the extrinsic pathways.[1]

The two distinct pathways are becoming increasingly blurred. Although the physiological importance of these new discoveries is not clear, it is apparent that the coagulation mechanism is overlapped and complex.

Common Pathway: Thrombin Generation

Factor X_a forms a complex with Factor V or V_m, platelet and tissue phospholipid, and calcium. Trace amounts of thrombin account for the presence of Factor V_m, a more active cofactor than Factor V. The Factor X_a complex is referred to as prothrombinase, the enzyme that converts prothrombin to thrombin.[17] The active site of the complex is located on the X_a molecule, as shown in the Figure 2-9.

Prothrombin has four cleavage sites and two attachment sites (Fig. 2-10). One attachment site is the area of γ-carboxyglutamic acid near the free amino terminus that binds calcium and a portion of the phospholipid molecule of the prothrombinase complex. The other attachment site, near the center of the molecule, binds Factor V or V_m. Once both sites are bound, Factor X_a cleaves the prothrombin molecule at site 1, producing one fragment called Prethrombin 2 and a smaller fragment called Fragment 1.2 that leaves the area of the reaction. Factor X_a next cleaves Prethrombin 2 at site 2, generating a dimeric thrombin the two chains of which are joined by disulfide bonds.

When thrombin becomes available, the reaction pattern changes. Thrombin autocatalytically cleaves a new prothrombin molecule at site 4, producing Prethrombin 1 and Fragment 1, the latter having no further role in the reaction. Now X_a acts on Prethrombin 1 at site 1 as before, producing Prethrombin 2 and Fragment 2, which also disappears. Prethrombin 2 is cleaved by X_a as before to form thrombin.

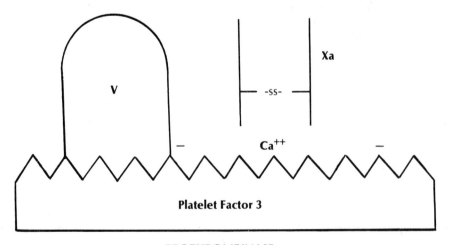

PROTHROMBINASE

FIG. 2-9. The prothrombinase complex.

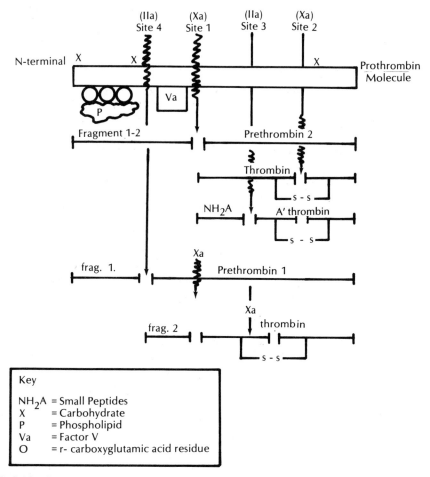

FIG. 2-10. Cleavage of prothrombin to form thrombin.

Thrombin is both autocatalytic and autoinhibitory. Following thrombin formation, free thrombin further cleaves Prethrombin 2 at site 3 to produce a shortened Prethrombin 2 and an amino-terminal peptide carrying several copies of γ-carboxyglutamic acid. Similarly, thrombin attacks the alpha chain of a neighboring thrombin molecule, releasing more amino-terminal peptides. This is shown in Figure 2-10. Loss of the peptide, with its calcium binding properties, inactivates the thrombin molecule. Figure 2-11 summarizes the reaction events of prothrombin cleavage.

Thrombin in high concentrations inhibits activation of Factors V and VIII. The mechanisms that explain why low levels of thrombin activate Factors V and VIII, while high levels inhibit, have not been determined.

Thrombin cleaves fibrinogen to produce fibrin monomers. It activates prothrombin by autocatalysis; it activates Factors V, VIII, and XIII and triggers platelet activation as described in Chapter 8. Thrombin's inhibitory roles include the cleavage of the

ROLES OF THROMBIN IN HEMOSTASIS

Initiates irreversible platelet plug formation
Enhances efficiency of Factors V and VIII
Inhibits Factors V and VIII
Converts fibrinogen to fibrin
Activates Factor XIII
Activates the fibrinolytic system by plasminogen/plasmin
Activates protein C
Cleaves prothrombin to form thrombin

γ-carboxyglutamic acid–carrying end of the prothrombin molecule, inhibition of Factors V and VIII when thrombin concentration is high, and activation of protein C.

Fibrin Formation

Thrombin cleaves fibrinogen at several sites, whereupon polymerization occurs in the final formation of fibrin. Figure 2-12 illustrates the three steps of fibrin formation.

Part I: Factor Complex Reactions

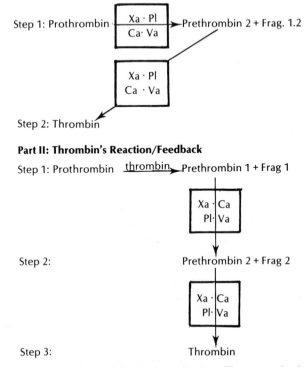

Step 1: Prothrombin · | Xa · Pl / Ca· Va | ► Prethrombin 2 + Frag. 1.2

| Xa · Pl |
| Ca · Va |

Step 2: Thrombin

Part II: Thrombin's Reaction/Feedback

Step 1: Prothrombin   thrombin ► Prethrombin 1 + Frag 1

| Xa · Ca |
| Pl· Va |

Step 2:   Prethrombin 2 + Frag 2

| Xa · Ca |
| Pl· Va |

Step 3:   Thrombin

FIG. 2-11. The thrombin generation and feedback mechanism. The terms platelet phospholipid (*Pl*) and platelet factor 3 are synonymous.

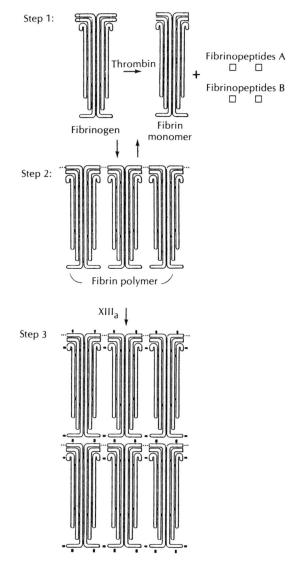

Step 1:

Thrombin

Fibrinopeptides A

Fibrinopeptides B

+

Fibrinogen

Fibrin monomer

Step 2:

Fibrin polymer

XIII$_a$

Step 3

FIG. 2-12. Fibrin formation. (Modified from Harker LA: Hemostasis Manual, 2nd ed, p 25. Philadelphia, FA Davis, 1976)

In step one, cleavage occurs at the carboxy terminals on the alpha and beta chains, producing *fibrin monomer* and two pairs of small peptides designated *fibrinopeptide A* and *fibrinopeptide B*.

In step two, free fibrin monomers spontaneously polymerize by hydrogen bonding to form *fibrin polymer*. The fibrin polymer is a gel and is the first visible clot. This clot is soft and friable.

The third step begins when Factor XIII$_a$, in the presence of calcium, catalyzes the formation of covalent linkages between the carboxy terminals of neighboring gamma chains. These linkages are between the ϵ-amino groups of lysine and the γ-amide groups of glutamine. In addition, XIII_a catalyzes inclusion of fibronectin and α-antiplasmin into the fibrin mesh, enhancing clot stability.

The clot formed at the end of step two is susceptible to rapid degradation by plasmin. Patients deficient in Factor XIII experience poor wound healing and chronic hemorrhage because of the inadequacy of the nonstabilized clot. Factor XIII_a imparts increased stability and resistance to degradation, preventing hemorrhage. Factor XIII deficiency may be detected by a laboratory test employing 5M urea solution, in which the noncrosslinked thrombus dissolves easily and the Factor XIII_a – modified thrombus remains undissolved. This test is described in Chapter 4.

The stabilized thrombus is the end point of the coagulation mechanism.

CONTROL MECHANISMS

There are five mechanisms that have been identified as factors that limit and control thrombus formation:

- Blood flow and endothelial factors
- Clearance mechanisms
- Feedback mechanisms of thrombin
- Fibrinolysis
- Naturally occurring inhibitors

Blood Flow and Endothelial Factors

The flow of blood washes away and dilutes active procoagulants and small fibrin clots from the site of clot formation. Unless venous stasis or a hypercoagulable state exists, thrombus formation is difficult in an intact vessel. This explains why more clots form in veins than in arteries, where the blood flow is rapid.

The vascular endothelium provides biochemicals that have antithrombotic properties, inhibiting thrombus formation. As already discussed in Chapter 1, those factors are prostacyclin, adenosine, serotonin, and thrombomodulin.

Clearance

Several organs and cells clear the circulation of clotting factors. The liver removes active coagulants, especially Factor X_a and plasminogen activator, from the circulation. It has been observed in animal studies that an inhibitor to X_a resides in the liver.[7] The monocytes and macrophages of the reticuloendothelial system (RES) remove particulate fibrin from the circulation.[34] Fibrinogen degradation products may also be removed by the RES.[22] Fibrinogen Fragments D and E are catabolized by the kidney.[16] Thrombin is cleared by binding slowly to endothelium, accelerating its own inactivation. This mechanism is described more fully under Protein C and Protein S, earlier in this chapter.

Feedback Mechanisms

Positive and negative feedback systems occur at several steps in the coagulation mechanism. Thrombin engages in the most complex series of feedback mechanisms. At low levels, thrombin catalyzes the modification of Factors V and VIII to V_m and VIII_m, as described in the previous section. This is an example of positive feedback. V_m and VIII_m are more active than their unmodified counterparts. However, at high levels of thrombin, the activity of V and VIII is inhibited in a negative feedback system. A similar situation arises in the autocatalytic reaction of thrombin, in which thrombin enhances and inhibits its own formation in both positive and negative feedbacks.

Factor XII_a converts prekallikrein to kallikrein. Kallikrein next enhances the formation of Factor XII_a, an example of positive feedback.

When fibrin gel is formed, other procoagulants are physically prevented from entering the reaction site. This is an example of negative feedback. Other interactions, including the effect of thrombin on Factor XIII, kallikrein activation of plasminogen proactivators, the effect of Factor X_a on Factor VII, and the effect of Factor VII_a on Factor XII activation, all play a role in coagulation control, although in many cases the role is obscure.

Fibrinolysis

The fibrinolytic system removes fibrin fragments and dissolves clots, ensuring a free-flowing vascular system. Plasmin is a proteolytic enzyme that digests fibrin. Fibrin degradation products (FDPs) are generated during fibrinolysis; certain FDPs are strong anticoagulants that interfere with platelet aggregation and fibrin polymerization.

Naturally Occurring Inhibitors

ATIII, α_2-macroglobulin, α_1-antitrypsin, α_2-plasmin inhibitor, C′1 inactivator, and protein C are plasma-borne inhibitors of coagulation. In most cases the concentration of these inhibitors in plasma exceeds the concentration of the procoagulants (see Table 2-2). Inhibitors actually constitute 20% of the globulin fraction of the plasma.[30b] Activation of procoagulants in the circulation is quickly neutralized by these inhibitors, ensuring that coagulation is limited to local sites.

The term *antithrombin* is used to designate activities and substances that inactivate thrombin. Originally it was thought that there were six antithrombins, all designated by roman numerals. Only two are now considered to be of importance, antithrombin I (ATI) and ATIII. The adsorption of thrombin to fibrin is considered to be a major control mechanism of inactivating thrombin. This activity is called ATI.

ATIII is the most important antithrombin. It is a glycoprotein that progressively inactivates thrombin. The reaction requires heparin as a cofactor. Natural or therapeutic heparin binds 1 : 1 at the lysine site on ATIII, causing a conformational change in the ATIII molecule that exposes the active arginine site (Fig. 2-13). The arginine-rich active site is exposed, combining covalently to the serine at the active site on thrombin. With the serine site bound, thrombin becomes inactive. The heparin – ATIII reaction is reversible, allowing for efficient reuse of the heparin molecule. The ATIII – thrombin reaction is irreversible. The heparin – ATIII complex can also inactivate Factors XII_a, XI_a, and X_a, kallikrein, and plasmin. Procoagulants that have formed a complex with phospholipid, cofactors, and calcium are protected from ATIII. The term *antithrombin VI* refers to the anticoagulant action of FDPs. The other antithrombins, ATII, ATIV, and ATV are insignificant, and their validity is questionable.

α_2-Macroglobulin is an antithrombin that is less potent than ATIII. It is postulated that α_2-macroglobulin inhibits thrombin in two steps. First, thrombin cleaves a small fragment off the α_2-macroglobulin molecule. Next, the large portion of the molecule

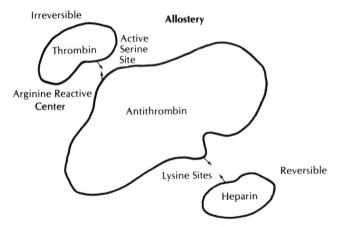

FIG. 2-13. Interaction of ATIII and heparin with thrombin. (Courtesy of George Fritsma)

undergoes a conformational change, trapping the thrombin inside in an irreversible reaction. α_2-Macroglobulin can also inactivate plasmin and kallikrein.

α_1-Antitrypsin inhibits Factor XI$_a$ and plasmin. Its inactivation of thrombin is still being debated.

α_2-Antiplasmin is the most important inhibitor of circulating plasmin. It forms a 1 : 1 complex at the active site of the enzyme that interferes with plasminogen binding to fibrin. This reaction slows down local fibrinolysis, enhancing clot retention. α_2-Antiplasmin inactivates any protease and is antithrombotic.

C1 inactivator (C1 esterase inhibitor) inhibits C1 esterase of the complement cascade and plasmin, kallikrein, Factor XII$_a$, and Factor XI$_a$.

Protein C, the vitamin K–dependent plasma glycoprotein, is an important regulator of the hemostatic mechanism. It circulates as a zymogen that is converted to a serine protease, when activated by thrombin. This reaction is greatly enhanced by thrombomodulin, a cofactor found on the surface of endothelial cells. Figure 2-14 illustrates how, in the presence of calcium, thrombin binds to thrombomodulin in a 1 : 1 complex with another cofactor, protein S. Protein S exists in two pools in the circulation, one bound to C4b-binding protein and the other free. It is the free pool that aids in the

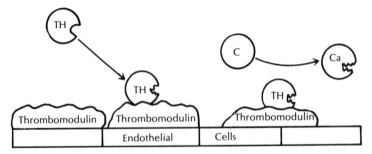

FIG. 2-14. Activation of protein C. (Modified from Comp PC, Clouse L: Plasma proteins C and S: The function and assay of two natural anticoagulants. Laboratory Management, December 1985)

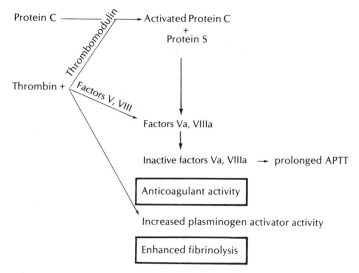

FIG. 2-15. Anticoagulant effects of protein C. (Davis GL, LaCroix KA: A review of protein C and its role in hemostasis. J Med Technol 2:2, 1985)

activation of protein C. As a complex, protein C–S destroys Factors V_a and VIII_a (VIII : C, specifically) through proteolysis. Protein C–S has also been shown to increase plasminogen activator activity by neutralizing the inhibitor of plasminogen activation. This enhances fibrinolysis (Fig. 2-15). The dual role of this protein, inhibiting coagulation and enhancing fibrinolysis, provides an overall anticoagulant effect.

FIBRINOLYSIS

The role of fibrinolysis in hemostasis is to digest and lyse the formed thrombus. Fibrinolysis prevents vessel occlusion at the site of trauma by reestablishing blood flow during the formation of granulation tissue. Plasmin is the enzyme that accomplishes fibrinolysis. Plasmin circulates as an inactive zymogen, plasminogen, that is converted upon contact with an activator such as tPA, urokinase, or streptokinase. The fibrinolytic system, diagrammed in Figure 2-16, includes cofactors and inhibitors.

During coagulation, plasminogen becomes bound to thrombin and is trapped within the thrombus. Here, activators, primarily tPA, cleave plasminogen to form plasmin. Plasmin hydrolyzes peptide bonds at sites of arginine and lysine, resulting in the production of FDPs. Activators will also convert circulating plasminogen, but free plasminogen is immediately inactivated by α_2-antiplasmin and other plasmin inhibitors.

Pathologic activation of free plasminogen in primary fibrinolysis or disseminated intravascular coagulation results in circulating levels of plasmin that supersede the inactivating capacity of the various antiplasmins. Pathologic fibrinolysis *(fibrinogenolysis)* constitutes a medical emergency because circulating fibrin monomers and FDPs can cause uncontrollable bleeding. Plasmin also catalyzes hydrolysis of Factors V and VIII.

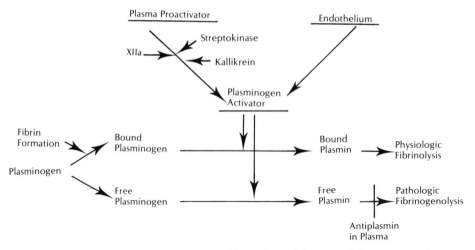

FIG. 2-16. Normal and abnormal pathways of fibrinolysis. (Courtesy of George Fritsma)

Activators

Plasminogen activators are intrinsic or plasma-borne, such as kallikrein or Factor XII$_a$, or extrinsic to plasma, such as tPA secreted by damaged endothelial cells. There are two exogenous activators, urokinase and streptokinase. Streptokinase is prepared from bacterial cultures of β-hemolytic streptococci, and urokinase is derived commercially from urine. Both are used therapeutically for clot dissolution (see Chap. 11).

Fibrin Clot Dissolution

Following plasminogen activation, plasmin cleaves fibrin to form smaller and smaller fragments that are removed by the RES and other organs.

There are three major domains on the fibrin molecule. Each domain consists of degradation Fragments D, E, and D. Each DD domain of the molecule is linked by a disulfide bond. The terminal ends have one domain each and represent the β and γ chains. Plasmin cleaves the fibrin at arginine–lysine bonds, of which there are more than 300 on the fibrin polymer. However, during degradation only 50 or 60 of these bonds are split.[15]

Plasmin digests fibrin (Fig. 2-17) by first cleaving the polymer centrally on the Aα chain at sensitive protease sites to produce fibrin strands (Fragment X) and A, B, and C split products. The main cleavage sites reside on the α chains of fibrin. This is stage 1 of fibrinolysis. All fragments of fibrin digestion are referred to as fibrin split products or fibrin degradation products (FSPs or FDPs).

In stage 2 the process of digestion continues by further action of plasmin on the fibrin strand (Fragment X) to produce Fragment Y and a smaller Fragment D. The cleavage here occurs at the central and terminal domains.

In stage 3 Fragment Y is then degraded into a Fragment E and a Fragment D (DED complex). This digestion proceeds until the fibrin is finally broken down into the D and E fragments and small peptides that can be cleared from the circulation.

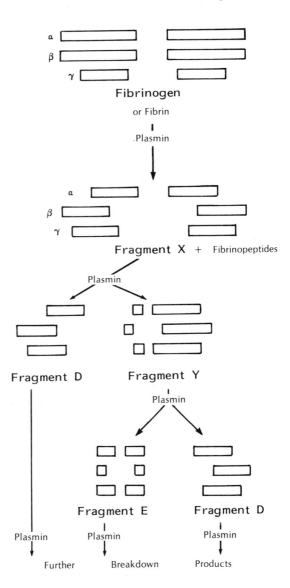

FIG. 2-17. Plasmin's proteolytic action on fibrin breaks fibrinogen down into smaller and smaller fragments. The D, E, and D fragments and polypeptides are the final degradation products that are removed from the circulation by the RES and liver and spleen. The larger fragments, X, Y, and D, if allowed to accumulate, have anticoagulant properties.

Degradation of fibrinogen by plasmin is more rapid than degradation of fibrin because there is no crosslinkage. FDPs from fibrinogen breakdown are different because of their lack of covalent bonding, holding the domains together.

When Fragments X and Y or intermediate FDPs accumulate, they can exert a strong anticoagulant effect. Fragments D and Y inhibit fibrin polymerization; Fragment E inhibits thrombin, while they all are thought to interfere with platelet function. Chapter 4 discusses the immunologic and paracoagulation tests to detect these FDPs.

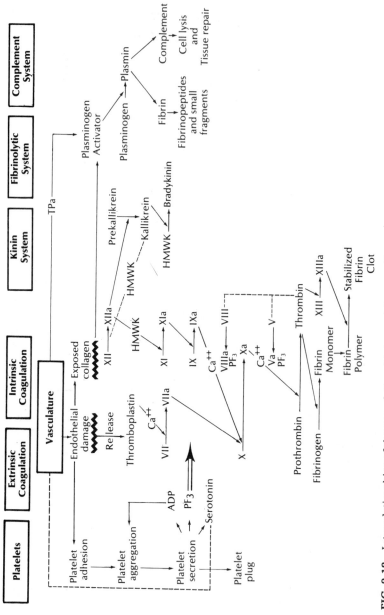

FIG. 2-18. Interrelationships of the coagulation, kinin, complement, fibrinolytic, and vascular systems. (Modified from Bishop ML, Duben-Von Laufen JL, Fody EP: Clinical Chemistry: Principles, Procedures, Correlations, p 509. Philadelphia JB Lippincott, 1985)

Inactivation: Control of Fibrinolysis

As stated previously, plasmin is rapidly inactivated by α_2-antiplasmin. This potent enzyme is of such concentration in the plasma that half of the total plasminogen concentration, if converted to plasmin, would be neutralized immediately. α_2-Antiplasmin is the major control mechanism of fibrinolysis. Free plasmin is rapidly inactivated.

In vitro studies have shown that α_2-macroglobulin, ATIII, and C1 inactivator do inhibit plasmin, although their significance *in vivo* is still not clear.

INTERACTION WITH OTHER MECHANISMS

In this textbook, coagulation, platelet activation, and vascular physiology are described as separate systems. An analytical approach is necessary for didactic reasons. In reality, there are many points of interaction among these systems. Some of these are illustrated in Figures 2-18 and 2-19.

The coagulation system and the vasculature interact in at least four places. First, contact activation of Factor XII requires exposure of negatively charged collagen. This is found in the basement membrane of the blood vessels, just outside the endothelial layer. Second, tissue thromboplastin is released from damaged vessel walls to activate Factor VII in the extrinsic mechanism. Third, tPA from endothelial and vascular

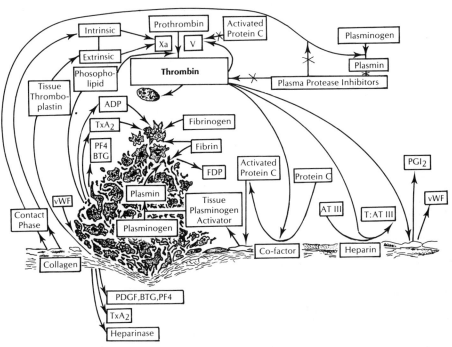

FIG. 2-19. Interactions among hemostatic components. (Thompson AR, Harker LA: Manual of Hemostasis and Thrombosis, 3rd ed, p 41. Philadelphia, FA Davis, 1983)

smooth muscle cells is needed to initiate fibrinolysis. Fourth, activation of protein C is mediated by thrombomodulin, a component of endothelial cell membranes.

Coagulation and platelet activation are intimately connected. Contact activation of Factor XII may be accomplished by certain platelet surface changes, including provision of XII$_a$ from the platelet itself. Furthermore, platelet phospholipid is part of at least three procoagulant complexes in the cascade mechanism. Platelets supply a variety of procoagulants, including platelet-specific substances like platelet factor 4 and β-thromboglobulin, that contribute to thrombus formation. Many investigators now consider the platelet to be the prime element of thrombus formation. Finally, platelets partially mediate clot retraction through an undefined mechanism.

Clots form at sites of trauma or injury. Consequently, coagulation must be perceived as an initial step in the inflammatory process that eventually includes infiltration by neutrophils, lymphocytes, and macrophages, the activators of the humoral amplification mechanisms of complement, kallikrein–bradykinin, mitogenesis, and granulation formation. The interaction between contact activation and formation of kinins is becoming clearer as research in this area continues. Activation of the complement cascade by Factor XII$_a$ and plasmin has been established. These systems also participate in coagulation at several points. Kallikrein, for example, activates several procoagulants, and HMWK serves as a cofactor in two enzymatic reactions. These two systems also interact to initiate fibrinolysis through activation of plasminogen to plasmin.

Hemostasis, like all humoral amplification mechanisms, seems unnecessarily complex, although it need not be. The system must be able to respond to physiologic and biochemical changes that can be extremely subtle. Amplification mechanisms involving multiple enzymes are able to produce a response, yet systems of this sort can be dangerous if the response is inappropriate. For this reason, each step requires internal and external feedback and controls. The control mechanisms ensure that coagulation proceeds only when necessary and in the appropriate amount.

REFERENCES

1. Altman R, Hemker HC: Contact activation in the extrinsic blood clotting system. Throm Diath Haemorrh 18:525, 1967
2. Bertino RM, Veltkamp JJ: Physiology and biochemistry of factor IX. In Bloom A, Thomas D (eds): Haemostasis and Thrombosis, pp 98–110. New York, Churchill Livingstone, 1981
3. Comp PC, Clouse L: Plasma protein C and S: The function and assay of two natural anticoagulants. Lab Man 23:29–32, 1985
4. Crois KA, Davis CL: A review of protein C and its role in hemostasis. J Med Technol 2:295–298, 1985
5. Crum ED: Abnormal fibrinogens. In Ogsten D, Bennett B (eds): Haemostasis: Biochemistry, Physiology and Pathology. London, John Wiley & Sons, 1977
6. Dahlbeck B: Human coagulation factor V purification and thrombin catalyzed activation. J Clin Invest 66:538, 1980
7. Dreykin D, Cochios F, Mosher D: An hepatic inhibitor of activated clotting factor X (Stuart). Biochem Biophys Res Commun 34:245, 1969
8. Doolittle RF: The structures of fibrinogen and fibrin. In Mahn KG, Taylor FB (eds): The Regulation of Coagulation, pp 501–514. New York, Elsevier, 1980
9. Edington TS, Plow EE: Conformational and structural modulation of the NH$_2$ terminal region of fibrinogen and fibrin associated with plasmin cleavage. J Biol Chem 250:3393, 1975

10. Francis CW, Marder VJ: Mechanisms of fibrinolysis. In Williams W, Beutler E, Erslev A, Lichtman MA (eds): Hematology, pp 1266–1273. New York, McGraw-Hill, 1983

11. Fujikawa K et al: Activation of bovine factor XII (Hageman factor) by plasma kallikrein. Biochemistry 19(1):322, 1980

12. Fujikawa K, Legaz M, Davies EW: Bovine factor X (Stuart factor): Mechanism of activation by a protein from Russell's viper venom. Biochemistry 11:4892, 1982

13. Hawn CV, Porter KR: The fine structure of clots formed from purified bovine fibrinogen and thrombin: A study with the electron microscope. J Exp Med 86:285, 1947

14. Hoyer LW: The factor VIII complex: Structure and function. Blood 58:1, 1981

15. Gralnick H: Congenital disorders of fibrinogen. In Williams W, Beutler E, Erslev A, Lichtman MA (eds): Hematology, pp 1399–1406. New York, McGraw-Hill, 1983

16. Iio A et al: The roles of renal catabolism and uremia in modifying the clearance of fibrinogen and its degradation fragments D and E. J Lab Clin Med 87:934, 1976

17. Jackson CM: Biochemistry of prothrombin activation. In Bloom A, Thomas D (eds): Haemostasis and Thrombosis, pp 140–159. New York, Churchill Livingstone, 1981

18. Kane WH, Majerus PW: Purification and characteristics of human coagulation factor V. J Biol Chem 256:1002, 1981

19. Kaplan AP: Initiation of the intrinsic coagulation and fibrinolytic pathways of man: The role of surfaces, Hageman factor, prekallikrein, high-molecular-weight-kininogen, and factor XI. Prog Hemost Thromb 4:127, 1977

20. Kerbiriou DM, Griffin JH: Human high molecular weight kinogen: Studies of structure, function relationships and of proteolysis of the molecule occurring during contact activation of plasma. J Biol Chem 254:12020, 1979

21. Keski-Oja J, Mosher DF, Vaheri A: Crosslinking of a major fibroblast surface-associated glycoprotein (fibronectin) catalyzed by blood coagulation factor XIII. Cell 9:29, 1976

22. Lee L: Reticuloendothelial clearance of circulating fibrin in the pathogenesis of the generalized Shwartzman reaction. J Exp Med 115:1065, 1962

23. Magnusson S: Primary structure studies on thrombin and prothrombin. Thromb Diath Haemorrh 54:31–35, 1973

24. Magnusson S, Sottrup JL, Pettersen TE et al: Principal structure of the vitamin K–dependent part of prothrombin. FEBS Lett 44:189–193, 1974

25. McMillan CR, Saito H, Ratnoff OD, Walton AG: The secondary structure of human Hageman factor (factor XII) and its alteration by activation agents. J Clin Invest 54:1312, 1974

26. Osterud B: Activation pathways of the coagulation system in normal haemostasis. Scand J Haematol 32:337–345, 1984

27. Radcliff R, Bagdasarian A, Colman R, Nemerson Y: Activation of bovine factor VII by Hageman factor fragments. Blood 50:611, 1977

28. Radcliff R, Nemerson Y: Mechanism of activation of bovine factor VII: Products of activation by factor Xa. J Biol Chem 251(4):749, 1976

29. Rosenberg RD: Hemorrhagic disorders. I. Protein interactions in the clotting mechanism. In Beck WS (ed): Hematology, 3rd ed, pp 373–400. Cambridge, MIT Press, 1981

30. Saito H: Normal hemostatic mechanisms. In Ratnoff OD, Forbes CD (eds): Disorders of Hemostasis, a, p 37; b, p 40. New York, Grune & Stratton, 1984

31. Saito H, Ratnoff OD, Marshall JS, Pensky J: Partial purification of plasma thromboplastin antecedent (factor XI) and its activation by trypsin. J Clin Invest 52:850, 1973

32. Shapiro SS, McCord S: Prothrombin. Prog Hemost Thromb 4:177, 1978

33. Silverberg M, Thompson R, Miller G, Kaplan AP: Initiation of the intrinsic coagulation pathway: Autoactivability of human Hageman factor and mechanisms by which the light chain derived from HMW-kininogen functions as co-factor in the activation of prekallikrein, factor XI, and Hageman factor. In Mann KG, Taylor FB (eds): The Regulation of Coagulation, p 531. New York, Elsevier, 1980

34. Spaet TH, Horowitz HI, Zucker-Franklin D et al: Reticuloendothelial clearance of blood thromboplastin by rats. Blood 17:196, 1961

35. Williams W: Biochemistry of plasma coagulation factors. In Williams W, Beutler E, Erslev A, Lichtman MA (eds): Hematology, pp 1202–1213. New York, McGraw-Hill, 1983
36. Wright IS: The nomenclature of blood clotting factors. Thromb Diath Haemorrh 7:381, 1962
37. Zimmerman T, Meyer D: Structure and function of Factor VIII/von Willebrand factor. In Bloom A, Thomas D (eds): Haemostasis and Thrombosis. New York, Churchill Livingstone, 1981
38. Zimmerman TS, Edington TS: Factor VIII related antigen: Multiple molecular forms in human plasma. Proc Natl Acad Sci USA 72:5121, 1975
39. Zur M, Nemerson Y: Tissue factor pathways of blood coagulation. In Bloom A, Thomas D (eds): Haemostasis and Thrombosis. New York, Churchill Livingstone, 1981

Specimen Collection and Quality Control   **3**

Harlene Stapf Palkuti

CASE STUDY   The technologist encounters an elderly patient with difficult veins and must draw a specimen for coagulation using a syringe. The specimen is obtained with the first syringe, and 4.5 ml of blood is squirted into a 10-ml Vacutainer tube containing 0.5 ml of buffered 3.8% sodium citrate anticoagulant. The technologist remains on the floor 1 hour to draw additional specimens before returning to the laboratory. Once back in the laboratory, the technologist, who works in the hematology department, is called to run some stat work on the Coulter S. While running complete blood counts (CBCs) on the stats, the technologist learns that her difficult draw has a hematocrit of 61%. Meanwhile, the coagulation technologist finally receives the coagulation tube that was drawn from this patient 3 hours before. Is it satisfactory to test the specimen, and would the results be valid after this period?

The handling of this specimen was less than optimal. First, all blood drawn for coagulation studies should be the second tube drawn; in the case of a syringe, two syringes are necessary. The first 2 ml to 3 ml of blood drawn would contain tissue thromboplastin that could activate the coagulation sequence and cause shortened results. Although it is best to place all specimens for testing on ice or in a cool block immediately, 2 hours is the maximum time allowed for specimens to be at room temperature prior to testing prothrombin times or activated partial thromboplastin times. This patient's hematocrit (the value of which was not known prior to specimen collection) would also affect the coagulation test result. The correct ratio of blood to anticoagulant should be 9 : 1. Therefore, 6.9 ml of blood should have been *gently* allowed to flow down the side of the 10-ml tube that contained 0.5 ml of sodium citrate. The specimen for this patient is unacceptable and should be redrawn.

The purpose of this chapter is to introduce the reader to techniques that ensure the validity of hemostasis test results. These techniques include collection, handling, and processing of hemostasis samples and quality assurance principles that ensure uniformity of testing.

Collection, handling, and processing whole blood and plasma samples for hemostatic tests require careful adherence to an established protocol. Coagulation and platelet function test procedures are especially sensitive to variations in these critical initial steps. During blood collection, for example, trauma may trigger activation of proteins, resulting in falsely shortened coagulation test results. During storage, exposure to negatively charged surfaces such as untreated glass may have the same effect. On the other hand, prolonged storage at room temperature diminishes the activity of Factors V and VIII, resulting in prolonged prothrombin times (PTs) or activated partial thromboplastin times (APTTs). Once blood is removed from the body and stored, *in vitro* changes are unavoidable. These changes vary in rate and intensity from individual to individual; thus, consistent application of blood handling protocols is essential if clinical conclusions may be reached through the use of hemostatic tests.

Each hemostasis laboratory may choose from among a variety of handling protocols, provided that certain standards are met. For example, collection for routine coagulation tests may be accomplished by syringe or evacuated tube. Storage times and temperatures vary from laboratory to laboratory, depending on the availability of facilities and clinical demands. Furthermore, each facility may select from a variety of anticoagulants, test procedures, reagent manufacturers, and clot detection devices. The most important fact that must be stressed is that once the laboratory has established protocols for specimen collection, handling, and processing, and for the performance of coagulation procedures, each technologist in that laboratory must *precisely adhere* to the guidelines. Deviation from established protocol will invalidate test results. Changes in protocol require careful study, clinical comparisons using a large number of normal and abnormal samples, and adjustment of mean values and normal ranges.

A working quality-control program is essential to ensure validity and correct clinical interpretation of test data. A particular test may be performed by one of several methods; furthermore, identical techniques produce varied results in different institutions because of ambient conditions and peculiarities of the patient population and laboratory personnel. Consequently, for test results to reflect the hemostatic condition of the patient, it is necessary that the individual laboratory establish a local normal range or reference limit.

Coagulation controls may be locally prepared or purchased commercially with previously determined reference results in both the normal and abnormal ranges. At least one control is incorporated into each group of specimens to be tested. Results of the control specimen are compared to the known value, and if they are in agreement, results of the unknown specimens are considered valid. Controls for platelet counting may be fresh or stored whole blood from healthy donors with preestablished results. Freshly drawn specimens from healthy donors are required for control of platelet function studies.

COLLECTION, HANDLING, AND PROCESSING OF WHOLE BLOOD SPECIMENS

Anticoagulants

Three anticoagulants are commonly used for the collection and preservation of whole blood specimens in the general hematology/hemostasis laboratory: ethylenediamine-tetraacetic acid (Sequestrene or EDTA), heparin, and sodium citrate in either of two concentrations, 3.2% or 3.8% (0.109M or 0.129M).

The anticoagulant chosen for whole blood collection for use in most coagulation and platelet function procedures is the dihydrate salt of sodium citrate ($Na_2C_6H_8O_7$-$2H_2O$). Sodium citrate and sodium oxalate (an anticoagulant previously used for coagulation testing) bind free plasma calcium to prevent clotting. Sodium citrate has replaced oxalate as the anticoagulant of choice for general coagulation procedures in most laboratories. Some advantages of citrate are that calcium ions are neutralized more rapidly in citrate than with oxalate, Factors V and VIII are more stable, and citrate has demonstrated increased sensitivity to the presence of heparin in the performance of APTTs.

Two concentrations of sodium citrate are available, although the choice of concentration provides no clear advantage. The International Committee for Standardization in Hematology (ICSH), the International Committee on Thrombosis and Haemostasis (ICTH), and the National Committee for Clinical Laboratory Standards (NCCLS) all permit the use of *either* 3.2% or 3.8% citrate for general coagulation assays such as the PT.[16,22] Sodium citrate is available in powder form; however, standard practice is to employ a liquid solution. No other type of anticoagulant is used for clot-based coagulation tests. Other forms of citrate anticoagulant that are used in the clinical laboratory are acid citrate dextrose (ACD) or citrate phosphate dextrose (CPD). These two solutions are used in storage of donor blood and derivatives such as platelet concentrates.

Heparin is a unique anticoagulant because of its ability to prevent coagulation both *in vivo* and *in vitro*. It is a naturally circulating anticoagulant, and synthetic heparin from various sources is commonly used as a therapeutic anticoagulant in thromboembolic disorders. Heparin is also used as an anticoagulant in the collection of blood specimens for the clinical chemistry laboratory and for certain specific hematologic applications including osmotic fragility tests and leukocyte alkaline phosphatase stain. Heparin is *unsuitable* as an anticoagulant for specimens submitted for hemostatic tests because it inhibits several coagulation factors (Fig. 3-1).[22] Acting as a catalyst for antithrombin III, heparin inhibits thrombin and Factors XII_a, XI_a, IX_a, and X_a.

Disodium or tripotassium EDTA also binds free plasma calcium, but it is unsuitable as an anticoagulant for the collection of specimens for hemostasis testing because Factor V is unstable in its presence. EDTA has been shown to inhibit the fibrinogen–thrombin reaction and to further bind the reagent calcium that is added to activate *in vitro* coagulation. EDTA is used for blood collected for routine hematologic workups and for platelet counting.

Blood Collection

Hemostatic tests require anticoagulated whole blood, platelet-rich plasma (derived from whole blood spun at low centrifugal force, enabling platelets to remain in the plasma for use in platelet function studies), platelet-poor plasma (platelets are removed by high centrifugal force), or platelet-free plasma (obtained by filtration). Blood sam-

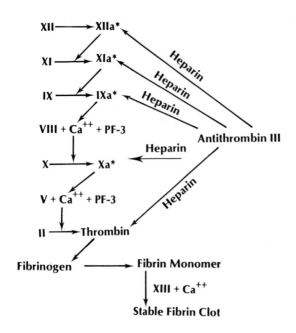

Intrinsic System

FIG. 3-1. Anticoagulant activity of heparin. (From Triplett DA: *Laboratory Evaluation of Coagulation*. Chicago: The American Society of Clinical Pathologists, © 1982. Used by permission)

PF₃ = Platelet Factor 3

* = Active serine protease

ples for hemostatic tests are collected using either evacuated tube systems such as Vacutainer or Venoject or syringes. Collection techniques must minimize trauma to tissue. Several general hematology textbooks provide stepwise protocols for blood collection that are suitable for the hemostasis laboratory. (One such text is Brown B: Hematology: Principles and Procedures, 4th ed. Philadelphia, Lea & Febiger, 1984.) Excess manipulation of the needle damages tissue and promotes release of coagulation-promoting interstitial tissue fluid, contaminating the specimen. Prolonged tourniquet application slows venous return. Slowed or stopped venous circulation is referred to as *stasis* and results in elevation of certain factors such as Factor VIII. Both stasis and tissue fluid contamination may result in false shortening of the various coagulation test results. Consequently, sparing use of a tourniquet and nontraumatic puncture are essential.

Large-bore collection needles provide the most reliable specimens; however, a 20-gauge or 21-gauge thin-wall needle may be employed for routine collections. These medium-bore needles provide reasonable comfort for the patient and do relatively little damage to the sample. Nineteen-gauge needles are recommended for obtaining specimens for special studies such as platelet aggregometry or factor assays. The bigger the bore of the needle, the less chance of mechanical disruption of red blood cells, commonly known as *hemolysis*. The presence of hemolysis interferes with coagulation tests and contributes to inaccurate results.

When specimens are collected by vacuum-tube apparatus, tubes must be composed of nonreactive material such as plastic, borosilicate, or siliconized glass. Specimens may not be collected or stored in containers made from soda lime or soft glass because these materials interact with and activate the coagulation system. Specimens for many *routine* coagulation tests may be collected in evacuated tubes provided that the first tube collected after venipuncture is never used. In most cases the coagulation test specimen is the last of the series of tubes collected. When only a coagulation specimen is needed, a "discard" tube must be drawn first, then the second tube collected for coagulation studies. Contaminating tissue fluid will be discarded with the first tube. Since evacuated tubes *always* cause some mechanical disruption during collection, they may not be used for special coagulation assays or platelet aggregometry.

The preferred collection technique employs the scalp vein infusion apparatus, commonly known as the "butterfly needle," with an attached syringe. Collection of blood through the butterfly tubing into syringes eliminates the activation of platelets and coagulation factors caused by the turbulence of evacuated tubes. Tissue fluid contamination is eliminated by allowing the first few drops of blood to flow from the end of the tubing onto an absorbent material or into a waste receptacle or by using a "two-syringe" approach. In the two-syringe approach, a small syringe is used to withdraw the first 2 ml to 3 ml of blood, then this syringe is removed from the tubing and discarded. The second syringe, or additional syringes, is (are) then attached to collect the test samples. The butterfly technique must be used for factor assays, platelet function studies, and other specialized hemostatic tests. Since butterfly needle collection creates additional expense and is time-consuming, it is impractical for routine coagulation testing.

Another more demanding technique is the two-syringe technique using a single hypodermic needle in place of the butterfly needle. A Luer-Lok (non-screw-tip) syringe is loosely fitted to a hypodermic needle to initiate venipuncture. A piece of absorbent material is placed between the needle hub and the arm, and the syringe is then carefully removed while the needle is immobilized. Additional syringes may be fitted to the needle as in the butterfly technique. Of course, care must be taken to prevent manipulation of the needle during syringe changes. There is some risk that additional tissue fluid may be released with each syringe change in this technique; thus it is recommended only when the butterfly approach is impractical.

Blood collected in a syringe is transferred to a tube for storage after the needle is removed from the syringe. It must be allowed to flow down the side of the tube, *never* directly squirted into the center, which would cause mechanical disruption or turbulence that results in hemolysis or activation. The blood must be added to the storage tube immediately after collection, and the tube gently inverted three to four times to mix with the anticoagulant. Vigorous mixing will also result in hemolysis or activation, affecting coagulation test results.

Although not recommended or advised, there are times when blood must be collected through an indwelling venous catheter. The first 20 ml are discarded or used in other laboratory tests. For pediatric patients with indwelling catheters, discard the first 5 ml to 10 ml. The sample is treated in the same fashion as any other syringe-collected sample.[16]

For most routine and special testing protocols, nine parts of whole blood are added to one part anticoagulant and gently mixed. This results in a final concentration of 10.9 mmol to 12 mmol of sodium citrate per liter of whole blood. For example, 4.5 ml of whole blood to 0.5 ml of sodium citrate or 2.7 ml of whole blood to 0.3 ml of sodium citrate are common mixtures. Commercially available evacuated tubes are designed to collect these precise volumes. Specimens submitted in vacuum tubes containing *less than 90%* of the expected volume are not suitable for hemostatic testing and must be rejected. Therefore, a tube designed to collect 4.5 ml of whole blood would be expected to contain 5 ml of blood – anticoagulant mixture and must contain a *minimum* of 4.5 ml of *mixture*. Likewise, a "2.7-ml draw" tube must collect a minimum *mixture* volume of 2.7 ml.

Visible hemolysis (pink tinge in plasma), severe lipemia (fatty cloudiness), and jaundice (yellowness) caused by a high bilirubin concentration may be reason to reject a specimen for coagulation testing. These factors may interfere with photo-optical clot detection instrumentation. If there is no alternative, the imperfect sample is tested and a note is appended to the report, indicating that results may be affected by the condition of the sample. For example, specimens collected during cardiovascular surgery may exhibit unavoidable hemolysis, and specimens from patients with hepatitis will usually exhibit jaundice.

Clotted specimens or specimens collected with inappropriate anticoagulants *cannot* be tested.

Specimen Handling and Processing

Specimens collected for coagulation testing must be fractionated by centrifugation within 60 minutes of the time of collection. Immediately after collection, samples are placed in a 4°C environment and maintained at that temperature until they can be transported back to the laboratory and centrifuged. A melting ice bath or cold rack such as a Kryorack is included on the specimen collection tray or cart for this purpose. The labile coagulation Factors V and VIII lose their activity during the first hour after specimen collection when held at room temperature, causing prolongation of various coagulation test results.

Many laboratories find the ice bath or cold rack to be cumbersome and impractical and must establish an alternative method of specimen handling. Tests of properly lined evacuated tube systems have demonstrated that specimens may be held for 2 hours at ambient temperature prior to centrifugation and testing without affecting the results of PT and APTT tests. This modification may be applied locally *after* experimental validation but is suitable only for routine testing.

Specimens collected for platelet function studies must be maintained at ambient temperatures (20°C), because cooling adversely affects results. Centrifugation must be started within 30 minutes of collection. Specimens collected for platelet counts can be held at ambient temperatures for up to 5 hours prior to performance of the count. Samples for counts can be held up to 24 hours at 4°C without significantly affecting the platelet count.

Most coagulation tests are performed on platelet-poor plasma. The specimen is placed in the centrifuge and spun at 4°C at a minimum of 1000 g for 10 minutes.[13,16] Tubes must remain capped during centrifugation to maintain pH. Failure to seal the tube results in loss of carbon dioxide and elevation of the pH. Plasma is transferred after centrifugation into a clean plastic, borosilicate, or siliconized test tube, and the tube is capped or sealed. A plastic pipet must be used for the transfer. Red cells and buffy coat are *not* transferred.

Platelet function tests are performed on platelet-rich plasma. The specimen is placed in the centrifuge and spun at *ambient* temperature at 50 g for 30 minutes.[13] A portion of the supernatant is transferred with a plastic pipet to a clean plastic, borosilicate, or siliconized test tube, and the tube is capped or sealed. The original specimen with its remaining supernatant is now centrifuged at 2000 g for a minimum of 10 minutes, to produce platelet-poor plasma.

Many laboratories may find the above methods of handling specimens for routine screening tests (*i.e.,* PT, APTT, thrombin time [TT]) impractical because of hospital size, number of employees, outpatient facilities, and so forth and must establish an alternative method of handling. Deterioration studies may be performed at *each* clinical laboratory to determine maximum times for transport and handling. Duplicate specimens from a variety of patients and from normal donors are collected and treated to various temperature conditions. They are tested at hourly intervals to determine when the labile factor activity becomes diminished. Maximum times are posted and printed in the laboratory manual. Specimens that are older than the published limits are not accepted for testing. The maximum transport and testing time should never exceed 4 hours in any case.

If testing of the specimen cannot be completed within the established time, the life of platelet-poor plasma for coagulation tests may be prolonged by freezing. This is often necessary for specialized coagulation tests such as factor assays and special coagulation panels that are performed infrequently. Multiple sample tubes should be collected, since these procedures require relatively large plasma volume. Samples are collected, transported, and fractionated in the same fashion as described in preceding paragraphs. Supernatant plasma from centrifuged tubes is withdrawn by plastic pipets and pooled into a single plastic vessel such as a beaker or flask. Once the pool is mixed, multiple small aliquots are withdrawn, placed in plastic vials, and sealed. Select the smallest aliquot volume possible to perform the test to facilitate rapid freezing and thawing and to extend the life of the sample. Single-tube specimens must also be aliquotted prior to freezing. Ensure that the seal will withstand cold temperatures. Special vials are available for this purpose from several manufacturers.

Samples must be frozen and stored at −70°C or below to preserve Factor VIII activity, which has demonstrated abrupt and unpredictable deterioration at various freezer temperatures.[17] Aliquots stored for coagulation procedures (in which Factor VIII will not participate) may be stored at −20°C or below, but not above. A frost-free freezer that automatically reaches warmer temperatures for brief cycles or freezers that are opened frequently should be avoided. Small aliquots and −70°C freezers with good circulation promote rapid freezing. Slow freezing causes formation of large ice crystals that denature the coagulation proteins. Rapid thawing is also important; aliquots from the freezer are placed in a 37°C incubator for 10 minutes to promote thawing. Slow thawing results in destruction of fibrinogen.[11,13] Always observe the specimen carefully after thawing. Turbidity indicates cryoprecipitation of Factor VIII, and the sample cannot be tested.

It cannot be stressed enough that each laboratory establish a procedure for handling of specimens throughout collection and testing periods based on their own constraints. These procedures should meet the majority of recommended guidelines for handling set forth by the NCCLS.[16] Once these protocols are established, they must be strictly adhered to.

Adjustment for Hematocrit

The standard 9 : 1 ratio of blood to anticoagulant produces altered hemostasis test results in patients with extremely high or low hematocrit levels. The change is an *artifact* of specimen collection and not indicative of the hemostatic condition of the patient. When the hematocrit is below 20%, the relative *increase* of plasma volume results in inadequate anticoagulation and shortening of coagulation test results. For example, an otherwise prolonged APTT may be falsely shortened into the normal range. When the hematocrit is above 55%, the relative *decrease* in plasma volume means excessive anticoagulation. In this case both the PT and the APTT values may be falsely prolonged, sometimes into the abnormal range. Platelet function tests are similarly affected. The ideal concentration in the blood–anticoagulant mixture must be maintained between 10.9 mmol and 12 mmol of sodium citrate per liter for accurate interpretation of test results.[8,11,20]

When hemostasis specimens are to be drawn from a patient known to be anemic or polycythemic, the ratio of anticoagulant to whole blood is adjusted according to the following formula:[13]

$$C = 1.85 \times 10^{-3} (100 - H) \times V$$

where

C = volume of 3.8% sodium citrate in milliliters

V = volume of whole blood in milliliters

H = hematocrit in percent

For example, to collect 4.5 ml of whole blood from a patient with polycythemia whose hematocrit is 60%,

$$C = 1.85 \times 10^{-3} (100 - 60) \times 4.5$$
$$C = 1.85 \times 10^{-3} \times (40) \times 4.5$$
$$C = 0.33 \text{ ml}$$

Therefore, in this example, 0.33 ml of 3.8% sodium citrate is used instead of 0.5 ml.

QUALITY CONTROL

A quality-assurance program is composed of three parts: (1) a standard protocol for specimen collection, handling, and processing; (2) specifications for glassware, pipets, and other measuring devices, reagent preparation, and instrument maintenance; and (3) a system of controls and normal values. Specimen handling is discussed in the first section of this chapter. Specifications for materials and instruments will be discussed next, followed by computation of controls and normal values.

Materials

Ordinary laboratory glassware has an adverse influence on hemostasis test results. Consequently, most reaction vessels, pipets, and storage containers are polypropylene plastic. Borosilicate glass or silicon-coated glassware may also be used. All materials are to be free of scratches and immaculately clean. Storage in closed containers prevents access by airborne dust. Any particulate matter will enhance contact activation, influencing hemostasis test results. To eliminate many sources of error in hemostasis testing, all materials must be disposable and should not be reused.

Specimens and reagents are measured with pipets that are calibrated to deliver the precise amount indicated. Semiautomated or automated hand-held pipettors are preferred to manual pipets. Pipets and pipet tips must be plastic and disposable. Pipettors are calibrated with a protocol described in any good reference book on quality assurance.

Most commercial reagents and controls in the hemostasis laboratory are in powder or lyophilized form ready for reconstitution with distilled or deionized water. Purity and pH of the water for reconstitution are specified in the manufacturer's package insert and must be observed. Water for reagent use must be regularly tested for purity and pH, or reagent-grade water can be purchased commercially.

Equipment

The following equipment may be found in the hemostasis laboratory: clot detection devices, aggregometers, platelet counters, centrifuges, water baths, heat blocks, and refrigerators. Since the production of a fibrin clot depends on a series of enzymatic reactions, the monitoring of time and temperature is very important and will be discussed throughout this section.

Wujastyk and Triplett have written an excellent review article concerning instrument selection and reagent use.[25] Which equipment and reagents a given coagulation laboratory chooses depends on the number and types of tests performed.

Clot-based assays are timed procedures in which certain reagents are added to plasma and the time to clot formation is measured. These clot times are compared to those of a normal population and controls, and recorded. Clot formation depends on the conversion of fibrinogen to fibrin, which is detected visually, electromechanically, or photo-optically. The first clot-based assays were manual techniques and relied on visual detection of the clot. Reagent was added to test plasma, and the mixture was observed for clot formation. Two approaches were used: the "tilt-tube" technique, in which the test tube containing the mixture was tilted at regular intervals until the gelatinous clot became evident, and the "wire-loop" technique, in which a metal loop similar to an inoculation loop was passed through the mixture at intervals until a clot was observed to cling to it. The technologist would simultaneously start a timer and introduce reagent, then stop the timer at the instant that the clot was observed. Manual methods were affected by individual bias, producing a wide range of error, and are no longer used clinically, although they are still used in some research-and-development situations and may serve as a backup method when instrumentation is unavailable.

One of the first semiautomated instruments introduced in the 1960s to the coagulation laboratory, and still widely used today, is the Fibrometer (BBL BioQuest Division, Becton, Dickinson and Co.). It is a fibrin strand clot detection system based on an electromechanical principle. A timer starts as reagent is dispensed by a hand-held pipet to test plasma. A head supporting two electrodes drops into the mixture. The first electrode remains submerged while the second sweeps through the mixture and withdraws from it at half-second intervals. During the period that the second electrode is out of the mixture, an electrical potential exists between the two electrodes. Upon clot formation, the moving electrode withdraws a fibrin strand as it leaves the mixture, the circuit is completed through the strand, and the timer stops. The time from initiation to completion is displayed and recorded.[7]

These electromechanical clot detectors eliminate observer bias and may provide good reproducibility when used for routine coagulation tests such as PT, APTT, and TT.

The permanent electrodes *must* be cleaned between each assay to prevent carryover of sample or reagent. Error may be introduced by erratic pipetting or mixing of reagent and plasma, by the presence of particulate matter in the reaction mixture, and by the action of the sweeping electrode, which may induce activation. Absolute precision is impossible because of the 0.5-second dwell time of the electrode, although the effect of this action is minimal.[22]

Photo-optical clot detection devices have become very popular because they enable the laboratory to rapidly test large numbers of individual patient specimens with improved precision. Light from a calibrated and focused light source passes through the sample contained in an optically neutral plastic cuvette. The beam falls on a photodetector and is converted into an electrical impulse. Changes in the intensity of the impulse are detected by electronic circuitry. The cuvette containing test plasma is placed in the light path, and the intensity of light passing through is recorded by the instrument. Reagent is added and a timer starts. As the clot forms, the mixture becomes more opaque, and the intensity of light falling on the photodetector decreases. The change is detected instantaneously, and the timer stops. The time is displayed and recorded.[14]

Photo-optical clot devices provide greater reproducibility than electromechanical devices because there is no possibility of carryover from sample to sample, and because detection is instantaneous. Because most photo-optical devices are automated, a series of test plasma cuvettes may be placed in a tray or wheel that advances the test sample to the reaction site, providing "walk-away" capability. Photo-optical devices may be interfaced with computers to facilitate handling of the data produced. Results from photo-optical devices are compromised when plasma samples are extremely cloudy because of the presence of fats (lipemia) or highly colored as in the case of severe hemolysis or jaundice. Such test samples must be tested on an electromechanical device or rejected. The presence of platelet aggregates or particulate material may also influence the consistency of results. Samples with fibrinogen levels below 50 mg/dl may not provide a sufficiently opaque clot to influence the detector.

Electronic and mechanical timers on semiautomated or automated instruments must be checked weekly for accuracy with a stopwatch. All clocks or stopwatches in the hemostasis laboratory must be checked weekly against a standard timer known to be in good condition. Both types of clot detection devices incorporate constant-temperature heat blocks and cooling blocks. These devices must reach the desired temperature for preservation of the specimen (4°C) and for enzymatic coagulation reactions (37° ± 1°C). Temperatures of constant temperature blocks must be checked and recorded daily and monitored during each test run.

Any constant-temperature incubators, refrigerators, or freezers must be checked for temperature daily and the temperature recorded.

Standard laboratory clotting measurements end with the formation of the first fibrin strands and are performed on isolated blood fractions. New methods of investigating the sequence of events that lead to this fibrin clot formation have emerged in the hemostasis laboratory and afford the possibility of directly measuring the activity of individual clotting factors and inhibitors. Synthetic chromogenic or fluorogenic substrate techniques and immune-based assays yield quantitative evaluations of enzyme activity and may supplant the clot-based assay.[5,6,23] Chapter 12 reviews these new approaches in detail.

All centrifuges must be tested at periodic intervals to establish the speed of rotation in revolutions per minute for each setting.

In addition to the usual piece of equipment, some laboratories view hemostasis by thromboelastography using either the Thromboelastograph or the Sonoclot. Both instruments measure the overall clotting process of *whole* blood, platelet-rich plasma, platelet-poor plasma, or platelet-free plasma from initiation to the final stages of clot lysis or retraction. Either instrument employs a transducer that measures changes in plasma elasticity. As clotting proceeds, a pen tracing representative of these changes is produced. Although thromboelastography cannot measure individual coagulation deficiencies, characteristic tracings have been reported in patients with factor deficiencies, hypercoagulation syndrome, and increased fibrinolysis.[4,26] These results are explored in Chapter 4.

Maintenance of the Thromboelastograph and Sonoclot includes monitoring the temperature of the constant-temperature block and ensuring that the mechanical devices such as stir bars and transducers are in proper working order. Normal fresh specimens are tested at specified intervals.

Normal Range (Reference Limits)

A normal range or, more accurately, a reference interval (RI) must be established for each procedure performed in the hemostasis laboratory. The RI means the interval that includes expected results for 95% of the normal population. Although this implies that 5% of normal subjects will generate "abnormal" results, the RI is essential to clinical interpretation of individual patient test results. To compute a normal range, a *minimum of 30* healthy individual donor specimens are required. The mean and standard deviation (SD) of the results are computed. Normal range is derived as the mean ±2 SD. The SD is a useful expression of dispersion of data points from the mean and is computed by squaring the difference from the mean of each data point and finding the square root of the sum.

$$SD = \sqrt{\frac{\Sigma(x - \bar{x})^2}{n - 1}}$$

where Σ = sum of

x = the individual observation or test

$\bar{x}$ = the average value of all tests

n = the total number of observations

Many large-scale studies have been conducted to determine the normal range for each clinically useful hemostasis procedure. The results of these studies have been published in journals and summarized in several textbooks, including this one (see Chap. 4). Such "textbook" normals are derived from large, mixed populations. Individual hemostasis laboratories *must* establish their own normal ranges. These may differ from published ranges because of the peculiarities of the local population, or because of particular conditions such as ambient temperature, altitude, type of equipment available, blood collection techniques, and blood storage techniques. Individual normal values are compared to published normals before adoption.

Donors for normal-range studies must be healthy. Persons scheduled for preemployment physical examinations, donors to the blood bank, patients scheduled for elective surgery, and institutional personnel may qualify. These donors must be receiving no medication, have no known illness, and fit the age range and sexual distribution required. Throughout, donor specimens are handled and processed in the same manner

---

GUIDELINES FOR ESTABLISHING A NORMAL RANGE

Throughout, donor specimens should be handled and processed in the same manner as the patient specimens.

A minimum of 30 individual donors should be used to generate test results. These donors must not be receiving any medication, have no known illnesses, and span the adult age range and sex distribution.

Data should be gathered over a period of several days to eliminate day-to-day variation.

The normal range should be reevaluated a minimum of once a year, when changing reagents or reagent lots, when changing instrumentation, or whenever modifying the collection or test procedure.

The test values should be compiled, and, using statistical analysis, the mean value should be determined and the SD derived.

The normal range is established as ±2 SDs from the mean.

Values falling within the third SD may or may not be normal and should be further evaluated.

---

as patient specimens, as outlined in the first half of this chapter. Data are gathered over a period of several days to incorporate day-to-day variations.

Collect all data and compute the mean and SD. The normal range is usually established as values within 2 SDs from the mean. For example, if the mean PT value were computed to be 11.5 seconds and one SD were 0.4 seconds, the limits of the normal range would then be 10.7 to 12.3 seconds. Any value above 12.3 seconds is then considered prolonged.

The normal range is reevaluated at least once a year, when changing lot numbers of reagents, when modifying the technique, or when changing instrumentation.

Platelet aggregometry procedures are qualitative or semiquantitative, and normal ranges are broadly defined or undefined. In aggregometry, a normal fresh sample is run each day or with each test run to ensure that the procedure is working correctly and to provide a reference value. This normal should be obtained from a healthy volunteer who does not smoke, has not taken aspirin for 10 days, and is not on other medications.

A protocol recommended for establishing a normal range is summarized under Guidelines for Establishing a Normal Range.

Controls

A control is a sample the value of which is previously determined by a reference method. Control samples are included at least once with each run of test samples to ensure the validity of results. Control samples for coagulation tests may be either locally or commercially prepared plasma pools. The local pools are usually frozen until use, and commercial pools are shipped in lyophilized (freeze-dried) or preserved liquid form. Commercially prepared platelet count controls are preserved single-donor whole blood.

Local plasma pools are prepared when large volumes of plasma are needed for expensive precision studies, when single-factor standard activity curves are prepared, or when a specialized new technique for which no commercial control is available is controlled. At least 50 ml of whole blood is collected by the butterfly technique from each of at least ten healthy adult donors—five men and five women. However, the more donors incorporated into the pool, the better the chances of representing a normal mean. Donors must be using no medication. Plasmas are pooled, filtered, or centrifuged, and routine PTs and APTTs are performed to ensure that the results are within the established normal range. After evaluation, the plasma pool is aliquotted into plastic, capped tubes and quickly frozen. Because deterioration is rapid and unpredictable, plasma pools are stored at −70°C and used within 3 months. Figure 3-2 demonstrates one deterioration study performed with Factor VIII: C.[17]

Commercially prepared plasma pools are available from several manufacturers. These commercial controls provide the following variety: normal citrated or heparinized plasma, plasmas assayed for specific factor activity levels, plasmas with moderate and prolonged coagulation test values, and plasmas with decreased activity of Factors II, VII, IX, and X (factors depressed in oral anticoagulant therapy).

The laboratory includes one normal control and at least one abnormal control in each run of test plasma. The results of unknowns tested in a run are reported *only* after the controls have been compared to the previously established results and found to be an acceptable match. The use of controls reflects how well the test can reproduce a result in the normal and abnormal range and verifies the accuracy of test results.

Each manufacturer performs repeated procedures on each lot of control plasmas to develop a mean value and limits of dispersion from the mean based on 2 SDs. The limits of dispersion are called *action limits* in most quality-assurance documentation. These

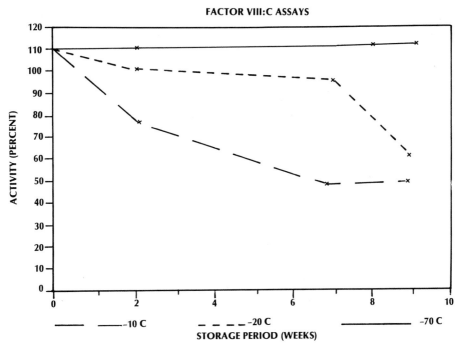

FACTOR VIII:C ASSAYS

FIG. 3-2. The stability of Factor VIII: C in plasma stored at −10°C, −20°C, and −70°C. (Redrawn from Palkuti H: Deterioration of Factor VIII: C in stored plasma for use in activity curves. Lab Med 15:41, 1984)

values are shipped with the plasmas and are marked in a package insert or stamped on the container. The laboratory does not use manufacturers' action limits directly but confirms them through a local assay procedure.

When a new lot number of control plasma is obtained, the first vial or vials are reconstituted with reagent-grade water and tested in runs with control plasmas that are already "in control." Daily testing of the new lot is performed on each shift, inserted in random order with each batch of specimens and tested under a variety of routine conditions. At least 30 determinations are made in this manner. The mean and SD are computed and compared to the manufacturer's previously derived values. These results should agree closely, and if they do, the newly computed action limits (mean, ± 2 SD) are put into service, and the new lot is used in place of the old lot of controls.

Most manufacturers of commercial control material provide a single lot number of control plasmas that remains unchanged over a period of 6 months to 1 year. The continued use of a single lot decreases the time required for establishing new control ranges and provides the technologist with familiar target values. This approach also enables the laboratory to participate in regional quality-control programs for comparison of interlaboratory results.

A control sample in the normal range and at least one in the abnormal range is included with each run of patient samples. As soon as a control value is generated, it is recorded in a table and on a Levy-Jennings chart and compared to the action limits (Fig. 3-3). When a control value falls outside the action limits, the control and the patient specimens within that run must be repeated. If the control plasma is still outside acceptable limits, the test is considered "out of control" and must be investigated. Investigation of out-of-control results is conducted as follows:

1. Because the action limits are based on the SD value, rules of random distribution require that 5% of all results fall outside the action limits. Therefore, repetition of the run is suggested before further troubleshooting is performed.
2. A new vial of control plasma is reconstituted with reagent-grade water and tested. Manufacturer's instructions must be followed rigorously. Some sources of error include water volume measurement, water purity, pH, or time for lyophilized plasma to go into solution.
3. Materials (plastic ware, pipets, transfer bulbs) should be investigated for contamination or scratches.
4. Instrumentation and equipment should be checked for errors in temperature, pinched or defective tubing, and contaminated or bent electrodes.
5. Contamination or deterioration of reagents could be the problem. Controls should be replaced and retested.

When the control values fall within the action limits, test results are "in control" and may be recorded and reported.

In addition to detection of within-run or within-day variation, controls are used to test for long-term variation, or *drift*. As soon as 30 results are generated over a period of days, a mean and SD are computed. These data should agree with the original assay values within 5%. If not, the procedure is evaluated with the troubleshooting steps listed above. Although within-day results of a control plasma may fall within the action limits, a procedure that has drifted may be out of control and easily detected visually by use of a Levy-Jennings chart (see Fig. 3-3). If the control value falls consistently on one side of the mean for eight or more determinations in a row, the procedure is investigated, even when the control has *never* fallen outside the action limits.

NORMAL CONTROL: PROTHROMBIN TIME (PT)

```
12.0
12.0 - - - - - - - - - - - - 1 - - - - - - - - - - - - - - - - -
11.7              1             1                        1
11.4      1 2 1 2 1       1   1 1            1 1   · 1      1   2 1
11.1        1 1   2   1 2       1              2 1 3 1   1   2 1
10.8 1   1   2 1     2 2 1 2   1 2 2   2     1 2 3 4   2   2 1 1
10.5 1 4 1 1 1 4 2 2 3 2 - - 1 3 1 2 1 1 1 2 2 4 3 2 2 - 2 2 2 2 1
10.2    1 1 2 2 1 2 2 2 1   2 1 1   3 2     5 2 5 4 3 1 1 2 3 2 1
9.9 2            1 3 7 4 3 1 3 1 2 6 2 1 1   6 5 3 4 3 2 2 5 7 6 8
9.6     3   1 1   1 4 2     2 3 2 3     3   1 4   1   1     6
9.3
9.0 - - - - - - - - - - - - - - - - - - - - - - - - - - - - - - -
9.0
```

```
                 1 1 1 1 1 1 1 1 1 1 2 2 2 2 2 2 2 2 2 2 3 3
Date 1 2 3 4 5 6 7 8 9 0 1 2 3 4 5 6 7 8 9 0 1 2 3 4 5 6 7 8 9 0 1
     Jan 80
```

Period	Mean	S.D.	C.V.	Observations
1/01/80 - 1/31/80	10.30	.521	5.057 G.F.	308
Oct 79 - Nov 79	10.34	.587	5.675 G.F.	577
Dec 79	10.50	.593	5.649 G.F.	286

Percentile Mean: 10.5 - Dev : 1.5

FIG. 3-3. A Levy-Jennings chart. The chart is an example of a computer-generated graph showing the quality-control program for a 1-month period. The test analyzed is the PT using a normal control plasma. The values plotted indicate (by numbers 1 through 8) the number of times that a test result yielded that time in seconds on that particular day. Time in seconds (9 to 12 seconds in a line on the left-hand side of the graph) represents the range interval calculated from the prior month's values (December, in this example). (Mean ± 2 SDs) Listed below are the mean SDs and CVs calculated for the new month and compared to those of the past 2 months. This allows for a computer statistical analysis, at a glance, of the quality-control system. For this month of January, the PT was considered to be in control and acceptable and verified by the technologist's initials recorded beside the CVs. *S.D.*, standard deviation; *C.V.*, coefficient of variation; *Dev.*, deviation. (Courtesy of Donna M. Corriveau)

Table 3-1 is an example of PT and APTT data derived from evaluating a new lot number of three commercial coagulation controls: one normal range, one moderately abnormal (level I), and one extremely abnormal (level II). Such a table lists

- The number of times each control was tested
- The mean value obtained for each level
- The derived SD
- The action limits, or the 2-SD range that determines the daily control range
- The coefficient of variation (CV), which is a measure of the precision of the method. The CV is derived by dividing the SD by the mean.

$$\%CV = \frac{SD}{\overline{x}} \times 100$$

TABLE 3-1
Evaluation of Commercial Control Plasmas for the PT and APTT

Parameter	Normal	Level I	Level II
PROTHROMBIN TIME			
Number of evaluations	63	64	53
Mean	11.1 sec	17.7 sec	26.8 sec
SD	0.12 sec	0.23 sec	0.28 sec
2-SD range	10.9–11.3	17.2–18.1	26.2–27.4
CV	1.1%	1.3%	1.0%
ACTIVATED PARTIAL THROMBOPLASTIN TIME			
Number of evaluations	56	35	32
Mean	31.3 sec	66.1 sec	99.2 sec
SD	0.89 sec	2.84 sec	4.52 sec
2-SD range	29.5–33.1	60.4–71.8	90.2–108.2
CV	2.8%	4.3%	6.5%

Controls for platelet counting consist of preserved whole blood with predetermined values. Typically, platelet count values are part of a series of whole blood values used together as a general hematology control substance. Results of platelet count controls are determined just like plasma pool controls, except that the materials are maintained in liquid form and have a maximum shelf life of 120 days.

There are no commercially available controls for platelet function studies. Common practice dictates the collection of fresh whole blood from a normal donor whenever platelet function studies are performed.

Validity

A laboratory test is valid when it is both precise and accurate. *Precision* represents the degree of agreement among individual measurements performed at a laboratory under their prescribed conditions and reflects the reproducibility of the test method. Precision must be determined by running repeated tests on the same samples in the normal as well as abnormal ranges. Precision is quantified by the SD that measures the spread in the individual laboratory results around the laboratory's mean, as demonstrated in this chapter under Controls. A low value for the SD indicates results that are closely scattered around the mean; conversely, a large SD value indicates a wide spread of results around the mean value. The terms *drift* and *scatter* further describe precision.

Accuracy is a more difficult condition to achieve in hemostasis laboratories. Accuracy is a measure of how near a test result is to the theoretical "correct" result. In the clinical chemistry laboratory, accuracy may be measured directly by employing standard substances containing precisely measured components. This approach is impossible in hemostasis because the components to be measured are either parts of a complex series of enzymatic interactions like the coagulation pathway or biological materials such as platelets. Locally prepared or commercial plasma controls are not standard materials because their components are not separately measured. The accuracy of a procedure may only be presumed through repeat measurements and a regular program of comparisons with external peer laboratories, commonly referred to as *surveys.* In a survey program, a central agency provides samples with known results that are not revealed to participant laboratories. Laboratories perform procedures on the samples and return the test results to the agency, which then statistically compares all data submitted. Laboratories may then examine their procedures and techniques for errors if their generated data are not in agreement with those of their peers.

When a laboratory procedure is reproducible but inaccurate, it is said to have a *systematic error.* When a test produces a mean near the real value but has a high degree of variation, it is said to possess *random error.* A valid procedure is one that incorporates no systematic error and has narrow limits of randomization.

General hematology laboratories and hemostasis laboratories must have established guidelines to aid in ensuring that results generated by the laboratory are valid, and that abnormal results are brought to the attention of the pathologist or the patient's physician in cases in which follow-up studies may be indicated. These guidelines are termed *limit check* and *delta check.*

Laboratories that are computerized have added the patient-based control mechanism called *delta check.* Patient values are expected to remain relatively constant from day to day or from measure to measure, and wide variation in values may indicate a testing error. The data processor is programmed to compare all patient results to any previous values collected within the past 48 hours. When the new result differs from the old by greater than a preset percentage, the new value is flagged. The operator will repeat the test on that patient sample or on the entire run if warranted. If the patient sample still differs by more than the preset percentage, the attending physician is consulted to discover the clinical reason for the change or to warn of possible complications.

To demonstrate the use of delta check, let us examine a patient's prolonged PT value of 15.5 seconds. The original PT was 12.3 seconds. The change over 24 hours is 26%, well above the established 20% delta check limit. The laboratory computer indicates this change by a warning system and alerts the technologist to recheck results by repeating the procedure. It is determined that this patient had been started on a course of oral anticoagulant therapy and that the change was anticipated. A delta check program controls for test variation and clerical errors.

The *limit check* is a procedure that was once done manually but now can routinely be computerized. It allows for the assessment of all test results outside a specified range for specified procedures on a given day. This provides the technologist an opportunity to review all out-of-range results and detect any quality-control problems. Each abnormal result should be verified with patient history or retested. The following guidelines are recommended to aid in establishing a limit check program.

1. The mean of duplicate determinations performed on all coagulation tests is reported. These duplicate results must have a CV of less than 5%.

    If the results are outside this 5% limit, the test is repeated in duplicate. If three of the four results agree within this 5% limit, the result can be reported.

    If no acceptable agreement occurs, obtain a new specimen for testing.

    If one tested value is within the normal range and the duplicate value is beyond the upper limit of normal, repeat the test in duplicate.

2. Normal clot times generated from patients known to be receiving oral anticoagulant or heparin therapy should be repeated. If they are verified, the physician should be alerted to these results.

3. Extremely prolonged clot times (beyond the terminal time of automated instruments) should be repeated or verified by an alternative clot detection system. The physician should also be alerted to these results and a new specimen requested for evaluation.

A valid laboratory test is *sensitive* and *specific*. Sensitivity of a test represents the smallest concentration or activity of the component that can be reliably measured. Specificity is the ability to be influenced by only the component intended to be measured and no other. Specificity and sensitivity are inversely related; the more sensitive a test, the less specific.[13,21,22] For example, there are two popular methods for determining the presence of fibrin (fibrinogen) degradation products (FDPs): the protamine sulfate paracoagulation test and the latex agglutination test (Thrombo-Wellcotest). Latex agglutination detects all degradation products (fibrin monomer, Fragments X, Y, D, and E), and it is positive in the presence of greater than 2 μg of any of these products. Paracoagulation detects only fibrin monomer and Fragment X and requires a concentration of greater than 20 μg. Thus, latex agglutination is more sensitive but less specific than paracoagulation. A screening test is designed with high sensitivity and low specificity and yields a high percentage of false-positive results. A definitive test is designed to be specific at the sacrifice of sensitivity, resulting in a high percentage of false negatives. Many test protocols combine a screening and a definitive test to reap the benefits of both.

Sensitivity and specificity may also be defined relative to their ability to predict disease. Thus, sensitivity is the frequency of positive test results in subjects defined as diseased by some other definitive system. For example, it was determined during a study of 100 people with hemophilia that 95% had prolonged APTTs. The sensitivity of the APTT test for hemophilia is then defined as 95%. This may be expressed in the working formula:

$$\text{Sensitivity} = \frac{\text{TP}}{\text{TP} + \text{FN}} \times 100 = \text{positivity in disease}$$

where

TP = true positives

FN = false negatives (those with disease for whom the test was negative)

Specificity becomes the frequency of negative test results in healthy subjects, calculated by the following formula:

$$\text{Specificity} = \frac{\text{TN}}{\text{FP} + \text{TN}} \times 100 = \text{negativity in health}$$

where

TN = true negatives

FP = false positives (healthy subjects for whom the test was positive)

Thus, if the APTT test is prolonged in four of 100 healthy subjects, the specificity is 96%.

The specificity and sensitivity of a test vary with the limits of normal. The values for a test result in a normal and diseased population always overlap; therefore, as the normal limits are set farther from the mean value, the test becomes more specific and less sensitive; conversely, as they are moved nearer the mean value, they become more sensitive and less specific. For example, when the upper limit of normal for an APTT is set at 1 SD above the normal mean, 99% of these hemophiliacs studied would have a positive APTT, but so would approximately 33% of all normal subjects. On the other hand, if the APTT limit were set at 3 SDs from the mean, only 1% of normal subjects would have a positive APTT, but about 30% of hemophiliacs would be negative. Therefore, the establishment of appropriate limits of normal has a major effect on diagnosis.

Sensitivity to Decreased Factor Levels

Since the APTT is used primarily as a general screening test to determine abnormalities in the intrinsic system of coagulation, it is important that this test be able to detect the clinically significant mild deficiencies of the coagulation factors (levels between 10% and 40% normal). Since there are various reagents commercially available for the performance of this test, each with different reported levels of sensitivity to decreased factor levels, it is important that each laboratory attempt to determine the sensitivity of the APTT test system used at their institution.[9,15]

Some insight into the ability of a particular APTT protocol to detect minor coagulopathies may be gained by conducting an *in vitro* investigation using mixtures of assayed normal plasma pools and known factor-deficient plasma. For example, a commercial source of normal plasma has an assayed value for Factor VIII:C of 100%. By making dilutions of this plasma in the appropriate deficient plasma (in this case, Factor VIII–deficient plasma), which is arbitrarily assigned a 0% value, various approximate factor levels can be obtained. An APTT is then performed on each mixture, and the lowest factor level that exceeds the established normal range is observed. This level will represent the point to which the patient's coagulation factor must decrease before the APTT test system will recognize the abnormality. An illustration of the results of such an investigation is shown in Table 3-2. These results show the sensitivity of the APTT for the Electra 700 (Medical Laboratory Automation) with the Automated APTT reagent (General Diagnostics/Organon Teknika) and an established normal range of 25 to 35 seconds.

TABLE 3-2
Sensitivity of the APTT to Various Levels of Factor VIII:C

Factor VIII Mixture	APTT
100% (0.5 ml PNP*)	32 sec.
50% (0.5 ml PNP + 0.5 ml DP†)	34 sec.
40% (0.4 ml PNP + 0.6 ml DP)	37 sec.
30% (0.3 ml PNP + 0.7 ml DP)	40 sec.
20% (0.2 ml PNP + 0.8 ml DP)	45 sec.
10% (0.1 ml PNP + 0.9 ml DP)	52 sec.
0% (0.5 ml DP)	>100 sec.

* Pooled normal plasma
† Factor-deficient plasma

Effects of Heparin

Heparin present in specimens submitted to the coagulation laboratory for monitoring heparin anticoagulant therapy or in specimens contaminated by drawing the specimen through a heparin-rinsed line (heparin lock) alters all laboratory procedures the end-points of which are determined by the formation of fibrin clots. Differences exist in the sensitivity of various laboratory tests to the concentration of heparin. Studies have been performed to determine the sensitivity of five popular laboratory techniques used to monitor the effectiveness of heparin: the Lee-White whole blood coagulation time test (L-W), the activated clotting time test (ACT), the PT, the APTT, and the TT.[18]

The L-W test measures the time required for whole blood to clot after it is drawn into a glass test tube.[12] Prolongation of the clot time is achieved with increasing concentrations of heparin for L-W test, as shown in Figure 3-4. However, there is considerable scatter in the clot times produced for each concentration of heparin, yielding large standard deviations.

In recent years the ACT (a bedside test) has been advocated for monitoring heparin therapy.[10] It requires a special collection tube containing diatomaceous earth to which whole blood is added and placed in a controlled-temperature unit. The time required for clot formation is recorded. Similar prolongation of clot times occurs with the ACT and

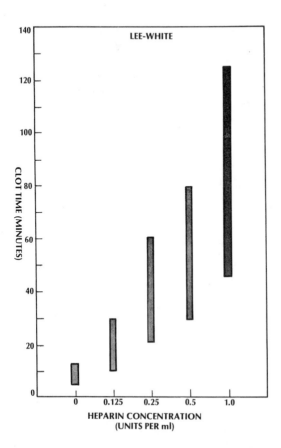

FIG. 3-4. Effect of heparin concentration on the L-W clotting time. (Palkuti H: Laboratory monitoring of anticoagulant therapy. J Med Technol 2[2]:82, 1985)

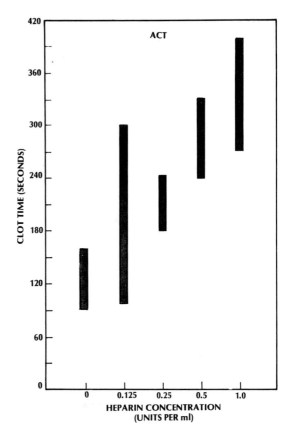

FIG. 3-5. Effect of heparin concentration on the ACT test. (Palkuti H: Laboratory monitoring of anticoagulant therapy. J Med Technol 2[2]:82, 1985)

the L-W coagulation time test, but there is less definition between the amount of heparin present and the clot time produced for the ACT (Fig. 3-5).

The APTT has become a useful, sensitive procedure for monitoring heparin therapy and for screening deficiencies of clotting factors included in the intrinsic coagulation system. It is used to determine the dose-effect of heparin within the therapeutic range of 0.2 to 0.5 units of heparin per milliliter. This procedure is sensitive to relatively small amounts of heparin, although considerable variation is exhibited in the presence of higher concentrations. The gradual prolongation of clot times in the "therapeutic range" falls within a range of clot times that current instrumentation can accurately reproduce (Figure 3-6).[19,24]

Unfortunately, the different thromboplastin reagents vary greatly in their sensitivity to heparin, and, therefore, certain reagents may fail to adequately detect therapeutic levels.[1,2,19] It is recommended that each hospital choosing to monitor heparin therapy with the APTT determine its own *in vitro* therapeutic range that reflects the specific laboratory reagents, instrumentation, and personnel. Similar problems are also found with the PT, used to monitor coumarin therapy.

Increasing concentrations of heparin can be added *in vitro* to a normal plasma pool, and their effects on the APTT, PT, and TT can be evaluated. The sensitivity of these tests to the concentration of heparin from one study is shown in Figure 3-7. The TT test

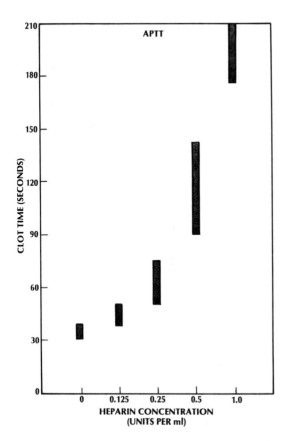

FIG. 3-6. Effect of heparin concentration on the APTT test. (Palkuti H: Laboratory monitoring of anticoagulant therapy. J Med Technol 2[2]:83, 1985)

demonstrates the most sensitivity to the presence of small amounts of heparin. Clot times produced in the range of 0.2 to 0.5 units of heparin per milliliter of plasma are from 94 to greater than 150 seconds. Unfortunately, it may be difficult to reproduce the extended clot times for values of heparin concentrations in the therapeutic range on current laboratory instrumentation. The PT shows the least sensitivity to therapeutic levels of heparin. A baseline (no heparin present) PT of 11 seconds increased to only 12.2 seconds in the presence of 0.6 units of heparin per milliliter of plasma. The progressive prolongation of the APTT test due to the presence of heparin is shown in Figure 3-7 for two photo-optical instruments, the Dual Channel Coagamate and the 2001 from General Diagnostics.[3] Since a gradual prolongation of clot time is produced with increasing concentrations of heparin, this test is useful to determine the dose-effect of heparin within the therapeutic range of 0.2 to 0.5 units of heparin per milliliter plasma.

By performing a heparin sensitivity curve to establish an *in vitro* heparin therapeutic range, the laboratory can evaluate various types of clot detection instrumentation and sensitivity of the APTT. An example of results generated from APTTs using a Fibrometer (BioQuest), an X-2 (Organon Teknika), and an Electra 700 (Medical Laboratory Automation) is shown in Figure 3-8. Results of the Fibrometer curve indicate that the APTT would not be an accurate test to monitor heparin at concentrations of heparin above 0.30 units per milliliter.

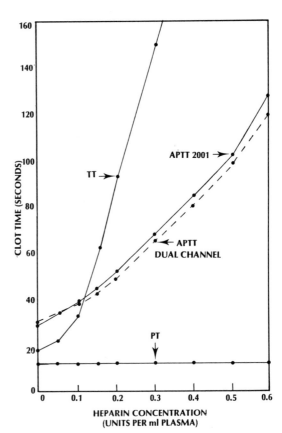

FIG. 3-7. Sensitivity of the PT, APTT, and TT to heparin concentration. (Palkuti H: Laboratory monitoring of anticoagulant therapy. J Med Technol 2[2]:83, 1985)

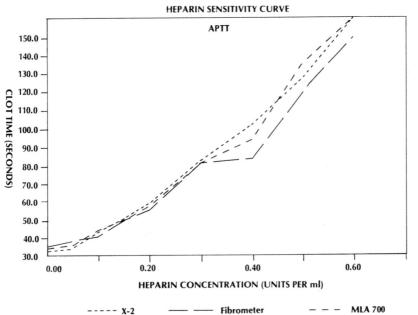

FIG. 3-8. Sensitivity of APTT to heparin concentration using the X-2, Fibrometer, and MLA Electra 700 instruments.

SUMMARY

The validity of a test result is the single largest issue that confronts the clinical laboratory on a daily basis. Any generated data that are not supported by proper technique and careful statistical analysis result in loss of confidence by the entire community served by the laboratory. Valid test results are achieved only when samples are collected, transported, and processed according to established protocol; tested using appropriate materials and calibrated equipment; and interpreted in the light of appropriate normal limits. Every laboratory should employ a systematic, documented quality-control program involving controls samples, daily inspection of action limits, and external comparison studies. All of these activities will yield reliable test results.

REFERENCES

1. Bain S et al: Heparin and the activated partial thromboplastin time — a difference between in-vitro and in-vivo effects and implications for the therapeutic range. Am J Clin Pathol 74:668–673, 1980
2. Brandt J, Triplett D: Laboratory monitoring of heparin: Effects of reagents and instruments on the activated partial thromboplastin time. Am J Clin Pathol 76(Suppl):530–537, 1981
3. Coagamate Dual Channel and 2001, Operators Manual, General Diagnostics, Division of Warner-Lambert Co., Morris Plains, NJ, 1979
4. Caprini J et al: The identification of accelerated coagulability. Thromb Res 9:167, 1976
5. Dade Division, American Hospital Supply Corporation: Protopath proteolytic enzyme detection system manual, December 1980
6. Duckert F et al: Chromogenic substrates in coagulation analysis. Diagnostics, 1977
7. Fibrometer Precision Coagulation Timer, Instructions and Technical Information, BBL Bio-Quest Division, Becton, Dickinson and Co., Cockeyesville, MD
8. Harker L: Hemostasis Manual, 2nd ed. Philadelphia, FA Davis, 1974
9. Hathaway W et al: Activated partial thromboplastin time and minor coagulopathies. Am J Clin Pathol 71:22–25, 1979
10. Hattersley P: Activated coagulation time of whole blood. JAMA 196(5):436–440, May 1966
11. Ingram GIC: Bleeding Disorders, Investigation and Management, 2nd ed, pp 243–328. Boston, Blackwell Scientific Publications, 1982
12. Lee R, White P: A clinical study of the coagulation time of blood. Am J Med Sci 145:495, 1913
13. Lenahan J, Smith K: Hemostasis, 17th ed, pp 12–15. Morris Plains, NJ, General Diagnostics, 1985
14. MLA 700, Operator's Manual, Medical Laboratory Automation, Mt. Vernon, NY, January 1984
15. Morin R, Willoughby D: Comparison of several activated partial thromboplastin time methods. Am J Clin Pathol 64:241, 1975
16. National Committee for Clinical Laboratory Standards: Tentative Guidelines for the Standardized Collection, Transport, and Preparation of Blood Specimens for Coagulation Testing, Vol 2, No. 4, pp 110–117. Villanova, PA, NCCLS, 1982
17. Palkuti H: Deterioration of factor VIII:C in stored plasma for use in activity curves. Lab Med 15(1):840–842, 1984
18. Palkuti H: Laboratory monitoring of anticoagulant therapy. J Med Technol 2(2):81, February 1985
19. Palkuti H et al: APTT-method for standardization in heparin therapy. American Society of Clinical Pathologists Summary Report, March 1976
20. Palkuti H, Kales A, Demeis F: Report on alterations in coagulation values due to hematocrit variations. Clotters Corner No. 15, Morris Plains, NJ, General Diagnostics, March 1977

21. Thomson J: Blood Coagulation and Haemostasis, 2nd ed, pp 330–350. Edinburgh, Churchill Livingstone, 1980
22. Triplett DA: Laboratory Evaluation of Coagulation, pp 349–366. Chicago, American Society of Clinical Pathologists Press, 1982
23. Triplett DA: Synthetic substrates present a breakthrough in coagulation assays. Boehringer Mannheim Diagnostics, June 1981
24. Triplett D: Anticoagulant therapy: Monitoring techniques. Lab Management 20(8):31–42, 1982
25. Wujastyk J, Triplett D: Selecting instrumentation and reagents for the coagulation laboratory. Pathologist, June 1983, pp 398–403
26. Zuckerman L et al: Comparison of Thromboelastography With Common Coagulation Tests. Evanston, IL, Northwestern University, 1981

Clot-Based Assays of Coagulation

4

George A. Fritsma

CASE STUDY

A 4-year-old boy with a history of streptococcal pharyngitis and tonsillitis was admitted to the hospital for a tonsillectomy. Routine admission laboratory work included a CBC with normal results and the following presurgical coagulation studies:

Bleeding time: 6.5 min. (normal: 2.75–8)
Prothrombin time: 11 sec. (normal: 10–13)
Activated partial thromboplastin time: 67 sec. (normal: 29–42)
Thrombin time: 20 sec. (normal: 18–25)

Surgery was postponed until investigation of the prolonged activated partial thromboplastin time (APTT) result was completed. The patient was apparently healthy and had no petechiae or purpura. The parents stated that the patient had been adopted at birth, that no family history was available, and that the child had had no bleeding episodes.

The prolonged APTT indicated a factor deficiency, so the test was repeated. In addition, mixing studies were performed using the APTT on patient plasma with fresh normal plasma, adsorbed plasma, and serum. Factor assays were also performed. Results of all coagulation tests were as follows:

APTT: 65 sec. (normal: 29–42)
APTT + fresh normal plasma: 45 sec.

APTT + adsorbed plasma: 43 sec.
APTT + serum: 46.5 sec.
Factor XI: 120% activity
Factor XII: 98% activity

These results eliminated possible deficiencies of all the numbered pro-coagulants, leaving Fletcher factor (prekallikrein) and Fitzgerald factor (high-molecular-weight kininogen, HMWK). The APTT was repeated with the modification of a prolonged (10-min.) activation incubation step. The result of the modified APTT was 39 seconds, yielding the presumptive diagnosis of Fletcher factor deficiency. Deficiency of Fitzgerald factor results in a prolonged APTT that remains prolonged upon extended activation.

Because Fletcher factor deficiency is not associated with a clinical bleeding disorder, surgery was performed without incident. The patient was dismissed the following day.

Fletcher factor (prekallikrein) is a glycoprotein with a molecular weight of 80,000 daltons. It is part of the contact activation mechanism and, in conjunction with Fitzgerald factor, activates Factor XII. Deficiency of Fletcher factor has been documented in about ten cases, in which it was inherited as an autosomal-dominant trait. The contact activation mechanism is essential to normal APTT results but is apparently bypassed *in vivo.* Patients with deficiency of Fletcher, Fitzgerald, or Hageman (Factor XII) factors have no clinical hemostatic symptoms. This is why the decision was made to proceed with surgery without special precautions.

Confirmation of Fletcher factor deficiency requires the use of specific deficient plasma (Fig. 4-1). Several weeks after surgery the hospital laboratory technologist obtained Fletcher-deficient plasma from a reference site and collected a fresh sample from this patient. The plasma sample was first tested using the kaolin clotting time technique in place of the APTT. Results were prolonged, and remained prolonged upon 60 minutes' incubation of patient plasma with kaolin. The patient plasma was then mixed with Fletcher deficient plasma and retested by kaolin clotting technique. The result was still prolonged, confirming Fletcher factor deficiency. The kaolin test was used in place of APTT to avoid the time-dependent correction phenomenon characteristic of Fletcher factor deficiency that was noted in the earlier testing sequence.

The *Lee-White whole blood coagulation time (WBCT)* test, first described in 1913, was the first laboratory procedure designed to assess clotting.[14] The Lee-White is now obsolete, but it was the first coagulation test procedure to employ an important principle: the time interval from initiation of coagulation to visible *in vitro* clot formation reflects the condition of the coagulation mechanism. A prolonged "clotting time" indicates serious coagulation inadequacy. The most commonly accepted battery of clinical, clot-based coagulation screening tests all use the clotting time principle: *prothrombin time (PT), activated partial thromboplastin time (APTT),* and *thrombin time (TT).* The more specialized tests, such as the *specific factor assays,* tests of *fibrinolysis, Stypven time, Reptilase time,* and *thrombin generation time (TGT)* are all based on the relationship between "time to clot formation" and ability of the coagulation system to function.

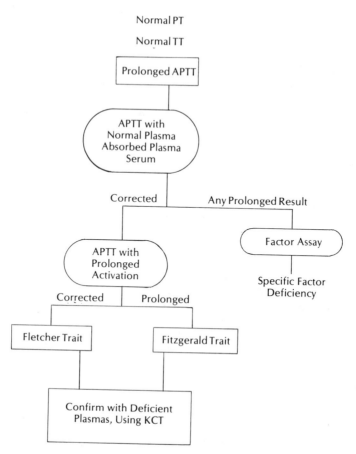

FIG. 4-1. Algorithm for distinguishing among Fletcher factor or prekallikrein deficiency (Fletcher trait), Fitzgerald factor or HMWK deficiency (Fitzgerald trait), and deficiencies of the numbered coagulation factors. *KCT,* kaolin clotting time.

A careful patient history and physical examination are necessary to diagnose a bleeding disorder. A short series of laboratory tests is then performed. Vascular integrity is assessed by the tourniquet test or petechiometry as described in Chapter 9. After a routine platelet count a bleeding time (BT) test is performed to determine platelet function and confirm that no vascular disease is present. Both platelet measurements are described in Chapter 9. At the same time, coagulation tests are performed.

The "routine" coagulation tests are designed to assess the function of each portion of the coagulation system, as described in Chapter 2. The PT detects procoagulant deficiencies in the *extrinsic* and *common* pathways and is sensitive to the effects of the commonly used oral anticoagulant coumarin. The APTT detects procoagulant deficiencies in the *intrinsic* and common pathways and is sensitive to the effects of intravenous or subcutaneous heparin therapy. The TT detects fibrinogen deficiency, dysfibrinogenemia, and antithrombic activity. The TT is also sensitive to the presence of heparin because heparin acts on antithrombin III to inhibit thrombin activity. All three tests are

TABLE 4-1
Procoagulants in the Factor Substitution Reagents

	Adsorbed Plasma	Aged Plasma	Serum
FACTORS PRESENT	I, V, VIII, XI, XII, XIII	I, II, VII, IX, X, XI, XII, XIII	VII, IX, X, XI, XII
FACTORS REMOVED	II, VII, IX, X	V, VIII	I, II, V, VIII, XIII

Definition and preparation:
   Adsorbed plasma: Fresh plasma treated with insoluble barium sulfate or aluminum hydroxide
   Aged plasma: Plasma that stood at 4°C for a minimum of 1 week
   Serum: Clotted whole blood; supernate serum is separated from the cells and incubated at 37°C for 2 hours.
(Courtesy of Donna M. Corriveau)

sensitive to the presence of circulating specific or nonspecific anticoagulants (inhibitors), but none is valuable for predicting a thrombotic condition. See Chapter 11 for a discussion of hypercoagulable or thromboembolic disorders.

The "special" clot-based coagulation tests are employed to detect the absence or inactivity of a single plasma procoagulant. *Factor substitution tests*, or *mixing studies*, employ the PT, APTT, and TT techniques on test plasma mixed with certain reagents. These reagents are fresh normal citrated plasma, barium sulfate $(BaSO_4)$– or aluminum hydroxide $(Al[OH]_3)$–adsorbed citrated plasma, and serum. The procoagulants in each reagent are known, so when a reagent is added to each test system, it is possible to isolate a procoagulant deficiency (Table 4-1). Stypven time and Reptilase time are snake venom–based procedures that also isolate single factor deficiencies. Mixing studies are also performed to detect the presence of circulating inhibitors or "anticoagulants" such as the lupus inhibitor or anti–Factor VIII.

Specific factor assays are also based on PT and APTT test principles. Here, *factor-deficient substrates*, plasmas from patients with congenital single coagulant deficiencies, are added to test plasmas. Specific factor assay test results confirm the results of mixing studies and provide the diagnosis of a congenital factor deficiency. Specific factor assays are also used to measure the activity level of the diminished procoagulant. Mixing studies and specific factor assays are seldom useful for diagnosis of acquired coagulation deficiencies when more than one procoagulant is deficient, and they cannot help isolate the identity of a circulating anticoagulant except in certain instances.

Tests of fibrinolysis assess the activation of plasminogen or the presence of fibrinogen/fibrin breakdown products (see Chap. 2). The *euglobulin lysis test* is clot based, but the test for *"fibrin split products"* is based on an immunologic agglutination reaction. Other tests of the fibrinolytic pathway are based on chromogenic assays and are discussed in Chapter 12.

All clot-based assays of coagulation may be performed manually. The technologist initiates coagulation in an optically clear plastic test tube and starts a timer, then observes the plasma–reagent mixture while repeatedly tilting the tube until a clot forms. The timer is then stopped and the time recorded. Most assays are now performed with automatic or semiautomatic instruments, described in Chapter 3. Instruments may be electromechanical, such as the Fibrometer (BBL BioQuest Division, Cockeysville, MD), or photo-optical, such as the Coag-a-Mate (Organon Teknika, Parsipanny, NJ 07054).

Specimen collection for coagulation studies is discussed in Chapter 3. The anticoagulant used in most cases is 3.2% or 3.8% sodium citrate in a final ratio of 1 : 10 (1 part anticoagulant plus 9 parts whole blood). The two-syringe or two-tube technique is essential, and the test sample must be refrigerated until the test is performed. All tests are performed on platelet-poor plasma (PPP) prepared by centrifugation of the sample of whole blood at 2000 g for at least 10 minutes. A uniform specimen collection protocol must be followed without deviation.

PHYSICAL EXAMINATION

Identification of any hemorrhagic disorder begins with a history and physical examination. Single procoagulant deficiencies are inherited disorders, so the patient history must include as much information as possible about his or her own hemorrhagic episodes plus bleeding experienced by parents, grandparents, siblings, and offspring. Sometimes, inheritance patterns may help diagnose an autosomal-dominant disorder such as von Willebrand disease or a sex-linked disorder like hemophilia A. Prolonged or excessive bleeding after trauma, surgery, or tooth extraction may be a sign of a coagulation disorder.

Physical findings of procoagulant deficiencies include inflamed joints caused by bleeding, peritoneal bleeding, urinary bleeding seen as fresh or occult blood in the urine, and bleeding into the gastrointestinal tract. Hemorrhages into skin and mucous membranes may be seen but are most often associated with platelet or vascular disorders rather than procoagulant deficiency. A complete description of the clinical symptoms and physical findings in the hemophilias is provided in Chapter 5. If suspicious symptoms exist, the routine screening assays are ordered.

SCREENING TESTS FOR EXTRINSIC PATHWAY DEFICIENCIES

Prothrombin Time

PRINCIPLE

Test plasma + tissue thromboplastin + $CaCl_2$ → fibrin clot

The PT is a screening test that detects deficiencies of procoagulants that participate in the extrinsic and common pathway except for *tissue thromboplastin*, for which no deficiency state has been described. The one-stage prothrombin time was developed by Armand Quick in 1935.[20] Deficiencies of prothrombin (Factor II) and Factors V, VII, or X (Fig. 4-2) result in prolonged PTs. The PT reagent consists of tissue thromboplastin of

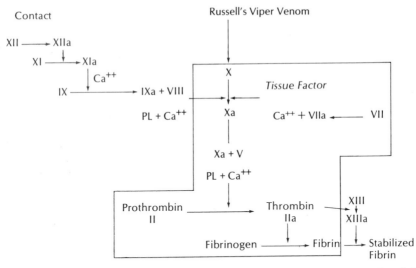

FIG. 4-2. Overview of the coagulation mechanism with the extrinsic and common portion circled. The circled portion represents factors measured by the PT test. PT reagents — tissue thromboplastin and ionic calcium — are in italics.

animal source suspended in a 0.025M solution of calcium chloride ($CaCl_2$). Commercially prepared tissue thromboplastin reagents are organic extracts of emulsified rabbit brain, lung, or brain–lung combination. Table 4-2 lists all commercial forms of tissue thromboplastin available to clinical laboratories, their source, and their relative sensitivity.

Figure 4-2 illustrates how tissue thromboplastin activates the coagulation reaction through the extrinsic pathway and demonstrates the participation of the extrinsic- and common-pathway procoagulants. Tissue thromboplastin first activates plasma Factor VII. Factor XII$_a$, if present from the contact activation portion of the intrinsic system, also activates a small amount of Factor VII, although this plays a minor role in the PT reaction.[12] Factor VII$_a$ from either source forms a complex with tissue thromboplastin that catalyzes the reaction of X to X$_a$. Factor X$_a$ subsequently forms a complex with Factor V, phospholipid (a component of the tissue thromboplastin reagent or from available platelet membrane material such as platelet factor 3), and free ionic calcium (Ca^{2+}) to catalyze the activation of prothrombin, forming thrombin. Thrombin in turn catalyzes the polymerization of fibrinogen to form fibrin. Fibrin is detected visually, photo-optically, or by electrical impedance.

For the PT, a whole-blood sample is collected with minimal trauma using the two-syringe or two-tube technique. Plasticware must be used throughout. The sample is immediately mixed with 3.2% or 3.8% sodium citrate anticoagulant in a ratio of 9 parts blood to 1 part sodium citrate solution. The fresh sample is centrifuged and the plasma stored between 2°C and 8°C until tested. Testing must be performed within 4 hours of

TABLE 4-2

Commercial Forms of Tissue Thromboplastin and Activated Partial Thromboplastin Available to the Coagulation Laboratory

Manufacturer	Product Name	Rabbit Brain	Rabbit Brain–Lung	Calcium
BRITAIN				
Manchester Comparative Reagent			Contains *human* brain.	
UNITED STATES				
Helena	Liquid Thromboplastin	X		
Boehringer-Mannheim	PT Reagent	X		
Pacific Hemostasis	Thromboscreen	X		X
Organon	Simplastin	X	X	X
Dade	Thromboplastin	X		
Dade	Thromboplastin C	X		X
Hyland	Thromboplastin	X		
Ortho	Ortho Brain Thromboplastin	X		X
Sigma	Thromboplastin	X		

(Courtesy of Donna M. Corriveau)

sample collection. If refrigeration is not available, the PT test must be performed within 2 hours of collection.

Thromboplastin–calcium chloride reagent is prewarmed to 37°C. An aliquot of test plasma, usually 0.1 ml, is transferred to the reaction vessel, which is also maintained at 37°C. The aliquot is incubated for a minimum of 3 minutes at 37°C and a maximum of 10 minutes. Aliquots that are incubated more than 10 minutes begin to deteriorate because of breakdown of the labile Factors V and VIII and because of evaporation. A premeasured volume of the reagent, usually 0.2 ml, is forcibly added to the plasma aliquot and a timer started. As soon as the clot forms, the timer stops, and the elapsed time is recorded. The procedure must be performed in duplicate, and duplicate values must be within 0.5 seconds of each other.

Each time a PT is performed alone or in a batch, a control plasma is tested. Preparation of pooled normal plasma (PNP) is described in Chapter 3, but lyophilized commercial controls are also available. The selected control is prepared in accordance with the provided instructions and tested by the same protocol as the patient plasma aliquot. If the control results match the premeasured time within 5%, the test results are presumed to be correct. See Chapter 3 for a more complete discussion of quality control.

The expected PT results for normal plasma fall between 10 and 14 seconds. The reference interval varies from site to site depending on the patient population, the type of tissue thromboplastin reagent used, the type of instrument used, the pH and ionic concentration (purity) of the water used, and the temperature. One midwestern medical center has established 11.5 to 12.5 seconds as its reference interval. This range is typical, but each center must establish its own range based on an adequate sample of normal donors. Day-to-day variation of a single lot of normal control plasma should not exceed 0.5 seconds, provided the same source of reagent is employed.[4]

PT results are prolonged in congenital single-factor deficiencies of prothrombin (II) or Factors V, VII, or X. They are also prolonged when the fibrinogen level is below 100 mg/dl, in *dysfibrinogenemia*, and in the presence of fibrinogen degradation products (FDPs) or fibrin degradation products (*also* referred to as FDPs).[26] Circulating specific inhibitors like anti–Factor VII and nonspecific inhibitors like *lupus anticoagulant* cause prolonged results that are not corrected by addition of fresh normal plasma.[24] Anti–Factor VIII, the most common of the specific inhibitors, has little effect on the PT. The effect of the lupus anticoagulant is increased in proportion to control values when tissue thromboplastin reagent is diluted 1 : 50 or 1 : 500 with buffer and used to test an aliquot of plasma. Therapeutic heparin gives variable effects.

The PT is prolonged in two important acquired coagulation disorders. *Disseminated intravascular coagulation* causes consumption of several factors in the extrinsic and common pathways, by production of FDPs, and by consumption of platelets. This combination of deficiencies profoundly prolongs the PT results.

Vitamin K deficiency is seen in malnutrition, during use of broad-spectrum antibodies that destroy gut flora, and in malabsorption syndromes. Vitamin K levels are low in the newborn, in whom bacterial colonization of the gut has not begun.[5] Clinical hemorrhage is likely, and the PT is the best indicator. Vitamin K is used for treatment.

Most orders for the PT are to monitor oral anticoagulant therapy using *coumarin* derivatives. The anticoagulant coumarin is available in several forms, but *sodium warfarin* is the form most commonly used. Coumarin blocks the *quinone–hydroxyquinone cycle* (see Chap. 6) and prevents the γ-carboxylation of *glutamic acid* residues near the N terminal of the vitamin K–associated *preprocoagulants* II, VII, IX, and X during synthesis. The *acarboxylated* preprocoagulants, acarboxy II, VII, IX, and X, called "proteins induced by vitamin K antagonists" *(PIVKAs)*, are nonfunctional and thus cannot participate in the coagulation cascade mechanism. The PT is sensitive to PIVKAs because Factors II, VII, and X participate in the PT reaction. Following the initiation of coumarin therapy, PT results are first affected by suppression of Factor VII activity. Factor VII is present in the plasma in the lowest concentrations of all the members of the vitamin K–dependent group, and its turnover rate is the greatest. Consequently, Factor VII activity drops rapidly upon initiation of treatment.[3]

A PT is performed prior to the start of therapy, and if it is prolonged, therapy is delayed until the cause of the lengthened PT result is determined. If the initial PT is within the normal range, the result is referred to as the *"baseline"* value, and therapy is initiated. Each day during the early stage of therapy a PT is performed and compared to the normal control. PT results during the first few days of therapy will change markedly from day to day. This is because conversion from active procoagulants to PIVKAs occurs at different intervals for each procoagulant. Factor VII activity is too low to measure within 6 hours and Factor X within 40 hours, and prothrombin (II) disappears in 60 hours (see Chap. 6). Results stabilize after a few days of therapy. The ratio of patient to control result reaches approximately 1.6 if tissue thromboplastin of animal origin is used. Exceeding the upper limit of the therapeutic range exposes the patient to the risk of hemorrhage. Vitamin K is administered intravenously to prevent hemorrhage after oral anticoagulant overdose.

PT results vary markedly with the source of tissue thromboplastin reagent. The ratio of expected times for warfarin-treated patient samples to expected times for normal control samples varies as well. For example, human brain extract reagent yields a ratio of patient PT to control PT of about 2.96. In contrast, reagent derived from rabbit heart and lung provides a ratio as low as 1.4 for the same patient and control combination. Because laboratories in the United States may choose from a variety of commercial tissue thromboplastin sources, variation in ratios exists among institutions, resulting in therapeutic confusion. For this reason an international standard human brain extract tissue thromboplastin is provided by the World Health Organization. The reagent, *British Comparative Thromboplastin (BCT)* is now available to various manufacturers to test in parallel with their own reagent against reference plasmas at many levels of activity. Comparisons in the form of ratios or graphs are available from the manufacturer for each reagent.[26] Chapter 6 provides a more detailed discussion of the current guidelines for anticoagulant therapy and varying reagent sensitivities.

PT results are severely affected by technical errors in sample collection, handling, and storage, and by the condition of plasticware materials. Samples that are icteric, hemolyzed, or lipemic may yield inaccurate results on photo-optical equipment. The concentration of sample collection anticoagulant is an important consideration, especially in the case of the patient with polycythemia vera whose hematocrit is above 60%. The small proportion of plasma available results in a relative increase in the ratio of anticoagulant to plasma, causing a prolonged PT result. The sources of error for the PT test are described in detail in Chapter 3.[16,18]

Russell Viper Venom Time (Stypven Time)

PRINCIPLE

Patient plasma + RVV* + $CaCl_2$ → fibrin clot

Stypven time is the name for a one-stage PT test using an alternate form of tissue thromboplastin derived from the venom of the *Russell's viper.* Russell's viper venom activates the common coagulation pathway at the level of Factor X, bypassing Factor VII. The Stypven time test is now obsolete because it has been replaced by single-factor assays, but in the past it was used to confirm congenital Factor VII deficiency. The Stypven time is prolonged in the case of congenital deficiency of Factors I (fibrinogen), II, (prothrombin), V, and X, but not in Factor VII deficiency. Therefore, the combination of a prolonged PT and a normal Stypven time indicates Factor VII deficiency. Russell's viper venom may be purchased from several distributors.

SCREENING TESTS FOR INTRINSIC PATHWAY DEFICIENCIES

Lee-White Whole Blood Coagulation Time

PRINCIPLE

Fresh whole blood + glass test tube → whole blood clot

---

* Russell's viper venom

The WBCT test was first developed in 1913 and serves as the forerunner of all "routine" clot-based coagulation tests.[14] The WBCT is based on the concept that the interval between initiation of clotting and formation of a visible clot depends on the integrity of the coagulation mechanism. This principle is now used for all routine clot-based assays. WBCT results are affected by each step of the intrinsic and common pathways (Fig. 4-3). Factors I (fibrinogen), II (prothrombin), V, VIII, IX, X, XI, XII, and XIII, prekallikrein (Fletcher factor), and HMWK (Fitzgerald factor) must all be active for clotting to proceed normally. The WBCT is affected by contact activation, but the extrinsic system plays no part. Heparin, coumarin, and circulating inhibitors may all cause a prolonged WBCT.

Prior to venipuncture, three 12-mm × 75-mm tubes are marked at approximately the 1-ml level and labeled #1, #2, and #3. A trauma-free venipuncture is performed using a "butterfly" infusion set (see Chap. 3). The first 1 ml to 2 ml of blood after venipuncture is allowed to flow into a tube and then discarded. Now 1 ml is placed in tube #3 as a stopwatch is started, then tube #2 and tube #1, respectively. After blood is placed in tube #1, the venipuncture is discontinued. After 3 minutes has elapsed, tube #1 is tilted 45°. This is repeated every 30 seconds until the blood has clotted. This is done with tube #2, then tube #3. When tube #3 clots, the watch is stopped and the time recorded.

The range of normal values for the WBCT in most institutions is 4 to 8 minutes at 37°C or 8 to 15 minutes at room temperature. The test result is prolonged in severe coagulation deficiencies and in the presence of heparin.

Intrinsic Pathway

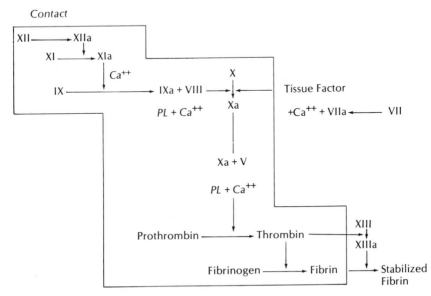

FIG. 4-3. WBCT and APTT. Overview of the coagulation mechanism with the intrinsic and common portion circled. The circled portion represents factors measured by the WBCT test and the APTT test. Italicized components are supplied in reagents. APTT reagents include contact activator, phospholipid, and ionic calcium.

The WBCT has been used to monitor heparin therapy, although the practice is no longer acceptable. The baseline WBCT result is determined, and therapy is begun. The goal of the therapy is to raise the WBCT to double the baseline value. For example, a patient with a WBCT of 6 minutes should receive sufficient heparin to reach a therapeutic WBCT range of 11 to 13 minutes. The WBCT is insensitive and affected by a variety of extraneous conditions such as venipuncture technique, size and material composition of the test tube, temperature, cleanliness of materials, and tilting technique. No control is used.

Clot Retraction

The tubes of blood from the WBCT are observed for *clot retraction*. After 1 hour the clot should be firm and should have withdrawn from the sides of the tube, occupying about half the original volume of the blood. Retraction is impaired in platelet abnormalities (see Chap. 10) such as *thrombocytopenia* and *thrombocytopathy*. Increased fibrinogen levels and *erythrocytosis* will also contribute to poor retraction. Clot retraction is increased in anemia and in abnormal fibrinolysis as seen in disseminated intravascular coagulation, increases in plasminogen activators, or antiplasmin deficiency. In these cases the clot is small and ragged and tends to disintegrate in 1 hour. The clot is also small in dysfibrinogenemia, hypofibrinogenemia, or afibrinogenemia.[16]

Activated Coagulation Time

PRINCIPLE

Fresh whole blood + particulate activator → whole blood clot

The *activated coagulation time (ACT)* is a modification of the WBCT introduced in 1966.[7] *Particulate activator* such as *diatomaceous earth, kaolin,* or *Celite* is placed in the sample tubes prior to the addition of blood. When blood is added, the tube is mixed thoroughly to disperse the activator throughout the blood. Normal ACT results are slightly below 100 seconds. Therapeutic heparin levels yield results of 150 to 190 seconds. The ACT is more sensitive and reproducible than the WBCT and is recommended by many clinicians as the preferred method for monitoring heparin therapy. It is simpler, more reproducible, and more linear than the APTT and may be performed at the patient's bedside.[8]

Dynamic Measure of Coagulation by Instrumental Analysis

Three instruments have been designed to measure physical changes in whole blood or plasma during coagulation. These are the *Thromboelastograph* (Haemoscope Corporation, Skokie, IL 60076), the *Sonoclot* (Sienco, Inc., Morrison, CO 80465), and the *Hemochron* (International Technidyne Corporation, Edison, NJ 08820).

The Sonoclot measures changes in viscosity over time in whole blood, platelet-rich plasma (PRP), or PPP (platelet-poor plasma) by a principle termed *dynamic impedance*. A cylindrical plastic probe attached to a transducer is suspended in the sample. The probe oscillates rapidly in a vertical motion parallel to the long axis of the cylinder. As plasma viscosity increases, greater internal voltage is required to maintain the period of oscillation of the probe. Changes in voltage required are recorded by pen on a graph, creating a Sonoclot "signature," as shown in Figure 4-4. The signature provides several measurable parameters: time to onset of clotting, rate of clot formation, time to peak of clot formation, and amplitude of peak clot viscosity. A reference interval has been computed for each of these parameters using whole blood, PRP, and PPP. A variety of reaction situations may be used, including simple recalcification, use of particulate activators such as kaolin or Celite, or use of no reagent, similar to the WBCT. Prolonged onset times, diminished clotting rate and peak amplitude, and delayed time to peak of clot formation are all associated with procoagulant deficiencies. The Sonoclot technique may be used to monitor heparin therapy.[21]

The Thromboelastograph (TEG) measures changes in clot "stiffness" of whole blood, PRP, and PPP by a principle termed "thromboelastography."[22] A disposable

SONOCLOT   SIGNATURE

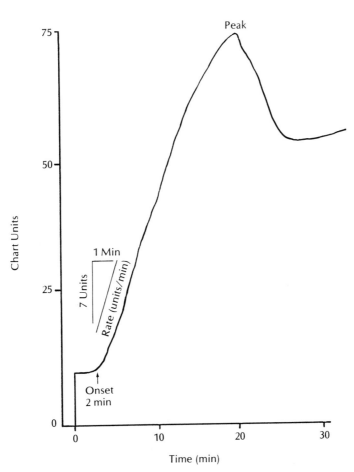

FIG. 4-4. A Sonoclot signature, the tracing produced by the Sonoclot dynamic impedance analyzer. Measurements include onset of clotting, rate of change in viscosity, and peak viscosity.

cylinder is suspended in a sample held in a stainless steel cup. The distance from the outer wall of the internal cylinder to the inner wall of the cup is 1 mm. The outer cup slowly oscillates 180° about its axis. As the clot forms, forces applied by the oscillating outer cup begin to drive the suspended cylinder in a similar motion. The motion is measured electronically and recorded by a pen recorder on a moving graph. Parameters similar to the Sonoclot parameters are measured, including time to onset, rate of clot formation, and peak amplitude of clot gelation. After several minutes the pattern amplitude becomes diminished. The rate at which this occurs is influenced by the fibrinolytic activity. Reagents include calcium chloride and particulate activators. Like the Sonoclot, the TEG is sensitive to heparin anticoagulant therapy and to procoagulant deficiencies. Both the Sonoclot and the TEG may provide results that correlate with hypercoagulability, or the thrombotic tendency. See Chapter 11 for a discussion of the hypercoagulable syndrome and its associated test results.

The Hemochron is the simplest of the three devices and is designed to detect only the ACT end point. A whole-blood sample is collected in a specially designed ACT tube containing particulate activator. A small cylindrical magnet is inserted into the tube. The tube is placed in a slanted well within the instrument and slowly rotated. When the clot forms, the magnet is displaced, and a proximity switch is activated to signal the end of the ACT.[9] The Hemochron-measured ACT is primarily used to monitor heparin therapy.

Activated Partial Thromboplastin Time

PRINCIPLE

Patient plasma + partial thromboplastin + particulate activator + $CaCl_2$ → fibrin clot

The APTT is used to detect deficiencies of the intrinsic and common coagulation pathways and to monitor the effects of heparin therapy. The APTT is a modern modification of the "recalcification time" test.[13] When whole blood is collected for either the recalcification time test or the APTT, sodium citrate anticoagulant forms a complex with plasma calcium. Free ionic calcium is necessary for coagulation to proceed, but calcium in the citrate complex is unavailable for the coagulation reaction. In the recalcification time test, citrated plasma is mixed with a solution of 0.025M $CaCl_2$. The interval from addition of the $CaCl_2$ solution to clot formation is measured. Prolonged recalcification times are caused by deficiencies of factors in the intrinsic or common pathways but not the extrinsic pathway. The recalcification time test is seldom used because the reference interval is unacceptably lengthy and broad. Clotting times using PRP range from 100 to 150 seconds, while PPP times range from 135 to 240 seconds. Variation in specimen storage and transport time, and poor regulation of most clinical-grade centrifuges make it impossible to control the actual concentration of platelets or platelet products in the plasma; thus, the reference interval is difficult to predict.

The APTT reagents include calcium chloride, "partial thromboplastin," and particulate activator. Partial thromboplastin is a chloroform extract of rabbit brain tissue phospholipid. Table 4-3 lists the various partial thromboplastin reagents commercially available. Partial thromboplastin mimics the effect of platelet phospholipid, also called platelet factor 3 (PF_3), by serving as the reaction site for Factor X activation and conversion of prothrombin to thrombin (see Chap. 2). The presence of partial thromboplastin in the reagent eliminates the need for platelets or intrinsic platelet substances in the test system and decreases the variation caused by uncontrolled concentration of platelet substance in the plasma. Particulate activator may be diatomaceous earth, kaolin, Celite, ellagic acid, or micronized silica. The activator provides a surface for attachment of Factor XII. When activator is present, contact activation is standardized because the uncontrolled effect of the reaction vessel surface is bypassed.[15]

In the APTT the coagulation reaction begins at the level of contact activation (see Fig. 4-3). Factor XII is converted to XII_a by the particulate activator. Both HMWK and prekallikrein take part in this reaction. XII_a reacts on XI to produce XI_a, which in turn converts IX to IX_a in what is traditionally termed the cascade reaction. IX_a forms a calcium-dependent complex with VIII and phospholipid (supplied in the reagent as partial thromboplastin) to catalyze the activation of X to X_a. This reaction is enhanced by the thrombin-mediated modification of Factor VIII to VIII_m. The remainder of the reaction from X to the formation of fibrin proceeds as described in the section on the PT, except that tissue thromboplastin and Factor VII are not involved. Procoagulants that participate in the APTT reaction are fibrinogen (I), prothrombin (II), V, VIII, IX, X, XI, XII, prekallikrein (Fletcher factor), and HMWK (Fitzgerald factor). Absent from the reaction are Factors III and VII, both part of the extrinsic mechanism, and XIII, which participates only in clot stabilization. The APTT is insensitive to platelet availability because the partial thromboplastin reagent bypasses the necessity for platelets.

Blood is collected, prepared, and stored the same as for the PT. To test the plasma, 0.1 ml of prewarmed (37°C) reagent consisting of partial thromboplastin and activator

TABLE 4-3
Partial Thromboplastin Reagents

Product Name	Manufacturer	Platelet Substitute	Activator
AAPTT	Hyland	Rabbit brain	Aluminum-coated silica
APTT Reagent	Helena Labs	Rabbit brain	Micronized kaolin
APTT Reagent	Boehringer-Mannheim	Rabbit brain	Ellagic acid
Rabbit Brain Cephalin	Sigma	Rabbit brain	
Thrombofax	Ortho	Bovine brain phospholipid	Ellagic acid
Actin	Dade	Rabbit brain cephalin	Ellagic acid
Actin FS	Dade	Rabbit brain cephalin	Ellagic acid and soy phosphatides
Platelin Plus	Organon	Rabbit brain phospholipid	Celite
Automated APTT	Organon	Rabbit brain phospholipid	Micronized silica
Thromboscreen Kontact	Pacific Hemostasis	Rabbit brain phospholipid	Mg^{2+}, Al^{2+} silicate

(Courtesy of Donna M. Corriveau)

is mixed with 0.1 ml of prewarmed plasma. The mixture is allowed to incubate for exactly 3 minutes. At the end of 3 minutes, 0.1 ml of prewarmed 0.025M $CaCl_2$ is forcibly added to the mixture, and a timer is started. When a clot forms, the timer is stopped, and the interval is recorded. Timing may be performed manually or automatically by using an electromechanical or photo-optical device. Like the PT, APTT tests are always performed in duplicate, and normal or elevated controls are tested with each unknown plasma. Patient and control results are reported simultaneously.

Like PT results, APTT results vary with the institution, locale, and population. In most cases normal APTT results will not exceed 45 seconds. In one typical midwestern institution the reference interval is 26 to 38 seconds. The relatively broad range reflects the influence of storage time and temperature, use of glass containers and tubes, type of reagent used, and type of clot detector employed.

The APTT result is prolonged in deficiency of one or more of the intrinsic or common factors: prothrombin (II), V, VIII, IX, X, XI, or XII, and when the fibrinogen (I) level is below 100 mg/dl. It is also prolonged in the presence of a specific inhibitor such as anti–Factor VIII or a nonspecific inhibitor such as the lupus anticoagulant. Antithrombic substances such as FDPs may also cause a prolonged APTT. Disseminated intravascular coagulation gives prolonged results because of consumption of procoagulants. Vitamin K deficiency results in diminished levels of procoagulant Factors II, VII, IX, and X; deficiency of II, IX, or X affects the APTT result. Because Factor VII does not affect the APTT, the test is not as sensitive to vitamin K deficiency or coumarin therapy as the PT. The APTT is not prolonged in deficiencies of Factors VII or XIII or platelet phospholipid (PF_3). The prothrombin consumption test (serum prothrombin) may be used as an estimate of platelet phospholipid availability. The prothrombin consumption test is described in Chapter 9.

The APTT is commonly used to measure heparin levels during therapy. Heparin potentiates the action of antithrombin III, which reacts covalently to neutralize thrombin and Factor X_a and suppress the coagulation mechanism. Heparin is administered clinically to prevent thromboembolic disorders in those at high risk, in the treatment of venous thrombosis and pulmonary embolism, in the treatment of disseminated intravascular coagulation, in the treatment of arterial thrombosis or embolism, and in patients undergoing surgery involving extracorporeal circulation. Heparin overdose results in hemorrhage and possible death; thus, continuous laboratory monitoring of heparin effectiveness is essential.[8]

The clinician orders an APTT test prior to initial administration of heparin. This "baseline" result should fall in the normal range. A prolonged APTT result may indicate a preexisting clinical coagulation condition that precludes the use of heparin. Once heparin administration is begun, the APTT result should reach a "target range" of about 1.5 to 2 times the normal control, or around 60 to 80 seconds.[2] When therapy is given in bolus form, the sample is drawn 3.5 hours after administration of heparin, or just $\frac{1}{2}$ hour prior to the next infusion. Subsequent doses are adjusted to achieve the desired APTT results.

In most cases of thromboembolic disease, heparin anticoagulation is tapered off after about 10 days. Oral coumarin therapy is begun after about 6 or 7 days, requiring that a PT be performed. As soon as the PT result reaches therapeutic levels, the heparin is discontinued.

Hematologists do not agree about which test is the most appropriate for measurement of heparin therapy. Besides the APTT, the ACT, TT, recalcification time, and anti–activated Factor X assay are recommended. While each provides advantages and disadvantages, it is clear that the APTT is currently the most popular clinical test. It is rapid, simple to perform, and universally available and offers good precision from day to day. Unfortunately, APTT results are not linear with heparin dosage, are affected by extraneous coagulation changes, and do not reliably predict hemorrhage. Many patients tend to bleed excessively even when the APTT is within the therapeutic range.

General reliability of APTT results depends on the consistent use of the same instrument, reagents, and materials. Glass containers tend to activate coagulation prior to performance of the test, often resulting in shortened APTT results. Plasma that is hemolyzed, icteric, or lipemic may not give reliable results in photo-optical devices.

SCREENING TESTS FOR FIBRIN FORMATION

Thrombin Time

PRINCIPLE

Test plasma + thrombin → fibrin clot

Thrombin is a protease produced in the activation of plasma prothrombin. Thrombin cleaves *fibrinopeptides A and B* from the α and β polypeptide monomers of circulating fibrinogen. Upon cleavage, individual fibrinogen molecules polymerize, forming insoluble fibrin, the protein of the visible clot. Cleavage and polymerization are described in Chapter 2. Thrombin may be harvested from human or bovine plasma, purified, and lyophilized for storage. In the TT test, reagent thrombin is mixed with test plasma. Prolonged results indicate fibrinogen deficiency, *dysfibrinogenemia,* or the presence of *thrombin inhibitors* or antithrombins.

The TT is the simplest of the clot-based screening tests (Fig. 4-5).[10] Reagent thrombin is prepared by diluting pharmaceutical bovine or human topical thrombin with normal saline solution to make a working dilution of about 2 units per milliliter. Although $CaCl_2$ enhances the TT reaction, it is not necessary and is not included in the test protocol. The reagent thrombin is warmed to 37°C for a minimum of 3 and a maximum of 10 minutes. Thrombin deteriorates during 37°C incubation and must be used within 10 minutes of the time that incubation is begun. An aliquot of PNP is allowed to incubate at 37°C for 1 minute. One-tenth milliliter of thrombin reagent is forcibly added to the PNP and a timer started. A clot should form between 25 and 35 seconds after addition of thrombin. If the interval is shorter, the reagent thrombin is further diluted and the step repeated. When the interval is reached, the reagent is ready for testing plasma.

Unknown plasma is tested in the same way as the PNP. Any plasma giving an interval of greater than 5 seconds above the PNP result when the PNP is in the 25- to 35-second range is considered to have a prolonged result. Prolongation may be the result of diminished fibrinogen levels. A fibrinogen level of less than 100 mg/dl will cause a prolonged TT result and is termed hypofibrinogenemia or *afibrinogenemia* (absence of fibrinogen). The presence of a biochemically abnormal, inactive form of fibrinogen is termed *dysfibrinogenemia,* a condition that also results in a prolonged TT. Prolongation may also be the result of the presence of circulating inhibitors or antithrombic substances. Three additional tests, the *toluidine blue* test, addition of PNP, and addition of *Reptilase* may be used to confirm or eliminate the presence of circulating inhibitors of coagulation and antithrombin. In most cases the substance is heparin.

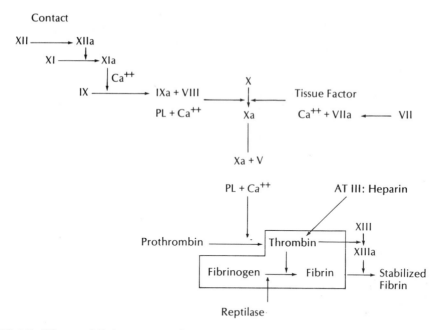

FIG. 4-5. TT test and fibrinogen assay. Overview of the coagulation mechanism with the action of thrombin circled. The circled portion represents factors measured by the TT test. Results are also affected by ATIII levels, heparin levels, and the presence of fibrin(ogen) degradation products. *PL,* phospholipid.

Toluidine Blue Test

PRINCIPLE

Test plasma + thrombin + toluidine blue → fibrin clot with heparin neutralization

The toluidine blue test is used only to confirm the presence of heparin. A 0.1% solution of toluidine blue in water is substituted for the normal saline solution in the TT test. If the TT result is corrected to within 5 seconds of the PNP result, the previous abnormal result was caused by the presence of heparin. When the toluidine blue test is performed, the test of PNP is always repeated with toluidine blue mixed with the plasma. The result of the PNP test is shortened to between 18 and 23 seconds by the dye. The plasma TT result must be within 5 seconds of this new PNP value.

PNP Addition Test

PRINCIPLE

Test plasma + thrombin + PNP → fibrin clot modified by antithrombin

TABLE 4-4
Differentiation of the Effects of Heparin and
Fibrin(ogen) Degradation Products Using the
Thrombin Time and the Reptilase Time

Test	Heparin	FDPs
Thrombin time	Prolonged	Prolonged
Reptilase time	Normal	Prolonged

(Courtesy of Donna M. Corriveau)

In another approach, test plasma that has given a prolonged TT result is mixed with PNP. If the result is still prolonged, the presence of an antithrombic substance such as heparin, FDPs, circulating fibrin monomers, or excessive antithrombin III is suspected. Confirmatory tests such as the test for FDPs must be performed.

Reptilase Test

PRINCIPLE

Test plasma + Reptilase (venom) → fibrin clot

The Reptilase time test is another variation of the TT whereby serine protease venom from the pit viper *Bothrops atrox* is substituted for thrombin. Reptilase hydrolyzes mainly fibrinopeptide A from the α monomer of fibrinogen to trigger fibrin formation. This reaction, unlike the thrombin reaction, is not affected by heparin, so the combination of a prolonged TT and normal Reptilase time result indicates the presence of heparin. A normal Reptilase interval is 18 to 22 seconds. A prolonged Reptilase time is seen in the presence of FDPs and other circulating inhibitors (Table 4-4).

The TT procedure may also be modified and used to determine the concentration of plasma fibrinogen by titration of the plasma and comparison to a standard. The fibrinogen determination is discussed in a subsequent section on specific factor assays.

The TT test is normally used in combination with the PT and APTT to screen for coagulation abnormalities. The TT is more sensitive to changes in fibrinogen concentration than either the PT or APTT and is preferred by many experts as a test for heparin therapy. However, the TT is not used in the laboratory as much as the APTT for this purpose.

SUBSTITUTION TESTS

Substitution tests, also called mixing studies, are PT, APTT, and TT tests performed on abnormal patient plasmas to which specific reagents have been added. Substitution reagents include fresh normal plasma collected from a healthy donor, PNP, BaSO$_4$- or

TABLE 4-5
Substitution Tests Using the PT and APTT in the Identification of Single Factor Deficiencies

Tests Without Substitutions		PT		APTT		
		Adsorbed Plasma Reagent	Serum Reagent	Adsorbed Plasma Reagent	Serum Reagent	
PT	*APTT*	*Adsorbed Plasma Reagent*	*Serum Reagent*	*Adsorbed Plasma Reagent*	*Serum Reagent*	**Factor Deficiency**
N	P			C	NC	VIII
N	P			C	C	XI, XII, HMWK Fletcher*
N	P			NC	C	IX
P	P	C	NC			V, I*
P	P	NC	C			X
P	P	NC	NC			II, circulating anticoagulant*
P	N	NC	C			VII

N, normal time; P, prolonged time; C, corrected; NC, not corrected
* Additional testing must be done to differentiate.

Al(OH)$_3$-adsorbed plasma, serum, and platelet neutralization reagent (Table 4-5). Substitution tests are used to detect congenital single factor deficiencies and circulating inhibitors (anticoagulants) but are not effective for identifying the missing factors in most acquired coagulation deficiencies with loss of more than one factor. One example of an acquired deficiency, described in Chapter 6, is vitamin K deficiency, in which prothrombin (II) and Factors VII, IX, and X are diminished.

A complete clinical history and physical examination are performed on the patient suspected of having a coagulation abnormality. Particular attention is given to a family history of bleeding tendencies or the presence of diseases such as lupus erythematosus that are associated with circulating inhibitors. Next, a battery of hemostatic tests including platelet count, bleeding time, platelet aggregometry, PT, APTT, and TT is performed. If the platelet parameters are normal and one, two, or all three of the coagulation screening tests are prolonged, substitution tests are performed.

Circulating Inhibitors

Hemophilia, autoimmune disease, long-term treatment with certain drugs, anemia, and collagen disorders are associated with the presence of circulating inhibitors. Anti–Factor VIII, the most common of the specific inhibitors, is detected in 10% of hemophiliacs who have been treated with factor concentrate, cryoprecipitate, or fresh-frozen plasma. Anti–Factor VIII may occasionally be present in nonhemophiliacs who have autoimmune disorders. The most common nonspecific inhibitor is the *lupus anticoagulant*. The lupus anticoagulant is an autoantibody directed against several types of phospholipid (Fig. 4-6). Its binding reactions impair the activation of Factor X and pro-

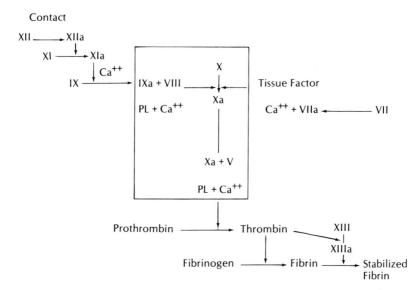

Contact

FIG. 4-6. Site of action of the lupus inhibitor. Overview of the coagulation mechanism with the two phospholipid-dependent reactions included. The inhibitor participates in an immune reaction with the membrane phospholipid to slow these reactions. *PL*, phospholipid.

thrombin. The APTT is usually prolonged in the case of either specific or nonspecific inhibitors. The PT results are unpredictable, and the TT results are usually normal.

Whenever the APTT, PT, or TT is prolonged, the first step is to mix the test plasma with fresh normal plasma or PNP in equal proportions (Fig. 4-7). In most cases, 0.1 ml of test plasma is added to 0.1 ml of reagent plasma, and the mixture is incubated at 37°C for several minutes. This mixture is tested using the protocol for the screen procedure that was prolonged. Only the system that demonstrated a prolonged result in the first screening test is used; in most cases this is the APTT. If the result of the test on the mixture is normal, "correction" has occurred, and a factor deficiency is suspected. Before a factor deficiency is confirmed, the mixing test is repeated with the incubation extended to 60 minutes at 37°C. Anti–Factor VIII is an IgG immunoglobulin that reacts more slowly than lupus anticoagulant, and its effect is enhanced by incubation. A control is incubated simultaneously. If the time interval of the control APTT is exceeded by the test sample–PNP mixture result, anti–Factor VIII may be suspected. If correction has occurred in both the 3-minute and 60-minute test sample–PNP mixture incubation steps, the original prolonged test result is most likely caused by a factor deficiency. If the prolongation is sustained in either case, a circulating inhibitor is suspected.

Although others are known, most instances of circulating inhibitor involve either lupus anticoagulant or anti–Factor VIII. It is important to distinguish between the two. If the clinical and familial history do not help to establish the distinction, two specialized laboratory procedures are used to identify lupus anticoagulant: the *tissue thromboplastin inhibition* test and the *platelet neutralization* test. Two others are used to confirm and quantitate anti–Factor VIII: the *Bethesda* and *New Oxford* procedures.

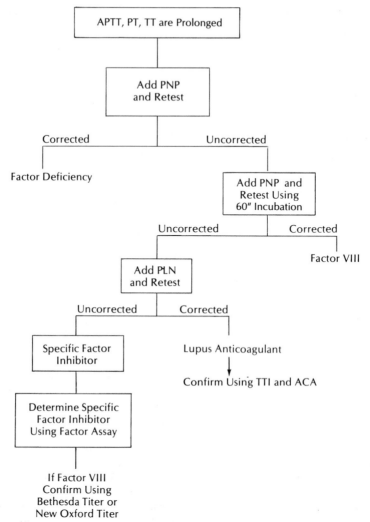

FIG. 4-7. Algorithm for detection of circulating inhibitor. When the screening test (APTT, PT, TT) is prolonged, retest after mixing test plasma with PNP. If the mixture gives a prolonged result, correction has not occurred. The test plasma is next mixed with PLN and the screening test repeated. If prolonged, a specific factor inhibitor is responsible for the prolongation. If corrected, the inhibitor is lupus anticoagulant. Specific factor inhibitors are identified using factor assays. In most cases the inhibitor is anti–Factor VIII. Anti–Factor VIII is then titered using the Bethesda or New Oxford technique. PLN, platelet neutralization reagent; TTI, tissue thromboplastin inhibition; ACA, anticardiolipin antibody.

Tissue Thromboplastin Inhibition

In the tissue thromboplastin inhibition test, PT reagent (tissue thromboplastin plus $CaCl_2$) is diluted 1 : 50 or 1 : 500 with saline.[24] The dilution is prewarmed, then 0.1 ml of dilute reagent is mixed with 0.1 ml of the test plasma, and the mixture incubated for 3 minutes. $CaCl_2$ (0.025 molar) is forcibly added and a timer started. PNP is tested at the same time, and the results are compared. If the ratio of patient plasma interval to PNP interval is 1.3 or greater, lupus anticoagulant is presumed to be present. A ratio of 1.1 or less is considered to be normal, and lupus anticoagulant is absent. The combination of a prolonged PNP–test plasma APTT result and a low tissue thromboplastin inhibition test ratio leads to the presumption that Factor VIII inhibitor is present. Confirmation of this presumption by the Bethesda or New Oxford titer is necessary.

Platelet Neutralization Test

Platelet neutralization reagent (PLN) is employed in the platelet neutralization test (*also* designated PLN).[24] The reagent is a lysate of platelet concentrate prepared in tris buffer, washed and frozen. The platelet neutralization test is an APTT substitution test wherein test plasma, prewarmed APTT reagent, and prewarmed PLN are mixed in equal quantities, usually 0.1 ml each. The mixture stands for 3 minutes at 37°C. $CaCl_2$ is forcibly added as in the usual APTT procedure, and the time is recorded. Lupus anticoagulant is neutralized by the phospholipid-rich PLN so that the APTT result is corrected. If another inhibitor is present, the result remains prolonged. The platelet neutralization test is more specific for the lupus anticoagulant than the tissue thromboplastin inhibition test. The combination of a prolonged PNP–test plasma APTT result and a prolonged platelet neutralization test result leads to the presumption that Factor VIII inhibitor is present. Confirmation of the presumption by the Bethesda or New Oxford titer is necessary.

Although clot-based assays are the accepted clinical approach to detection of the lupus anticoagulant, recent experiments have shown that enzyme immunoassay using cardiolipin as the solid-phase antigen will detect anticardiolipin antibody. The presence of this antibody correlates with the presence of lupus anticoagulant as defined by the clot-based assays and is associated with systemic lupus erythematosus in about the same proportions as the anticoagulant. Anticardiolipin antibody also correlates clinically with thromboembolic disorders. It is likely that the immunoassay will supplant the less specific clot-based assays in the future.

Bethesda Titer for Factor VIII Inhibitor

The presence of Factor VIII inhibitor may be confirmed by titration of the inhibitor by the Bethesda method.[11] In the *Bethesda* method, 0.2 ml of test plasma suspected of containing Factor VIII inhibitor is incubated with 0.2 ml of PNP for 2 hours at 37°C. A control sample consisting of 0.2 ml of imidazole buffer at *p*H 7.4 mixed with 0.2 ml of PNP is incubated simultaneously. During the incubation period, anti–Factor VIII from the test plasma neutralizes a percentage of PNP Factor VIII activity. The proportion of Factor VIII activity neutralized is related to the level of inhibitor activity. Following incubation, residual Factor VIII level in the PNP test plasma mixture is measured by specific factor assay as described later in this chapter. The level of inhibitor in the sample is expressed as a percentage of the control. If the test sample–PNP mixture retains more than 75% of the residual Factor VIII of the control, there is no significant Factor VIII inhibitor in the test plasma. If the residual VIII level is less than 25% of control, the test plasma Factor VIII inhibitor level is titered by use of several dilutions of the test sample mixed with PNP. One Bethesda unit of activity is that amount of antibody that leaves 50% residual Factor VIII in the mixture.

New Oxford Titer for Factor VIII Inhibitor

The *New Oxford* method of titration employs a series of dilutions of test plasma in imidazole-buffered saline. In the New Oxford technique, 0.4 ml of test serum–buffer solution are mixed with 0.1 ml of Factor VIII concentrate and allowed to incubate for 4 hours at 37°C. The Factor VIII concentrate is first adjusted to a potency of 3 to 6 international units per milliliter. The dilutions of plasma chosen are those that will span the point at which 50% of the initial Factor VIII is destroyed. A control sample using 0.4 ml of buffer alone, substituted for the test sample dilution, is incubated and tested simultaneously. Residual Factor VIII is determined in sample dilutions and controls by specific factor assay, and the test sample result is expressed as a percentage of control. The exact level of Factor VIII in the control sample is also measured and expressed in international units. A graph of residual Factor VIII as a percentage of control is plotted against the dilution of the test plasma. The level of dilution required to leave 50% residual Factor VIII is defined as a New Oxford unit.[11]

Acquired inhibitors specific for fibrinogen (I) and Factor V, IX, XI, and XIII have been described. In most cases an inhibitor develops in persons lacking the specific procoagulant, but anti–Factors IX and XI have been detected in systemic lupus erythematosus. Factor V inhibitor has been demonstrated postoperatively and is usually transient.

Fibrinogen activation is suppressed by the presence of circulating fibrin monomer, FDPs, and heparin. Heparin measurement has been described in the use of the WBCT, APTT, and TT. Detection of fibrin monomer and degradation products will be described in the section on fibrinolysis.

Congenital Single Factor Deficiencies

When the prolonged APTT, PT, or TT is corrected by addition of PNP, a single factor deficiency is suspected. BaSO$_4$- or Al(OH)$_3$-adsorbed plasma and serum are used to identify the deficiency. Adsorbed plasma provides fibrinogen (I) and Factors V, VIII, XI, XII, and XIII. Serum provides Factors VII, IX, X, XI, and XII (see Table 4-1).

Combinations of APTT, PT, and TT results in the presence of each of the substitution reagents are used to determine what procoagulant is deficient.[23] These combinations are described below and summarized in Figure 4-8.

If the APTT and TT are normal and PT is prolonged, Factor VII is deficient. There is no case recorded of tissue thromboplastin (III) deficiency, because abundant procoagulant is released from all body tissues. No further substitution studies are necessary.

If the APTT is prolonged and both PT and TT are normal, the problem is in the intrinsic pathway. The deficient factor is VIII, IX, XI, XII, prekallikrein, or HMWK. Correction of the APTT by adsorbed plasma but not by serum indicates Factor VIII deficiency. Correction by serum but not adsorbed plasma indicates that Factor IX is deficient. These findings may be confirmed by specific factor assay. Correction by both adsorbed plasma and serum indicates that the deficiency is in the contact activation mechanism: XI, XII, prekallikrein, or HMWK. Further delineation requires specific factor assay. Note that the prolongation of the APTT by prekallikrein (Fletcher factor) deficiency reverts to normal if the test plasma alone is incubated with APTT reagent for 1 hour (review the case study at the beginning of this chapter).

If both the APTT and PT are prolonged, the problem is in the common pathway. Fibrinogen (I), prothrombin (II), Factor V, or Factor X may be deficient. If the TT is prolonged, the missing or diminished factor is fibrinogen. If the TT is normal, prothrombin (II), Factor V, or Factor X is suspected. Correction of both the APTT and PT by adsorbed plasma alone indicates that Factor V is deficient. Correction by serum alone indicates that the problem is Factor X. If neither corrects, prothrombin (II) is the

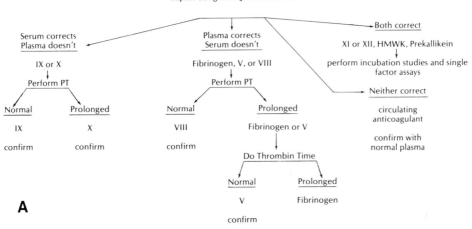

A

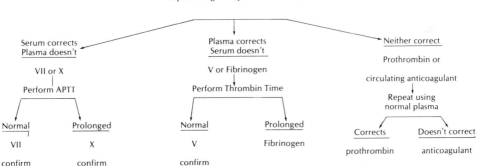

B

FIG. 4-8. Substitution studies. *(A)* When the APTT is prolonged, repeat using serum and adsorbed plasma. If serum corrects but plasma does not, the deficiency is in IX or X. If plasma corrects but serum does not, the deficiency is in fibrinogen, V, or VIII. If both correct, the deficiency is in XI, XII, HMWK, or prekallikrein. *(B)* When the PT is prolonged, repeat using serum and adsorbed plasma. If serum corrects and plasma does not, the deficiency is in VII or X. If plasma corrects but serum does not, the deficiency is in V or fibrinogen. If neither corrects, the deficiency is prothrombin, or there may be a circulating anticoagulant.

deficient factor. Every conclusion is confirmed by single factor assay. Factor X deficiency may also be confirmed by the Stypven time test, as described previously.

While factor substitution is essential for the detection of circulating anticoagulants, its value for detecting single factor deficiencies is limited. The results of substitution assays described above are confounded by multiple factor deficiencies that are typical of acquired disorders, circulating inhibitors, and the presence of FDPs. In most deficiency cases, the history and physical condition of the patient indicate the probable deficiency. Confirmation may be based on the results of APTT, PT, and TT screens plus one or two specific factor assays. Thus, factor substitution for single factor deficiencies is used only when the clinical information is inadequate to lead the laboratory investigator to a conclusion.

SPECIFIC FACTOR ASSAYS

Factor Assays Based on the APTT

Quantitative assays of Factors VIII, IX, XI, and XII, prekallikrein, and HMWK are performed using the APTT test whenever a deficiency of one of these factors is suspected.[23] Test plasma is mixed with reagent *factor-deficient plasma* and tested using the APTT system. Factor-deficient plasma is a reagent plasma collected by commercial suppliers from a hemophiliac and processed for distribution. Specific factor-deficient plasma provides normal activity of all procoagulants but the one specified. As expected, reagent plasmas deficient in Factors VIII, IX, XI, and XII, prekallikrein, or HMWK give prolonged APTT results. When test plasma is mixed with factor-deficient plasma and the mixture is tested using the APTT system, a normal result indicates that the activity of the procoagulant missing from the reagent plasma is supplied by the test plasma, implying that the activity of the procoagulant in question is normal in the patient. A prolonged result implies that the factor activity is absent from the test plasma as well as the reagent plasma. The APTT time interval of the test plasma – factor-deficient plasma mixture is compared to a previously prepared standard curve that plots time interval against percentage activity (Fig. 4-9). The mean time interval is assigned the value 100%, and a result between 50% and 150% of normal is considered to be acceptable.

In humans, plasma procoagulants are present at an activity level ten times that necessary for normal coagulation. Consequently, quantitative factor assays are customarily performed using a 1 : 10 dilution of test plasma. By convention, the normal range is established using this 10% dilution, not undiluted plasma. This approach ensures that the factor assay is sensitive to subtle changes in factor activity. Thus a 100% APTT result for factors VIII, IX, XI, and XIII, prekallikrein, and HMWK actually represents the normal time interval obtained on a 10% solution of plasma. This dilution step also diminishes the effect of circulating inhibitors, when present. In preparation of a curve, a 1 : 20 dilution represents 50% activity, 1 : 40 is 25%, 1 : 80 is 12.5%, and so on, with the ultimate dilution giving an activity level of 0.8%. Dilutions greater than 1 : 1280 give extremely long APTT time intervals, so the titer becomes relatively insensitive.

In the Factor VIII assay a 10% solution of test plasma in *imidazole-buffered normal saline* is mixed with undiluted Factor VIII – deficient plasma. Factor VIII – deficient plasmas are collected from patients with hemophilia A who have complete absence of Factor VIII. To this mixture is added partial thromboplastin reagent. In most cases, 0.1 ml of partial thromboplastin is mixed with 0.1 ml each of test plasma and factor-de-

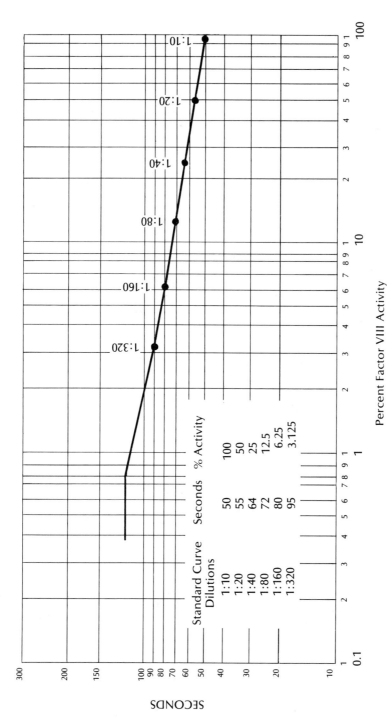

Standard Curve Dilutions	Seconds	% Activity
1:10	50	100
1:20	55	50
1:40	64	25
1:80	72	12.5
1:160	80	6.25
1:320	95	3.125

Percent Factor VIII Activity

FIG. 4-9. Factor VIII assay standard curve (APTT-based). (Courtesy of Donna M. Corriveau)

ficient plasma. After incubation for 3 to 5 minutes at 37°C, 0.1 ml of 0.025-molar CaCl$_2$ is added and a timer started. The interval to clot formation is compared with a standard curve, and the result is reported as a percentage of normal. All dilutions are made using imidazole-buffered saline at pH 7.3. Tests may be performed on either electromechanical or photo-optical devices. When using an electro-mechanical device such as the Fibrometer, a 0.4-ml probe is necessary to measure clotting in the total reaction mixture.

The standard curve is prepared using serial dilutions of PNP. A twofold serial dilution starting with 10% PNP (arbitrarily set at 100% activity as described above) is used in most applications, and the percentage activity levels for each dilution are 100, 50, 25, 12.5, 6.25, 3.125, 1.6, and 0.8. Eight dilutions and a blank are customarily used, and the curve is prepared on log–log graph paper. Higher dilutions yield longer time intervals. The dilutions are mixed with factor-deficient plasma, and the interval between the addition of CaCl$_2$ and clot formation is recorded as in the original test above.

Figure 4-9 demonstrates a typical standard curve. When patient plasma is tested, the time interval obtained is entered on the vertical coordinate and converted to a percentage. The percentage is reported. When the time interval is shorter than the time of the 100% standard, the curve is extrapolated to provide a percentage value greater than 100.

Tests for Factors IX, XI, and XII, prekallikrein, and HMWK may be performed using the same approach, except that the appropriate factor-deficient plasma is substituted for Factor VIII.

A simple modification of the APTT screening test helps distinguish among deficiencies of the contact activation procoagulants prekallikrein (Fletcher factor), HMWK (Fitzgerald factor), and Factor XII (Hageman factor). Deficiency of any of these three results in a prolonged APTT without significant hemorrhagic symptoms. If prekallikrein is the deficient procoagulant, incubation of the test sample plasma and partial thromboplastin reagent at 37°C for 10 to 60 minutes results in reversion of the APTT result to normal. This is because prolonged contact activation in the presence of normal Factor XII and HMWK activity bypasses the need for prekallikrein. If Factor XII or HMWK is absent, the APTT result does not revert to normal. Once the prolonged incubation modification of the APTT has been performed, specific factor assay is used for confirmation of the suspected deficiency.

Quantitation of von Willebrand Factor

Von Willebrand factor (vWF) is the macromolecular portion of the Factor VIII molecule that is essential for normal platelet adhesion. In von Willebrand disease (vWD) the molecule is diminished in concentration or defective in structure (see Chap. 5). vWD is characterized by a decrease in Factor VIII levels, as measured above, diminished Factor VIII–related antigen (VIIIR : Ag) levels, and vWF activity as quantitated here.

Ristocetin agonist reacts with formalin-preserved normal platelets in the presence of normal levels of vWF to cause platelet agglutination, assessed by visual inspection or in an aggregometer. Both the rate of agglutination, as determined by aggregometry, or the time to formation of 4+ agglutination, as detectable visually, are proportional to vWF availability. Formalin-fixed platelets retain the vWF receptor site.

To perform the visual test, 0.1 ml of formalin-treated platelets (Organon Teknika, Parsipanny, NJ 07054) is placed on a glass slide. A total of 0.25 ml of ristocetin and

0.005 ml of undiluted plasma sample are added. A timer is started and the slide rocked until 4+ agglutination is observed, whereupon the timer is stopped. The elapsed time is proportional to the level of vWF. The results are compared with a previously prepared standard curve that uses four dilutions of PNP: 0, 1:2, 1:4, and 1:8.[1]

The test may also be performed using aggregometry and the process described in Chapter 9.

The reference interval for normal results is 50% to 136%. Any result less than 50% may indicate vWD.

Factor Assays Based on the PT

Quantitative assays of prothrombin (II) and Factors V, VII, and X are performed with the PT test whenever one of these procoagulants is thought to be deficient. Test plasma is mixed with reagent factor-deficient plasma, and the mixture is tested with the PT system. A normal PT result indicates that the procoagulant missing from the reagent plasma is present in the test plasma. A prolonged result implies that the procoagulant is absent from the test plasma. Like the factor assays based on the APTT, assays of II, V, VII, and X use a standard curve in which the mean for the normal population is assigned the value 100% and the reference interval extends from 50% to 150%. Another similarity between APTT- and PT-based factor assays is 1:10 dilution of the test plasma with imidazole-buffered saline. The 10% PNP dilution PT interval is assigned the value 100% and used as the 100% standard.

In the Factor VII assay, a prewarmed 10% solution of test plasma in imidazole-buffered saline is mixed with an equal proportion of prewarmed Factor VII–deficient plasma. In most cases 0.1 ml of each plasma is used. Now 0.2 ml of tissue thromboplastin–$CaCl_2$ reagent is forcibly added to the mixture, and a timer is started. The timer is stopped when the clot is formed, and the interval is observed. The interval is compared with the standard curve, and plasma activity of Factor VII is reported as a percentage of normal. Tests may be performed on either electromechanical or photo-optical devices. When an electromechanical device such as the Fibrometer is used, a 0.4-ml probe is necessary to measure clotting in the total reaction mixture.

The standard curve is prepared using serial dilutions of PNP. A twofold serial dilution starting with 10% PNP (arbitrarily set at 100% activity) is used in most applications, and the percentage activity levels for each dilution are 100, 50, 25, 12.5, 6.25, 3.125, 1.6 and 0.8. Eight dilutions and a blank are customarily used, and the curve is prepared on log–log graph paper. Higher dilutions yield longer time intervals. The dilutions are mixed with factor-deficient plasma, and the interval between addition of tissue thromboplastin–$CaCl_2$ and clot formation is recorded as in the original test above.

Figure 4-10 demonstrates a typical standard curve. When patient plasma is tested, the time interval obtained is entered on the vertical coordinate and converted to a percentage. The percentage is reported. When the time interval is shorter than the time of the 100% standard, the curve is extrapolated and used to provide a percentage value greater than 100.

Tests for prothrombin or Factors V and X may be performed in the same fashion except that the appropriate factor-deficient plasma is substituted for Factor VII–deficient plasma. These three procoagulants may also be measured with the APTT test procedure.

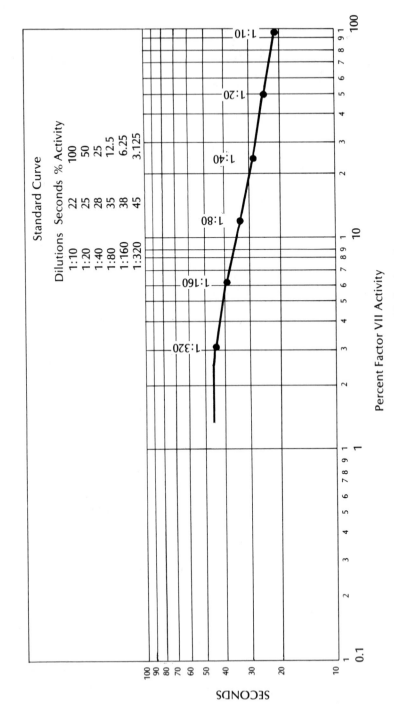

FIG. 4-10. Factor VII assay standard curve (PT-based). (Courtesy of Donna M. Corriveau)

Fibrinogen Assays

Dysfibrinogenemia, afibrinogenemia, and hypofibrinogenemia cause prolonged PT, APTT, and TT results. The screening test most sensitive to fibrinogen deficiency is the TT. Results of the TT are prolonged whenever the fibrinogen level is below 100 mg/dl of plasma. Diagnostic demands often require that the exact level of fibrinogen be determined. When this is the case, one of two assay procedures is commonly employed: the modified TT, commercially known as the Data-Fi (Dade Division, American Hospital Supply, Hialeah, FL), and the Ellis-Stransky turbidimetric procedure.

In the *modified TT*, thrombin reagent is used at a concentration of 100 units per milliliter. The *TT screen* (described previously) employs a much smaller concentration, approximately 2 units per milliliter. In the modified TT the plasma to be tested is diluted 1 : 10 with *Owren's veronal buffer,* so that the functional level of fibrinogen is diluted to 20 mg/dl to 40 mg/dl instead of the normal 200 to 400, the levels detected by the TT screen performed on undiluted plasma. The modifications of higher reagent concentration and lower plasma concentration provide a linear relationship between elapsed time to clot formation and concentration of fibrinogen when the concentration is between 100 mg/dl and 400 mg/dl. Beyond these limits the results are not linear. Dilution of plasma also minimizes the effects of antithrombins such as heparin, FDPs, and dysproteinemias. Heparin levels below 0.6 units per milliliter and FDP levels below 100 μg/dl will not affect the results of the modified TT so long as the 1 : 10 sample plasma dilution is employed.[19]

Before patient specimens are tested, a standard curve is prepared (Fig. 4-11). Fibrinogen standard, available commercially (Dade Division, American Hospital Supply, Hialeah, FL), is reconstituted with 1 ml of distilled water. Using veronal buffer, three dilutions of the standard are prepared: 1 : 5, 1 : 15, and 1 : 40. Dilutions are converted to fibrinogen concentration in milligrams per deciliter using the original concentration of fibrinogen value supplied with the reagent. For each dilution 0.2 ml is transferred to a reaction tube, warmed to 37°C, and tested by adding 0.1 ml of thrombin reagent. Time from addition of thrombin to clot formation is recorded and plotted on a graph against concentration.

Patient plasma is tested as follows. A 1 : 10 dilution of plasma is prepared using veronal buffer. In most cases, 0.1 ml of plasma is mixed with 0.9 ml of buffer. Then, 0.2 ml of the mixture is warmed to 37°C in a reaction vessel. Next, 0.1 ml of thrombin reagent is added, a timer is started, and the mixture is observed until a clot forms. The timer is stopped and the interval compared with the graph. Results are reported in milligrams per deciliter of fibrinogen. A control consisting of PNP is always tested with the patient plasma and the result compared to a predetermined value. The control result must be within 5% of the preassayed value.

Several modifications become necessary if the result is outside the range of 200 mg/dl to 400 mg/dl. If the clotting time of the 1 : 10 dilution indicates a fibrinogen level above 400 mg/dl, a 1 : 20 dilution is prepared and tested. The resulting fibrinogen concentration must be multiplied by two to compensate for the curve, which is designed for 1 : 10 dilutions. If the clotting time of the 1 : 10 dilution is excessively long, indicating less than 200 mg/dl of fibrinogen, a 1 : 5 dilution of the test plasma is prepared. The resulting fibrinogen concentration must be divided by 2 to compensate for the curve. Care must also be taken that the thrombin reagent is pure and has not degenerated. Exposure to sunlight or oxidation will result in rapid breakdown of thrombin.

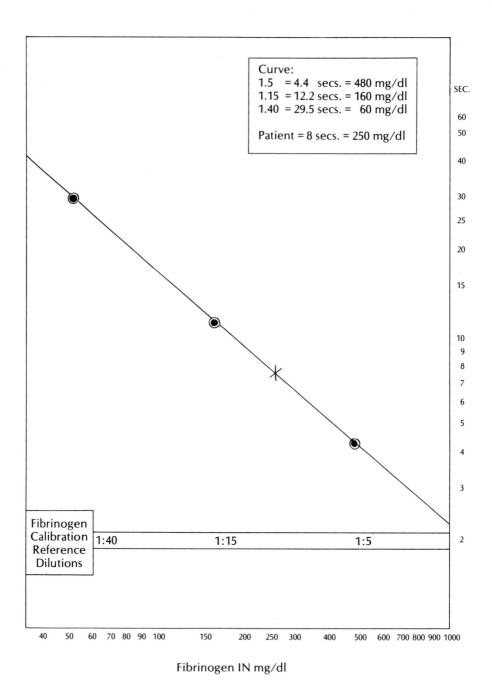

Curve:
1.5 = 4.4 secs. = 480 mg/dl
1.15 = 12.2 secs. = 160 mg/dl
1.40 = 29.5 secs. = 60 mg/dl

Patient = 8 secs. = 250 mg/dl

SEC.

Fibrinogen
Calibration
Reference
Dilutions

1:40   1:15   1:5

Fibrinogen IN mg/dl

FIG. 4-11. Fibrinogen assay standard curve (TT-based). Three dilutions of the fibrinogen reference are made: 1 : 5, 1 : 15, and 1 : 40. These dilutions are tested against thrombin reagent and the times recorded. Test samples are diluted 1 : 10 and tested using the same reagent. The results in time elapsed are read on the graph and translated into fibrinogen dilution or concentration in mg/dl. Dots indicate the point on the curve where a certain dilution's concentration falls. For instance, a 1 : 5 dilution has a test time of 4.4 seconds and a concentration of 480 mg/dl. The patient's (X) fibrinogen concentration can then be determined. (Courtesy of Donna M. Corriveau)

The reference interval for fibrinogen concentration is 200 mg/dl to 400 mg/dl at all ages, including the full-term and premature infant.[5] Hypofibrinogenemia is usually associated with disseminated intravascular coagulation, severe liver disease, or, rarely, primary fibrinolysis. Dysfibrinogenemia will give the same results as hypofibrinogenemia by this test method because abnormal fibrinogen is hydrolyzed more slowly by thrombin than normal fibrinogen. Immunologic and turbidimetric (Ellis-Stransky) measures of fibrinogen indicate normal concentrations in dysfibrinogenemia. Although antithrombic effects are minimized by the dilution of plasma samples, heparin levels above 0.6 units per milliliter and FDP levels above 100 μg/ml prolong the results and give falsely lowered fibrinogen level results.

A number of colorimetric and turbidimetric fibrinogen assays have been developed. While technically less demanding, none of these techniques is as sensitive or accurate as the Dade fibrinogen assay. The Ellis-Stransky technique is an illustrative turbidimetric method.[6] A mixture of thrombin and $CaCl_2$ is prepared so that the final concentration of thrombin is approximately 50 units per milliliter and the concentration of $CaCl_2$ is 0.025M. A 1:10 dilution of test or control plasma is prepared with *barbitone* buffer at a *p*H of 7.2. One drop of the thrombin–$CaCl_2$ solution is added to 3 ml of plasma dilution, and the reaction mixture stands for 20 minutes while precipitation of the fibrinogen occurs and turbidity develops. The turbidity is measured in a photometer against a blank consisting of plasma dilution alone. The results are compared with a standard curve and reported in milligrams per deciliter.

Interpretation of turbidimetric and colorimetric methods is similar to the Dade fibrinogen assay, except that the numeric result must be considered semiquantitative, since the tests are less precise.

Qualitative Factor XIII Assay

Factor XIII is also termed *fibrin stabilizing factor*. During polymerization of fibrinogen, fibrin strands are first held together by weak hydrogen bonds. The clot is unstable. Factor XIII, activated by thrombin to XIII_a, is a transpeptidase that catalyzes the formation of lateral covalent bonds between fibrin strands. Clots acted on by Factor XIII_a are stable. Patients with congenital or acquired absence of Factor XIII experience a variety of hemorrhagic symptoms like poor wound healing, ecchymoses, hematomas, menorrhagia, and umbilical bleeding. Routine coagulation screening tests do not detect Factor XIII deficiency; the TT, PT, and APTT results are all normal, provided that the remainder of the coagulation system is intact. Thus the decision to perform the Factor XIII assay must be based on clinical symptoms. Factor XIII inhibitors have been reported.

The unstable clot that forms in the absence of Factor XIII or in the presence of Factor XIII inhibitor dissolves in a 5M urea solution or a 2% solution of monochloracetic acid. A Factor XIII–stabilized clot will remain intact for at least 24 hours.[17]

Three tubes are prepared. The first tube receives 0.3 ml of test plasma. The third tube receives 0.3 ml of PNP. Tube #2 receives 0.2 ml of test plasma and 0.1 ml of PNP. Then, 0.1 ml of 0.025M $CaCl_2$ is transferred to each of the three tubes. After clot formation, all three are incubated at 37°C for 30 minutes. Now 3 ml of 5M urea solution is transferred to each of the three tubes, and the tubes are tapped gently to dislodge the clots from the sides. The tubes are capped and incubated at ambient temperature for 24 hours but are observed for evidence of clot dissolution at 1, 2, 4, and 24 hours. Decreasing size of clot, fragmentation, and increasing turbidity of the urea solution are evidence for clot dissolution. The test plasma tube (tube #1) is compared to the PNP (#3) in detection of dissolution, and results are reported as "Factor XIII present" or "Factor XIII absent." If a Factor XIII inhibitor is present in the test plasma, dissolution will be seen in both the first and the second tubes, the one in which patient plasma and PNP were mixed.

Factor XIII deficiencies are usually acquired in metastatic carcinoma, leukemia, hypergammopathy, collagen disease, and liver disease, but congenital Factor XIII deficiencies have been described.

TESTS OF FIBRINOLYSIS

The direct measurement of plasminogen or plasmin levels and plasminogen activators uses chromogenic substrates and is described in Chapter 12. The only clot-based assay used to test the fibrinolytic mechanism is the somewhat nonspecific *euglobulin lysis* test.

Tests of fibrinogen and fibrin catabolism include the immune-based fibrinogen/fibrin degradation products procedure and tests of circulating fibrin monomer, also termed *paracoagulation* tests.

Euglobulin Lysis

Excessive fibrinolytic activity occurs under a variety of conditions. Inflammation and trauma may be reflected in a radical increase in plasmin that causes hemorrhage. Bone trauma, fractures, and surgical dissection of bone as in cardiac surgery may result in increases in fibrinolysis. A time-honored approach to measurement of fibrinolytic activity is the euglobulin lysis test.[25]

Test plasma is diluted and acidified with 1% acetic acid until the solution reaches the pH of 5.35 to 5.40. Upon refrigeration a precipitate forms that contains fibrinogen, plasminogen, active plasmin, and plasminogen activators. This precipitate is termed the *euglobulin fraction*. Excluded from the precipitate are most plasma antiplasmins, so that fibrinolysis may proceed unchecked. The tubes are centrifuged and the supernate decanted completely. The precipitate is redissolved in borate buffer or phosphate-buffered saline, and reagent thrombin is added. A clot should form immediately. A timer is started at the time of thrombin addition, and the clot is observed periodically for dissolution over a period of 90 minutes. Normal fibrinolysis proceeds slowly in the euglobulin system, so that a firm clot is present after 90 minutes. Disappearance of the clot prior to 90 minutes indicates increased fibrinolysis.

Because the euglobulin lysis test is fraught with technical error, both positive and negative plasma controls are included. PNP is used as the negative control, while PNP plus streptokinase is used as the positive control. Streptokinase is a humoral activator of plasminogen. Clot dissolution of the test fraction is compared with both the positive and negative controls. Another control, the *patient activated control* is also prepared. This is a sample of patient euglobulin fraction with streptokinase added. This control ensures against patient sample plasminogen depletion. When plasminogen levels are diminished, such as in a long-term case of disseminated intravascular coagulation, clot dissolution will not occur. The euglobulin lysis time will appear normal because of the lack of plasminogen. The patient activated control indicates when this condition exists. Streptokinase-activated plasma from the patient should cause rapid clot dissolution. When plasminogen is depleted, the streptokinase-activated control will give no dissolution, and the euglobulin lysis time will appear normal. Thus a normal result in the patient activated control means that the actual test result is untrustworthy.

Hypofibrinogenemia and Factor XIII deficiency affect the euglobulin lysis time. In hypofibrinogenemia there is less fibrin to be lysed, and a short lysis time may be seen without a genuine increase in fibrinolytic activity. In Factor XIII deficiency the original clot quality is poor, and dissolution by normal levels of plasmin is more rapid.

Fibrinogen and Fibrin Degradation Products

The catabolic pathways of fibrin and fibrinogen are biochemically identical, as described in Chapter 2. Normal fibrinolysis yields the FDPs X, Y, C, D, and E in concentrations below 2 µg/ml of plasma. The level of the degradation products is suppressed by the low rate of the degradation reaction and the high rate of clearance. Pathologic degradation of fibrin and fibrinogen, a result of increased plasma-borne plasminogen activation, yields FDPs at levels of 2 µg/ml to 40 µg/ml or more. Increased plasminogen activation is characteristic of acute and chronic disseminated intravascular coagulation and primary fibrinolysis.

The Thrombo-Wellcotest (Wellcome Reagents, Ltd., Beckenham, England) is an immunologic measure of the plasma concentration of FDPs. Purified Fragments D and E are administered to laboratory sheep, which respond with production of specific immunoglobulins. The immunoglobulins are harvested, extracted, and purified by affinity column chromatography to yield specific antisera at controlled concentrations. A 0.5% suspension of polystyrene latex particles in glycine saline buffer is coated with the anti-FDP globulin standardized to be sensitive to FDPs at 2 µg/ml.

Two milliliters of whole blood are collected by syringe venipuncture and immediately mixed with 20 units of bovine thrombin and 3600 units of soybean trypsin inhibitor. The thrombin promotes rapid and complete clotting, while the trypsin inhibitor neutralizes plasmin, preventing fibrin breakdown *in vitro*. All FDPs present in the plasma may be assumed to be produced in the body in advance of sample collection. If heparin is present in the sample, its antithrombic activity thwarts these preparations. In this case, Reptilase is added to the sample to bypass the antithrombic effect of the heparin, as described in this chapter in the section on the TT test. The clotted sample is centrifuged and supernatant serum separated from the clot immediately after collection. Correct handling of the sample ensures that the serum FDP level is not inappropriately elevated by *in vitro* degradation.

A portion of the test serum is diluted 1:5 with glycine-buffered saline, and another portion is diluted 1:20. One drop each of undiluted serum, 1:5, and 1:20 dilutions is placed in a labeled circle on a clean glass slide. One drop of well-mixed latex suspension is added to each drop of sample or dilution and mixed. The slide is rocked for 2 minutes and the mixture observed for agglutination. Negative and positive sera, supplied by the manufacturer, are always tested with each unknown test serum. The positive test serum contains an FDP concentration of 5 µg/ml to 10 µg/ml (Fig. 4-12).

Results of the Thrombo-Wellcotest are semiquantitative and may be reported in micrograms per milliliter. If only the undiluted serum mixture demonstrates agglutination, the FDP concentration is reported as greater than 2 µg/ml and less than 10 µg/ml. If the undiluted and 1:5 circles show agglutination, the result is reported as greater than 10 µg/ml and less than 80 µg/ml, and if all three wells clump, the result is greater than 80 µg/ml. A negative result—absence of agglutination in all three wells—is reported as less than 2 µg/ml. Control results are observed and recorded.

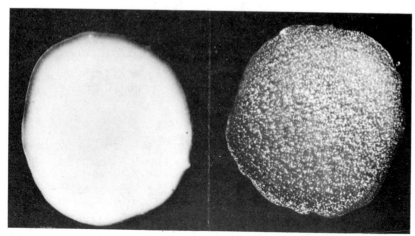

FIG. 4-12. Results of the Thrombo-Wellcotest for FDPs. *(Left)* Nonagglutinated pattern. The FDP concentration is less than 2 μg/ml. *(Right)* Agglutinated pattern. The FDP concentration is greater than 2 μg/ml. (Photographs provided by The Wellcome Foundation, Ltd, 183 Euston Road, London NW1 2BP. © 1986, The Wellcome Foundation Ltd)

Plasma Paracoagulation Tests

Fibrin monomers, mostly in the form of degradation products X and Y, circulate in the plasma of patients with acute disseminated intravascular coagulation or primary fibrinolysis. The monomers are present as a result of unchecked plasma fibrinolysis and fibrinogenolysis and possess antiplatelet and antithrombic properties. Monomers are also termed *paracoagulants*. The circulating fibrin monomers are detected by mixing a milliliter of PPP to 0.1 ml of 1% protamine sulfate at 37°C. The protamine sulfate induces polymerization and formation of visible white fibrin threads. The test is simply reported as positive or negative.

The presence of platelet materials, a delay of mixing sample with anticoagulant, and a failure to incubate the reaction mixture at 37°C all cause false-positive results.

REFERENCES

1. Allain JP, Cooper HA, Wagner RH et al: Platelets fixed with paraformaldehyde: A new reagent for assay of von Willebrand factor and platelet aggregating factor. J Lab Clin Med 85:318–328, 1975
2. Basu D, Gallus A, Hirsh J, Cade J: A prospective study of the value of monitoring heparin treatment with the activated partial thromboplastin time. N Engl J Med 287:325–327, 1972
3. Biggs R, Denson KWE: The fate of prothrombin and factors VIII, IX, and X transfused to patients deficient in these factors. Br J Haematol 11:532–547, 1963
4. Biggs R, Denson KWE: Standardization of the one-stage prothrombin time for the control of anticoagulant therapy. Br Med J 1:84–88, 1967
5. Bleyer WA, Hakami N, Shepard TH: The development of hemostasis in the human fetus and newborn infant. J Pediatr 79:838–853, 1971
6. Ellis BC, Stransky A: A quick and accurate method for the determination of fibrinogen in plasma. J Lab Clin Med 58:477–480, 1961

7. Hattersley P: Activated coagulation time of whole blood. JAMA 136:436–440, 1966

8. Hattersley PG: Heparin anticoagulation. In Koepke JA (ed): Laboratory Hematology. New York, Churchill Livingstone, 1984

9. Hill JD, Dontigny L, de Leval M, Mielke CH: A simple method of heparin management during prolonged extracorporeal circulation. Ann Thorac Surg 17:129–134, 1974

10. Jim RTS: A study of the plasma thrombin time. J Lab Clin Med 50:45–60, 1950

11. Kasper CK, Aledort LM, Counts RB et al: A more uniform measurement of factor VIII inhibitors. Thromb Diath Haemorrh 34:869–872, 1975

12. Kisiel W, Fujikawa K, Davie EW: Activation of bovine factor VII (proconvertin) by factor XIIa (activated Hageman factor). Biochemistry 16:4189–4193, 1979

13. Langdell RD, Wagner RH, Brinkhous KM: Effect of antihemophilic factor on one-stage clotting tests: A presumptive test for hemophilia and a simple one-stage antihemophilic factor assay procedure. J Lab Clin Med 41:637–641, 1953

14. Lee RI, White PD: A clinical study of the coagulation time of blood. Am J Med Sci 243:279–285, 1913

15. Lenahan JG, Phillips GE: Some variables which influence the activated partial thromboplastin time assay. Clin Chem 12:269–273, 1966

16. Lenahan JG, Smith K: Hemostasis, 17th ed. Parsipanny, NJ, Organon Teknika, 1985

17. Losowsky MS, Hall R, Goldie W: Congenital deficiency of fibrin stabilizing factor. Lancet ii:156–158, 1965

18. National Committee for Clinical Laboratory Standards NCCLS H28-P: Proposed guidelines for the one-stage prothrombin time test (PT). Villanova, PA, NCCLS, 1980

19. National Committee for Clinical Laboratory Standards NCCLS H30-P: Proposed guidelines for a standardized procedure for the determination of fibrinogen in biological samples. Villanova, PA, NCCLS, 1982

20. Quick AJ: The prothrombin in hemophilia and obstructive jaundice. J Biol Chem 109:LXXIII, 1935

21. Sienco Sonoclot Coagulation Analyzer Model DP-1546 Manual. Sienco, Inc. Morrison, CO 80465

22. Sugiura K, Ono IF, Watanabe K, Ando Y: Detection of hypercoagulability by the measurement of dynamic loss modulus of clotting blood. Thromb Res 27:161–166, 1982

23. Triplett DA: Laboratory Evaluation of Coagulation. Chicago, American Society of Clinical Pathologists, 1982

24. Triplett DA, Brandt JT, Kaczor D, Schaeffer J: Laboratory diagnosis of lupus inhibitors: A comparison of the tissue thromboplastin inhibition procedure with a new platelet neutralization procedure. Am J Clin Pathol 79:678–682, 1983

25. von Kaulla KN, Schultz RL: Comparative studies for evaluating fibrinolysis: Studies with two combined techniques. Am J Clin Pathol 29:104–109, 1985

26. Williams WJ, Beutler E, Erslev AJ, Lichtman MA: Hematology, 3rd ed. New York, McGraw-Hill, 1983

The Hemophilias **5**

Andrew E. Weiss

CASE STUDY* A 16-year-old black girl was evaluated for a possible bleeding disorder. She had had spontaneous nosebleeds since the age of 3 years. Her clinical history indicated easy bruising, iron therapy to treat anemia, mucosal bleeding, hematuria, and heavy menstrual periods. She sometimes had painful, swollen, and tender joints. She reported that her uncle had frequent, severe nosebleeds that required transfusion.

LABORATORY FINDINGS	PATIENT	NORMAL
Template bleeding time	13.5 min. (excessive blood)	2 – 8 min.
Prothrombin time (PT)	11.4 sec.	11.5 – 14 sec.
Activated partial thromboplastin time (APTT)	33 sec.	22 – 36 sec.
Platelets	339,000/μl	150,000 – 400,000/μl
Platelet function studies:		
Retention	40%	31% – 83%

* Case study from Corriveau DM: Chemical assessment of coagulation. In Bishop ML, Duben-Von Laufen JL, Fody EP: Clinical Chemistry: Principles, Procedures, Correlations, pp 519 – 520. Philadelphia, JB Lippincott, 1985

128

Aggregation curves

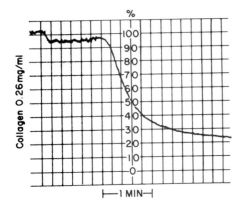

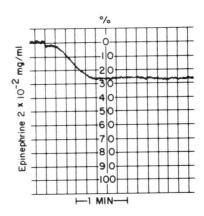

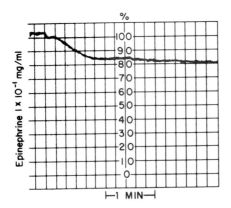

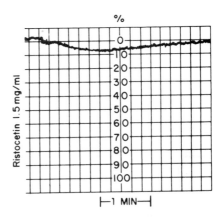

Factor VIII : C	80%	
Factor VIII – related antigen	40%	45%–185%
Plasma ristocetin von Willebrand factor (vWF)	23%	45%–140%

This is a classic case of von Willebrand disease (vWD) with a defective response of platelet aggregation to ristocetin. Decreased levels of Factor VIII – related antigen and vWF are seen. The prolonged bleeding time with excessive bleeding is a strong indicator of a vascular or platelet problem. vWD is an autosomal-dominant disorder with severe symptoms. Several variants of the disease have also been found to exhibit mild depression of Factor VIIIR:Ag.

The Factor VIII molecule is a large, multimeric structure composed of two distinct parts. Factor VIII : C is the procoagulant portion, and its synthesis is sex linked. Where it is produced has yet to be determined. The larger portion, which is autosomal in inheritance, consists of Factor VIII : Ag and

VIIIR:RCo, or vWF. The latter is produced by endothelial cells and megakaryocytes.

Factor VIII:C is normal in this case, but it can be decreased in some cases, usually ranging from 24% to 40%. The other portions of the Factor VIII molecule would not be decreased if a diagnosis of hemophilia were entertained. Only the procoagulant, Factor VIII:C portion of the molecule is defective in hemophilia A. When a hemophilia A patient is given cryoprecipitate, the Factor VIII:C level remains elevated 8 to 12 hours, whereas the vWF-infused patient will have a prolongation of 2 to 4 days.

Table 5-1
Nomenclature of the Hemophilias

| Deficient Factor | Hereditary Deficiency State | |
	Preferred Term	*Synonyms*
Factor I (fibrinogen)	Hereditary hypofibrinogenemia or afibrinogenemia	
Factor II (prothrombin)	Factor II deficiency	Hypoprothrombinemia
Factor V	Factor V deficiency	Parahemophilia Owren's disease
Factor VII	Factor VII deficiency	Hypoproconvertinemia Serum prothrombin conversion accelerator deficiency
Factor VIII	Hemophilia A	Classic hemophilia Factor VIII deficiency Antihemophilic factor deficiency
vWF	vWD	Vascular hemophilia Pseudohemophilia Angiohemophilia
Factor IX	Hemophilia B Factor IX deficiency	Christmas disease Plasma thromboplastin component deficiency
Factor X	Factor X deficiency	Stuart factor deficiency Stuart-Prower factor deficiency
Factor XI	Factor XI deficiency	Hemophilia C Plasma thromboplastin antecedent deficiency
Factor XII	Factor XII deficiency	Hageman factor deficiency Hageman trait
Factor XIII	Factor XIII deficiency	Fibrin stabilizing factor deficiency
Prekallikrein	Prekallikrein deficiency	Fletcher factor deficiency
High-molecular-weight kininogen	HMWK deficiency	Fitzgerald factor deficiency Flaujeac factor deficiency Fujiwara factor deficiency Williams factor deficiency

The hemophilias are a group of hereditary bleeding disorders caused by a deficiency in activity of one or another of the plasma "clotting factor" proteins necessary for normal blood coagulation. Table 5-1 shows the designated clotting factors and their corresponding hereditary deficiency states.

PATHOPHYSIOLOGY

The process of blood coagulation involves a series of biochemical reactions (Fig. 5-1), with each reaction requiring one or more of the plasma clotting factors and dependent on and using the product(s) of the preceding reaction. If any one of the clotting factors is deficient, the reaction that requires that factor cannot proceed at its normal rate, the initiation of subsequent reactions is delayed, and the time required for formation of a clot is greatly prolonged. Consequently, bleeding from injured blood vessels continues for a much longer time, and more blood is lost into the joint, muscle, or other site of injury.

The other hemostatic mechanisms of the hemophiliac are entirely normal, and the blood vessels are no more fragile or easily broken than vessels of normal people. The platelets are normal in number and function. This mechanism is usually adequate to produce hemostasis for small lacerations and puncture wounds. Exceptions to this general rule are seen in congenital afibrinogenemia (where the lack of fibrinogen impairs normal platelet aggregation) and vWD (where deficiency in Factor VIII complex results in impaired platelet adhesion to wound surfaces). Also, ingestion of platelet-inhibiting drugs by hemophiliacs add a second, acquired hemostatic defect that potentiates the bleeding tendency and complicates the diagnostic evaluation.

There are different degrees of clinical severity of the hemophilias, which generally correspond to the degree of clotting factor deficiency.[109] Except in vWD, however, all affected members of a family are affected to the same degree. *Severe* hemophilia is defined as 1% or less of normal activity of the clotting factor. Severely affected patients are constantly troubled by bruises, hematomas, hemarthroses, and other forms of bleeding from minimal, often unrecognized traumas. *Moderate* hemophilia is defined as 1% to 5% of normal clotting factor activity, with such patients suffering less frequent and less severe bleeding episodes. *Mild* hemophiliacs, with more than 5% of normal activity, generally have few bleeding problems, except with surgery, dental extractions, or major traumas. At that time, they may bleed as much as severe hemophiliacs. Clearly, even a small amount of clotting factor can provide a significant amount of hemostatic protection when present at the time of injury, just as a parked car can be prevented from rolling by a small wheel-chock that would be rolled over by a moving car. By the same token, just as it takes a roadblock to stop the moving car, much higher levels of clotting factor are necessary to control active bleeding.

The hemophilias are "low prevalence" disorders, but they are far from rare. A number of surveys conducted in the United States, in various European countries, and by the World Health Organization (WHO) have shown that approximately one in every 10,000 males has severe hemophilia A (due to deficiency in Factor VIII) or hemophilia B (due to deficiency in Factor IX), with hemophilia A occurring four to five times more frequently than hemophilia B.[109] Furthermore, the milder forms of hemophilia A and B have been shown to occur with equal or greater frequency than the severe form. Thus, about one in every 5,000 males, or 10,000 total population, has hemophilia A or B. These two disorders account for about 90% to 95% of all patients with hemophilias

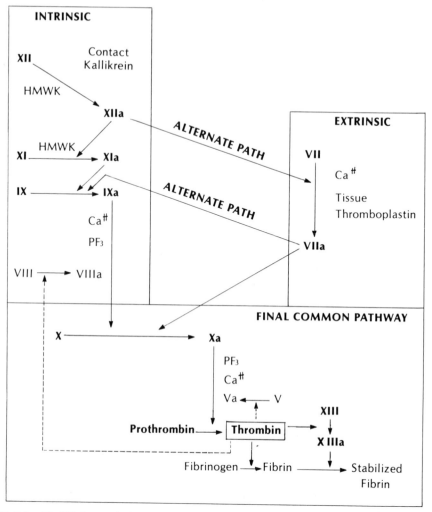

FIG. 5-1. Modified coagulation reaction cascade. *HMWK,* high-molecular-weight kininogen. (Courtesy of Donna M. Corriveau)

other than vWD. The autosomal-recessively inherited deficiencies in Factors I, II, V, VII, X, XI, and XIII are very rare, with individual prevalence estimates ranging from less than one to at most five to six per million population. Together they constitute only 5% to 10% of cases other than vWD. The prevalence of vWD is now recognized to be far greater than previously thought, with estimates ranging as high as one in 200 persons.[20,79]

PATHOGENESIS

Hemophilia A and B

Hemophilia A (Factor VIII deficiency) and hemophilia B (Factor IX deficiency) are inherited as X-linked recessive traits, occurring almost exclusively in males (Fig. 5-2). It is probable that a series of allelic genes exist for both hemophilia A and hemophilia B, with each allele determining a more or less severe degree of deficiency.[43] Since there are no opposing genes on the Y chromosome, the recessive hemophilia A and B traits are expressed in the male (XY).

Female (XX) carriers of hemophilia A or B are generally asymptomatic, being protected by the production of sufficient clotting factor by cells under the control of the X-chromosome bearing the normal factor VIII or IX gene. According to the Lyon hypothesis, only one of the two X chromosomes is active; however, extreme "lyonization" of the hemophilic and normal gene-bearing X chromosomes occasionally results in a "symptomatic carrier." Low clotting factor levels and bleeding symptoms similar to

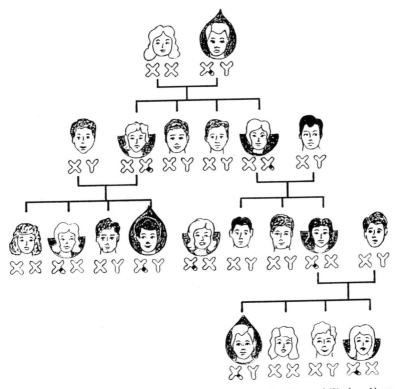

FIG. 5-2. Pattern of inheritance of X-linked recessive traits, such as hemophilia A and hemophilia B. The trait is transmitted by unaffected female carriers. Male offspring who receive the abnormal gene will have hemophilia; female offspring who receive the gene will be carriers. Hemophiliacs are indicated by a blood drop and carriers by a half blood drop.

those of a mild hemophiliac occur because of the inactive normal gene. True hemophilia A or B in a female is extremely rare but can result from (1) a union (often consanguineous) between a hemophiliac and a carrier, (2) a spontaneous hemophilic gene mutation on the normal gene-bearing X chromosome of a daughter of a hemophiliac or carrier, or (3) a chromosomal abnormality that allows hemizygous expression of the trait in a phenotypic female (XO).

Some 25% to 40% of newly diagnosed cases of hemophilia A and B have no known family history of the disease.[109] It is often inferred that these cases are the result of spontaneous gene mutations. The rate of spontaneous gene mutations in hemophilia is relatively high, being estimated at 1.3×10^{-5} for hemophilia A and 6×10^{-7} for hemophilia B.[56] Such mutations probably do account for a significant number of new cases each year. However, a large number of the apparently sporadic cases may be due to silent passage of the recessive gene through several generations of females or families becoming separated so that one branch of the family is unaware of the hemophiliacs in another branch.

For many years hemophilia A and B were considered to be due to quantitative deficiencies in the respective clotting factor proteins. But in 1956 Fantl and co-workers reported that the plasma of some hemophilia B patients contained a substance that could neutralize the human Factor IX inhibitor antibody to the same extent as normal plasma, while plasma from other patients did not.[34] They postulated that some hemophiliacs produce qualitatively abnormal molecules with reduced or absent clotting factor activity. Patients have either reduced or absent production of normal clotting factor protein or produce a molecule so abnormal that the antigenic sites are affected.

About 10% of hemophilia B patients have been shown to have this cross-reacting material (CRM).[84] These CRM+ dysfunctional variants have been subdivided further into those who have prolonged PTs when an ox brain thromboplastin is used (hemophilia^{BM}) and those with normal ox brain PTs (hemophilia B$_{Chapel Hill}$ and hemophilia B$_{Alabama}$).[25,28] Patients who are completely devoid of cross-reacting material (CRM−) or have reduced immunologically detectable protein in proportion to their reduced Factor IX activity levels (CRM^{R}) represent genetically deficient production of the protein. A fifth genetic variant (hemophilia B$_{Leyden}$), in which Factor IX levels tend to increase with age, has been described.[100] Inactive but immunologically detectable Factor VIII coagulant antigen (VIII:C Ag) has been found in about 10% of hemophilia A patients through the use of homologous human Factor VIII inhibitor antibody.[109] However, almost all of these CRM+ patients were mild or moderately affected, with measurable levels of Factor VIII activity. The absence of VIII:C Ag in the vast majority of severe hemophilia A patients has allowed for the use of a Factor VIII:C Ag immunoassay for prenatal detection of hemophilia A.[36]

von Willebrand Disease

vWD results from quantitative and qualitative deficiencies in a plasma protein that is necessary for the normal, rapid adhesion of platelets to exposed subendothelial collagen at sites of vascular injury. The protein (vWF protein) also serves as a carrier protein, stabilizing the clotting Factor VIII. Consequently, deficiencies in this vWF protein result in a mixture of clinical and laboratory findings reflecting impaired platelet function, impaired coagulation, or both.

vWF is a large-molecular-weight multimeric glycoprotein synthesized in platelets and vascular endothelial cells.[52,77] Circulating vWF consists of a series of multimers ranging in size from approximately M_r 800,000 to greater than M_r 12×10^6. The hemostatic efficacy of the vWF multimers is directly proportional to their size, the largest multimers being more effective in binding platelets to subendothelium and the smallest multimers being least effective.[112]

vWD is not a single disease but a heterogeneous group of quantitative and qualitative disorders that result in decreased levels of vWF in the plasma. Several subtypes have been recognized.[112] In *type I* vWD there is a quantitative deficiency in all multimeric sizes of vWF, both in plasma and in the cells of origin (megakaryocytes and endothelial cells). This defect produces a reduced capacity to synthesize the basic vWF subunits. In *types IIA and IIB* there is absence of large and intermediate-sized multimers, although the plasma levels of small vWF multimers are normal or increased. In type IIA the larger multimers are also absent from platelets, indicating defective ability to form the larger multimers from normally produced subunits. In type IIB the larger multimers are present in and released from platelets and endothelial cells but disappear rapidly from the plasma. This is possibly due to a qualitative abnormality that causes increased avidity for binding to tissue sites. In the rare, severe *type III* disease there is virtual absence of all sizes of multimers from both plasma and cells of origin, indicating almost complete inability to synthesize vWF subunits. Another condition, called pseudo-vWD, has been described in a few patients. In this condition the platelets have increased avidity for binding vWF, resulting in the rapid removal of vWF from the plasma.

vWF synthesis is controlled by genes on chromosome 5 (Fig. 5-3). All types of vWD are inherited as autosomal traits.[112] Types I, IIA, and IIB, the most common forms of vWD, are inherited as dominant traits transmitted by either parent (Fig. 5-4). The rare, severe type III is inherited from both parents and may represent either a homozygous recessive inheritance of a distinct severe defect or a more severe expression of the dominant types I, IIA, and/or IIB in a homozygous or doubly heterozygous inheritance of two dominant genes.

Other Hemophilias

Hereditary Afibrinogenemia and Hypofibrinogenemia

Hereditary afibrinogenemia and hypofibrinogenemia, rare quantitative deficiencies in fibrinogen, are transmitted in an autosomal-recessive manner, affecting both males and females. Afibrinogenemic patients have no demonstrable fibrinogen by either functional or immunologic methods, while hypofibrinogenemic patients have comparably reduced levels of immunologically detectable and clottable fibrinogen. It is likely that afibrinogenemia represents the homozygous-recessive state, in which no fibrinogen is synthesized, while hypofibrinogenemic persons are heterozygous for the trait, synthesizing only about half the normal amount of fibrinogen.[72]

Dysfibrinogenemia

More than 85 different inherited qualitative abnormalities of the fibrinogen molecule have been reported, each being named for the city in which it was identified. However, fewer than half of these cause a hemorrhagic tendency.[72] All appear to be inherited as autosomal-dominant traits, with both males and females affected. The functional defect may result from amino acid substitutions that (1) impair cleavage of fibrinopeptides by thrombin (22 variants), (2) impair polymerization of fibrin monomers (41 variants), or (3) impair stabilization of the fibrin polymer (6 variants).[72]

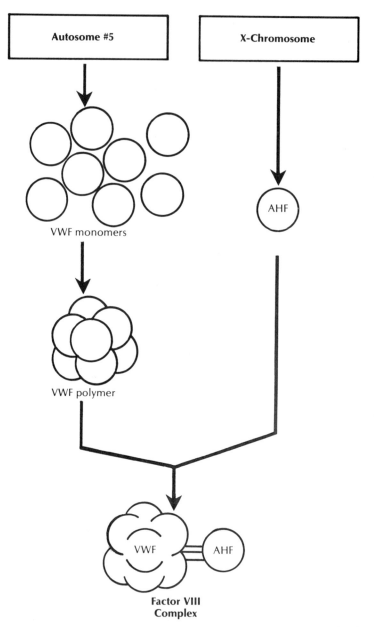

FIG. 5-3. The vWF molecular complex is synthesized in endothelial cells and platelets under the direction of genes location on autosome 5. The Factor VIII clotting factor molecule is synthesized under the direction of genes on the X chromosome and becomes bound to the vWF to form the Factor VIII complex. A genetic defect in vWF synthesis results in von Willebrand disease; a genetic defect in Factor VIII clotting factor synthesis results in hemophilia A.

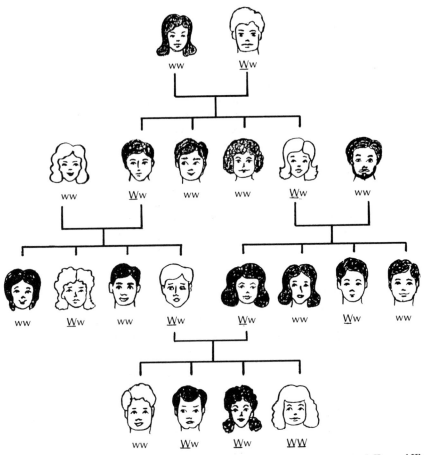

FIG. 5-4. Pattern of inheritance of autosomal-dominant disorders such as types I, IIa, and IIb von Willebrand disease. Both males and females are affected, and the trait is transmitted directly from one generation to the next. The dominant von Willebrand disease gene is shown as a <u>W</u>, while the recessive normal gene is shown as a w.

Congenital Hypoprothrombinemia

Hereditary deficiency in Factor II is probably the rarest of the hemophilias. It is inherited as an autosomal-recessive trait, affecting both males and females. In true congenital hypoprothrombinemia the amount of immunologically detectable Factor II protein is reduced in proportion to the Factor II activity level (CRM$^-$ or CRM^R), but *dysprothrombinemias*, with normal or disproportionately higher immunologically detectable Factor II protein, have been described.[71]

Factor V Deficiency

Also known as "parahemophilia," hereditary Factor V deficiency is inherited as an autosomal-recessive trait and affects both males and females. Mild, moderate, and severe degrees of deficiency are seen in homozygous-recessive patients. Heterozygous carriers tend to have reduced Factor V levels in the range of 50% to 60% of normal activity. Dysfunctional protein variants have not been described.

Factor VII Deficiency

Factor VII deficiency is inherited as an autosomal-recessive trait, affecting both males and females. Homozygous-recessive patients may have mild, moderate, or severe deficiencies in Factor VII activity, and heterozygotes tend to have about half-normal levels. Both "hypo-" (reduced/absent production; CRM⁻ or CRMᴿ) and "dys-" (dysfunctional protein; CRM⁺) forms have been described.

Factor X Deficiency

Hereditary Factor X deficiency is transmitted as an autosomal-recessive trait, affecting both males and females. Homozygous-recessive patients may have mild, moderate, or severe deficiencies. Heterozygotes tend to have about half-normal levels. Both hypo- and dys- forms have been described. It is interesting that of the two index cases of "Stuart-Prower factor" deficiency, Mr. Stuart was shown to have a true absence of synthesis of Factor X protein, while Miss Prower was found to have a nonfunctional variant.[31]

Factor XI Deficiency

Also known as hemophilia C, hereditary Factor XI deficiency is rare in the general population but relatively common among people of Jewish descent. It has been estimated that the prevalence among Ashkenazi Jews may be as high as 3%.[88] The disorder is inherited as an autosomal-recessive trait, and both males and females are affected. The vast majority of homozygous-recessive patients have mild to moderate deficiencies and bleeding tendencies, but severely affected patients are rare. All patients who have been studied have shown proportionately decreased levels of the Factor XI protein and activity. No dysfunctional variants have been described.

Factor XIII Deficiency

Hereditary Factor XIII deficiency is inherited as an autosomal-recessive trait, affecting both males and females. Since plasma Factor XIII levels of 1% to 2% or more are adequate for fibrin stabilization, only those homozygous-recessive patients with severe deficiencies have clinical bleeding tendencies.[62] Factor XIII deficiency is detected with the clot solubility test. Patients with milder deficiencies (and heterozygous carriers with half-normal levels) can be detected with quantitative Factor XIII assays, but these cases usually go undetected. Thus, the overall frequency of Factor XIII deficiencies is unknown. The active site for Factor XIII activity resides on subunit a of the two-subunit molecule. All patients who have been studied with antibodies specific for the a and b subunits have shown absence of the *subunit a* protein, while *subunit b* protein levels may be normal, reduced, or absent.[70] No cases with dysfunctional a subunits have been described.

Deficiencies in Contact Factors

Initiation of clotting via the intrinsic pathway involves the interaction of Factor XII (Hageman factor), prekallikrein (Fletcher factor), and high-molecular-weight kininogen (HMWK; Fitzgerald, Flaujeac, Fujiwara, or Williams factor). Hereditary deficiencies in each of these factors have been described. Deficiency states appear to be inherited as autosomal-recessive traits, although autosomal-dominant transmission of

Factor XII deficiency has been reported.[14] Homozygous-recessive patients may have mild, moderate, or severe deficiencies, although most reported patients have had severe deficiencies. All of the patients with HMWK deficiency and most of the patients with deficiencies in Factor XII or prekallikrein have had no immunologically detectable protein. This represents absent or decreased factor synthesis. Dysfunctional variants of Factor XII and prekallikrein have been described. Prekallikrein and HMWK circulate as a complex. Some patients with HMWK deficiency also have a deficiency of prekallikrein. A deficiency in any one of these factors causes prolongation of the partial thromboplastin time (PTT) and other tests of intrinsic pathway clotting. *None of these contact factor deficiency states results in a clinical bleeding tendency.* The interaction of these three factors also involves the activation of the fibrinolytic system. Thus, thromboembolic tendencies have been described in both Factor XII and prekallikrein-deficient patients.

Combined Factor Deficiencies

Although acquired coagulation factor deficiency states often involve deficiencies in two or more factors, *hereditary deficiencies are almost always single-factor deficiencies.* Nevertheless, a number of familial combined factor deficiencies have been described, including Factor VIII deficiency plus a deficiency in Factors V, VII, IX, X, and XI, or XII; Factor IX deficiency plus a deficiency in Factors XI or XII; deficiencies in both Factors XII and XIII; and various combinations of deficiencies in Factors II, VII, IX, and X.[94] Factor VIII deficiency has also been described in combination with a hereditary dysfibrinogen (fibrinogen$_{St. Louis}$).

Many of these combined deficiency states have been found in only one or two families. Often the individual deficiency states could be demonstrated in other family members, suggesting a chance mating of persons carrying the genes for both diseases. This is particularly likely with combinations involving Factor VIII, where the Factor VIII deficiency may stem from the very highly prevalent, autosomal-dominant, vWD. In other cases, however, the combined deficiencies tend to be transmitted together as autosomal-dominant traits distinct from the X-linked or autosomal-recessive patterns associated with the individual factor deficiency states. The most common is the combined deficiency of Factors V and VIII. It has been suggested that many of these cases result from uncontrolled enzymatic degradation of these factors by activated protein C, due to an autosomal-dominantly inherited deficiency in protein C inhibitor.[74] Familial combined deficiencies in Factors II, VII, IX, and X appear to be due to production of dysfunctional proteins, which may be the common product of a single hereditary defect (*e.g.*, in an enzyme involved in the metabolism of vitamin K or the γ-carboxylation of glutamic acid residues necessary for the normal binding of these factors onto phospholipid surfaces in the clotting reactions).

CLINICAL MANIFESTATIONS

Hemophilia A and B

Hemophilia A and hemophilia B are inherited as X-linked recessive traits that exhibit the mild, moderate, or severe degrees of factor deficiency. Clinically, they are indistinguishable. The clinical problems of hemophilia A and B are related to bleeding and to the residual and consequential effects of bleeding. The first indication that a bleeding disorder is present may be bleeding after circumcision or from the umbilical cord, although these signs need not be present. Otherwise, there may be few if any symptoms during the first 6 to 9 months of life.[12] Severe hemophilia A was diagnosed in infants who presented at the age of 6 weeks with small "fingerprint" bruises on their backs and chests where parents had gripped them in lifting and playing with them. However, once the infant began to crawl, bruises, hematomas, and other bleeding episodes were common.

The term *spontaneous bleeding* is often used when a patient cannot recall a specific antecedent trauma. Such bleeding is not truly spontaneous, since the clotting factor deficiency causes prolonged bleeding from an injured blood vessel. Therefore, some trauma—unrecognized or unremembered—must have occurred to cause the vascular injury.

In the milder forms of hemophilia there may be no symptoms, and the bleeding disorder may go unsuspected for years, until excessive or prolonged bleeding is encountered after a surgical or dental procedure or major trauma. Adenoid-tonsillectomy and dental extractions seem to be particularly stressful hemostatic challenges; even the mildest hemophiliacs usually experience abnormal bleeding with these procedures.

A common misconception is that the hemophiliac will bleed profusely, perhaps to death, from a small cut. Actually, patients with hemophilia A and B usually do not have serious bleeding from minor lacerations and puncture wounds, since platelet hemostasis is usually adequate to control bleeding from such injuries. Similarly, platelet hemostasis is sufficient to control bleeding from mucous membranes. Nosebleeds can be controlled quickly by proper local measures, and significant gingival bleeding is uncommon. Hematuria is a frequent clinical manifestation in hemophiliacs. It results from rupture of glomerular capillaries during straining in heavy lifting, pushing, or pulling. Transfusion therapy is used to control hematuria, although urologic investigation is not usually indicated. Gastrointestinal bleeding, on the other hand, rarely if ever occurs without underlying gastrointestinal lesions. The cause should always be investigated thoroughly, the problem determined, and treatment begun.

Small, superficial bruises and other minor soft tissue hemorrhages are quite common, but of little consequence. These are usually self-limited and resolve spontaneously. The most serious problems in hemophiliacs stem from internal hemorrhages into joints, muscles, and deep soft tissues. Bleeding into the soft tissues of the neck, the lower part of the face, the tongue, or the floor of the mouth constitutes an emergency situation because the hematomas may enlarge and spread very rapidly through these loose tissues. Airway compression and asphyxiation can occur within a matter of hours.

Hemorrhages into large muscles such as the buttocks, thigh, calf, or forearm result in considerable blood loss with formation of hematomas and compression of underlying nerves and blood vessels. Untreated hemorrhages into the forearm can cause permanent damage to nerves supplying the hand. Permanent nerve injuries with footdrop result from hemorrhages in the calf. Bleeding into the iliopsoas muscle and retroperitoneal soft tissues may be particularly serious. This large, relatively unrestricted area can accommodate large quantities of blood, and the expanding retroperitoneal hematoma may compress emerging spinal nerve roots, resulting in sensory and motor denervation of the lower extremity. The symptoms of a retroperitoneal hemorrhage are quite pleomorphic. It may present as pain in the abdomen, back, flank, hip, or groin or as a nerve compression syndrome. It may be so severe as to mimic a ruptured intervertebral disc or acute surgical abdomen. Numerous emergency appendectomies, exploratory laparotomies, and myelograms have been performed on patients with unrecognized retroperitoneal hemorrhages. Another hemorrhagic problem mimicking an acute abdomen in the hemophiliac is intestinal intramural hematoma.

The major cause of death in hemophilia is intracranial hemorrhage.[33] Lasting neurologic impairment results from intracranial hemorrhages that are not diagnosed and treated in the early stages. These result from trauma to the head or, perhaps more often, from shaking injuries to the brain. There is no correlation between severity of the head trauma and the occurrence of an intracranial hemorrhage in hemophiliacs. Hemorrhages often result from trivial injuries. In about half of all cases there is no history of a preceding head trauma. Even when there is a known head injury, only half of the patients develop symptoms within the first 24 hours. In the remaining cases there may be a lag period between trauma and symptoms ranging from 2 days to as long as 6 weeks.[33] For these reasons, all head injuries should be treated, no matter how trivial, even if a few days have lapsed. All symptoms compatible with an intracranial hemorrhage should be treated as such until proven otherwise.

The most frequent problem and major cause of disability in severe hemophilia A and B is bleeding into joints. The large weight-bearing joints are the most frequently affected, with hemarthroses of the knees accounting for about half of all joint hemorrhages and ankle and elbow hemarthroses for about 20% each.[108] The shoulders, wrists, and hips are affected even less. Hemarthroses are not common during the first year of life but occur with increasing frequency once the child begins to walk.[12] The majority of severely affected hemophiliacs suffer 20 to 30 hemarthroses per year, although there is great variation among patients, with some experiencing only two to three joint hemorrhages per year and others suffering 50 or more.

An acute hemarthrosis causes swelling, pain, inability to move or bear weight on a joint, and absence from school or work. Depending on the type and degree of injury, the symptoms of an untreated hemarthrosis vary from mild to moderate, with pain, stiffness, slight swelling, and limitation of motion to an excruciatingly painful, tensely swollen joint that cannot be moved or bear weight. Mild symptoms resolve within days, while moderate symptoms may persist for several weeks. Regardless of the severity of symptoms, however, the presence of blood in the joint induces an acute inflammatory reaction. The resultant thickened, hypervascular synovium makes the joint particularly vulnerable to reinjury until the inflammation has resolved.[108] Moreover, the proteolytic enzymes released from platelets and phagocytic cells during the inflammatory reaction cause further damage to the joint tissues.

The first few hemorrhages into a joint may appear to resolve without significant damage. But, with repeated hemarthroses, the processes of injury, inflammation, and healing lead to progressive joint damage and, eventually, crippling deformities. Early changes are characterized by hemosiderosis, hypertrophy, and hyperplasia of the synovial membrane. With further hemorrhages and inflammation, the synovium and joint capsule become fibrotic. With continuing degeneration there is erosion of the articular cartilage and changes in the subchondral bone.[108] During this process there is progressive loss of range of motion in the affected joints, with secondary wasting of muscles that move joints, particularly the extensor muscles. Flexion contractures result from maintenance of the joint in a flexed position to minimize pain during an acute hemarthrosis, and from the decreased ability of the wasted muscles to extend the joint. The contracted joint is subject to abnormal stresses; therefore, it is more vulnerable to trauma, creating a vicious cycle of repeated hemarthroses and increasing joint damage. Such crippling hemarthropathy is not an inevitable consequence of hemarthroses in hemophiliacs. Prompt, aggressive transfusion therapy of every hemarthrosis can reduce the amount of bleeding and inflammation, thereby reducing the amount of joint damage and crippling deformities.

Hemophiliacs and their families also suffer many indirect emotional, social, and economic effects from the disorder. Hemophilia is typical of most chronic diseases in that these secondary problems may greatly influence the course of the disease.

Hemophilia has a great emotional impact on the functioning of a family.[4] Parental guilt feelings and fears that even normal activities may result in injury lead to extreme overprotectiveness, as seen in the case study in Chapter 1. Similar fears and tendencies toward overprotection may also extend to teachers, physicians, and others charged with the care of the child who do not understand the true nature of the disease. Antagonism may develop between the parents or toward others, with each antagonist criticizing the other's methods of caring for the child and blaming the other for the child's injuries.

The hemophilic child suffers not only the direct emotional traumas of pain and separation from family and friends but also the additional impact of excessive restriction of activities at home, play, or school. A hemophiliac has the same needs for social contact and interaction as any other child, yet excessive restriction from participation and competition with other children fosters feelings of difference and inferiority. The child may react to these emotional stresses in a variety of ways, ranging from complete withdrawal and fearful passivity, to denial of his condition with rebellion against the restriction and varying degrees of the "daredevil reaction" (excessively competitive and aggressive participation in activities with high risk of injury). Adolescent and adult hemophiliacs often hesitate to assume responsibilities, because an unpredictable injury might prevent the fulfillment of commitments or cause embarrassment over breaking a social engagement. Many hemophiliacs conceal their disorder to gain acceptance from peers and avoid rejection by social contacts and potential employers.

Hemophiliacs often experience great difficulty in finding appropriate employment. The hemophiliac requires a vocation that emphasizes intellectual abilities and skills rather than physical labor. However, a completely sedentary occupation tends to promote muscle wasting, the development of joint contractures, and frequent hemorrhages. In our technological society, opportunities for professional, "white collar," clerical, and other suitable jobs are closely linked to education and training. Frequent absences from school, progressively increasing educational deficits, and discouragement often lead to premature termination of the educational process. A national survey found that one third of adult hemophiliacs had not completed high school, and one fourth had only a grade school education.[60] Consequently, although most hemophiliacs are able to find employment, they are often employed in jobs ill-suited to their disease. This contributes to further hemorrhages, greater disability, and absenteeism that may cost them their jobs. Also, employers who have little knowledge and understanding of the hemophilias may fear placing hemophiliacs in positions of responsibility; therefore, employment levels and incomes are often well below those of nonhemophiliacs with equivalent education and training.

Compounding the problem, families of hemophiliacs suffer many economic problems. Treatment is expensive, ranging from $6,000 to more than $15,000 per year (the cost of the factor concentrates to treat acute bleeding episodes).[93] Thus, another vicious cycle is formed. With a more severe bleeding tendency, more episodes require treatment, and more expenses are incurred. Moreover, those with limited education and training, who are unemployed or underemployed, have even less financial resources, and less reimbursement from health insurance is received.

von Willebrand Disease

The clinical manifestations of vWD differ in many respects from those of hemophilia A and B. In patients with hemophilia A or B the clotting factor levels remain constant from one time to another (unless raised by a transfusion), while in patients with vWD the levels vary widely from one time to the next.[3,13] There may be long symptom-free periods interspersed with periods of frequent bleeding symptoms. Also, the hemophilias tend to be characterized by bleeding into soft tissues, while the bleeding manifestations of vWD usually involve the skin and mucous membranes, reflecting the impaired platelet function more than the deficiency in Factor VIII coagulant activity.[112]

The common, dominant forms of vWD (types I, IIA, and IIB) result in mild to moderate bleeding tendencies that are clinically indistinguishable. The frequency and severity of bleeding symptoms are extremely variable, both from one patient to another and from one time to another in the same patient. In a study of 56 affected persons in two large vWD families, one third of the children, one third of the adult males, and half of the adult females had significant bleeding symptoms.[76] Sons or daughters of symptomatic parents often had symptomatic children, yet the parents had no bleeding symptoms.

Bruising, excessive and prolonged bleeding from cuts, epistaxis, gum bleeding, and excessive and prolonged menstrual bleeding are common problems. Hematuria, gastrointestinal bleeding, and hematomas in muscles and deep soft tissues occur less often, while hemarthroses are unusual. Symptoms may disappear entirely during pregnancy, but severe postpartum hemorrhaging may occur. There is usually excessive and prolonged bleeding after severe traumas or surgeries (especially dental extractions, tonsillectomies, and gynecologic surgeries), which may be life-threatening. This is not always true; many patients have undergone one surgical procedure without bleeding yet hemorrhaged profusely with a later procedure.

Patients with severe type III disease suffer frequent and severe bleeding episodes. Common bleeding manifestations include epistaxis, gingival bleeding, hematuria, gastrointestinal bleeding, large ecchymoses, deep hematomas, profuse bleeding from lacerations, and memorrhagia in affected women. Recurrent hemarthroses may lead to crippling joint deformities similar to those in hemophilia A or B.

Other Hemophilias

The autosomal-recessively inherited factor deficiencies exhibit bleeding problems similar to those of hemophilia A and B. The frequency and severity of bleeding episodes generally correlate with the degree of factor deficiency. The types of bleeding problems that occur reflect the impairment of the coagulation process, with primarily soft tissue bleeding. Bleeding from the umbilical stump or circumcision wound are common in affected newborns. Intracranial hemorrhage may also occur. Ecchymoses, intramuscular and soft tissue hematomas, and epistaxis are common problems in older children and adults. Hemarthroses may occur in severely affected patients. Menorrhagia is a serious problem in affected females. Gingival bleeding, hematuria, gastrointestinal bleeding, and bleeding from cuts occur less often. Serious bleeding may complicate surgical procedures, dental extractions, and the postpartum period. A unique symptom of Factor XIII deficiency is a tendency toward poor wound healing and excessive scar formation that is seen in 25% of patients.[70]

Inhibitors

The development of a circulating inhibitor is a serious complication of hemophilia. These inhibitors are highly specific antibodies that inactivate the corresponding clotting factor. Although inhibitors are seen most often in hemophilia A and B, they have also been reported in patients with vWD, congenital afibrinogenemia, and hereditary deficiencies of Factors II, V, VII, X, XI, and XIII.[90]

The inhibitors of Factor VIII and Factor IX are IgG immunoglobulins that are highly specific for their respective target factors. Immunoneutralization techniques have shown great homogeneity of the inhibitor antibody species within a hemophilic patient. Most have had only a single light-chain type (usually κ, although some have contained a mixture of κ and λ light chains), and many have had only a single heavy chain (often IgG4).[104] However, studies using isoelectric focusing have shown much greater heterogeneity of the immunoglobulin populations, both in structure and Factor VIII–neutralizing capacity.[53]

The inactivation of Factor VIII by inhibitor antibodies is time and temperature dependent. Factor VIII inhibitors in hemophilia A patients almost always show "type I" reaction kinetics, in which there is a rapid, progressive loss of Factor VIII activity over 2 to 4 hours, with complete inactivation when there is antibody excess.[15,16] It has been suggested that the type I antibody recognizes an antigenic site(s) on the Factor VIII molecule, located very close to the Factor VIII activity site. The binding of the inhibitor antibody blocks activation of Factor VIII or inhibits its interaction with activated Factor IX in the coagulation reaction sequence.[39] The inactivation of Factor IX by its inhibitor occurs almost instantaneously.[85]

Two types of Factor VIII inhibitors can be distinguished on the basis of their immunologic response to reexposure to the antigen (i.e., Factor VIII).[8] In the classic type there is an anamnestic rise in antibody titer after infusion of even trace amounts of Factor VIII. Patients with this type of inhibitor are referred to as "high responders." Other patients, however, show little or no rise in titer after Factor VIII infusions and are referred to as "low responders." The consistently very low antibody titers of low responders can be overcome by high doses of Factor VIII, allowing for more effective treatment of acute bleeding episodes. This also increases the chance that the inhibitor may go undetected both clinically and with in vitro screening tests.

High-responder inhibitors develop in about 10% ± 5% of severe hemophilia A and B patients.[104] The incidence of the more-difficult-to-detect low responders is unknown but may be equal to or greater than that of the high-responder type. Inhibitors develop almost exclusively in severely affected patients, although a few cases of inhibitors in moderately affected patients have been reported.[104] Inhibitors tend to appear at an early age, but Strauss showed that the correlation is not precisely to age but rather to transfusion exposure.[96] Fifteen of 17 patients in Strauss's study, and 11 of 12 in Weiss's series, developed their inhibitors after more than 20 but less than 100 "exposure days" (i.e., a day on which one or more infusions of Factor VIII–containing blood products were administered). This suggests that patients who are prone to develop inhibitors will do so after a critical amount of antigenic stimulation.

The very first reports of inhibitors in hemophiliacs suggested that the inhibitor was an antibody that developed in response to transfusion of a protein foreign to the patient's immune system.[30] There is little question that exposure to the normal factor protein plays a role in the development of an inhibitor. With one questionable exception, all hemophiliacs who have developed inhibitors have had infusions of normal factor–containing blood products prior to the appearance of the antibody.[104] However, as Strauss recognized, the majority of hemophiliacs receive equal or greater exposures yet do not develop inhibitors.[96] This suggests that some hemophiliacs may have an immunologic predisposition that permits development of an inhibitor antibody after exposure to the factor antigen, while other hemophiliacs lack the immunologic susceptibility and thus will not develop inhibitors no matter how much Factor VIII they receive. The occurrence of inhibitors in several, but not all, hemophiliacs within a family supports the concept of an inherited immunologic predisposition.[37,104] Also, breeding studies in dogs with hemophilia A have indicated that the capacity to develop an inhibitor is transmitted separately and independently from the hemophilia gene.[40]

DETECTION AND DIAGNOSIS

A careful, complete history is of major importance in the detection of hemophilia. In severely affected patients, recurrent bleeding episodes usually make the condition apparent within the first few years of life. However, the condition often goes undetected in mildly affected patients, since there may be few or no bleeding symptoms unless the patient is subjected to a significant hemostatic challenge such as surgery, dental extraction, or major trauma. This is not only a most unfortunate way to detect a bleeding disorder, but under such circumstances laboratory diagnosis may be complicated by emergency blood transfusions. Presurgical screening of all patients with a platelet count, Ivy or template bleeding time, PT, and APTT is advocated. Over the years, some 10% of the hemophiliac patients at one midwestern hemophilia center have been detected and diagnosed as a result of such presurgical/predental screening. Unfortunately, nearly twice as many of the patients suffered significant postoperative, postextraction, or postpartum bleeding prior to recognition of their bleeding disorder.

Detection and diagnosis of hemophilia in the newborn poses special problems. Collection of a "clean" sample of venous blood with an appropriate plasma:citrate ratio is essential for coagulation tests. In the neonate it can be particularly difficult to obtain because of small, hard-to-find veins, poor blood return, and a physiologically high hematocrit. Cord blood samples are usually contaminated by thromboplastic substances from the cord matrix, which leads to partial activation and false-shortening of coagulation screening tests.

Also, the PT and APTT are often prolonged in the newborn because of physiologically low levels of Factors II, VII, IX, and X. These factor levels are only half the normal level in full-term infants and lower in prematures. The normal, adult levels are not reached until 6 to 12 months of age.[18,89,113] Severe hemophilia B and all degrees of hemophilia A can be diagnosed by factor assays on very carefully obtained samples. Screening tests may fail to detect congenital bleeding disorders in the newborn because interpretation of slightly low Factor IX levels may be quite difficult when mild hemophilia B is suspected. For these reasons, and because of the difficulty in obtaining a clean venous blood sample in newborns and small infants, it is best to defer circumcision in infants of known or possible carriers until 6 to 9 months of age before testing.

In older children and adults a few simple clotting tests can effectively screen the coagulation process. The whole blood clotting time, however, has long been recognized as an extremely poor test for clotting factor deficiencies.[32] It is poorly reproducible, nonspecific (being prolonged by thrombocytopenia and platelet dysfunctions as well as clotting factor deficiencies), and very insensitive (giving normal results with Factor VIII or IX levels as low as 4% to 5% of normal).[32]

The PT measures clotting by the extrinsic coagulation pathway (see Fig. 5-2) and will be prolonged by deficiencies in Factors VII, X, and V, prothrombin, and fibrinogen. The PTT screens the intrinsic coagulation pathway (see Fig. 5-2). Whether performed by the original method or accelerated by the addition of kaolin, ellagic acid, Celite, or other inert earth metals, the PTT/APTT will be prolonged by deficiencies in the intrinsic factors (Factors XII, XI, IX, or VIII) or deficiencies of the common path (Factors X or V, prothrombin, or fibrinogen).

The sensitivity of PT and APTT tests varies with the reagent used. Several studies have shown that the various commercial APTT reagents differ greatly in their ranges of normal results, slopes of factor dilution curves, sensitivity to various factors, and so forth.[11,91,106] Most APTT reagents are standardized against dilution curves of Factor VIII, and recognizably prolonged results are obtained with Factor VIII levels of 25% to 30% or less. Sensitivity to other factors is less consistent, with some reagents not giving recognizably prolonged results until Factor IX, X, or XII levels are as low as 15%.[106]

Because of slight variations in reagent concentration and test system variations in normal plasma, control results vary between days and within days. The slope of factor dilution curves, however, remains constant from day to day in spite of fluctuations (Fig. 5-5).[106] Therefore, maximum sensitivity and specificity of PT and APTT test results requires interpretation in terms of a concurrently tested normal control. Interpretation of APTT results using an inflexible normal range might give false "abnormal" or false "normal" results.

Used together, the PT and APTT can help to pinpoint clotting factor deficiencies. A prolonged APTT and normal PT suggest a deficiency in one of the factors of the intrinsic pathway (prekallikrein, HMWK, or Factor XII, XI, IX, or VIII), while a prolonged PT and a normal APTT suggest a deficiency in Factor VII, the one factor unique to the extrinsic pathway. Prolongation of both tests suggests a deficiency in one of the common pathway factors (X, V, prothrombin, or fibrinogen). This scheme of differentiation holds true when the PT, the APTT, or both are markedly prolonged, as in a severe deficiency. However, depending on the reagents used, one or the other test system may be more or less sensitive to the factors in the common pathway. A mild deficiency of one of these factors may be manifest as a slight prolongation in the more sensitive test but not in the other. It must also be emphasized that such a scheme of differentiating factor deficiencies is valid only for hereditary single-factor deficiencies. Acquired clotting factor deficiencies almost always involve multiple factors and both coagulation pathways.

Further qualitative differentiation of single factor deficiencies is accomplished with substitution tests. This is best done by mixing the patient plasma with a plasma specifically deficient in a single clotting factor. Failure of the patient's plasma to correct the clotting time of the mixture indicates that it too is deficient in that factor. Correction of the clotting time is evidence against a deficiency in that factor. An older system of substitution testing employs aged normal serum (deficient in Factors V and VIII, prothrombin, and fibrinogen) and adsorbed normal plasma (deficient in Factors VII, IX, and X and prothrombin). Although such tests were useful in the early days of coagulation studies, they are of no value when multiple deficiencies are present, since these usually involve deficiencies in both "consumable" and "adsorbable" factors, and neither reagent will correct the clotting time of the test plasma. They are also of little help, and can be misleading, with mild single factor deficiencies when the patient's APTT is prolonged 10 to 20 seconds. Partial correction is then difficult to interpret. Neither type

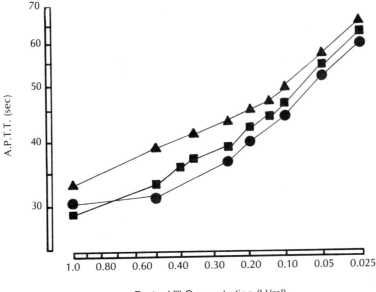

FIG. 5-5. Variations in PT and APTT reagent systems result in variations in normal control values between and even within days. When daily factor dilution curves are performed, a series of parallel curves emanating from the 100% normal control value are found. Maximum sensitivity to clotting factor deficiencies requires interpretation in terms of the concurrent normal control.

of substitution test can be used when inhibitor antibodies are present, since the antibody will inactivate the corresponding clotting factor.

LABORATORY FINDINGS

The patterns of coagulation screening test results seen with each type of hemophilia are shown in Table 5-2. Definitive diagnosis requires specific clotting factor assays. This is necessary for quantitation of the degree of the factor deficiency. Sometimes it is the only means of detecting milder deficiencies. Assay results are expressed as a percentage of normal activity or as units per milliliter, where 1 unit is defined as the amount of factor activity present in 1 ml of average normal human plasma and is equivalent to 100% of normal activity.

Factor assay methods vary widely from one coagulation center to another. While most centers have excellent reproducibility with their assays in house, there is great variability among centers in the assay values on identical test samples. A recent collaborative study showed that the concentration of the factor in the reference standard to which a test sample is compared is a critical variable.[67] Most commercial normal plasma controls are intended for use only as controls for PT and APTT tests and are prepared so as to give consistently normal clotting times in these tests without regard to the concentrations of individual factors. Unless a control plasma has been preassayed and certified to contain a stated factor concentration, it cannot be assumed to contain

Table 5-2
Coagulation Screening Test Results in the Hemophilias

Screening Test	I	II	V	VII	VIII	vWF	IX	X	XI	Contact Factors	XIII
Platelet count	N	N	N	N	N	N	N	N	N	N	N
Bleeding time	N	N	N	N	N	N-↑	N	N	N	N	N
Prothrombin consumption test	N		↓		↓	↓	↓		↓	↓	N
Whole blood clotting time	N-↑	N-↑	N-↑	N	N-↑	N-↑	N-↑	N-↑	N-↑	N-↑	N
PT	N-↑	↑	↑	↑	N	N	N	↑	N	N	N
APTT	N-↑	↑	↑	N	↑	N-↑	↑	↑	↑	↑	N
Thrombin time	↑-N	N	N	N	N	N	N	N	N	N	N
Clot solubility	N	N	N	N	N	N	N	N	N	N	↑

N, normal; ↑, increased; ↓, decreased

100% of normal activity, or even close to it. Marked differences in Factor VIII have been found among commercial control plasmas. Lot-to-lot variation arises within products, with some containing as little as 50% and others more than 200% Factor VIII activity. In-house pools of normal plasma may also vary widely from one pool to another, particularly in their concentrations of Factors V and VIII, vWF, and fibrinogen. All are acute-phase reactants that are increased in response to many stimuli. The optimal Factor VIII normal control is a preassayed standard that has been standardized against the WHO factor standard. Between-laboratory variation affects the ability of a laboratory to diagnose vWD or carriers of hemophilia A or B. In-house reproducibility is essential for the management of hemophilic patients undergoing surgery or procedures requiring therapy and careful monitoring of factor levels.

DETECTION AND DIAGNOSIS OF VON WILLEBRAND DISEASE

vWD can be one of the most challenging, often frustrating, diagnoses to establish. Despite the high prevalence of the disease, bleeding symptoms are usually so mild and variable that only a small percentage of vWD patients are referred for evaluation. Furthermore, there are no simple, sensitive laboratory tests capable of detecting more than a small fraction of affected persons. Detection and diagnosis require a high index of suspicion by physicians, application of a full battery of tests, and very careful interpretation of results in concert with the genetic and clinical histories (Table 5-3). Even then, it is often necessary to repeat the battery of tests on one or more occasions to document sufficient abnormal results to establish the diagnosis.

The only direct test for vWD is correction of the bleeding time by infusion of platelet-free, vWF-rich plasma products (i.e., cryoprecipitate).[112] Some authors consider demonstration of the typical "delayed rise" in Factor VIII clotting activity after infusion (see below) to be equally diagnostic.[80] This procedure is both cumbersome and

Table 5-3
Laboratory Expression of Hemophilia A and von Willebrand Disease

	Hemophilia A	von Willebrand Disease		
		Type I	*Type IIA*	*Type IIB*
VIII:C	↓	N–↓	N–↓	N–↓
VIIIR:Ag	Normal	N–↓	N–↓	N–↓
VIII:RCoF	Normal	N–↓↓	N–↓	N–↓
Ristocetin-induced PRP aggregation	Normal	N–↓	N–↓	N–↓
Bleeding time	Normal	N–↑	N–↑	N–↑
Analysis of FVIII/vWF structure	Normal	Normal	Loss of high- and intermediate-molecular-weight multimeric forms	Loss of highest-molecular-weight multimeric forms
Therapy	Cryoprecipitate or Factor VIII concentrate	Cryoprecipitate or DDAVP	Cryoprecipitate	Cryoprecipitate

N, normal; ↑, increased; ↓, decreased; *PRP*, platelet-rich plasma

expensive, involving serial Factor VIII assays before and at intervals after infusion. The infusion also carries the risk of transmission of hepatitis or acquired immune deficiency syndrome (AIDS). It is generally agreed that infusions for purely diagnostic purposes are not warranted, although, when there are therapeutic indications for an infusion, the opportunity should be seized to document correction of the bleeding time or delayed rise in Factor VIII activity.

Indirect tests for vWD involve assessment of the several properties of the Factor VIII complex. Von Willebrand's original description of the disorder was that of an autosomal-dominantly inherited bleeding disorder with a prolonged Ivy bleeding time.[101] Later the association of reduced Factor VIII clotting activity was recognized.[78] Until the early 1970s, these two tests were the sole criteria for the diagnosis. However, by that time it was already recognized that bleeding time and Factor VIII levels varied greatly from one time to another, and independent of each other, so that on any given day either or both could be normal or abnormal.[13] If both were normal on the day of testing, the diagnosis could be missed. If low Factor VIII activity were the only abnormality, a misdiagnosis of mild hemophilia A or hemophilia A carrier might be made. If only the bleeding time were abnormal, a platelet dysfunction might be suspected. Then, two new tests were added to the diagnostic armamentarium. Zimmerman and colleagues showed that patients with vWD had reduced levels of Factor VIII–related protein, which tended to be proportional to or lower than the Factor VIII activity level.[111] At the same time, Howard and Firkin reported that aggregation of human platelets by ristocetin required a plasma cofactor that was deficient in patients with vWD.[51]

Each of these four tests (Ivy bleeding time, Factor VIII activity assay, Factor VIII–related antigen immunoassay, and ristocetin cofactor activity) suffers from problems of insensitivity, nonspecificity, and irreproducibility, as well as from the variability inherent in the disorder itself. Bleeding times are abnormal in the hereditary and acquired platelet disorders and vascular purpuras. Factor VIII activity is reduced in hemophilia A, Protein C inhibitor deficiency, and disseminated intravascular coagulation. The level is stimulated to normal or increased levels in patients with vWD during pregnancy, estrogen therapy, acute inflammation, adrenaline responses, and so forth. Ristocetin-induced aggregation is decreased or absent in Bernard-Soulier syndrome and may be normal or increased in type IIB vWD. Factor VIII–related antigen may be quantitatively normal, despite a significant deficiency in the hemostatically effective large multimers, due to high concentrations of small multimers.

Most frustrating of all, however, is the peculiar variability of the disease itself in patients with heterozygous dominant types I and II. The laboratory findings, like the bleeding tendency, vary from one patient to another and from one time to another in the same patient. A study of 56 proven vWD patients from two large families found that at a single testing, 26% had prolonged bleeding times, 48% had low Factor VIII activity, 52% had low Factor VIII–related antigen, and 71% had low ristocetin cofactor activity.[76] Furthermore, 12% of patients showed all four tests abnormal, 23% showed three or more abnormal results, and 40% showed two or more abnormal tests, while in 17% all four tests were normal. These findings were supplemented by those of Abildgaard and colleagues,[3] who performed serial tests on 50 patients from 25 families. Every possible combination of results was seen, and some patients showed five to six different combinations of results during the course of the study. Thirty percent showed normal results for all tests on at least one occasion, and 18% never showed more than one abnormal result on any single test day.

The implications of these studies are sobering, particularly in view of the high prevalence of the syndrome. Half to two thirds of affected persons may have clinically inapparent disease activity under everyday conditions, yet have the potential for serious bleeding from trauma or surgery. There is no single, simple test for detection and diagnosis of vWD. As a single screening test the bleeding time could be expected to give false-negative (i.e., normal) results in 50% to 75% of patients. Even when a battery of four tests is used, on any given day, 15% to 20% of affected persons might show all-normal results, making it virtually impossible to state that a patient does not have vWD on the basis of a single battery of tests. Only when all-normal results are found repeatedly can the possibility of vWD be excluded.

The diagnosis of severe, type III vWD is less complicated. Since these patients consistently have very low levels of vWF, the bleeding time is almost always greatly prolonged, there is essentially no ristocetin cofactor activity, and both Factor VIII activity and Factor VIII–related antigen are severely deficient, usually to the level of 5% ± 4%.

DETECTION AND QUANTITATION OF INHIBITORS

Screening tests for detection of inhibitors are based on the failure of normal plasma to correct the clotting time of a test plasma. The APTT is used in screening tests for inhibitors of factors of the intrinsic pathway, and the PT is used for detection of inhibitors against factors of the extrinsic pathway. Since inhibitors in hemophiliacs are directed against the specific clotting factor in which the patient is already deficient, and since this inhibition does not affect other factors, the results of routine coagulation screening tests are no different from those of a patient with the same deficiency but no inhibitor. The presence of an inhibitor can be detected only by mixing tests. The addition of normal plasma to Factor VIII (or IX)–deficient plasma should shorten the APTT, but if an inhibitor is present, it will inactivate the Factor VIII (or IX) of the normal plasma so that its corrective effect on the APTT will be reduced. The extent to which the Factor VIII (or IX) of the normal plasma is inactivated, and therefore the degree to which the corrective effect is reduced, is a function of the antibody titer and kinetics and the conditions of the test system.

The reaction between Factor VIII and its inhibitor is progressive. In type I inhibitors, there is a log-linear relationship between the amount of Factor VIII remaining after a given period of incubation and the initial concentration of both Factor VIII and antibody.[104] When an inhibitor is present in high concentration, a significant portion of the Factor VIII in the normal plasma can be rapidly inactivated. The mixing test may be prolonged even without incubation. When the antibody titer is low, enough Factor VIII activity may be present in the early stages of the reaction to correct an unincubated APTT. Without sufficient incubation, low levels of inhibitor may not be detected.[86] Consequently, mixing tests for detection of Factor VIII inhibitors should be incubated for 1 to 2 hours at 37°C. The inhibitor–Factor IX reaction, on the other hand, is immediate, and mixing tests for detection of Factor IX inhibitors can be performed without incubation.[85]

The sensitivity of inhibitor screening tests also depends on the "normality" of the normal plasma used in the mixture and the sensitivity of the APTT or PT reagent systems used to test for residual factor activity. As mentioned before, APTT and PT reagents may vary greatly in their sensitivity to deficiencies in different clotting factors. If a reagent system gives significant, recognizable prolongations at factor concentrations of 25% of normal activity or less, then inhibitor concentrations that inactivate half or more of the factor in a starting mixture with 50% factor activity could be detected. However, if the reagent system does not give recognizable prolongations until a factor level is reduced to 12% or less, the same inhibitors would not be detected unless present in a concentration that would inactivate three fourths of the factor in a 50% starting mixture. Since the relationship between residual Factor VIII activity and initial inhibitor concentration is log-linear, this would represent a twofold difference in sensitivity to inhibitor.

For the same reason, the concentration of factor in the starting mixture is a critical variable. If a pooled normal plasma contains exactly 100% Factor VIII, a one-plus-one mixture of normal and patient plasma will contain 50% of the factor prior to any inhibitor effect. However, if the normal plasma contains 75% or 150% Factor VIII, the equal-parts mixtures would contain 38% or 75%, respectively. A reagent system sensitive to 25% factor levels detects inhibitor concentrations that inactivate as little as one third of the factor and up to two thirds of the factor. Thus, to ensure maximal sensitivity of inhibitor screening tests, both the sensitivity of the reagent system to the factor under study and the concentration of the factor in the normal plasma must be controlled, either through pretest selection or by varying the ratio of normal to patient plasma in the starting mixture.

The concentration of inhibitor may be quantitated by titers or assays. The inhibitor titer may be determined by incubating mixtures of normal plasma plus serially diluted test plasma and determining the APTT or residual Factor VIII or IX concentration of each mixture. The titer may be interpreted as the highest dilution at which the APTT is still significantly prolonged or as the transition from antibody excess to antigen excess (*i.e.*, the lowest dilution at which residual Factor VIII or IX activity is found).[83,85,86]

Inhibitor assays are based on quantitation of residual factor activity after incubation with a test plasma dilution. The antigen/factor is in slight excess, so there is a log-linear relationship between residual factor activity and initial inhibitor concentration. The standard unit of measurement of inhibitor concentration is the Bethesda unit.[59] One Bethesda unit is the amount of inhibitor that will inactivate 50% of the Factor VIII in a mixture of equal parts of normal plasma (1 U/ml) and inhibitor plasma or dilution during incubation for 2 hours at 37°C.

The standard procedure for inhibitor assay involves the incubation of a mixture of equal parts of test plasma (or diluted test plasma) and normal plasma (containing 100% of the factor to be assayed) for 2 hours at 37°C.[59] The residual factor is then tested with a one-stage (APTT) factor assay. A control mixture of equal parts of the normal plasma and imidazole buffer is also incubated and the residual factor activity assayed. To correct for nonspecific loss of factor activity during incubation, the residual/factor concentration of the test sample is divided by that of the control, with the result expressed as a percentage of the control value. A standard curve is constructed such that 50% of the control value equates to 1 unit of inhibitor and 25% of the control value to 2 units of inhibitor. The inhibitor concentration of the test sample is read directly from the standard curve.

DETECTION OF CARRIERS OF THE HEMOPHILIAS

In autosomal-dominantly inherited types of vWD there is no true "silent carrier" state, since the disease is manifest in heterozygotes. However, as discussed previously, most affected persons have few or very mild symptoms. It is quite common for an asymptomatic person to escape recognition until a diagnosis of vWD in another member of the family leads to studies of the whole family.

True silent carrier states are seen with the recessively inherited hemophilias. In the autosomal-recessively inherited deficiency states (hypofibrinogenemia, hypoprothrombinemia, and Factor V, VII, X, XI, or XIII deficiency), only homozygous-recessive persons who have received a recessive gene from *each* parent are affected. One or both parents could be homozygous (*i.e.*, have the disease), and a spontaneous mutation in a gene from a noncarrier parent is possible, but most often both are silent-carrier heterozygotes. Silent carriers can often be detected by their approximately half-normal levels of the factor.[106] It must be recognized, however, that laboratory imprecisions, variations in gene expression and stimulation of factor synthesis by acute-phase reactions, and so forth may result in the finding of a normal level of the factor on some occasions. Therefore, great care must be taken, both before testing and in interpretation of the results, to avoid serious misunderstandings and emotional disruption in the family.

The most common types of hemophilia, hemophilia A and hemophilia B, are both inherited as X-linked recessive disorders (see Fig. 5-3). The recessive gene is carried on the X chromosome and is the only gene present for expression in males (XY). All of the daughters of a hemophilia A or B patient must receive their father's X chromosome and therefore be "obligatory carriers." A carrier female contributes either her normal or her hemophilia gene – bearing X chromosome to each offspring, regardless of sex. There is a 50/50 chance that each son will have hemophilia and a 50/50 chance that each daughter will be a carrier. Because these genes have relatively high mutation rates, the mother of a single hemophilic son cannot be assumed to be a carrier if there are no other affected relatives. If she bears a second hemophilic son, however, a carrier state is certain. Thus, carrier testing for genetic counseling is not necessary in the obligate carrier daughter of a hemophiliac or in mothers who have more than one hemophilic son or one hemophilic son plus other affected relatives. When a carrier state cannot be established on purely genetic grounds, "carrier testing" is indicated.

Carriers of hemophilia A or B tend to have approximately half-normal levels of Factor VIII or IX activity.[43,99] This is in keeping with the Lyon hypothesis that only one X chromosome is functioning in each cell of a female, while the other is nonfunctioning.[69] Random chance would be expected to place about half of the Factor VIII– or IX – producing cells of a hemophilia A or B carrier under control of the hemophilic gene – bearing X chromosome and half under control of the normal gene – bearing X chromosome, resulting in half-normal factor levels. In some carriers, however, the chance distribution of normal and hemophilic gene – bearing X chromosomes might be 60:40, 25:75, and so forth, and, in fact, the levels of Factor VIII or IX found in carriers describe a distribution curve centered at 50% of normal activity.[99] Since the Factor VIII and IX activity levels of noncarrier women also describe a distribution curve, centered at about 100% and with the lower limit of normal reaching as low as 50%, there is substantial overlap between the ranges of carrier and noncarrier women. Thus, when a Factor VIII or IX activity level of 50% or less is found in a potential carrier, a carrier state can be assumed. But, a carrier state cannot be excluded when higher levels are found, even levels over 100%.

The cells capable of producing normal Factor VIII are subject to stimulation by estrogens, by epinephrine, and by acute-phase reactions. Serial testing of obligate carriers has shown predictable cyclic variations in Factor VIII levels in the same patient during the menstrual cycle, with levels peaking at 100% and falling to 25% at the nadir of estrogen effect. Similarly, two potential carriers tested elsewhere had been told that they were not carriers. When taken off oral contraceptives and at the end of their menstrual cycles, these women were found to have levels below 50%. Both had been taking oral contraceptives at the time of the first testing. Factor IX production is less affected by these variables, but extremes of lyonization still result in a wide range of Factor IX levels in carriers of hemophilia B.

Maximum capacity to detect hemophilia A carriers is obtained with concurrent testing and comparison of Factor VIII activity and Factor VIII – related antigen.[46,63,69] Studies of known carriers have shown Factor VIIIR:Ag levels similar to those of noncarrier women, but Factor VIII activity levels averaging only about half the VIIIR:Ag.[46,69,111] When the ratio of Factor VIII activity to VIIIR:Ag is used, some 90% of carriers can be detected, even when their levels of Factor VIII activity are high.[63] The sensitivity and specificity of this method depend on the methods used for quantitation of the two variables and, particularly, on the statistical methods used to relate the ratio to the probability of carriership. In general, the lower the probability assigned per ratio value, the lower the sensitivity to detecting carriers and the higher the specificity in distinguishing noncarriers.

MANAGEMENT OF THE HEMOPHILIAS

Coordinated Comprehensive Care

The total management of the hemophilic patient requires attention to all of his orthopaedic, dental, emotional, social, educational, vocational, and financial problems, as well as the treatment of acute bleeding episodes. Such care is beyond the knowledge, skills, and available time of any single physician. A coordinated comprehensive approach is required, with a multidisciplinary team of specialists in each of these areas working together to correct existing problems, prevent others, and provide each patient the maximum opportunity for a normal, productive life. In such team management, close communication and coordination of activities are essential. All too often the involvement of multiple specialists without close coordination and communication has resulted in fragmentation of care, with patients being shuffled from one specialist to another. True comprehensive hemophilia care requires all of the participating specialists to function as a coordinated team, each member knowing what every other member is doing, so that each specialist's treatment *complements* rather than *complicates* the treatments by the others.

Treatment of Bleeding Episodes

The treatment of bleeding in hemophilia depends on replacement of the missing clotting factor by infusion of appropriate factor concentrates or plasma. The clotting reactions can then proceed normally to form a clot and control the bleeding. Rational replacement therapy requires an accurate diagnosis of the type and degree of clotting factor deficiency, knowledge of the biochemical characteristics of the deficient factor, and knowledge of availability and potency of factors in various concentrates and plasma products (Table 5-4).

Therapeutic Agents

Fresh-frozen plasma was introduced in 1950 as a means of replacing the missing clotting factors, and it remained the primary agent for treatment of hemophilia for nearly two decades. The effectiveness of plasma transfusions, however, is limited by the large volumes needed to raise clotting factor levels even slightly. Fresh-frozen plasma contains approximately 250 units of each clotting factor in a volume of 300 ml. The maximum volume that can be infused at one time without causing circulatory overload, approximately 15 ml per kilogram of body weight, raises clotting factor levels by only about 25% to 30% activity. Such levels are not adequate to control severe hemorrhages or to provide hemostasis for surgery. Even hemarthroses or other moderately severe hemorrhages may not be controlled by these levels, necessitating additional plasma transfusions and/or hospital admission for sustained therapy.

Effective treatment became a reality with the development of highly purified clotting factor concentrates. With these concentrates, factor levels of 100% or more can be attained so that even the most severe bleeding episodes can be controlled, and major surgery can be performed without excessive bleeding. As shown in Table 5-4, concentrates are available for fibrinogen, vWF, and Factors II, VII, VIII, IX, and X. No concentrated forms of Factors V, XI, or XIII are available. Cryoprecipitate is prepared from single units of plasma and is rich in fibrinogen, Factor VIII activity, and vWF. The exact content of each factor varies from bag to bag, depending on donor levels and a variable

Table 5-4
Factors Provided by the Coagulation Factor Concentrates

Concentrate	Factor(s) Provided
Cryoprecipitate	Factor VIII vWF Fibrinogen
Antihemophilic factor (AHF) concentrates	Factor VIII
Prothrombin complex concentrates	Factor IX Factor VII Factor X Prothrombin
No concentrate available	Factor V Factor XI Factor XIII

amount of loss during preparation. On the average, each bag contains about 100 to 120 units of Factor VIII activity and about 200 mg of fibrinogen. The vWF content is generally assumed to be proportionate to the Factor VIII activity. Highly purified lyophilized concentrates of Factor VIII are available from several manufacturers. These are concentrated about 30 times greater than plasma, with about 25 units of Factor VIII activity per milliliter of reconstituted volume. These concentrates are preassayed, and the Factor VIII content of each vial is indicated on the label. Factor VIII concentrates produced by monoclonal antibody capture or genetic engineering will soon be available. These concentrates will be free of risk of blood-transmissible diseases. Concentrates of Factor IX are available as *prothrombin-complex concentrates (PCCs)*, which also contain Factors II, VII, and X. Usually only the Factor IX content is indicated on the label, but the Factor II, VII, and X content can be obtained from the manufacturer. In general, Factors II and X are present in amounts similar to that of Factor IX, but the Factor VII content may be much lower.

Administration and Dosage

Plasma and concentrates must be given intravenously. The amount given depends on the patient's plasma volume, the plasma concentration of the factor before infusion, and the concentration desired after infusion. Dosage calculations are based on the definition of a "unit" of factor activity: *1 unit is the amount present in 1 ml of average normal plasma* and is synonymous with 100% of normal activity. The desired level after infusion (in units/ml), less the preinfusion factor level (in units/ml), equals the "desired rise" in units/ml. The desired rise (in units/ml) multiplied by the patient's plasma volume (in milliliters) equals the number of units that must be given to achieve the desired rise.

$$\text{Units to be given} = \text{desired rise (U/ml)} \times \text{plasma volume (ml)}$$

The patient's plasma volume can be estimated from his weight and hematocrit. The blood volume is usually about 65 ml/kg body weight for adults and about 75 ml/kg for children. Thus, the plasma volume can be calculated by multiplying the blood volume by the plasmacrit $(1 - HCT)$. When the hematocrit is in the normal range, the plasma volume may be estimated directly as 4% (adults) or 5% (children) of the body weight in grams or, more simply, 40 ml to 50 ml/kg. Another rule of thumb that can be used in a patient with a normal hematocrit is that 1 unit of Factor VIII/kg will give a 2% rise in Factor VIII concentration (1 U in 50 ml/kg = 0.02 U/ml/kg).[2] With Factor IX, however, 1 U/kg results in only about 1% rise in Factor IX activity.[57]

The clotting factor levels necessary to control various bleeding episodes depend on several variables: (1) the type and severity of injury, (2) the location of the hemorrhage, and (3) the time the bleeding has been in process. When bleeding is just from a minor injury, low factor levels may be able to control it; mild to moderately severe hemophiliacs suffer far fewer bleeding episodes requiring treatment than do severe hemophiliacs. However, once the hemorrhage is under way, much higher levels are needed to control it. The presence of swelling in a joint indicates that the bleeding is either progressing very rapidly or has been in process for some time. In either event, higher levels will be required than if treatment had been given earlier in the course of the bleeding. Hemorrhages into critical areas, such as the neck, retroperitoneal soft tissue, or central nervous system, require sustained high levels for several to many days.

In general, the doses recommended by various authors have been derived empirically over years of treating hemophiliacs. Some advocate low doses, in the range of 10 U/kg, for the early treatment of joint hemorrhages,[10,24,82] while others recommend doses of 20 U to 25 U/kg.[7] In a study of some 500 promptly treated joint hemorrhages, Weiss found that doses of 8 U to 11 U/kg were successful in controlling the hemarthrosis 90% of the time, while 10% required additional infusions or absence from school or work.[107] This was in agreement with other reports.[10,24,81] However, 30% of the patients who were successfully treated with these doses had rebleeding in the same joint within 10 days. Treatment with doses of 15 U to 18 U/kg reduced the failure rate to 4% and the rebleeding rate to 13%. This was in agreement with the reported results of treatment with doses of 20 U to 25 U/kg.[7] Treatment with doses of 11 U to 15 U/kg gave intermediate results. Thus, there is a dose–efficacy relationship in which prompt treatment with low doses successfully controls the bleeding in 90% of cases but apparently does not allow sufficient healing to prevent rebleeding if normal activities are resumed. Higher doses not only successfully control a higher percentage of hemorrhages but also allow for better healing and less frequent rebleeding. The doses routinely used at one midwestern hemophilia center and cooperating hemophilia emergency treatment centers are shown in Table 5-5.

Prompt Aggressive Treatment

The availability of concentrates led to recognition of two important concepts of modern hemophilia care: that most bleeding episodes can be treated on an outpatient basis and that the sooner the factor infusions are given, the better the outcome. During the era of plasma therapy, the limited effectiveness of single outpatient infusions and the incon-

Table 5-5
Therapeutic Levels and Doses for Treatment of Bleeding Episodes

Type of Hemorrhage	Desired Level (%)	Doses (U/kg)	
		FVIII	*FIX*
Hemarthrosis			
Early treatment; no swelling	30	15	30
Rapidly evolving or delayed treatment; swelling present	50	25	50
Muscle or soft tissue hematoma			
Mild, but impairing joint movement	30	15	30
Extensive, with vascular or nerve compression	50–100*	25–50	50–100
Bleeding into neck, lower part of face, tongue, or floor of mouth	50–100*	25–50	50–100
Retroperitoneal, proven or suspected	50–100*	25–50	50–100
Lacerations requiring sutures	30	15	30
Intracranial hemorrhage (proven or suspected), all head injuries, and tumbling/shaking injuries	100*	50	100

* Sustained therapy indicated

venience of treatment in the hospital emergency room led many patients to delay seeking treatment for many hours or even days in the hope that the bleeding would cease without treatment. This "wait and see" attitude resulted in the development of crippling joint deformities.

The greater effectiveness, rapidity, and convenience of administration of concentrates has greatly changed these attitudes and consequences. Hemophilia centers throughout the world began to train parents, wives, friends, or the patients themselves to prepare and administer concentrate infusions at home. In this way an infusion can be completed within 30 to 45 minutes after the very first suspicion of bleeding. Moreover, the concentrates and infusion supplies can be taken to work, on family outings, on vacations, and on business trips. Prompt, aggressive treatment is always immediately available.

Together, prompt, aggressive treatment of bleeding episodes and coordinated comprehensive hemophilia care have reduced absenteeism from school or work by more than 70%. Hospitalization for treatment of bleeding is down by 85% to 90%, and the costs of hemophilia care have been reduced by about half.[65,93,105] Most importantly, the prompt, aggressive treatment of joint hemorrhages is reducing the development of joint damage so that today's hemophilic children have far less need for joint replacements and physical rehabilitation.[6,23]

Sustained Therapy

Treatment of serious life- or limb-threatening acute hemorrhages or chronic hemorrhagic synovitis, prophylactic hemostatic management during surgical procedures, and vigorous physical rehabilitation programs require sustained therapy to maintain appropriate hemostatic levels for many days or weeks. Hemostatic levels can be maintained for prolonged periods by either repeated "booster" injections at regular intervals or a continuous infusion of clotting factor. When intermittent injections are used, an initial "loading" dose is given to raise the factor concentration to twice the minimum level desired, and "booster" doses equal to half the loading dose are given at intervals determined by the rate of disappearance of the factor from the plasma.

Most clotting factors behave as "two-compartment drugs," with biphasic exponential disappearance curves (Fig. 5-6). The rapid-phase disappearance represents the combined effects of equilibration between the intravascular and extravascular fluid compartments plus the biologic degradation or alteration of the molecule. The more gradual, second-phase disappearance represents only the rate of metabolism of the molecule after equilibrium has been reached. Numerous studies of Factor VIII disappearance after infusions of plasma, Cohn fraction I, cryoprecipitate, intermediate- and high-potency concentrates, and animal Factor VIII concentrates to hemophilia A patients have shown a first-phase half-disappearance time ($T_{1/2}$) of 5 to 7 hours and a second-phase half-disappearance time of about 12 hours.[17,106,110] In hemophilia B, infused Factor IX has a more rapid first-phase disappearance ($T_{1/2} = 1.5-4$ hours) but a

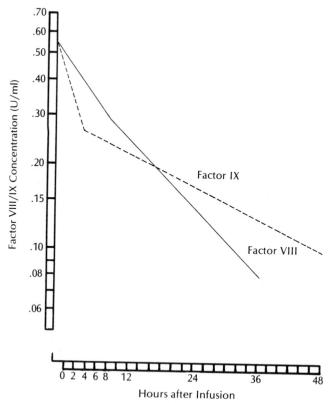

FIG. 5-6. Disappearance of coagulation factor activity from the plasma after an infusion follows a two-compartment model. An early rapid fall-off represents the combined effects of equilibration with extravascular fluids and of molecular decay. The slower second-phase disappearance represents true molecular decay.

much slower second-phase disappearance ($T_{1/2}$ = 24 hours).[17,21,57] As shown in Figure 5-6, the net result is that 12 hours after an infusion of either Factor VIII or Factor IX, the level has fallen to about 40% of that achieved immediately after the infusion.

First and second booster injections should be given to hemophilia A patients at 6-hour intervals, to allow for saturation of the extravascular compartment. Then, 12-hour-interval doses are continued to maintain levels above the desired minimum at all times. We also administer booster infusions to hemophilia B patients at 12-hour intervals during the 4 to 5 days necessary to saturate the extravascular compartment, and then change to 24-hour-interval booster doses.[106]

A desired Factor VIII or IX level can be maintained by a continuous infusion of concentrate.[75] Although the kinetics of a two-compartment system are beyond the scope of this chapter, the amount that must be infused per unit of time is equal to the amount eliminated from the plasma in that time. Based on a series of 18 Factor VIII disappearance studies with multiple samples in each phase,[110] the elimination constant for Factor VIII has been calculated to be 0.068/hr.[106,110] Therefore, the amount of Factor VIII that must be infused per hour (at a constant rate) may be calculated as

$$U/hr = 0.068/hr \times plasma\ volume\ (ml) \times desired\ level\ (U/ml)$$

Usable data on the kinetics of Factor IX are limited and show wide variation. However, based on one disappearance curve, Hermens calculated an elimination constant of 0.048/hr for Factor IX.[48]

Other Hemophilias

In *congenital hypofibrinogenemia* the critical minimum level seems to be about 100 mg/dl, and a loading dose of fibrinogen to achieve a 200 mg/dl level would be

$$Milligrams\ of\ fibrinogen\ to\ be\ infused = desired\ rise\ (mg/dl) \times plasma\ volume\ (dl)$$

Since the plasma volume is approximately 50 ml/kg in children and 40 ml/kg in adults, the plasma volume can be estimated at 1 dl/2 kg in children and 1 dl/2.5 kg in adults. The number of bags of cryoprecipitate required to provide this dose is calculated as

$$Bags = fibrinogen\ to\ be\ infused\ (mg)\ divided\ by\ 200\ mg\ to\ 250\ mg/bag$$

Fibrinogen has a long half-life of 3 to 5 days,[98] and booster infusions would be needed approximately every 3 to 5 days. Because of the several variables involved, it is recommended that fibrinogen levels be monitored immediately after infusion and daily thereafter. Booster infusions should be given when the level falls to 100 mg/dl.

Congenital deficiencies in Factors II, VII, and X can be replaced with PCCs (prothrombin-complex concentrates). Except for single-infusion, low-level treatment for mild to moderate acute bleeding episodes, in which plasma infusions may suffice, PCC is the only product capable of achieving and maintaining high levels of Factor VII. Plasma can be used to raise Factors II and X to high levels by the stepwise manner described below for Factors V and XI and can be used for booster infusions to maintain levels attained with either PCC or plasma. Factor II and Factor X have very long half-lives of 60 to 80 hours and 40 hours, respectively. High levels can be sustained with booster doses at 24- to 48-hour intervals.[17] Factor VII, however, disappears very rapidly after infusion, with a $T_{1/2}$ of 3 to 4 hours.[17] Consequently, high levels can be attained only with a high-potency concentrate, and booster doses must be given at 4-hour intervals.

No concentrated preparations of *Factor V* or *Factor XI* are currently available. The only product for replacement therapy for these disorders is fresh-frozen plasma. The volume limitations of plasma prevent attainment of high levels with a single infusion. However, both Factor V and Factor XI have relatively long half-lives of about 36 hours.[103,106] High levels can be achieved through stepwise elevations with repeated plasma infusions at 12-hour intervals over several days preoperatively.[106] Because of the variable content of Factors V and XI per bag, the preinfusion and postinfusion levels should be assayed with each plasma infusion. The patient must also be monitored closely for fluid overload because of the progressively rising oncotic pressure of the accumulating total protein load. Restriction of nonplasma fluids and diuretic therapy may be needed.

Factor XIII deficiency can be replaced by infusion of cryoprecipitate or plasma. Plasma Factor XIII levels of 10% of normal activity appear to provide adequate hemostasis.[70] A loading dose to achieve a 20% level can be accomplished by a single infusion of either 15 ml/kg of plasma or one bag of cryoprecipitate per 6 kg ± 2 kg. The half-life of Factor XIII is very long, with estimates ranging from 7 to 14 days, so that booster infusions would be needed only weekly. Furthermore, since levels above 2% appear to prevent a serious bleeding tendency, administration of one bag of cryoprecipitate per 3 kg to 5 kg at monthly intervals provides prophylaxis for severely deficient patients.[62]

TREATMENT OF BLEEDING IN VON WILLEBRAND DISEASE

Bruises, bleeding from cuts, and nosebleeds are often amenable to direct local measures. Excessive or prolonged menstrual bleeding in women with vWD can often be ameliorated by cyclic therapy with combination estrogen–progesterone oral contraceptive agents.[106] This not only helps to control the menstrual cycle but also stimulates increased synthesis and/or release of Factor VIII and vWF. More serious bleeding requires replacement of the missing Factor VIII complex by infusion of appropriate plasma products.

The product of choice for replacement therapy in all types of vWD is cryoprecipitate. Cryoprecipitate contains 40% to 60% of the Factor VIII activity and vWF, including almost all of the most active large multimers, from the original plasma concentrated into 5% to 10% of the original volume. This allows infusion of the multiple units necessary to raise the Factor VIII complex to high levels. Cryoprecipitate or plasma from hemophilia A patients is also effective in shortening the bleeding time, even though it has no Factor VIII clotting activity.[29] The highly purified lyophilized Factor VIII concentrates, however, do not contain the large and intermediate vWF multimers and, therefore, have little effect on the bleeding time.[112]

Infusion of sufficient amounts of vWF quickly shortens the bleeding time.[29,106] It appears that vWF levels of about 20% to 30% are adequate for rapid platelet plug formation and a normal bleeding time. As the vWF concentration falls below the 20% to 30% hemostatic level, the bleeding time becomes progressively prolonged.[44] vWF disappears relatively rapidly after infusion, with a half-disappearance time of Factor VIII–related antigen and ristocetin cofactor activity in the range of 6 to 8 hours.[26,61]

The response of Factor VIII clotting activity after infusion is quite different from that of the other Factor VIII complex properties and from the Factor VIII clotting activity response in patients with hemophilia A. Infusion of cryoprecipitate into a patient with hemophilia A results in an immediate and predictable dose-related rise in Factor VIII

activity followed by the biphasic disappearance described above. Infusion of cryoprecipitate to a patient with vWD, however, results in a rise in Factor VIII activity that is
often considerably less than that predicted from the dose given. The Factor VIII activity
subsequently rises to an even higher level within the next 12 to 24 hours.[112] As shown
in Figure 5-7, some patient levels rise progressively to a peak at about 12 hours, then

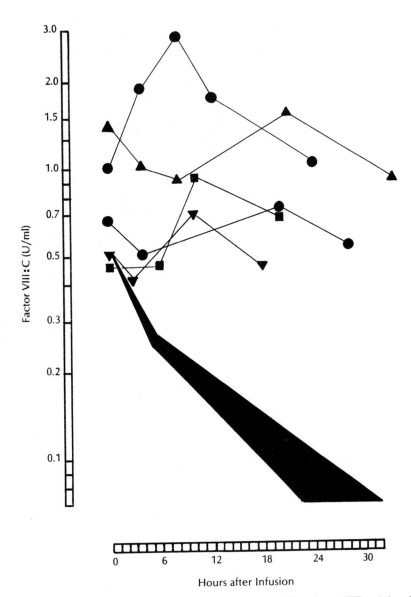

FIG. 5-7. A characteristic feature of vWD is the "delayed rise" in Factor VIII activity after an
infusion. The shaded area shows the normal biphasic disappearance of Factor VIII after infusion
into patients with hemophilia A. In vWD the levels continue to rise or rise again after some fall-off.

begin to fall, while in other patients the levels may begin to fall off from the immediate postinfusion peak and then show a "secondary" (or "delayed") rise. Infusion of cryoprecipitate from a hemophilia A patient produces no immediate rise in Factor VIII activity, but there is a subsequent progressive increase to a peak at 12 to 24 hours as the vWF molecules from the hemophiliac bind and stabilize Factor VIII coagulant activity molecules produced by the patient with vWD.[26]

Because the several hemostatic properties of the Factor VIII complex vary so much from one time to another in patients with vWD, and because the available assay methods are time-consuming and valuable hours would be wasted in performing assays on which to base precise dosage calculations, most acute bleeding episodes are treated with empirically determined doses. There is little correlation between the occurrence of bleeding episodes and the presence of particularly low levels of vWF or Factor VIII activity at the time. On any given day, 80% of heterozygous vWD patients have vWF and Factor VIII levels between 25% and 75% of normal activity, and only 10% of patients have levels below 25% of normal activity. Therefore, infusions of cryoprecipitate sufficient to raise the Factor VIII level by 50% (i.e., one bag per 4–5 kg) should achieve levels of 50% or higher in even the most severely deficient patients, with most patients attaining levels in the range of 75% to 125%.

When sustained therapy is required, booster infusions must be timed to maintain hemostatically adequate levels of both vWF and Factor VIII activity. This depends on the preinfusion levels and continuing endogenous production of each, as well as the doses administered and the disappearance rates of the infused vWF and Factor VIII activity. The secondary rise in Factor VIII activity usually results in sustained high levels for 24 hours or more, but the vWF's rapid falloff can result in subhemostatic levels, prolonged bleeding times, and active bleeding despite high Factor VIII activity levels. Bleeding times should be performed at 6- to 8-hour intervals and Factor VIII activity monitored at 12- to 24-hour intervals during sustained therapy. Booster doses are administered whenever either parameter falls outside the desired hemostatic range.

Recently, a new modality of therapy has become available for treatment of type I vWD and mild hemophilia A. An analogue of the posterior pituitary hormone vasopressin, 1-desamino-8-D-arginine-vasopressin, or DDAVP, stimulates the release of Factor VIII and vWF from endothelial cell and platelet stores.[73,102] This can result in a twofold to threefold increase in plasma levels.[73,102] DDAVP infusions can be effective for treatment of acute bleeding episodes in patients with type I vWD, who have the capacity to produce all sizes of vWF multimers.[50,87] It is ineffective in patients with type III disease, who cannot produce any vWF, and in those with type IIA, who do not form the larger multimers. Its use is contraindicated in patients with type IIB and pseudo-vWD because the sudden outpouring of large vWF molecules with increased binding avidity has been shown to result in serious thromboembolic complications or severe thrombocytopenia.[50,87] Because DDAVP-induced release may deplete the intracellular stores of vWF, repeated infusions of DDAVP may not be effective in maintaining hemostatic levels.[73,102]

MANAGEMENT OF PATIENTS WITH INHIBITORS

Since inhibitor antibodies are directed against a factor that is already congenitally absent, the presence of an inhibitor does not increase the frequency or severity of bleeding episodes. However, an inhibitor greatly impairs the ability to treat bleeding episodes with replacement therapy by inactivating the infused factor. When low-responder inhibitors are present in low titers (*i.e.*, less than 8 – 10 Bethesda U/ml), it is possible to infuse sufficient factor to achieve antigen excess with hemostatically effective levels of factor activity.[8,9] With higher inhibitor levels the volume requirements of even the highest-potency concentrates would be prohibitive. Procedures such as exchange transfusion and plasmapheresis to lower the antibody titer are of temporary value.[9,81,86,96] Immunosuppressive therapy has been universally unsuccessful in hemophiliacs with inhibitors.[9,54,81]

Some inhibitors are less reactive with animal Factor VIII than with human Factor VIII.[9] In such instances, therapy with animal Factor VIII concentrates may provide effective hemostasis. However, the heterologous Factor VIII is antigenic, and within about 7 days after exposure, antibodies to the animal Factor VIII appear and quickly rise to high levels. Also, to the extent that there is cross-reactivity between the anti – human Factor VIII antibody and the animal Factor VIII, the human inhibitor will also inactivate the animal Factor VIII in proportion to the inhibitor titer. The animal Factor VIII will also stimulate a rise in the anti – human Factor VIII inhibitor level.[9]

The observation that early PCCs (prothrombin-complex concentrates) contained varying levels of activated factors led to the use of these products in an attempt to bypass Factor VIII inhibitors.[1,27,35,42,64] Several clinical trials have shown that PCCs may be effective in controlling 50% or more of acute bleeding episodes.[1,9,27,35,42,49,54,64,66,68,81,92] There are a few reports of their successful use to provide hemostasis for surgery.[42,47,49,55] More purified PCCs lack some of the inhibitor bypassing activity of the earlier preparations but are still effective in about half of treatments for joint hemorrhages and other mild to moderately severe acute bleeding episodes.[1,9,27,35,42,54,64,66,68,82,92] Activated prothrombin-complex concentrates (APCCs) are available and may be effective in a greater percentage of bleeding episodes.[49,66,92] The effects of the inhibitor bypassing activity are transient and not subject to laboratory monitoring. There are no correlations among the doses administered, shortening (if any) of the APTT, and/or the clinical outcome of treatment.[1,27,49,92] Infusion of these activated factors poses risks for thrombotic complications, particularly in patients with impaired liver function. There have been several reports of myocardial infarctions, disseminated intravascular coagulation, and venous thromboembolic complications associated with prolonged high-dose therapy with both PCCs and APCCs.[5,38,45,58,68,95,97]

A most promising approach to inhibitor management is the induction of tolerance. Several investigators have reported that continuing, daily high-dose treatment with Factor VIII concentrates for prolonged periods has resulted in decreased levels and sometimes disappearance of Factor VIII inhibitors.[19,22,41] The mechanism of this inhibitor suppression is unknown, but it has been suggested that high concentrations of antigen may stimulate a suppressor response or, perhaps, facilitate the development of anti-idiotypic antibodies against the inhibitor.[41]

REFERENCES

1. Abildgaard CF, Britton M, Harrison J: Prothrombin complex concentrate (Konyne) in the treatment of hemophilic patients with factor VIII inhibitors. J Pediatr 88:200–205, 1976
2. Abildgaard CF, Cornet JA, Fort E, Schulman I: The *in vivo* longevity of antihemophilic factor (factor VIII). Br J Haematol 10:225–237, 1964

3. Abildgaard CF, Suzuki Z, Harrison J et al: Serial studies in von Willebrand's disease: Variability versus "variants." Blood 56:712–716, 1980

4. Agle DP, Mattsson A, Weiss AE: Psychological Factors in Hemophilia. New York, The National Hemophilia Foundation, 1980

5. Agrawal BL, Zelkowitz L, Hletko P: Acute myocardial infarction in a young hemophiliac patient during therapy with factor IX concentrate and epsilon aminocaproic acid. J Pediatr 98:931–933, 1981

6. Ali AM, Gandy RH, Britten MI, Dormandy K: Joint hemorrhage in hemophilia. Br Med J 3:828–831, 1967

7. Allain J-P: Dose requirement for replacement therapy in hemophilia A. Thromb Haemost 42:825–831, 1979

8. Allain J-P, Frommel D: Antibodies to factor VIII. V. Patterns of immune response to factor VIII in hemophilia A. Blood 47:973–982, 1976

9. Allain JP, Roberts HR: Treatment of acute bleeding episodes in hemophilic patients with specific factor VIII antibodies. In Brinkhous KM, Hemker HC (eds): Handbook of Hemophilia, pp 659–671. Amsterdam, Excerpta Medica, 1975

10. Ashenhurst JB, Langehenning PL, Seeler RA: Early treatment of bleeding episodes with 10 u/kg of factor VIII. Blood 50:181–182, 1977

11. Babson AL, Babson SR: Comparative evaluation of a partial thromboplastin reagent containing a nonsettling, particulate activator. Am J Clin Pathol 62:856–860, 1974

12. Baehner RL, Strauss HS: Hemophilia in the first year of life. N Engl J Med 275:524–528, 1966

13. Barrow EM, Graham JB: Von Willebrand's disease. Prog Hematol 4:203–221, 1964

14. Bennett B, Ratnoff OD, Holt JB, Roberts HR: Hageman J. (factor XII deficiency): A probable second genotype inherited as an autosomal dominant characteristic. Blood 40:412–415, 1972

15. Biggs R, Austin DEG, Denson KWE et al: The mode of action of antibodies which destroy factor VIII. I. Antibodies which have second-order concentration graphs. Br J Haematol 23:125–136, 1972

16. Biggs R, Austin DEG, Denson KWE et al: The mode of action of antibodies which destroy factor VIII. II. Antibodies which give complex concentration graphs. Br J Haematol 23:137–155, 1972

17. Biggs R, Denson KWE: The fate of prothrombin and factor VIII, IX and X transfused to patients deficient in these factors. Br J Haematol 9:532–547, 1963

18. Bleyer WA, Hakami N, Shepard TH: The development of hemostasis in the human fetus and newborn infant. J Pediatr 79:838–853, 1971

19. Bloom AL: Factor VIII inhibitors revisited. Br J Haematol 49:319–324, 1981

20. Bowie EJW: Von Willebrands disease. XXX National Hemophilia Foundation Medical–Scientific Symposium, Indianapolis, 1981

21. Bowie EJW, Thompson JH, Didisheim P, Owen CA: Disappearance rates of coagulation factors: Transfusion studies in factor-deficient patients. Transfusion 7:174–184, 1967

22. Brackmann HH, Gormsen J: Massive factor VIII infusion in a hemophiliac with factor VIII inhibitor high responder. Lancet 2:933, 1977

23. Brettler DB, Cederbaum AI, Forsberg AD et al: A long term study of hemophilic arthropathy of the knee on a program of factor VIII given at time of each hemarthrosis. Blood 60(Suppl 1):208a, 1982

24. Britton M, Harrison J, Abildgaard CF: Early treatment of hemophilic hemarthroses with minimal dose of new factor VIII concentrate. J Pediatr 85:245–247, 1974

25. Brown PE, Hougie C, Roberts HR: The genetic heterogeneity of hemophilia B. N Engl J Med 283:61–64, 1970

26. Buchanan GR: Von Willebrand's disease: A confusing disorder. Pediatr Ann 9:328–342, 1980

27. Buchanan GR, Kevy SV: Use of prothrombin complex concentrates in hemophiliacs with inhibitors: Clinical and laboratory studies. Pediatrics 62:767–774, 1978

28. Chung KS, Goldsmith JC, Roberts HR: Purification of characterization of an abnormal Factor IX Alabama (abstr.). XVII Congress of the International Society of Haematology, Paris, 1978
29. Cornu P, Larrieu MJ, Caen J, Bernard J: Transfusion studies in von Willebrand's disease: Effect on bleeding time and factor VIII. Br J Haematol 9:189–202, 1963
30. Craddock CG, Lawrence JS: Hemophilia: A report of the mechanism of the development and action of an anticoagulant in two cases. Blood 2:505–518, 1947
31. Denson KWE, Lurie A, DeCataldo F et al: The factor X defect: Recognition of abnormal forms of factor X. Br J Haematol 18:317–327, 1970
32. Didisheim P, Lewis JH: Congenital disorders of the mechanism for coagulation of blood. Pediatrics 22:478–493, 1958
33. Eyster ME, Gill FM, Blatt PM et al: Central nervous system bleeding in hemophiliacs. Blood 51:1179–1188, 1978
34. Fantl P, Sawers RJ, Marr AG: Investigation of a hemorrhagic disease due to beta-prothrombinase deficiency complicated by a specific inhibitor of thromboplastin formation. Australas Ann Med 5:163–176, 1956
35. Fekete LF, Holst SL, Peetoom F et al: "Auto"–factor IX concentrate: A new therapeutic approach to treatment of hemophilia A patients with inhibitors. XIV Congress of the International Society of Hematology, São Paulo, Brazil, 1972
36. Firshein SI, Hoyer LW, Lazarchik J et al: Prenatal diagnosis of classic hemophilia. N Engl J Med 300:937–941, 1979
37. Frommel D, Allain J-P: Genetic predisposition to develop factor VIII antibody in classic hemophilia. Clin Immunol Immunopatholol 8:34–38, 1977
38. Fuerth JH, Mahrer P: Myocardial infarction after factor IX therapy. JAMA 245:1455–1456, 1981
39. Gawryl MS, Hoyer LW: Inactivation of factor VIII coagulant activity by two different types of human antibodies. Blood 60:1103–1109, 1982
40. Giles AR, Tinlin S, Hoogendoorn H et al: Development of factor VIII:C antibodies in dogs with hemophilia A (factor VIII:C deficiency). Blood 63:451–456, 1984
41. Gomperts ED, Jordan S, Church JA et al: Induction of tolerance to factor VIII in a child with a high-titer inhibitor: *In vitro* and *in vivo* observations. J Pediatr 104:70–75, 1984
42. Goodnight SH, Common HH, Lovrien EW: Factor VIII inhibitor following surgery for epidural hemorrhage in hemophilia: Successful therapy with a concentrate containing factors II, VII, IX and X. J Pediatr 88:356–357, 1976
43. Graham JB, McLendon WW, Brinkhous KM: Mild hemophilia: An allelic form of the disease. Am J Med Sci 225:46–53, 1953
44. Griggs TR, Brinkhous KM: Porcine von Willebrand factor: In vivo survival and relationship to bleeding time. Fed Proc 34:222, 1975
45. Gruppo RA, Bove KE, Donaldson VH: Fatal myocardial necrosis associated with prothrombin complex concentrate therapy in hemophilia A. N Engl J Med 309:242–243, 1983
46. Hathaway HS, Lubs ML, Kimberling WJ, Hathaway WE: Carrier detection in classical hemophilia. Pediatrics 57:251–254, 1976
47. Heisel MA, Gomperts ED, McComb JG, Hilgartner M: Use of activated prothrombin complex concentrate over multiple surgical episodes in a hemophilic child with an inhibitor. J Pediatr 102:951–954, 1983
48. Hermens WTh: Dose calculation of human factor VIII and factor IX concentrates for infusion therapy. In Brinkhous KM, Hemker HC (eds): Handbook of Hemophilia, pp 569–589. Amsterdam, Excerpta Medica, 1975
49. Hilgartner MW, Knatterud GL, the FEIBA Study Group: The use of factor eight inhibitor by-passing activity (FEIBA, Immuno) product for treatment of bleeding episodes in hemophiliacs with inhibitors. Blood 61:36–40, 1983
50. Holmberg L, Nilsson IM, Borge L et al: Platelet aggregation induced by 1-desamino-8-arginine vasopressin (DDAVP) in type IIB von Willebrand's disease. N Engl J Med 309:816–821, 1983

51. Howard MA, Firkin BG: Ristocetin — a new tool in the investigation of platelet aggregation. Thromb Diath Haemorrh 26:362–369, 1971
52. Hoyer LW, de los Santos RP, Hoyer JR: Antihemophilic factor antigen: Localization in endothelial cells by immunofluorescent microscopy. J Clin Invest 52:2737–2744, 1973
53. Hultin MB, London FS, Shapiro SS, Yount WJ: Heterogeneity of factor VIII antibodies: Further immunochemical and biologic studies. Blood 49:807–817, 1977
54. Hultin MB, Shapiro SS, Bowman HS et al: Immunosuppressive therapy of factor VIII inhibitors. Blood 48:95–108, 1976
55. Hutchinson RJ, Penner JA, Hensinger RN: Anti-inhibitor coagulant complex (Autoplex) in hemophilia inhibitor patients undergoing synovectomy. Pediatrics 71:631–633, 1983
56. Inherited Blood Clotting Disorders. Report of a WHO Scientific Group. World Health Organization Tech. Rep. Ser. No. 504, Geneva, 1972
57. Kasper CK: Surgical operation in hemophilia B: Use of factor IX concentrate. Calif Med 113:4–8, 1970
58. Kasper CK: Clinical use of factor IX concentrates: Report on thromboembolic complications. Thromb Diath Haemorrh 33:640–644, 1975
59. Kasper CK, Aledort LM, Counts RB et al: A more uniform measurement of factor VIII inhibitors. Thromb Diath Haemorrh 34:869–872, 1975
60. Katz AH: Hemophilia: A Study In Hope. Springfield, IL, Charles C Thomas, 1970
61. Kernoff PB, Rizza CR, Kaelin AC: Transfusion and gel filtration studies in von Willebrand's disease. Br J Haematol 28:357–370, 1974
62. Kitchens CS, Newcomb TF: Factor XIII. Medicine (Baltimore) 58:413–429, 1979
63. Klein HG, Aledort LM, Bouma BN et al: A co-operative study for the detection of the carrier state of classic hemophilia. N Engl J Med 296:959–962, 1977
64. Kurczynski EM, Penner JA: Activated prothrombin concentrate for patients with factor VIII inhibitors. N Engl J Med 219:164–167, 1974
65. Levine PH, Britten AFH: Supervised patient-management of hemophilia: A study of 45 patients with hemophilia A and B. Ann Intern Med 78:195–201, 1973
66. Lusher JM, Blatt PM, Penner JA et al: Autoplex vs Proplex: A controlled, double-blind study of effectiveness in acute hemarthroses in hemophiliacs with inhibitors to factor VIII. Blood 62:1135–1138, 1983
67. Lusher JM, Ofosu FA, Edson JR et al: North American study of factor VIII concentrate potency. Scand J Haematol Suppl 40(33):149–160, 1984
68. Lusher JM, Shapiro SS, Palascak JE et al: Efficacy of prothrombin complex concentrates in hemophiliacs with antibodies to factor VIII. N Engl J Med 303:421–425, 1980
69. Lyon MF: Chromosomal and subchromosomal inactivation. Annu Rev Genet 2:31, 1968
70. Mammen EF: Factor XIII deficiency. Semin Thromb Hemost 9:10–12, 1983
71. Mammen EF: Factor II abnormalities. Semin Thromb Hemost 9:13–16, 1983
72. Mammen EF: Fibrinogen abnormalities. Semin Thromb Hemost 9:1–9, 1983
73. Mannucci PM, Canciani MT, Rota L, Donovan BS: Response of factor VIII/von Willebrand factor to DDAVP in healthy subjects and patients with haemophilia A and von Willebrand's disease. Br J Haematol 47:283–293, 1981
74. Marlar RA, Griffin JH: Deficiency of protein C inhibitor in combined factor V/VIII deficiency disease. J Clin Invest 66:1186–1189, 1980
75. McMillan CW, Webster WP, Roberts HR, Blyth WB: Continuous intravenous infusion of factor VIII in classic hemophilia. Br J Haematol 18:659–667, 1970
76. Miller CH, Graham JB, Goldin LR, Elston RC: Genetics of classic von Willebrand's disease. I. Phenotypic variation within families. Blood 54:117–136, 1979
77. Nachman RL, Jaffe EA: Subcellular platelet factor VIII antigen and von Willebrand factor. J Exp Med 141:1101–1113, 1975
78. Nilsson IM, Blomback M, von Francken I: On an inherited autosomal hemorrhagic diathesis with antihemophilic globulin (AHG) deficiency and prolonged bleeding time. Acta Med Scand 159:35–57, 1957

79. Nilsson IM, Holmberg L: Von Willebrand's disease today. Clin Haematol 8:147–168, 1979
80. Owen CA, Bowie EJW, Didisheim P, Thompson JH: The Diagnosis of Bleeding Disorders, p 135. Boston, Little, Brown & Co, 1969
81. Penner JA, Kelly PE: Management of patients with factor VIII or IX inhibitors. Semin Thromb Hemost 1:386–399, 1975
82. Penner JA, Kelly PE: Letter: Lower doses of factor VIII for hemophilia. N Engl J Med 297:401, 1977
83. Robboy SJ, Lewis EJ, Schur PH, Coleman RW: Circulating anticoagulants to factor VIII: Immunochemical studies and clinical response to factor VIII concentrates. Am J Med 49:742–752, 1970
84. Roberts HR, Grizzel JE, McLester WD, Penick GD: Genetic variants of hemophilia B: Detection by means of a specific PTC inhibitor. J Clin Invest 17:360–365, 1968
85. Roberts HR, Gross GP, Webster WP et al: Acquired inhibitors of plasma factor IX: A study of their induction, properties and neutralization. Am J Med Sci 251:81–88, 1966
86. Roberts HR, Scales MB, Madison JT et al: A clinical and experimental study of acquired inhibitors to factor VIII. Blood 26:805–818, 1965
87. Ruggeri ZM, Mannucci PM, Lombard R et al: Multimeric composition of factor VIII/von Willebrand factor following administration of DDAVP: Implications for pathophysiology and therapy of von Willebrand's disease subtypes. Blood 59:1272–1278, 1982
88. Seligsohn U, Modan M: Definition of the population at risk of bleeding due to factor XI deficiency in Ashkenazi Jews and the value of activated partial thromboplastin time in its detection. Isr J Med Sci 17:413–415, 1981
89. Sell EJ, Corrigan JJ: Platelet counts, fibrinogen concentrations and factor V and factor VIII levels in healthy infants according to gestational age. J Pediatr 82:1028–1032, 1973
90. Shapiro SS, Hultin M: Acquired inhibitors to blood coagulation factors. Semin Thromb Hemost 1:336–385, 1975
91. Sibley C, Singer JW, Wood RJ: Comparison of activated partial thromboplastin reagents. Am J Clin Pathol 59:581–586, 1973
92. Sjamsoedin LJM, Heijnen L, Mauser-Bunschoten EP et al: The effect of activated prothrombin complex concentrate (FEIBA) on joint and muscle bleeding in patients with hemophilia A and antibodies to factor VIII. N Engl J Med 305:717–721, 1981
93. Smith PS, Levine PH: The benefits of comprehensive care in hemophilia: A five year study of outcomes. Am J Publ Health 74:616–617, 1964
94. Soff GA, Levin J: Familial multiple coagulation factor deficiencies. Semin Thromb Hemost 7:112–148, 1981
95. Stenbjerg S, Jorgensen J: Disseminated intravascular coagulation and infusion of factor VIII inhibitor bypassing activity. Lancet 1:360, 1977
96. Strauss HS: Acquired circulating anticoagulants in hemophilia A. N Engl J Med 281:866–873, 1969
97. Sullivan DW, Purdy LJ, Billingham M, Glader BE: Fatal myocardial infarction following therapy with prothrombin complex concentrates in a young man with hemophilia A. Pediatrics 74:279–281, 1984
98. Tytgat GN, Collen D, Vermylen J: Metabolism and distribution of fibrinogen. II. Fibrinogen turnover in polycythemia, thrombocytosis, haemophilia A, congenital afibrinogenemia and during streptokinase therapy. Br J Haematol 22:701–717, 1972
99. Veltkamp JJ, Drion EF, Loeliger EA: Detection of the carrier state in hereditary coagulation disorders. Thromb Diath Haemorrh 18:403–422, 1968
100. Veltkamp JJ, Meilof J, Remmelts HG et al: Another genetic variant of haemophilia B: Haemophilia B Leyden. Scand J Haematol 7:82–90, 1970
101. Von Willebrand EA: Uber hereditaere pseudohaemophilie. Acta Med Scand 76:521–550, 1931
102. Warrier AI, Lusher JM: DDAVP: A useful alternative to blood components in moderate hemophilia A and von Willebrand disease. J Pediatr 102:228–233, 1983

103. Webster WP, Roberts HR, Penick GD: Hemostasis in factor V deficiency. Am J Med Sci 248:194–202, 1964
104. Weiss AE: Circulating inhibitors in hemophilia A and B: Epidemiology and methods of detection. In Brinkhous KM, Hemker HC (eds): Handbook of Hemophilia, pp 629–646. Amsterdam, Excerpta Medica, 1975
105. Weiss AE: Modern management of hemophilia. Res Staff Physician 23:74–87, 1977
106. Weiss AE: The Hemophilias. Miami, Dade Monograph, 1978
107. Weiss AE: Dosage–efficacy relationship in single-dose replacement therapy for acute bleeding episodes in hemophilia. Thromb Haemost 46:124, 1981
108. Weiss AE, Brinkhous KM: Hemarthroses and hemarthropathy in hemophilia A and B: Pathologic alterations and their amelioration by prompt transfusion therapy. In McCollough NC (ed): Comprehensive Management of Musculoskeletal Disorders in Hemophilia, pp 23–32. Washington, National Academy of Science, 1973
109. Weiss AE, Brinkhous KM: Pathogenesis and incidence of the hemophilias. In McCollough NC (ed): Comprehensive Management of Musculoskeletal Disorders in Hemophilia, pp 3–16. Washington, National Academy of Science, 1973
110. Weiss AE, Webster WP, Strike LE, Brinkhous KM: Survival of transfused factor VIII in hemophilic patients treated with epsilon aminocaproic acid. Transfusion 16:209–214, 1976
111. Zimmerman TS, Ratnoff OD, Powell AE: Immunologic differentiation of classic hemophilia (factor VIII deficiency) and von Willebrand's disease. J Clin Invest 50:244–254, 1971
112. Zimmerman TS, Ruggeri ZM: Von Willebrand's disease. Prog Hemost Thromb VI:203–236, 1982
113. Zipursky A, deSa D, Hsu E et al: Clinical and laboratory diagnosis of hemostatic disorders in newborn infants. Am J Pediatr Hematol Oncol 1:217–226, 1979

Acquired Coagulation Disorders

6

Andrew E. Weiss

Clinical bleeding is frequently encountered as a complication of a wide variety of acute and chronic diseases. Furthermore, many diseases can cause several hemostatic abnormalities. Severe liver disease, for example, may be associated with thrombocytopenia, impaired platelet function, coagulation factor deficiencies, intravascular coagulation, or excessive systemic fibrinolysis. The bleeding diathesis may be the result of one or another of these abnormalities or, as is most often the case, the combined effect of several hemostatic defects. Thus, in any given patient it is necessary to be aware of all of the hemostatic defects that can occur in his particular disease and to evaluate the status of each potentially abnormal mechanism before the cause of the bleeding can be determined and specific treatment(s) instituted.

VITAMIN K DEFICIENCY

CASE STUDY

Hemostatic Profile of Vitamin K Deficiency

PARAMETER	RESULT
Platelet count	412,500/μl
Ivy bleeding time	4 min.
Prothrombin time (PT)*	>60/12/14 sec.

(Continued)

169

Hemostatic Profile of Vitamin K Deficiency *(Continued)*

PARAMETER	RESULT
Activated partial thromboplastin time (APTT)*	>100/32/33 sec.
Thrombin time (TT)*	13/12/— sec
Fibrinogen	387 mg/dl
Factor II	0.04 U/ml
Factor V	0.89 U/ml
Factor VII	0.01 U/ml
Factor VIII	1.08 U/ml
Factor IX	0.25 U/ml
Factor X	0.01 U/ml

* Patient/control/mix

Biochemistry

Natural vitamin K is a fat-soluble vitamin obtained primarily through the diet, particularly in green leafy vegetables, fish, and liver. Bile salts are necessary for its absorption, which occurs primarily in the proximal small intestine.[39,121] Vitamin K is also synthesized by intestinal bacteria such as *Bacteroides fragilis* and some strains of *Escherichia coli*.[6] These organisms reside primarily in the jejunum and ileum, beyond the site of maximal vitamin K absorption; therefore, bacterial vitamin K contributes very little after the neonatal period.[90] It has generally been held that body stores of vitamin K are quite limited and quickly exhausted when dietary sources are interrupted. However, there is some evidence to suggest that vitamin K deficiency may evolve more slowly than predicted from studies of vitamin K turnover.[40,115] It may be that when dietary supplies of vitamin K are adequate, the turnover rate is high; but as body stores diminish, the recycling mechanism described below may be used to a greater degree, thereby extending the time before stores are completely exhausted.

Role in Factor Synthesis

Vitamin K is an essential cofactor for the production of functional clotting factors II, VII, IX, and X. These four factors are very similar; they are all synthesized in liver parenchymal cells and circulate as single-chain proenzymes that are activated to two-chain active serine proteases through cleavage of an arginyl bond by the active enzyme of the preceding clotting reaction.[107] There are close structural homologues between these factors, including the presence of unique γ-carboxyglutamic acid residues at the first 10 to 12 glutamic acid positions from the N-terminal end of the protein chain.[42,43,107] Only eight proteins are known to possess γ-carboxyglutamic acid residues, four of which are Factors II, VII, IX, and X, and two others, proteins C and S, are involved with hemostasis as modulating natural inhibitors.[42] The presence of the γ-carboxyglutamic acid residues is essential for the normal binding of these proteins to phospholipid surfaces in the presence of calcium ions (Fig. 6-1).[33] Since phospholipid binding is necessary for physiologic activation of the proenzyme to its active enzymatic state, failure to perform the γ-carboxylation reaction results in nonfunctional proteins

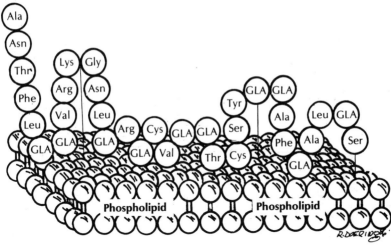

FIG. 6-1. Binding of vitamin K–dependent clotting factors to the phospholipid surface through γ-carboxyglutamic acid residues.

(*i.e.*, acarboxy-II, acarboxy-VII, acarboxy-IX, and acarboxy-X). These not only cannot participate in the clotting reactions, but also exert a slight inhibitory effect on the reactions of normally functional molecules.[60]

The γ-carboxylation reactions are posttranslational modifications of preformed precursor proteins.[43,101] The enzyme that mediates the conversion of the glutamic acid residues to γ-carboxyglutamic acid residues, γ-glutamyl carboxylase, requires reduced vitamin K quinone (vitamin K hydroquinone) as a cofactor (Fig. 6-2). The reduction of vitamin K to the hydroquinone state is mediated by various vitamin K quinone reductases in the presence of NADH or NADPH. In the carboxylation reaction, vitamin K hydroquinone is converted to an inactive epoxide form, which is reduced back to the original vitamin K quinone state by vitamin K epoxide reductase. This latter reaction allows for continuous recycling of the limited vitamin K stores in the liver.

As the supply of vitamin K becomes depleted and the production of normally functional, γ-carboxylated factors decreases, the plasma levels of previously produced normal factors fall in accordance with the biologic half-lives of each factor. Factor VII has a very short half-life of only about 3 to 4 hours, falling to levels at which bleeding may occur within 24 to 28 hours after complete cessation of new factor synthesis.[102,128] Factor IX has a half-life of about 24 hours but does not fall to subhemostatic levels for 3 to 4 days.[10,102,128] Factors II and X have half-lives in the range of 2 to 3 days, and severe deficiencies do not develop for 5 to 10 days after cessation of synthesis.[102] At the same time, there is a progressive increase in nonfunctional acarboxy-II, -VII, -IX, and -X in the plasma, which may exert an inhibitory effect on the coagulation reactions. (These nonfunctional precursor proteins were formerly called PIVKAs, for protein induced by vitamin K absence (or antagonists), but this term has been replaced by the new "acarboxy-" terminology assigned by the International Committee on Thrombosis and Haemostasis.[107])

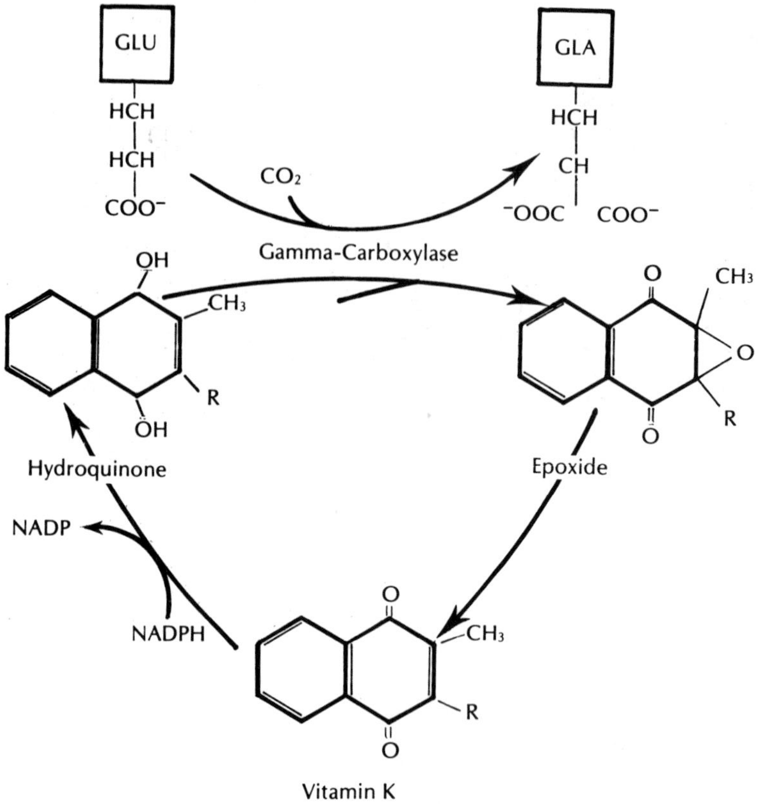

FIG. 6-2. The vitamin K cycle.

Etiology and Pathogenesis

The causes and pathophysiology of vitamin K deficiency are quite predictable from the metabolism of the vitamin. Vitamin K is so ubiquitous in foods, and the daily requirement so small, that pure dietary deficiency is rarely a cause. However, body stores are limited and become exhausted when dietary intake is interrupted, so that hospitalized patients receiving intravenous fluids and no oral feedings for prolonged periods may become vitamin K deficient. Also, since bile salts are necessary for absorption of the fat-soluble vitamin, biliary atresia or obstruction, fat malabsorption syndromes, and chronic diarrhea may result in vitamin K deficiency. On the other hand, for the reasons stated above, broad-spectrum antibiotics that disrupt the vitamin K–synthesizing intestinal flora should not cause a significant reduction in the vitamin K available for absorption when adequate dietary sources are continued.

"Hemorrhagic disease of the newborn" was a common problem in the United States until routine administration of vitamin K to all newborns was instituted in the 1960s. It remains a problem in developing countries today. The full-term newborn has physiologically low levels of Factors II, VII, IX, and X (in the range of 40%–50% of normal adult levels), and premature infants may have levels as low as 20% to 30%.[13,149]

Also, minimal stores of vitamin K are received from the mother.[73] In classic hemorrhagic disease of the newborn, insufficient vitamin K for Factor II, VII, IX, and X production leads to further decreases in the levels of these factors and development of bleeding symptoms by 2 to 5 days of life.[75] Breastfed infants are more prone to developing hemorrhagic disease,[130] both because human milk contains very little vitamin K and because it is rich in immunologic factors that retard establishment of vitamin K–synthesizing bacterial flora.[58,70] Maternal ingestion of anticonvulsants and some antimicrobial drugs may induce an early-onset, severe vitamin K deficiency with life-threatening hemorrhages developing within hours after birth.[75]

Dysfunctional acarboxy–Factors II, VII, IX, and X may also result from inhibition of the γ-carboxylation reaction and/or vitamin K utilization. The coumarin oral anticoagulant drugs inhibit the γ-carboxylation reaction through inhibition of the vitamin K epoxide reductase and, to a lesser extent, the vitamin K quinone reductase reactions.[42,43,107] Deficiency in functional vitamin K–dependent factors can result from therapeutic overdosage or accidental, intentional, or felonious ingestion of coumarin drugs, coumarin-containing rat poisons, and so forth. I have seen one case of surreptitious ingestion of coumarin by a psychiatrically ill patient, and similar cases have been described in the literature.[37] Also, several newer antibiotics, including carbenicillin, moxalactam, cephamandole, cefoxitin, and cefoperazone, have been reported to cause a deficiency in the vitamin K–dependent factors. This may be related to inhibition of the γ-carboxylation reaction by N-methylthiotetrazole side-chain–containing metabolites of these drugs.[80] Aspirin, tetracyclines, and sulfonamides have also been reported to inhibit vitamin K directly, although deficiency in vitamin K–dependent clotting factors usually occurs only with long-term, high-dose use.[54]

Diagnosis and Treatment

The diagnosis of vitamin K deficiency has generally been based on the documentation of decreased levels of Factor II, VII, IX, and X activity, without deficiencies in other liver-produced factors, and the subsequent correction of these deficiencies following administration of vitamin K. As shown in the case study, the typical pattern of laboratory findings is one of a prolonged PT and APTT (reflecting the multiple factor deficiencies in both intrinsic and extrinsic pathways), correction by mixing with normal plasma (thereby excluding inhibitors), and specific deficiencies in the four vitamin K–dependent clotting factors, with normal levels of Factor V and other liver-produced factors.

Several immunoassays have now been developed to measure the levels of nonfunctional, acarboxy precursors in plasma. Through the use of antibodies equally reactive to both normal γ-carboxylated Factor II and its acarboxy precursor, the presence of nonfunctional precursor can be detected by the discrepant results of functional and immune assays on a patient's plasma.[26] The presence of residual acarboxy-II in plasma after absorption of normally binding γ-carboxylated Factor II onto barium sulfate and the presence of two peaks (*i.e.,* normal and acarboxy) on crossed electrophoresis demonstrate nonfunctional forms.[84,91] Also, non–cross-reacting antibodies to both γ-carboxylated and acarboxy Factor II have been prepared and used for radioimmunoassay of each.[12]

Specific therapy for vitamin K deficiency is the administration of vitamin K. The route of administration depends on the severity of the factor deficiencies and hemorrhagic manifestations and the rapidity with which correction is required. When the deficiencies and bleeding tendency are mild and slow correction over several days is acceptable, oral vitamin K can be used if there is no impairment of absorption. When the deficiencies and bleeding manifestations are severe, requiring prompt correction, or if there is impaired absorption of orally administered vitamin K, the vitamin can be administered parenterally. With intramuscular administration of vitamin K, correction of the PT is usually seen within 24 hours. With intravenous administration, PT correction usually begins within a few hours.[90] In cases of life-threatening hemorrhage it may be necessary to replace the deficient factors directly, through infusions of plasma or prothrombin-complex concentrates.

LIVER DISEASE

Diseases of the liver can produce a variety of hemostatic defects:

- Deficiencies in clotting factors and natural protease inhibitors synthesized in hepatic parenchymal cells
- Production of clotting factor and antiprotease proteins with abnormal structure and/or function
- Impaired clearance of circulating activated clotting factors
- Accumulated plasminogen activators causing or contributing to the development of disseminated intravascular coagulation (DIC) and/or excessive systemic fibrinolysis, thrombocytopenia, and platelet dysfunction

Some 85% of patients with liver disease have at least one hemostatic abnormality. Fifteen percent have a clinical bleeding tendency.[29]

Pathogenesis and Pathophysiology

The liver is the major site of synthesis of nonimmunoglobulin proteins, including almost all of the clotting factors, plasminogen, antithrombin III, antiplasmin, and proteins C and S. The four vitamin K–dependent clotting factors (II, VII, IX, and X) are synthesized in liver parenchymal cells.[69,100] This function is affected by even very mild degrees of hepatocellular disease, since plasma levels of Factors II, VII, IX, and X may decrease before there is any other evidence of liver disease.[113] Factor V is also produced in hepatic parenchymal cells,[100] but its levels do not seem to fall unless liver disease is moderately severe. Factor XIII is also produced in the liver and may become deficient in moderate and severe hepatocellular disease.[113]

The liver is also the primary site of synthesis of fibrinogen.[27,38] The Factor VIII coagulant protein may be synthesized in specialized hepatic endothelial cells rather than hepatocytes.[140,141] However, fibrinogen and Factor VIII levels are usually not decreased except in very severe liver disease, and Factor VIII is more often increased. Decreased levels of fibrinogen may be due to decreased synthesis or to consumption or degradation in DIC, systemic fibrinolysis, or both. Fibrinogen and Factor VIII are both acute-phase reactants. In inflammatory liver disease, decreased synthesis of these factors by affected cells may be obscured by the increased output from stimulated, unaffected cells. This proceeds until there are too few unaffected cells left or an additional element of consumption/degradation exceeds the capacity for synthesis.

Antithrombin III and antiplasmin, the major natural protease inhibitors modulating the coagulation and fibrinolytic mechanisms, and protein C and protein S, which inactivate activated Factor V and Factor VIII, are all synthesized in the liver and have been reported to become deficient in hepatocellular diseases.[77,113] Deficiencies in natural inhibitors tend to be proportionate to the severity of the liver disease.[113] The greater deficiencies seen in severe liver disease may predispose to development of DIC and/or systemic fibrinolysis. They may also be the result of consumption in DIC and/or fibrinolysis.

Patients with liver disease may produce structurally and/or functionally abnormal clotting factor proteins. Dysfibrinogens with impaired fibrin monomer polymerization and prolonged TTs have been described in a variety of liver diseases, including acute and chronic hepatitis, cirrhosis, and, most commonly, hepatocellular carcinoma.[53,77,113,123,139] The abnormal monomer polymerization has been shown to be due to the presence of an excess of sialic acid residues.[123] When these are removed, the fibrin monomers polymerize normally.[86] The presence of small amounts of acarboxy-II in the plasma of vitamin K–replete patients with liver disease has been described.[12] Discrepant results between functional assays and immunoassays for antithrombin III are also reported.[1,31]

The liver also functions to clear circulating plasminogen activators and activated clotting factors from the plasma. When these clearance activities are impaired in patients with cirrhosis or fulminant hepatitis, plasminogen activators and/or activated clotting factors may accumulate to levels at which excessive systemic fibrinolysis or DIC results.[30,36] The hemostatic abnormalities and difficulties in distinguishing between DIC and fibrinolysis are discussed below. In liver disease this differentiation may be even more difficult. Perhaps the only means of diagnosing DIC in patients with liver disease is the demonstration of improvement in the levels of fibrinogen and platelets after treatment with heparin.[22,136,138] The risks and benefits of such a diagnostic/therapeutic trial must be weighed carefully.

Thrombocytopenia is another common cause of bleeding in patients with liver disease.[113] The thrombocytopenia may result from platelet sequestration in an enlarged spleen from concomitant folic acid deficiency in alcoholics, consumption in secondary DIC, or toxic effects of various uncleared metabolites on the bone marrow. Various combinations — perhaps additive — of several of these mechanisms can also be at fault. Abnormal platelet function with impaired aggregation and platelet factor 3 release has been described in liver disease.[113,133] This is seen particularly in patients with evidence of intravascular coagulation and fibrinolysis. Elevated levels of fibrin degradation products cause platelet dysfunction.[133]

Laboratory Evaluation

With the wide variety of hemostatic abnormalities that occur in patients with liver disease, examination of the hemostatic mechanism is diagnostically and prognostically valuable. Deficiencies in Factors II, VII, IX, and X may develop in patients with very mild liver disease, sometimes before there is other evidence of liver disease. The PT has been advocated as a highly sensitive test of liver function.[50] Trace levels of acarboxy-II may appear even before the PT is prolonged.[12] It has been suggested that this may be the "most sensitive early marker for hepatocyte disease."[134]

There is good correlation between the degree of deficiencies in antithrombin III and clotting Factors II, VII, IX, and X and other tests of hepatic protein synthesis (*e.g.*, serum albumin, cholinesterase). These provide a sensitive index of the functional state of the liver.[77] Several authors have reported that the PT is a better index of prognosis in acute viral or toxic hepatitis than are transaminases, albumin, or bilirubin.[20,73] PT ratios less than 1.8 indicate a favorable prognosis and ratios of 1.8 and above a poor prognosis.[48] Factor V levels also correlate well with other tests of protein synthesis, but they do not become deficient until there is more severe liver damage. Deficiency in fibrinogen indicates severe liver disease or the development of DIC or fibrinolysis.

The TT provides important diagnostic and prognostic clues. A prolonged thrombin clotting time in patients with liver disease suggests hypofibrinogenemia (usually less than 50–75 mg/dl) or impaired fibrin monomer polymerization due to dysfibrinogens or the inhibitory effect of fibrin(ogen) degradation products (FDPs). The addition of normal plasma should correct a TT prolongation that is due solely to hypofibrinogenemia. The inhibitory effects of dysfibrinogens and FDPs are only partially corrected by the addition of normal plasma. The Reptilase time provides similar information, helping to exclude an inhibitory effect of heparin or showing a more dramatic prolongation by dysfibrinogens.[106] Prolongation of the TT in the presence of a normal fibrinogen level and low levels of FDPs suggests the presence of a dysfibrinogen.

Hemostatic Management

There is no good correlation between the presence or severity of single hemostatic abnormalities and clinical bleeding. Most often, bleeding results from a combination of seemingly mild to moderate hemostatic defects that, by themselves, would not cause bleeding. Impaired hemostasis may potentiate bleeding from local lesions such as esophageal varices or gastric or duodenal ulcers. Correction of the hemostatic defects may be helpful as part of the overall management of such lesions. Deficient clotting factors can be replaced by infusions of fresh-frozen plasma (which contains fibrinogen, clotting Factors II, V, VII, VIII, IX, X, XI, and XIII, antithrombin III, antiplasmin, and plasminogen). The amount of correction that can be achieved is limited by the volume of plasma that can be infused at one time without risk of circulatory overload. A dose of 15 ml of plasma per kilogram of body weight will usually raise clotting factor levels by only about 15% to 25% of normal activity. However, the long in vivo half-lives of most of these factors allow for progressive stepwise increases to higher levels through repeated infusions of plasma at 12-hour intervals. Use of prothrombin-complex concentrates to replace Factors II, VII, IX, and X in these patients is not advocated, because these concentrates are known to contain activated clotting factors that cause DIC or thromboembolic complications. Patients with impaired hepatic function do not clear activated factors, and DIC or other thromboembolic complication may result.[67,82] Thrombocytopenia due to impaired platelet production is corrected by infusions of platelet concentrates, but platelet infusions provide only very short-lived corrections when platelets are sequestered in an enlarged spleen or consumed in DIC.

When there is strong evidence suggesting DIC, a trial of heparin therapy may be considered. Although some studies have shown increased levels of fibrinogen and platelets when heparin therapy is given for DIC in liver disease, other studies have shown no benefit.[22,47,136,138] A trial of antifibrinolytic therapy has been advocated in patients with evidence of excessive systemic fibrinolysis.[113] Since there is no test or combination of tests to distinguish primary fibrinolysis from secondary fibrinolysis of DIC, antifibrinolytic therapy without concurrent heparin therapy is not advocated. Blocking the protective fibrinolysis in DIC results in widespread thrombosis.

RENAL DISEASE

Altered hemostatic mechanisms play a role in the pathogenesis of many renal vascular and glomerular diseases. In hemostatic disorders such as DIC, hemolytic–uremic syndrome, and thrombotic thrombocytopenic purpura, there is fibrin deposition in the renal microvasculature. The fibrin produces acute glomerular disease, renal cortical/tubular necrosis, or renal vein or artery thrombosis. Fibrinogen, and in some cases Factor VIII, has been demonstrated in glomerular fibrin deposits, suggesting active participation of the clotting process in the fibrin deposition.[63] Elevated FDPs are found in the plasma and urine of patients with glomerulonephritis from a variety of causes.[59,126] The level of urine FDPs (but not serum FDPs) correlates well with disease activity.[49] Thus, the pathogenesis of many renal disorders may involve localized coagulation or platelet-mediated thrombosis, perhaps triggered by metabolic or immune complex–induced endothelial cell injury.

Not only can the hemostatic processes be direct or intermediate mechanisms in the pathogenesis of renal diseases, but some renal diseases *cause* hemostatic disorders.

Nephrotic Syndromes

A variety of renal diseases can cause a disruption of the normal barriers between blood and urine in the glomeruli, resulting in the loss of low-molecular-weight proteins, such as albumin, into the urine. Clotting Factors II, VII, IX, X, and XII, antithrombin III, and protein C are all small proteins, with molecular weights in the range of 50,000 to 80,000 daltons. All of these proteins have been demonstrated in the urine of nephrotic patients.[95,131,137,145] Plasma deficiencies have been reported for only clotting Factors VII, IX, and XII and antithrombin.[32,61,68,95] However, most studies have shown normal or elevated plasma levels of these factors despite demonstrable urinary losses, suggesting compensatory increased factor synthesis.[71,137] Factors V and VIII are often markedly elevated, a finding attributed to increased synthesis, but possibly resulting from persistence of activated V and VIII due to deficiencies in protein C.[66,137] The degree of factor deficiency(ies) correlates with the degree of proteinuria.[68,137] It is recommended that a PT and APTT be performed on all nephrotic patients before renal biopsy or other invasive procedures are performed. If prolonged, specific factor assays should be performed to identify the factor(s) that is(are) deficient. Then, appropriate factor replacement therapy can be administered to correct the deficiencies and permit the surgery to be performed without excessive bleeding.

Although significant clotting factor deficiencies and bleeding tendencies are uncommon in patients with nephrotic syndromes, thrombotic complications occur in some 25% of patients.[66,68,71,81] A causal relationship between this thrombotic tendency and deficiency in antithrombin III has been inferred, but not established. Antithrombin III has been demonstrated in the urine of nephrotic patients in amounts that correlate with urine protein levels. There is a strong correlation between the degrees of deficiency in the plasma and the daily urinary protein excretion. In one study, thrombosis occurred in more than 40% of patients with decreased antithrombin III levels, but in only 3% of those with normal level.[68] However, antithrombin III is consumed in the formation of thrombin–antithrombin complex during clotting, and the observed deficiencies might have been, at least partially, the result rather than the cause of the thrombosis.

Renal Failure (Uremia)

Pathogenesis and Pathophysiology

Prior to the 1970s, when the inhibiting effect of aspirin on platelet function became recognized, bleeding complications had been reported to occur in up to 60% of patients with acute and chronic renal failure.[108] Today such bleeding is rare because aspirin is contraindicated in uremic patients. Bleeding is due not just to aspirin-induced platelet dysfunction but rather to the superimposition of this hemostatic defect on other uremia-induced platelet and coagulation defects. A variety of hemostatic defects have been described in uremic patients. Thrombocytopenia is present in up to 50% of patients, although there is very poor correlation between the platelet count and bleeding in uremic patients.[19,79,112] Marked prolongation of the TT with slight prolongation of the

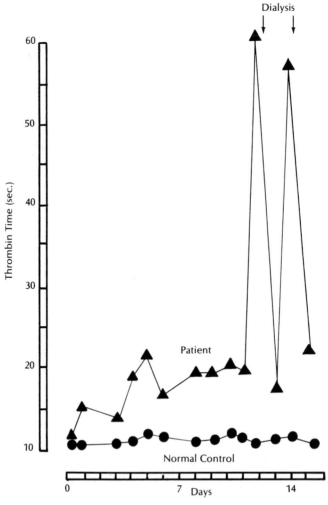

FIG. 6-3. Prolongation of the TT by uremic inhibitor and its correction following dialysis.

PT and APTT is seen in 25% to 50% of patients.[64] The presence of a normal fibrinogen level, accompanied by failure of normal plasma to correct the prolonged TT in mixing tests and reversion of the TT to normal following dialysis, indicates a circulating, dialyzable inhibitor of fibrin monomer polymerization (Fig. 6-3).

The most significant abnormality, however, is impaired platelet function, with prolongation of the bleeding time, decreased platelet adhesion to glass beads and wound surfaces, impaired platelet shape change, and decreased/absent release in platelet aggregation and platelet factor 3 availability tests.[16,18,79,109] These abnormalities are also corrected by dialysis, indicating a circulating inhibitor.[18,109,127] Several metabolites that are increased in the serum and urine of uremic patients have been shown to inhibit platelet function. Horowitz and co-workers found that guanidinosuccinic acid (GSA), at concentrations similar to those in the sera of uremic patients, inhibited platelet shape change and aggregation.[62] Dialysis reduces the serum GSA levels and corrects the platelet abnormalities. Rabiner and Molinas showed similar effects from phenolic acids.[110] These substances appear to affect platelets through different mechanisms.[108] The varying types and degrees of platelet dysfunction seen in uremic patients reflect various levels of several inhibiting substances. There is no correlation, however, between the presence or degree of platelet dysfunction and elevations of serum creatinine or urea nitrogen.[14,109,127]

Diagnosis and Management

Table 6-1 shows the hemostasis laboratory findings of two patients with acute renal failure. Both had disproportionately prolonged bleeding times relative to their mild to moderate degrees of thrombocytopenia, indicating impaired platelet function. They also had disproportionate retardation of prothrombin consumption, indicating impaired platelet factor 3 availability, and impaired platelet aggregation in response to epinephrine, weak adenosine diphosphate (ADP), and collagen. Patient A had a slightly prolonged TT, with normal PT and APTT. Patient B had a marked prolongation of the

TABLE 6-1
Hemostatic Profile of Two Patients With the Uremic Inhibitor

Test	Case A	Case B
Platelet count/μl	108,000	98,000
Ivy bleeding time (min.)	>15	>15
PT (sec.)*	13/12	12/12
APTT (sec.)*	39/33	32/30
TT (sec.)*	18/12	14/11
Fibrinogen (mg/dl)	264	684
Factor V (U/ml)	1.40	2.37
Factor VIII (U/ml)	5.07	3.60
Factor IX (U/ml)	1.49	2.42
Factor X (U/ml)	1.28	

* Patient/control

TT, with only partial correction on mixing with normal plasma, and mild prolongation of the PT and APTT, indicating significant inhibition of fibrin monomer polymerization. The diagnosis of a uremic inhibitor rests on the demonstration of inhibition of platelet function or fibrin monomer polymerization in a patient with uremia. The correction of these abnormalities after dialysis should be demonstrated whenever possible. The only means of treatment available is the removal of the inhibition by dialysis or plasmapheresis.

INHIBITOR AUTOANTIBODIES

Inhibitor autoantibodies are a well-documented cause of hemorrhagic disease. They may be divided into two general categories: (1) antibodies directed against and forming complexes with a specific clotting factor, preventing its participation in the coagulation reaction sequence or causing its rapid removal from the circulating plasma, and (2) nonspecific antibodies that do not bind or destroy specific clotting factors but block their interaction in the clotting process.

Specific Inhibitors

Specific inhibitors are highly specific immunoglobulins that bind and inactivate only the clotting factor against which they are directed. Specific inhibitors directed against Factors II, V, VII, VIII, IX, X, XI, and XIII and the von Willebrand factor have developed in patients with the corresponding congenital deficiency state, but inhibitors to Factors II, V, VIII, IX, and XIII and von Willebrand factor have also been described in nonhemophiliacs.

The most common specific inhibitor in nonhemophiliacs is directed against Factor VIII. These inhibitors have been reported to develop (1) in women during the latter half of pregnancy and up to 6 months postpartum; (2) in patients with a variety of autoimmune diseases (systemic lupus erythematosus (SLE), rheumatoid arthritis, Crohn's disease, ulcerative colitis, drug reactions, and various immune-mediated dermatologic conditions); (3) in patients with lymphoproliferative disorders; and (4) in person with no apparent underlying disease.[119] Inhibitors to Factors IX and XI are far less common but are also associated with systemic lupus, other autoimmune disorders, and pregnancy. Inhibitors against Factors V and XIII are rare. The majority of reported cases have been in patients under treatment for tuberculosis with isoniazid or streptomycin.[119] Acquired von Willebrand disease is discussed below.

The specific inhibitor of Factor VIII differs from other specific inhibitors in that the binding of antibody to Factor VIII is time and temperature dependent. Studies of the kinetics of Factor VIII inactivations by inhibitor have shown two patterns, type I and type II. In type I, there is a rapid, progressive loss of Factor VIII activity over 2 to 4 hours, with complete inactivation at antibody excess. Type II has "complex" kinetics, with an early rapid loss of Factor VIII followed by a plateauing, with residual Factor VIII activity remaining even in the presence of inhibitor.[8,9] Type I inhibitors are seen in patients with hemophilia A and in some nonhemophiliacs with autoantibodies to Factor VIII, but the type II inhibitors occur almost exclusively as autoantibodies in nonhemophiliacs. It has been suggested that these two kinetic patterns reflect antibodies directed against different antigenic sites on the Factor VIII molecule. The type I antibody recognizes an antigen located very close to the Factor VIII activity site, while the type II antibody is directed against an antigen remote from the active site, partially blocking the Factor VIII binding to von Willebrand factor.[45] These two types of reaction kinetics also carry implications for laboratory detection and quantitation, as discussed below.

The occurrence of a deficiency in Factor II in some patients with SLE has been known for years, but only recently has its pathogenesis been clarified. It occurs in a disease state characterized by the development of multiple autoantibodies, yet an absence of any evidence of vitamin K deficiency, liver disease, or urinary losses. Mixing tests show no evidence of inhibitor of Factor II activation or activity.[35,76] Recently, however, Bajaj and co-workers[2,3] have demonstrated the presence of antibodies that bind to Factor II without neutralizing its coagulant activity. The antibodies are directed against an antigenic site on the prothrombin portion of the Factor II molecule, not against Fragments 1 or 2, which contain the phospholipid binding and Factor V_a binding sites. The resulting immune complex retains all of the properties essential to prothrombin activation. Moreover, the antibodies do not interfere with the active sites of the α-thrombin formed when Fragments 1 and 2 are cleaved from the complex by X_a. This accounts for the lack of evidence of an inhibitor with *in vitro* mixing tests. *In vivo*, however, the immune complexes are cleared rapidly from the circulation, resulting in a quantitative deficiency in Factor II.

Detection and Quantitation

The methods of detection and quantitation of specific inhibitors are discussed in Chapter 5. Only those differences encountered in non-hemophiliacs will be discussed here. The presence of an inhibitor should be suspected in any patient who has a condition known to be associated with inhibitor development (*i.e.*, autoimmune diseases, lymphoproliferative disorders, pregnancy, etc.) and in any person who has the sudden onset of a severe bleeding tendency. Autoimmune phenomena such as thrombocytopenia, thrombotic tendencies, and inhibitors may appear months or even years before other manifestations lead to the recognition of underlying systemic lupus. Inhibitors are known to develop in persons with no apparent underlying disease.

The first indication of an inhibitor is usually the failure of normal plasma to correct a prolonged APTT or PT in mixing tests. However, it must be remembered that the Factor VIII inhibitor is time and temperature dependent. When the inhibitor is present at high titer, sufficient Factor VIII in the normal plasma may be neutralized rapidly enough to prolong the mixing test without incubation, but lower levels of inhibitor will not be detected unless the patient – normal plasma mixture is incubated for two hours at 37°C. Also, the complex reaction patterns of type II Factor VIII inhibitors result in varying amounts of residual Factor VIII activity, even when the incubation is prolonged or the inhibitor is in excess. This further complicates interpretation of even incubated mixing tests. Type II inhibitors are difficult to quantitate, since the first-order kinetic relationship between inhibitor concentration and residual Factor VIII activity does not pertain.

Inhibitors of Factors IX, XI, and V are not time and temperature dependent and have type I kinetic patterns. This results in prolonged mixing tests without incubation and allows quantitation by the standard methods.

Factor XIII inhibitors are quite difficult to document. The only test for Factor XIII available in most laboratories is the urea solubility screening test, which is sensitive only to Factor XIII levels of approximately 2% or less. The test may not show the rapid dissolution indicative of a severe Factor XIII deficiency in patients with inhibitor-mediated deficiencies of this magnitude. Unless the inhibitor is present in high concentrations to neutralize almost all of the Factor XIII present in a normal plasma–patient plasma mixture, it may be difficult to establish that an inhibitor is present.

Management of Specific Inhibitors

The management of bleeding episodes in patients with inhibitors is discussed in Chapter 5. However, in contrast to the situation in hemophiliacs, in nonhemophiliacs autoantibody production can often be suppressed. Inhibitors developing in pregnant or postpartum women or spontaneously in persons with no apparent disease often disappear spontaneously in a period of months to years. Inhibitors in patients with autoimmune disorders usually remit as the underlying disease is brought under control. Corticosteroids or immunosuppressive agents are used. Such therapy may also be effective in suppressing antibody production in other nonhemophilic inhibitor patients.

Nonspecific Inhibitors

Nonspecific inhibitor antibodies are not directed against specific clotting factor proteins, but rather interfere with the interaction of clotting factors on a phospholipid surface. The interactions of Factors VIII, IX_a, and X plus those of Factors V, X_a, and II take place on a negatively charged phospholipid surface. The later reaction results in thrombin-modified Factor V (V_m or V_a) that binds to specific sites on the platelet phospholipid membrane.[135] The membrane-bound Factor V_a serves as a receptor for Factor X_a,[93,94] which also attaches to the phospholipid through calcium-dependent binding of its γ-carboxyglutamic acid residues. This complex of Factors V_a and X_a on the phospholipid surface constitutes the "prothrombinase complex." Factor II binds to the surface through its γ-carboxyglutamic acid residues and calcium. The relationship of the factors allows for Factor X_a cleavage, converting the Factor II zymogen into thrombin.[28,94] Numerous studies have suggested that the nonspecific inhibitors bind to the phospholipid surface in such a way as to inhibit the binding of Factor II, and possibly also X_a, to the surface.[8,28,35,76]

Nonspecific inhibitors were first reported in patients with SLE. These are often referred to as *lupus inhibitors.* About 10% of SLE patients have nonspecific inhibitors, accounting for about half of all patients with nonspecific inhibitors.[116,120] In a study of 58 patients with nonspecific inhibitors, Schleider and his colleagues[116] found that 29 (50%) met the American Rheumatism Association criteria for the diagnosis of lupus, and seven (12%) had other autoimmune disorders or lymphoreticular neoplasms. The remaining patients had a wide variety of diseases with no apparent common denominator. However, nonspecific inhibitors may develop months or even years before other manifestations of SLE. Also, a number of drugs (*e.g.,* procainamide, chlorpromazine, hydralazine) have been shown to induce a lupus-like state or development of nonspecific inhibitors.[5,17,146]

The nonspecific inhibitor, as an isolated hemostatic defect, rarely if ever causes a clinical bleeding tendency, even with major surgery. When a bleeding diathesis is present, there are usually additional hemostatic defects, such as thrombocytopenia, the antibody-mediated Factor II deficiency, specific inhibitors or platelet dysfunctions, uremic inhibitors, or drug-induced inhibition.

Detection and Diagnosis

Since the nonspecific inhibitor interferes with clotting factor interactions on phospholipid surfaces in both the intrinsic and common pathways, both the APTT and PT tests may be affected. Table 6-2 shows the APTT, PT, and TT results of six patients with nonspecific inhibitors. The APTT is almost always affected to a much greater degree than the PT, which often shows little or no prolongation despite marked prolongation of the APTT. That the prolongations are the result of an inhibitor, rather than deficiencies, is demonstrated by the failure of normal plasma to correct the prolongations in mixing tests. The sensitivity of both tests to nonspecific inhibitors varies greatly with the APTT and PT reagents used — possibly reflecting their phospholipid composition. The TT is not affected.

The prothrombin consumption test (PCT; serum prothrombin time) also tests clotting via the intrinsic pathway, with the patient's platelets supplying the phospholipid surface. The PCT is usually normal. This suggests that the nonspecific inhibitor retards the rate of the clotting reactions, affecting tests that measure the rate of clotting, but that it does not prevent the ultimate completion of the reactions during the hour allowed for clotting in the PCT. It may also reflect the observations of Thiagarajan and co-workers that a purified monoclonal lupus inhibitor binds to free negatively charged phospholipids, but does not bind to the same phospholipids in the membranes of washed platelets.[132] This suggests that the nonspecific inhibitors may have far less effect on clotting *in vivo* than *in vitro*.

The diagnosis of a nonspecific inhibitors rests on the demonstration of (1) the inhibitory effect on coagulation screening tests and (2) the presence of normal concentrations of all clotting factors. In documenting the latter, it is important that the factor assay test several dilutions of the test plasma. The nonspecific inhibitor will tend to inhibit the APTT or PT reactions in one-stage assays. Typically, the assay curves will indicate progressively higher factor concentrations with more diluted samples. Patient curves that start out showing a deficiency and cross the control line to indicate more than 100% activity at higher dilutions are almost pathognomonic for nonspecific inhibitors.

TABLE 6-2
Effect of Nonspecific Inhibitors on Coagulation Screening Tests

Case	PT (sec.)*	APTT (sec.)*	TT (sec.)*
1	23/12/17	76/32/74	10/12/
2	13/12/	93/29/68	10/11/
3	15/12/	88/31/86	12/11/
4	17/12/16	>80/34/>80	14/13/
5	14/12/14	60/32/59	12/12/
6	15/12/	79/30/57	14/12/

* Patient/control/mix

Acquired von Willebrand Disease

Acquired deficiency in von Willebrand factor (vWF), resulting in a bleeding disorder similar to congenital von Willebrand disease, has been described in association with autoimmune disorders, lymphoproliferative disorders, myeloproliferative disorders, benign monoclonal gammopathies, and a variety of other disorders such as intestinal angiodysplasia, Wilms' tumor, congenital heart disease, and hemolytic–uremic syndrome.[148] In some cases the presence of a specific neutralizing inhibitor antibody could be demonstrated, but in other cases no such inhibitor could be found.[56,125,148] Mannucci and colleagues studied seven patients who did not have neutralizing inhibitors.[85] They found normal synthesis and release of vWF by megakaryocytes, including a full normal spectrum of large and small multimers. There was a rapid disappearance of vWF from the plasma. Two mechanisms have been proposed to explain this rapid disappearance of vWF: (1) autoantibodies that bind to vWF without blocking active sites but result in rapid clearance of the antibody–vWF complex[44,107] and (2) selective absorption of vWF onto abnormal cell surfaces.[65,92,117,147] The former mechanism is identical to one that results in the specific Factor II deficiency in some lupus patients. It seems particularly likely for all seven of Mannucci's patients, since they had lymphoproliferative disorders in which secretion of abnormal monoclonal or polyclonal antibodies is common. It may be that different pathogenetic mechanisms with a common result are involved in the different diseases. In autoimmune and lymphoproliferative disorders a nonneutralizing antibody may be involved, while selective absorption may be the mechanism in angiodysplasia, solid tumor, congenital heart disease, or DIC, in all of which abnormal surfaces may be present.

Most of the neutralizing anti-vWF antibodies react primarily with the vWF component of the Factor VIII complex, but different patterns of inhibition of vWF-related activities are seen in different patients. In some patients there is inhibition of ristocetin-cofactor activity, with little or no effect on Factor VIII coagulant activity or Factor VIII–related antigen levels.[52,56,114] In others, various combinations of these three activities were inhibited.[41,46,88,125] Even when the anti-vWF antibody has specificity for sites that neutralize only one or more vWF-related activities, all activities become reduced as the antibody–vWF complexes are cleared rapidly from the plasma.

Most of the reported cases of acquired von Willebrand disease have had moderate to severe bleeding into or from the skin or mucous membranes or from operative wounds. This is in contrast to congenital von Willebrand disease, in which the vast majority of patients have very mild bleeding tendencies. This reflects the much lower levels of vWF-related activities found in patients with the acquired syndrome, whereas patients with congenital von Willebrand disease tend to have varying levels of vWF-related activities, often falling well within the normal range. Rarely do they fall below 10% of normal activity except in the severe, type III von Willebrand disease. Patients with acquired von Willebrand disease usually have levels below 20%, and often below 10% of normal activity.

Detection and Diagnosis

Acquired von Willebrand disease should be suspected in any person with the recent onset of moderate to severe bleeding, especially in patients who have undergone surgery, dental extraction, or other significant hemostatic challenge in the past without excessive bleeding. The suspicion should be even greater when such a scenario occurs in a patient with an autoimmune or lymphoproliferative disorder or other condition in which acquired von Willebrand disease is known to occur. The platelet count, PT, and TT are not affected in congenital or acquired von Willebrand diseases, and the APTT may or may not be prolonged. However, the Ivy bleeding time has been prolonged in more than half of all reported cases of acquired von Willebrand disease. The diagnosis of von Willebrand disease can be extremely difficult to establish, as described in Chapter 5, but the levels of vWF-related activities in the acquired syndrome are generally much lower and the likelihood of establishing the diagnosis greater. The full battery of Factor VIII: C, VIIIR: Ag and VIII: RCo should always be performed. The tests should all be done on the same blood sample, so that there can be no question about variation in levels from one day to another. Treatment, illness, or other factors in the interval between samples may offset test values. The most difficult differentiation is between an acquired von Willebrand disease and a previously unrecognized congenital von Willebrand disease. A past history of uncomplicated surgery or dental extraction points to an acquired state, as does the finding of very low levels of vWF-related activities. But the variability of congenital von Willebrand disease is such that many patients report uncomplicated surgery at one time yet have severe bleeding following a lesser procedure. Tests of vWF-related activities on the patient's parents may help. For the reasons described above, it may not be possible to demonstrate the presence of the inhibitor antibody. Normal plasma mixing tests of Factor VIII: C, VIIIR: Ag, and VIII: RCo should be performed to evaluate for neutralizing antibodies.

Dysproteinemias

Hemorrhagic complications occur frequently in patients with multiple myeloma, Waldenström's macroglobulinemia, hypergammaglobulinemia, and other dysproteinemias. The bleeding may be due to a variety of hemostatic defects, including thrombocytopenia, platelet dysfunction, inhibition of fibrin formation, hyperviscosity, or a combination. The defect most often responsible for bleeding is impaired platelet function due to nonspecific adsorption of the abnormal protein onto the platelet membrane.[111] The coating of protein blocks fibrinogen binding sites and other receptors, resulting in prolonged bleeding times and impaired/absent adhesion, platelet factor 3 availability, and aggregation.[74,104,105] Impaired fibrin formation is seen more often than the platelet dysfunction but correlates poorly with the presence of clinical bleeding.[96] Through nonspecific protein-to-protein interactions, the abnormal proteins form nonimmune complexes with fibrinogen that interfere with thrombin cleavage or fibrin monomer polymerization.[21,23] Figure 6-4, *B*, shows the grossly abnormal pattern of fibrin formed in a thrombin-clotted mixture of normal fibrinogen and myeloma protein. This defect results in prolongation of the TT and sometimes also the PT and APTT. There is a general correlation between the concentration of dysprotein in the plasma and the presence and degree of impaired platelet function and fibrin formation.[74,104]

Detection and Diagnosis

Table 6-3 shows the hemostatic profile of a patient with IgG myeloma. This patient presented with recurrent colonic bleeding, and the diagnosis of multiple myeloma was unsuspected. Routine coagulation studies revealed the markedly prolonged TT, with poor correction by normal plasma. Of the six common causes of a prolonged TT, the patient was not receiving heparin (sample contamination was excluded by repeat sampling), the plasma fibrinogen level was normal, FDPs were not elevated, and the patient was not uremic, leaving dysproteinemias and a dysfibrinogen in consideration. A pro-

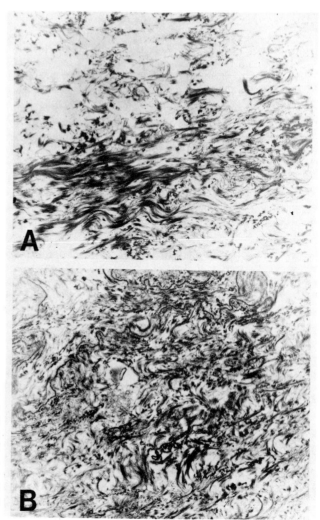

FIG. 6-4. Disruption of normal fibrin monomer polymerization by myeloma protein. *(A)* Normal polymerization of a thrombin-clotted mixture of human fibrinogen and saline. *(B)* Grossly abnormal polymerization of a thrombin-clotted mixture of human fibrinogen and myeloma protein.

tein electrophoresis provided the diagnosis. Fibrinogen electrophoresis showed no reaction, since the antigenic sites were blocked by the coating of myeloma protein. Platelet aggregation studies showed impaired aggregation with all agonists.

DISSEMINATED INTRAVASCULAR COAGULATION

The syndrome of DIC is also called "defibrination syndrome," "consumption coagulopathy," "intravascular coagulation," "fibrinolysis syndrome," and "paradoxical hem-

TABLE 6-3
Hemostatic Profile of Multiple Myeloma

Test	Result
Platelet count/μl	207,500
Ivy bleeding time (min.)	>15
PT (sec.)*	15/12/
APTT (sec.)*	33/32/
TT (sec.)*	52/12/25
Fibrinogen (mg/dl)	696
FDPs (μg/ml)	<32
Fibrinogen immunoelectrophoresis	No reaction

* Patient/control/mix

orrhage with thrombosis syndrome." It is not a primary disease state, but rather an "intermediary" disease process that is triggered by an underlying primary disease, which in turn may cause serious hemorrhagic or thrombotic manifestations.[89] The wide variety of diseases in which DIC may occur is shown under Disorders Associated With Intravascular Coagulation.

DISORDERS ASSOCIATED WITH INTRAVASCULAR COAGULATION

OBSTETRIC COMPLICATIONS

Abruptio placentae
Retained placental fragments
Retained dead fetus
Amniotic fluid embolism
Eclampsia and preeclampsia
Septic abortion
Intra-amniotic hypertonic saline–induced abortion

MALIGNANT NEOPLASMS

Carcinoma: prostate, pancreas, lung, breast, stomach, colon, gallbladder, etc.
Malignant melanoma; rhabdomyosarcoma
Leukemia, especially promyelocytic; neuroblastoma

INFECTIONS

Bacterial: meningococcemia; gram-negative sepsis; pneumococcal sepsis; tuberculosis; other
Viral: herpes simplex; cytomegalovirus; variola; hemorrhagic measles; varicella
Rickettsial: Rocky Mountain spotted fever; typhus
Fungal: histoplasmosis; candidiasis; aspergillosis
Protozoal: malaria

(Continued)

IMMUNOPATHOLOGIC DISORDERS

Hemolytic transfusion reactions
Purpura fulminans
Hemolytic–uremic syndrome (some cases)

MISCELLANEOUS

Shock
Cardiopulmonary bypass surgery
Extensive trauma or burns
Giant hemangiomas
Aortic aneurysms
Cyanotic congenital heart disease
Heatstroke
Spider bite (brown recluse)
Hyaline membrane disease
Snakebite

Trigger Mechanisms

Pathogenesis

As shown in Figure 6-5, the trigger stimulus from the underlying disease may be the release of tissue thromboplastin from cells damaged by trauma, surgery, burns, or hemolysis, resulting in activation of the coagulation process via the extrinsic pathway. DIC is seen frequently in women with complications of pregnancy such as abruptio placentae, amniotic fluid embolism, and retained dead fetus. In each case, tissue factor or other thromboplastic substances enter the maternal bloodstream and activate the clotting process. In abruptio placentae, activated clotting factor from the retroplacental hemorrhage also enters the fetal circulation, causing intravascular coagulation or thrombosis in the newborn. Many malignant tumors actively produce and secrete thromboplastic substances, activating the coagulation process at various levels.

Other disease states trigger DIC through damage to vascular endothelial cells and exposure of subendothelial surfaces to contact activation of the intrinsic coagulation pathway. Injury to endothelial cells results in disruption of intercellular bridges and retraction of the cells, leaving gaps with exposed subendothelial collagen between the cells.[83] With more extensive damage, the cells may slough, leaving large surfaces exposed for contact activation. Many viruses and rickettsiae tend to invade and damage endothelial cells directly. Bacterial toxins and circulating antigen–antibody complexes also cause endothelial damage indirectly through the immune or complement reactions against the toxins or complexes attached to these "innocent bystander" endothelial cells.

DIC is very frequently associated with shock. It may be either the result or the cause of the shock. Studies of trauma victims have shown evidence of DIC in up to 38% of patients who were or had been in shock, compared with 24% of patients without shock.[122] As blood pressure falls, compensatory vascular responses shunt the blood

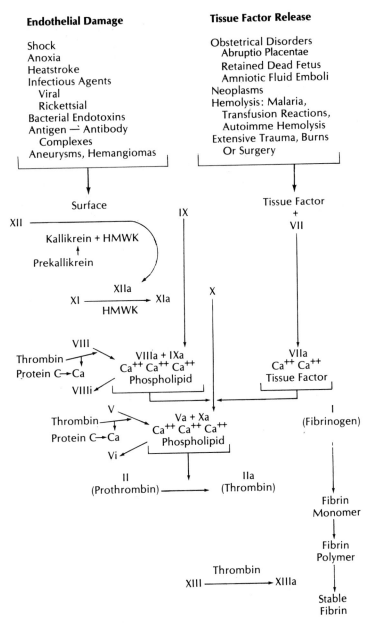

FIG. 6-5. Initiation of DIC by diseases that cause endothelial damage and activation of clotting via the intrinsic pathway and by diseases that cause release of tissue factor from injured tissues and clotting via the extrinsic pathway.

flow to the brain, lungs, and heart, with decreased flow to the skin, extremities, and viscera. The resulting stasis and progressively greater hypoxia and acidemia in the underperfused tissues leads to anoxic damage to endothelial cells, surface activation of contact factors and platelets, and perhaps also liberation of tissue thromboplastin from severely damaged cells.[57] In the relatively static blood, the activated coagulation process rapidly generates thrombin, causing extensive and progressive local thrombosis. The process can extend into the general circulation to produce DIC. There is also evidence that DIC causes shock by contact or feedback activation of Factor XII, resulting in excessive activation of prekallikrein, leading to generation of bradykinin, widespread vasodilation, and hypotension.[87]

Regardless of whether the underlying disease triggers intravascular coagulation by means of tissue thromboplastin release and activation of the extrinsic pathway or through endothelial damage with contact activation of the intrinsic pathway, both pathways lead to the generation of thrombin. Moreover, because of the crossover and feedback mechanisms, it is likely that both pathways ultimately become involved to some extent.

Pathophysiologic Effects

The pathophysiology of the clinical and laboratory manifestations of DIC is outlined in Table 6-4. The many abnormalities are primarily the result of the process of thrombin

---

TABLE 6-4
Thrombin and Plasmin in the Pathophysiology of DIC

Pathophysiologic Event	Observed Effect
GENERATION OF THROMBIN	
"Consumption" of Factors V and VIII and prothrombin	Decreased Factors V and VIII
	Decreased prothrombin
ACTIONS OF THROMBIN	
Destruction of Factors V and VIII	Decreased Factors V and VIII
Conversion of fibrinogen to fibrin monomers	Decreased fibrinogen
	Circulating fibrin monomers
Activation of Factor XIII	Decreased Factor XIII
Aggregation of platelets and formation of platelet thrombi	Decreased platelets
Formation of thrombin– antithrombin complexes	Decreased antithrombin
ACTIVATION OF FIBRINOLYSIS	
Conversion of plasminogen to plasmin	Decreased plasminogen
ACTIONS OF PLASMIN	
Destruction of Factors V and VIII	Decreased Factors V and VIII
Proteolysis of fibrin and fibrinogen to FDPs	Decreased fibrinogen

---

generation. The subsequent action of thrombin, the secondary activation of fibrinolysis and actions of plasmin, and the actions of the antiproteases and other normal control mechanisms restrain the coagulation and fibrinolytic processes.[142] During the generation of thrombin, the "consumable" Factors V and VIII are first activated by small amounts of thrombin. Subsequently, they are degraded to inactive forms by thrombin-activated protein C, resulting in reduced levels of Factor V and Factor VIII activity. Prothrombin-to-thrombin conversion results in reduced levels of prothrombin. Thrombin cleaves fibrinogen to fibrin monomers, liberating fibrinopeptides A and B, thus reducing the fibrinogen level. The resulting fibrin monomers may polymerize and progress to form localized thrombi or may diffuse as fibrin deposits throughout the microvasculature. They can form soluble complexes with fibrinogen or fibrin(ogen) degradation products and remain in the circulation. Thrombin activates Factor XIII, which becomes depleted in the process of catalyzing the crosslinking of fibrin strands. Thrombin is also a potent platelet aggregating agent. The aggregation of platelets into platelet thrombi, as well as their incorporation into intravascular clots, results in thrombocytopenia. As thrombin is generated within the circulation, antithrombin III acts to neutralize it through the formation of thrombin–antithrombin complexes. However, in the absence of heparin, antithrombin activity is slowly progressive, and, if the rate of thrombin generation exceeds the capacity of antithrombin to neutralize it, the available antithrombin is consumed in complex formation, leaving the thrombin activity unchecked.

Secondary activation of the fibrinolytic mechanism occurs rapidly as a protective mechanism to maintain the patency of blood vessels. If fibrinolysis is not quickly activated, or if the rate of formation of fibrin and platelet thrombi in the microcirculation exceeds the capacity of the fibrinolytic system to dissolve them, vaso-occlusion and infarction of tissues and organs may result. This leads to the thrombotic manifestations of DIC. Activation of fibrinolysis is initiated by the release of tissue plasminogen activator from endothelial cells in response to protein C, Factor XII$_a$–mediated activation of the kinin systems, stasis, anoxia, and other stimuli. Tissue plasminogen activator cleaves specific arginine–valine bonds in the single-chain plasminogen molecule, converting it to the active, two-chain enzyme plasmin. Plasmin is a potent and nonspecific proteolytic enzyme capable of degrading many proteins besides fibrin, including native fibrinogen and Factors V and VIII. High levels of both antiplasmin and antiactivator enzymes normally act to neutralize free plasmin in the circulation, restricting its formation and action to sites of thrombi. However, as with antithrombin, generation of plasmin at rates and amounts exceeding the capacity of the available antiprotease can result in excessive systemic fibrinolysis. Such unrestricted plasmin action can lead to further decreases in the levels of fibrinogen and Factors V and VIII, as well as depletion of antiplasmins in plasmin–antiplasmin complex formation and depletion of plasminogen by conversion to plasmin.

Degradation of fibrin and fibrinogen by plasmin liberates a series of progressively smaller fibrin(ogen) degradation products (FDPs), which serve as valuable markers of the presence of fibrinolytic activity. The large, early degradation products may form soluble complexes with fibrin monomers or fibrinogen.[7] Circulating FDPs also interfere with normal fibrin monomer polymerization and inhibit platelet aggregation.[7] It has been suggested that these inhibitory effects may explain the presence of bleeding symptoms in many patients whose platelet counts and clotting factor levels are above those at which bleeding might be expected.

DIC frequently causes a microangiopathic hemolytic anemia. This results from the fragmentation of erythrocytes during passage through microvessels encrusted by fibrin deposits.[15] Schistocytes are present in the peripheral blood smear in more than two thirds of cases of DIC.[124,144] This morphologic finding serves as a valuable indicator of intravascular fibrin deposition when other causes can be excluded.

Thus, the pathogenesis and pathophysiology of DIC involve an activation of the coagulation process by some trigger from an underlying disease, leading to generation of thrombin activity and conversion of fibrinogen to fibrin within the vascular system. In the process, platelets, fibrinogen, Factors II, V, and VIII, and other procoagulants become depleted, resulting in a hemorrhagic tendency. Fibrin deposits in the microvasculature produce a microangiopathic hemolytic anemia, progressing to occlusive thrombi and infarction of tissues and organs. Prompt activation of fibrinolysis prevents thrombotic complications but also contributes to the hemorrhagic tendency through further depletion of clotting factors and the inhibitory effects of FDPs.

Clinical/Laboratory Findings

The classic clinical and laboratory picture of DIC would include clinical signs of hemorrhage or thrombosis; laboratory findings of a microangiopathic hemolytic anemia; clearly deficient levels of platelets, fibrinogen, Factors II, V, VIII, and XIII, and antithrombin III, with resulting prolongations of the PT, APTT, and TT; elevated levels of FDPs; and demonstrable circulating fibrin monomers. Unfortunately, such a clear-cut picture is rarely seen.

DIC is a dynamic process, and the clinical and laboratory manifestations are affected by several interacting factors. These include the platelet and clotting factor levels prior to the onset of the DIC; the rate and amount of the trigger stimulus; the adequacy of the natural control mechanisms; the capacity of the bone marrow, liver, and endothelial cells to compensate for platelet and clotting factor consumption through increased production; and the effectiveness of the fibrinolytic mechanism in dissolving fibrin deposits and maintaining vessel patency.

Recognition of a significant drop in platelet count or clotting factor levels requires comparison of the observed level to a measured or presumed level prior to the onset of their consumption in DIC. In most instances there is no measured baseline level for comparison; decreases are recognized only when the levels fall below the lower limit of normal. However, platelet counts and levels of fibrinogen, Factor V, and Factor VIII rise to well above the normal range during pregnancy and in acute-phase responses to inflammation, trauma, or neoplasm, and marked drops from these supernormal levels may go unrecognized if the observed levels still fall within the normal range. This was well illustrated by a study of the DIC in women undergoing therapeutic abortion by intra-amniotic infusion of hypertonic saline.[143] As shown in Figure 6-6, there were highly significant decreases in platelets, fibrinogen, and Factors V and VIII from their preinfusion levels, and the level of FDPs increased. The presence of DIC was confirmed by demonstration of an increased rate of turnover of radiolabeled fibrinogen (from a half-life of 4.8 days prior to hypertonic saline infusion to 2 days after infusion). Thus, the procedure clearly triggered DIC, with a significant decrease in platelets, fibrinogen, and Factors V and VIII. These decreases would not have been recognized without reference to the baseline levels, since none of the postinfusion levels fell below the normal range. This probably accounts for the fact that recognizably decreased levels of fibrinogen and Factor V are found in only 50% to 60% of patients with DIC; recognizably decreased levels of Factor VIII are seen in fewer than 20% of cases.[124,144]

The clinical and laboratory manifestations of DIC also depend on the rate and

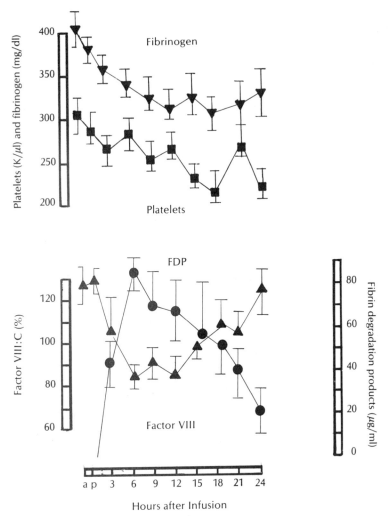

FIG. 6-6. Changes in the levels of platelets, fibrinogen, Factor VIII, and FDPs in subclinical DIC following intra-amniotic saline–induced abortion. Despite the significant decreases in platelets, fibrinogen, and Factor VIII from their baseline levels, absolute values were within normal limits.

amount of trigger stimulus from the underlying disease. Cooper and colleagues induced DIC in dogs by infusions of tissue thromboplastin.[24] When several strengths of thromboplastin were used, it was observed that continuous infusions of low and intermediate doses not only were well tolerated but increased the levels of fibrinogen and clotting factors. With high doses of thromboplastin, however, the rate of intravascular coagulation and clotting factor consumption was too rapid to be compensated by increased factor synthesis, and the fibrinogen and Factors V and VIII fell to very low levels. Marked platelet consumption occurred even with very low doses, reflecting a slower response of compensatory thrombocytopoiesis. This is in keeping with the finding of recognizable thrombocytopenia in more than 90% of cases of DIC.[124,144]

A closely related pathophysiologic variable is the ability of the natural hemostatic control mechanisms to contain the intravascular coagulation. Normally flowing blood washes tissue thromboplastin, activated factors, and so forth away from the site(s) of liberation/activation, diluting them and transporting them to clearance sites. Particulate matter, such as tissue thromboplastin and FDPs, is cleared from the blood by the reticuloendothelial system, and activated clotting factors, plasminogen activators, and plasmin are cleared by the liver.[78,99] Normal blood flow is disrupted, however, in patients in shock or immobilized due to trauma, surgery, serious infections, tumors, or complications of pregnancy. The clearance mechanisms are impaired by reduced blood flow to the liver and spleen or in hepatocellular disease. Antithrombin III, antiplasmin, and other protease inhibitor proteins are produced in the liver. Their synthesis or release is impaired in hepatocellular disease. Antithrombin III levels are also reduced in late pregnancy and in newborn infants, possibly accounting for the high frequency of DIC in sick neonates and in complicated pregnancies.

The development of severe deficiencies in platelets and clotting factors, resulting in a hemorrhagic tendency, depends not only on the rate of platelet and clotting factor consumption in the intravascular clotting (which depends on the rate and amount of trigger stimulus and the adequacy of control mechanism to contain the clotting process), but also on the ability of normal platelet and clotting factor production mechanisms to compensate for the consumption by increased production. This compensation requires a healthy status of bone marrow, liver, and endothelial cell production systems. It also depends on the abruptness of onset of the DIC and the rate and amount of platelet and clotting factor consumption relative to both the rapidity with which a response can be mounted and the maximal rate and amount of platelet and clotting factor produced. A previously healthy person who suffers an acute injury or illness and develops DIC will be able to compensate for platelet and clotting factor consumption far better than the patient who is severely debilitated and cachectic from terminal cancer with marrow and liver involvement. This is well illustrated by a study of the course of DIC after implantation of glioblastomas into the brains of guinea pigs.[99] During the early phase of tumor growth the animals were able to fully compensate for platelet and clotting factor consumption, and normal or elevated platelet counts and levels of fibrinogen and Factors V and VIII were seen. However, as tumor growth progressed, the animals became progressively debilitated and unable to compensate for the presumably increasing stimulus for DIC and platelet and clotting factor consumption. The platelet, fibrinogen, Factor VIII, and Factor V levels fell to subnormal levels.

Thus, when DIC develops suddenly, a strong trigger stimulus induces rapid, widespread intravascular clotting and consumption. It is unlikely that a compensatory increase in platelet and clotting factor production can be mounted quickly enough or to a degree sufficient to offset the consumption. However, with a slowly evolving or low-grade DIC, the rate of platelet and clotting factor consumption is fully or at least partially compensated for by an increase in platelet and clotting factor production.[103] The normal capacity to increase production may be reduced, however, by the effects of disease on the general health status and, particularly, the function of the platelet- and clotting factor–producing organs.

The clinical and laboratory manifestations of DIC also depend on how quickly the fibrinolytic mechanism becomes activated and the extent to which it can dissolve intravascular fibrin deposits to maintain vascular patency and blood flow to tissues and organs. The extremely important role of fibrinolysis in lysing thrombi and preventing tissue damage and death in DIC was demonstrated dramatically by animal experiments in which fibrinolysis was blocked by administration of ε-aminocaproic acid (EACA).[99] The animals died within minutes after EACA administration. On postmortem examination, not only were the small vessels occluded by thrombi, but also the great vessels and the heart! When the onset of DIC is abrupt and the process rapidly progressive with massive, widespread fibrin deposition, death occurs within a short time after the onset, and fibrin thrombi are found throughout the microcirculation. More localized manifestations of the thrombotic component of DIC may include dermal thrombosis and gangrene, usually in the extremities (*e.g.*, purpura fulminans), and organ dysfunctions due to the occluded blood supply (*e.g.*, renal vein thrombosis, renal cortical necrosis). In most cases, however, prompt activation of fibrinolysis results in rapid dissolution of intravascular fibrin deposits, and there is little or no evidence of tissue damage.

Spectrum of Clinical and Laboratory Manifestations

In view of this highly dynamic pathophysiologic process, with multiple interacting variables, it is not surprising that there is a spectrum of clinical manifestations that extends from totally asymptomatic patients with fully compensated consumption to the classic, acute, fulminant DIC, with widespread hemorrhagic or thrombotic manifestations. The spectrum of laboratory findings is equally broad, as illustrated by the findings in the five cases shown in Table 6-5. All five patients presented with acute onset of symptoms. Cases 1 and 2 presented with bleeding, case 4 with thrombosis and gangrene, and case 3 with both hemorrhage and thrombotic organ impairment. Nevertheless, their laboratory findings varied widely. All had elevated FDPs, prolonged PTs and TTs, and low Factor V levels. Four of the five had clearly low platelet counts, while the other's was within the normal range. Three had prolonged APTTs and low fibrino-

TABLE 6-5
Laboratory Findings in Five Cases of DIC

Test	Case 1	Case 2	Case 3	Case 4	Case 5
Platelet count ($\times 10^3/\mu$l)	40	15	180	55	75
PT (sec.)[†]	19/12	18/12	34/12	19/12	19/12
APTT (sec.)[†]	48/32	33/31	98/32	49/33	28/30
TT (sec.)[†]	20/12	35/12	60/12	30/12	ND*
Fibrinogen (mg/dl)	153	93	178	80	47
Factor V (U/ml)	0.29	0.49	0.12	0.43	0.43
Factor VIII (U/ml)	0.45	0.85	0.33	0.77	0.59
FDPs (μg/ml)	32–64	32–64	64–128	32–64	>256
Euglobulin lysis time (hr.)	>2	>2	1.5	>3	ND*
Fibrin monomer test	+	+	ND*	ND*	ND*

* Not done

† Patient/control

+, positive test result

gen and Factor VIII levels. Moreover, there was no consistent pattern, each of the patients showing one or two normal results among the consumable factors and low levels of others.

Table 6-6 combines the results of three studies, showing the spectrum of laboratory findings in DIC.[25,124,144] Thrombocytopenia, with platelet counts below 150,000/μl, is the most consistent abnormal finding. Elevated FDPs and fragmented red cells on the peripheral blood film were also frequent findings, being seen in 68% to 82% and 75% to 86% of cases, respectively. Positive fibrin monomer tests and low antithrombin III levels were found in about 75% of cases. On the other hand, despite the name "defibrin-ation syndrome," hypofibrinogenemia (below 150 mg/dl in newborns and 200 mg/dl in older children and adults) is found in only 57% of cases. Factor V deficiency is seen in only 58% of cases; low Factor VIII levels are found in only 15% to 20% of cases. Among the coagulation screening tests, the PT and TT are prolonged in about two thirds of patients, while the APTT is prolonged in about half.

Clearly, there is no single laboratory test — or even a small battery of tests — that can reliably detect or exclude the presence of DIC. Moreover, those tests that most consistently show abnormal results are not specific. The list of causes of thrombocyto-penia is extensive. Elevated FDP levels result from lysis of intravascular thrombi in any venous or arterial thromboembolic state, from resolution of extravascular hematomas or surgical wounds, and from primary excessive systemic fibrinolysis. Fragmented red cells (schistocytes) are seen in patients with artificial heart valves, burns, glomerulo-nephritis, thrombotic thrombocytopenic purpura, and hemolytic–uremic syndrome not mediated by DIC. Antithrombin III levels are physiologically low in the newborn and are reduced to varying degrees in hepatocellular disease, in late pregnancy, in some patients taking estrogen–progesterone combination oral contraceptives, and in many cases of venous thrombosis. The PT and APTT may be prolonged because of physiologic deficiencies in the newborn, congenital or acquired single or multiple factor deficiency states, or specific or nonspecific coagulation inhibitors. The TT is prolonged in congeni-

TABLE 6-6
Frequency of Abnormal Laboratory Tests in DIC

Test	No. Abnormal/ No. Tested	Percentage Abnormal
↓ Platelet count (<150,000/ml)	390/410	95%
↑ FDPs (>10 μg/ml)	301/397	76%
Fragmented red cells	246/353	70%
↓ Factor II (<75%)	266/391	68%
↑ TT (>control + 3 sec.)	254/377	67%
+ Fibrin monomer test	183/277	66%
↓ Factor V (<55%)	224/389	58%
↓ Fibrinogen (<200 mg/dl)	224/390	57%
↑ PT (>control + 3 sec.) and APTT (>control + 6 sec.)	204/363	56%
↓ Factor VIII (<50%)	29/181	16%

tal or acquired hypofibrinogenemia and dysfibrinogenemia, heparin therapy, dysproteinemias, and uremia, as well as with the severe hypofibrinogenemia or inhibition by FDPs in both DIC and primary systemic fibrinolysis.

Diagnostic Criteria

There are no well-defined, generally accepted criteria for the diagnosis of DIC. The criteria described in studies from various medical centers have varied from rigid requirements of documented deficiencies in specific consumable factors, elevated FDPs, positive monomer tests, and so forth, to liberal criteria documenting several but not all possible abnormalities, to scoring systems. In view of the great variability of the syndrome, the fewer tests performed or the more demanding the criteria, the fewer cases will be recognized. The frequency with which the diagnosis is made depends on both the awareness of physicians of the possibility of DIC occurring in various underlying diseases and the use of appropriate laboratory evaluations as follow-up.

The ideal means of diagnosis is through demonstration of circulating thrombin, or a circulating product of a specific action of thrombin on fibrinogen. Several "fibrin monomer" tests have been developed, including the ethanol gelation and protamine paracoagulation tests.[51,58,72,118] The ethanol gel test has limited sensitivity, particularly when fibrinogen levels are low, giving positive results in fewer than half of cases with fibrinogen levels below 50 mg/dl and 75% of cases with higher fibrinogen levels.[124] The protamine test has high sensitivity but low specificity. Radioimmunoassays of fibrinopeptides A and B have been developed but are not widely available.[11,98] Fibrinopeptide A is rapidly cleared from the circulation and may not be present if blood collection is delayed or if DIC is low grade or intermittent.[97] Fibrinopeptide B is cleared slowly and may be detected even after the DIC has ceased.

In the absence of specific tests for DIC, several authors have proposed scoring or point systems that combine clinical and laboratory findings to reach an arbitrary score necessary to support a diagnosis. One such system, described by Whaun and Oski, assigns two points for each of the following: presence of thrombocytopenia, elevated FDP levels, and fragmented red cells.[141] One point is given for each clinical finding of sepsis, bleeding, thrombosis, or gangrene and laboratory findings of hypofibrinogenemia, hypoprothrombinemia, decreased Factor V, decreased Factor VIII, prolonged TT, and prolongation of both the PT and the APTT. A total score of seven points is required for diagnosis of DIC. Such a system is useful to prevent a premature diagnosis of DIC based on too little evidence through clinical symptoms only. Achievement of the required point score provides only the necessary support for the diagnosis. It *does not* establish a specific diagnosis. For example, a bleeding patient (1 point) is found to have thrombocytopenia (2 points), prolongations of the TT (1 point) and both the PT and the APTT (1 point), slightly elevated FDPs (2 points), and low levels of Factors II (1 point) and V (1 point). This totals to a score of 9 points, more than enough to support a diagnosis of DIC. However, he also has low levels of Factors VII, IX, and X, an accelerated euglobulin lysis time, and severe liver disease, with splenomegally and excessive systemic fibrinolysis.

Differentiation between DIC and liver disease may be quite difficult. DIC has been described as a complication of severe liver disease.[22,136,138] As discussed earlier, the hemostatic abnormalities associated with hepatocellular disease include thrombocytopenia, decreased synthesis of many clotting factors (including Factors II and V and antithrombin), and impaired clearance of plasminogen activators, leading to systemic fibrinogenolysis. Destruction of fibrinogen and Factor VIII and the formation of FDP occurs. Thus, almost all of the laboratory findings of DIC can be seen with liver disease.

Differentiation between primary excessive systemic fibrinolysis and DIC with secondary fibrinolysis is also difficult. As described above, excessive fibrinolysis causes deficiencies in fibrinogen and Factors V and VIII and elevated FDPs. Thrombocytopenia is often considered a distinguishing feature of DIC. However, thrombocytopenia may also occur in primary fibrinolysis as a result of platelet clumping by FDPs.[4] Fibrin monomer tests should provide the differential point, but the limited sensitivity and specificity of the available tests make this too unreliable for making potentially life-or-death decisions. From a clinical standpoint, excessive systemic fibrinolysis is more likely to be due to secondary fibrinolysis of DIC than primary activation of plasmin.

Treatment

The most important aspect to the management of DIC is treatment of the underlying disease. Once the trigger stimulus is removed, the intravascular coagulation will cease. With moderate and low-grade DIC, no further treatment may be needed. Some acute, fulminant DIC syndromes quickly resolve once the trigger is removed. In abruptio placentae, for example, the trigger for DIC ceases upon evacuation of the uterus. In some instances (e.g., severe infections, malignancies) it may not be possible to bring the underlying disease under control for some time. If there are significant hemorrhagic or thrombotic complications, symptomatic treatment of the DIC may be necessary. Specific treatment for the DIC may be directed at (1) interruption of the intravascular coagulation process, (2) replacement of deficient clotting factors, platelets, antithrombin, and so forth, or (3) augmentation or control of fibrinolysis.

If interruption of the coagulation process (i.e., anticoagulation) is needed at all, it is needed immediately, and the anticoagulant agent of choice is heparin. Heparin acts as a cofactor for antithrombin, converting it from a slow, progressive inhibitor to an immediate-acting inhibitor of thrombin and other activated clotting factors. The decision to administer heparin must be considered carefully. It has been estimated that only about 5% of patients need and benefit from heparin therapy, while in the vast majority of patients it is not helpful and can be harmful.[34] Four criteria can be used to determine whether heparin should be administered in DIC:

There is a definite diagnosis of DIC with evidence that the process is ongoing
The underlying disease cannot rapidly be brought under control
There is significant hemorrhage or thrombosis that warrants intervention
There are no contraindications to using heparin in that particular case

There are many different schemes for heparin therapy in DIC. It has been noted that there is great individual variation in responsiveness to heparin in patients with DIC.[142] A major reason for this is the varying degrees of deficiency in antithrombin III in patients with DIC. Since heparin has no anticoagulant effect in the absence of antithrombin III, the degree of anticoagulation achieved with heparin therapy is a function of both the heparin and antithrombin III levels. Before this fact was appreciated, it was not uncommon for patients to receive multiple, massive doses of heparin with little or no effect. Then they would receive an infusion of plasma (intended to replace clotting factors, but also replacing antithrombin), causing a dramatic swing to hyperheparinemia with more hemorrhaging than before. Today, antithrombin levels are often obtained as part of the DIC evaluation, or in conjunction with the decision to anticoagulate. Therefore, potential "heparin resistance" is recognized, and antithrombin is given before or with the heparin.

When the trigger mechanism is removed or is interrupted by anticoagulant therapy, the intravascular coagulation ceases, and clotting factor levels rise rapidly toward normal.[142] Fibrinogen and Factors V and VIII may return to hemostatic levels within hours, although platelet recovery is much more gradual. If the platelet- and clotting factor–producing tissues and organs are impaired, the levels remain low. If bleeding is a significant problem, replacement therapy may be indicated. Replacement therapy with appropriate blood components should be specifically targeted to the deficiencies identified. Platelets should be replaced through infusions of platelet concentrates; fibrinogen and Factor VIII by infusions of cryoprecipitate; and Factor V, prothrombin, antithrombin, or other factors by infusions of fresh-frozen plasma.

In the early 1970s, Weiss and colleagues wrote, "Replacement therapy should not be administered until the DIC has been halted because the administration of additional coagulation factors merely fuels the fire, providing more substrate for further clotting."[142] This remains true, but the rule that "heparin should always be given prior to or together with the replacement therapy" is not. Many underlying diseases have short-lived trigger mechanisms, and, by the time the various deficiencies indicating DIC are documented, the process may have ceased.[34] If there is ongoing DIC, replacement therapy fuels the fire, leading to more fibrin deposition, quickly consuming the infused clotting factors. If the DIC has ceased, replacement therapy provides sustained hemostatic levels without further fibrin deposition and without the need for anticoagulant therapy. Thus, the key is whether the DIC process is ongoing or halted. One approach to this question has been to administer a diagnostic/therapeutic trial of replacement therapy, then to observe the rate of disappearance of the infused platelets and clotting factors. Platelet counts and clotting factor assays should be performed immediately after infusion and at close intervals thereafter. If excessively rapid disappearance is seen, ongoing DIC can be inferred, and anticoagulant therapy may be indicated before any further replacement therapy is given.

Occasionally, there may be a significant thrombotic component to DIC, with suboptimal fibrinolytic response. This results from depletion of plasminogen, requiring plasma replacement therapy, or from inadequate activation, requiring augmentation by infusions of streptokinase, urokinase, or tissue plasminogen activator. On other occasions there may be evidence of excessive systemic fibrinolysis, with serious hemorrhaging and severe hypofibrinogenemia. The latter requires consideration of antifibrinolytic therapy. In general, antifibrinolytic therapy is almost never indicated. The secondary fibrinolysis is a major protective mechanism, and, as described above, when this is blocked in the presence of ongoing DIC, extensive, perhaps life-threatening thrombosis can result.[99] Therefore, even when there is evidence of excessive fibrinolysis, antifibrinolytic agents should never be administered until effective anticoagulant therapy has been established.

REFERENCES

1. Abildgaard U, Fagerhol MK, Egeberg O: Comparison of progressive antithrombin activity and the concentrations of those thrombin inhibitors in human plasma. Scand J Clin Lab Invest 26:349–354, 1970
2. Bajaj SP, Rapaport SI, Barclay S, Herbst KD: Acquired hypoprothrombinemia due to nonneu-

tralizing antibodies to prothrombin: Mechanism and management. Blood 65:1538–1543, 1985

3. Bajaj SP, Rapaport SI, Fierer DS et al: A mechanism for the hypoprothrombinemia of the acquired hypoprothrombinemia–lupus anticoagulant syndrome. Blood 61:684–692, 1983

4. Barnhart MI, Cress DC, Henry RL et al: Influence of fibrinogen split products on platelets. Thromb Diath Haemorrh 17:78–98, 1967

5. Bell WR, Boss GR, Wolfson JS: Circulating anticoagulant in the procainamide-induced lupus syndrome. Arch Intern Med 137:1471–1473, 1977

6. Bentley R, Meganathan R: Biosynthesis of vitamin K (menaquinone) in bacteria. Microbiol Rev 46:241–280, 1982

7. Bick RL: The clinical significance of fibrinogen degradation products. Semin Thromb Hemost 8:302–330, 1982

8. Biggs R, Austin DEG, Denson KWE et al: The mode of action of antibodies which destroy factor VIII. I. Antibodies which have second-order concentration graphs. Br J Haematol 23:125–136, 1972

9. Biggs R, Austin DEG, Denson KWE et al: The mode of action of antibodies which destroy factor VIII. II. Antibodies which give complex concentration graphs. Br J Haematol 23:137–155, 1972

10. Biggs R, Denson KWE: The fate of prothrombin and factors VIII, IX and X transfused to patients deficient in these factors. Br J Haematol 9:532–547, 1963

11. Bilezikian SB, Nossel HL, Butler VP Jr et al: Radioimmunoassay of human fibrinopeptide B and kinetics of fibrinopeptide cleavage by different enzymes. J Clin Invest 56:438–445, 1975

12. Blanchard RA, Furie BC, Jorgensen M et al: Acquired vitamin K–dependent carboxylation deficiency in liver disease. N Engl J Med 305:242–248, 1981

13. Bleyer WA, Hakami N, Shepard TH: The development of hemostasis in the human fetus and newborn infant. J Pediatr 79:838–853, 1971

14. Bonnin JA, Cheney K: The PTF test: An improved method for estimation of platelet thrombo-plastic function. Br J Haematol 7:512–522, 1961

15. Brain MC, Dacie JV, Hourihane DO'B: Microangiopathic haemolytic anemia: The possible role of vascular lesions in pathogenesis. Br J Haematol 8:358–374, 1962

16. Cahalane SF, Johnson SA, Monto RW, Caldwell MJ: Acquired thrombocytopathy: Observations on the coagulation defect in uremia. Am J Clin Pathol 30:507–513, 1958

17. Canoso RT, Hutton RA, Deykin D: A chlorpromazine-induced inhibitor of blood coagulation. Am J Hematol 2:183–191, 1977

18. Castald PA, Rozenberg MC, Steward JH: The bleeding disorder of uremia. Lancet 2:66–69, 1966

19. Cheney K, Bonnin JA: Haemorrhage, platelet dysfunction and other coagulation defects in uremia. Br J Haematol 8:215–222, 1962

20. Clark R, Rake MD, Flute PT: Coagulation abnormalities in acute liver failure: Pathogenetic and therapeutic implications. Scand J Gastroenterol (Suppl) 19:63–70, 1973

21. Cohen I, Amir J, Ben-Shaul Y et al: Plasma cell myeloma associated with an unusual myeloma protein causing impairment of fibrin aggregation and platelet function in a patient with multiple malignancy. Am J Med 48:766–776, 1970

22. Coleman M, Finlayson N, Bettigole RE et al: Fibrinogen survival in cirrhosis: Improvement by "low dose" heparin. Ann Intern Med 83:79–81, 1975

23. Coleman M, Vigliano EM, Weksler ME, Nachman RL: Inhibition of fibrin polymerization by lambda myeloma globulins. Blood 39:210–223, 1972

24. Cooper HA, Bowie EJW, Owen CA: Chronic induced intravascular coagulation in dogs. Am J Physiol 225:1355–1358, 1973

25. Corrigan JJ: Heparin therapy in bacterial septicemia. J Pediatr 91:695–700, 1977

26. Corrigan JJ, Kryc JJ: Factor II (prothrombin) levels in cord blood: Correlation of coagulant activity with immunoreactive protein. J Pediatr 97:979–983, 1980

27. Crane LJ, Miller DL: Synthesis and secretion of fibrinogen and albumin by isolated rat hepato-cytes. Biochem Biophys Res Commun 60:1269–1277, 1976

28. Dahlback B, Nilsson IM, Frohm B: Inhibition of platelet prothrombinase activity by a lupus anticoagulant. Blood 62:218–225, 1983

29. Deutsch E: Blood coagulation changes in liver disease. Prog Liver Dis 2:69–83, 1965

30. Deykin D: The role of liver in serum induced hypercoagulability. J Clin Invest 45:256–263, 1966

31. Duckert F: Behavior of antithrombin III in liver disease. Scand J Gastroenterol (Suppl) 19:109–112, 1973

32. Epstein O, Bevan G, Sidiqui N et al: Factor VII deficiency associated with nephrotic syndrome. Br Med J 2:1361, 1976

33. Esmon CT, Suttie JW, Jackson CM: The functional significance of vitamin K action: Difference in phospholipid binding between normal and abnormal prothrombin. J Biol Chem 250:4095–4099, 1975

34. Feinstein DI: Diagnosis and management of disseminated intravascular coagulation: The role of heparin therapy. Blood 60:284–287, 1982

35. Feinstein DI, Rapaport SI: Acquired inhibitors of blood coagulation. Prog Hemostasis Thromb 1:75–95, 1972

36. Fletcher AP, Biederman O, Moore D et al: Abnormal plasminogen–plasmin system activity (fibrinolysis) in patients with hepatic cirrhosis: Its cause and consequences. J Clin Invest 43:681–695, 1964

37. Forbes CD, Prentice CRM, Sclare AB: Surreptitious ingestion of warfarin. Br J Psychiatry 125:245–247, 1974

38. Foreman WB, Barnhart MI: Cellular site for fibrinogen synthesis. JAMA 187:128–132, 1964

39. Forsgren L: Studies on the intestinal absorption of labeled fat-soluble vitamins (A, D, E, K) in the thoracic duct lymph in the absence of bile in man. Acta Chir Scand (Suppl) 399:1–29, 1969

40. Frick PG, Riedler G, Brogli H: Dose response and minimal daily requirement for vitamin K in man. J Appl Physiol 23:387–389, 1967

41. Fricke WA, Brinkhous KM, Garris JB, Roberts HR: Comparison of inhibitory and binding characteristics of an antibody causing acquired von Willebrand syndrome: An assay for von Willebrand factor binding by antibody. Blood 66:562–569, 1985

42. Friedman PA: Vitamin K–dependent proteins. N Engl J Med 310:1458–1460, 1984

43. Gallop PM, Lian JB, Hauschka PV: Carboxylated calcium-binding proteins and vitamin K. N Engl J Med 302:1460–1466, 1980

44. Gan TE, Sawers RJ, Koutts J: Pathogenesis of antibody-induced acquired von Willebrand syndrome. Am J Hematol 9:363–371, 1980

45. Gawryl MS, Hoyer LW: Inactivation of factor VIII coagulant activity by two different types of human antibodies. Blood 60:1103–1109, 1982

46. Gazengel C, Prieur AM, Jacques C et al: Antibody-induced von Willebrand syndrome: Inhibition of VIII vWf and VIII AGN with sparing of VIII AHF by the autoantibody. Am J Hematol 5:355–363, 1978

47. Gazzard BG, Clark R, Borirakchanyavat V, Williams R: A controlled trial of heparin therapy in the coagulation defect of paracetamol-induced hepatic necrosis. Gut 15:89–93, 1974

48. Gazzard BG, Henderson JM, Williams R: Early changes in coagulation following paracetamol overdose and a controlled trial of fresh frozen plasma. Gut 16:617–620, 1975

49. George CRP, Slichter SJ, Quadracci LJ: A kinetic evaluation of hemostasis in renal disease. N Engl J Med 291:1111–1115, 1974

50. Glueck HI, Will RM, McAdams AJ: Measurement of prothrombin: A neglected liver function test in infancy and childhood. J Pediatr 76:914–922, 1970

51. Godal HC, Abildgaard U: Gelation of soluble fibrin in plasma by ethanol. Scand J Haematol 3:342–350, 1966

52. Gouault-Heilmann M, Dumont MD, Intrator L et al: Acquired von Willebrand's syndrome with IgM inhibitor against von Willebrand's factor. J Clin Pathol 32:1030–1035, 1979

53. Green G, Thompson JM, Poller L, Dymock IW: Abnormal fibrin monomer polymerization in liver disease. Gut 16:827, 1975

54. Green J: Antagonists of vitamin K. Vitam Horm 24:619–632, 1966
55. Gurewich V, Hutchinson E: Detection of intravascular coagulation by a serial dilution prot-amine gelation test. Ann Intern Med 75:895–902, 1971
56. Handin RI, Martin V, Moloney WC: Antibody-induced von Willebrand's disease: A newly defined inhibitor syndrome. Blood 48:393–405, 1976
57. Hardaway RM: Disseminated intravascular coagulation in experimental and clinical shock. Am J Cardiol 20:161–173, 1967
58. Haroon Y, Shearer MJ, Rahim S et al: The content of phylloquinone (vitamin K_1) in human milk, cow's milk and infant formula foods determined by high-performance liquid chroma-tography. J Nutr 112:1105–1117, 1982
59. Hedner U: Urinary fibrin/fibrinogen derivatives. Thromb Diath Haemorrh 34:693–708, 1975
60. Hemker RE, Miller AD: Kinetic aspects of the interaction of blood coagulation inhibition by the protein induced by Vitamin K absence (PIVKA). Thromb Diath Haemorrh 20:78–87, 1968
61. Honig GR, Lindley A: Deficiency of Hageman factor (factor XII) in patients with the nephrotic syndrome. J Pediatr 78:633–637, 1971
62. Horowitz HI, Stein IM, Cohen BD, White JG: Further studies on the platelet-inhibiting effect of guanidinosuccinic acid and its role in uremic bleeding. Am J Med 49:336–345, 1970
63. Hoyer JR, Michael AF, Hoyer LW: Immunofluorescent localization of antihemophilic factor and fibrinogen in human renal diseases. J Clin Invest 53:1375–1384, 1974
64. Hutton RA, O'Shea MJ: Haemostatic mechanism in uraemia. J Clin Pathol 21:406–411, 1968
65. Joist JH, Cowan JF, Zimmerman TS: Acquired von Willebrand's disease: Evidence for a quan-titative and qualitative factor VIII disorder. N Engl J Med 298:988–991, 1978
66. Kanfer A, Kleinknetch D, Broyer M et al: Coagulation studies in 45 cases of nephrotic syn-drome without uremia. Thromb Diath Haemorrh 24:562–571, 1970
67. Kasper CK: Clinical use of factor IX concentrates: Report on thromboembolic complications. Thromb Diath Haemorrh 33:640–644, 1975
68. Kauffmann R, Veltkamp J, van Tilburg N, van Es L: Acquired antithrombin III deficiency and thrombosis in the nephrotic syndrome. Am J Med 65:607–613, 1978
69. Kazmier FJ, Spittell JA, Bowie EJW et al: Release of vitamin K–dependent coagulation factors by isolated perfused rat liver. Am J Physiol 214:919–922, 1968
70. Keenan WJ, Jewett T, Gluek HI: Role of feeding and vitamin K in hypoprothrombinemia of the newborn. Am J Dis Child 121:271–277, 1971
71. Kendall AG, Lohmann RC, Dossetor JB et al: Nephrotic syndrome: A hypercoagulable state. Arch Intern Med 127:1021–1027, 1971
72. Kidder WR, Logan LJ, Rapaport SI, Patch MJ: The plasma protamine paracoagulation test: Clinical and laboratory evaluation. Am J Clin Pathol 58:675–686, 1972
73. Koller F: Theory and experience behind the use of coagulation tests in diagnosis and prog-nosis of liver disease. Scand J Gastroenterol (Suppl) 19:51–61, 1973
74. Lackner H: Hemostatic abnormalities associated with dysproteinemias. Semin Hematol 10:125–133, 1973
75. Lane PA, Hathaway WE: Vitamin K in infancy. J Pediatr 106:351–359, 1985
76. Lechner K: Acquired inhibitors in nonhemophilic patients. Haemostasis 3:65–93, 1974
77. Lechner K, Niessner H, Thaler E: Coagulation abnormalities in liver disease. Semin Thromb Hemost 4:40–56, 1977
78. Lee L: Reticuloendothelial clearance of circulating fibrin in the pathogenesis of the general-ized Shwartzman rection. J Exp Med 115:1065–1082, 1962
79. Lewis JH, Zucker MB, Ferguson JH: Bleeding tendency in uremia. Blood 11:1073–1076, 1956
80. Lipsky JJ: N-methyl-thio-tetrazole inhibition of the gamma-carboxylation of glutamic acid: Possible mechanism for antibiotic-associated hypoprothrombinemia. Lancet 2:192–193, 1983
81. Llach F: Renal Vein Thrombosis. New York, Futura, 1983

82. Lusher JM, Shapiro SS, Palascak JE, Blatt PE: Letter: Hazards of prothrombin complex concentrates in treatment of hemophilia. N Engl J Med 304:671, 1981
83. Majno G: Two endothelial "novelties": Endothelia contraction; collagenase digestion of the basement membrane. Thromb Diath Haemorrh (Suppl) 40:23, 1970
84. Malia RG, Preston FE, Mitchell VE: Evidence against vitamin K deficiency in normal neonates. Thromb Haemost 44:159–160, 1980
85. Mannucci PM, Lombardi R, Bader R et al: Studies of the pathophysiology of acquired von Willebrand's disease in seven patients with lymphoproliferative disorders or benign monoclonal gammopathies. Blood 64:614–621, 1984
86. Martinez J, MacDonald KA, Palascak JE: The role of sialic acid in the dysfibrinogenemia associated with liver disease: Distribution of sialic acid on the constituent chains. Blood 61:1196–1202, 1983
87. Mason JW, Kleeberg V, Dolan P et al: Plasma kallikrein and Hageman factor in gram negative bacteremia. Ann Intern Med 73:545–551, 1970
88. McGrath KM, Johnson CA, Stuart JJ: Acquired von Willebrand disease associated with an inhibitor to factor VIII antigen and gastrointestinal telangiectasia. Am J Med 67:693–696, 1979
89. McKay DG: Disseminated Intravascular Coagulation: An Intermediary Mechanism of Disease. New York, Hoeber, 1965
90. McMillan CW, Weiss AE, Johnson AM: Acquired coagulation disorders in children. Pediatr Clin North Am 19:1029–1045, 1972
91. Meguro M, Yamada K: A simple and rapid test for PIVKA-II in plasma. Thromb Res 25:109–114, 1982
92. Meyer D, Frommel D, Larrieu MJ, Zimmerman TS: Selective absence of large forms of factor VIII/von Willebrand factor in acquired von Willebrand's syndrome: Response to transfusion. Blood 54:600–606, 1979
93. Miletich JP, Jackson CM, Majerus PW: Interaction of coagulation factor Xa with human platelets. Proc Natl Acad Sci USA 74:4033, 1977
94. Miletich JP, Jackson CM, Majerus PW: Properties of the factor Xa binding sites on human platelets. J Biol Chem 253:6908, 1978
95. Natelson EA, Lynch EC, Hettig RA, Alfrey CP: Acquired factor IX deficiency in nephrotic syndrome. Ann Intern Med 73:373–378, 1970
96. Nilehn J-E, Nilsson IM: Coagulation studies in different types of myeloma. Acta Med Scand (Suppl) 445:194–199, 1966
97. Nossel HL: Radioimmunoassay of fibrinopeptides in relation to intravascular coagulation and thrombosis. N Engl J Med 295:428–432, 1976
98. Nossel HL, Younger LR, Wilner GD et al: Radioimmunoassay of human fibrinopeptide A. Proc Natl Acad Sci USA 68:2350–2353, 1971
99. Odom MH, Hurt JP, Krigman MR: Induction of thrombosis in guinea pigs by a brain tumor. Lab Invest 27:550–556, 1972
100. Olson JP, Miller LL, Troup SB: Synthesis of clotting factors by the isolated perfused rat liver. J Clin Invest 45:690–701, 1966
101. Olson RE, Suttie JW: Vitamin K and gamma carboxyglutamate biosynthesis. Vitam Horm 35:59–108, 1978
102. O'Reilly RA, Aggler PM: Studies on coumarin anticoagulant drugs: Initiation of warfarin therapy without a loading dose. Circulation 38:169–177, 1968
103. Owen CA, Bowie EJW: Chronic intravascular coagulation and fibrinolysis (ICF) syndromes (DIC). Semin Thromb Hemost 3:268–290, 1977
104. Penny R, Castaldi PA, Whitsed HM: Inflammation and haemostasis in paraproteinemias. Br J Haematol 20:35–44, 1971
105. Perkins HA, Mackenzie MR, Fudenberg HH: Hemostatic defects in dysproteinemias. Blood 35:695–707, 1970
106. Prentice CRM: Acquired coagulation disorders. Clin Haematol 14:413–442, 1985

107. Prydz H: Vitamin K–dependent clotting factors. Semin Thromb Hemost 4:1–14, 1977
108. Rabiner SF: Uremic bleeding. Prog Hemost Thromb 1:233–250, 1972
109. Rabiner SF, Hrodek O: Platelet factor 3 in normal subjects and patients with renal failure. J Clin Invest 47:901–912, 1968
110. Rabiner SF, Molinas F: The role of phenol and phenolic acids on thrombocytopathy and defective platelet aggregation of patients with renal failure. Am J Med 49:346–351, 1970
111. Rao AK, Walsh PN: Acquired qualitative platelet disorders. Clin Haematol 12:201–238, 1983
112. Rath CW, Maillard JA, Schreiner GE: Bleeding tendency in uremia. N Engl J Med 257:808–811, 1957
113. Roberts HR, Cederbaum AI: The liver and blood coagulation: Physiology and pathology. Gastroenterology 63:297–320, 1972
114. Sampson BM, Greaves M, Malia RG, Preston FE: Acquired von Willebrand's disease: Demonstration of a circulating inhibitor to the factor VIII complex in four cases. Br J Haematol 54:233, 1983
115. Sann L, Leclercq M, Bourgeois J et al: Pharmacokinetics of vitamin K, in newborn infants (abstr). Pediatr Res 17:155A, 1983
116. Schleider MA, Nachman RL, Jaffe EA, Coleman M: A clinical study of the lupus anticoagulant. Blood 48:499–509, 1976
117. Scott JP, Montgomery RR, Tubergen DG, Hays T: Acquired von Willebrand's disease in association with Wilm's tumor: Regression following treatment. Blood 58:665–669, 1981
118. Seaman AJ: The recognition of intravascular clotting: The plasma protamine paracoagulation test. Arch Intern Med 125:1016–1021, 1970
119. Shapiro SS, Hultin M: Acquired inhibitors to the blood coagulation factors. Semin Thromb Hemost 1:336–385, 1975
120. Shapiro SS, Thiagarajan P: Lupus anticoagulants. Prog Hemost Thromb 6:263–285, 1982
121. Shearer MJ, Barkhan P, Webster GR: Absorption and excretion of an oral dose of tritiated vitamin K in man. Br J Haematol 18:297–308, 1970
122. Simmons RL, Collins JA, Heisterkamp GA et al: Coagulation disorders in combat casualties. Ann Surg 169:455–481, 1969
123. Soria J, Soria C, Samama M et al: Dysfibrinogenemies acquises dans les atteintes hepatiques severes. Coagulation 3:37–44, 1970
124. Spero JA, Lewis JH, Hasiba U: Disseminated intravascular coagulation: Findings in 346 patients. Thromb Haemost 38:28–33, 1980
125. Stableforth P, Tamagnini GL, Dormandy KM: Acquired von Willebrand syndrome with inhibitors both to factor VIII clotting activity and ristocetin-induced platelet aggregation. Br J Haematol 33:565–573, 1976
126. Steihm ER, Trygstad CW: Split products of fibrin in human renal disease. Am J Med 46:774–786, 1969
127. Stewart JH, Castaldi PA: Uraemic bleeding: A reversible platelet defect corrected by dialysis. Q J Med 36:409–423, 1967
128. Strauss HS: Surgery in patients with congenital factor VII deficiency (congenital hypoconvertinemia). Blood 25:325–334, 1965
129. Sun NCJ, Bowie EJW, Kazmier FJ et al: Blood coagulation studies in patients with cancer. Mayo Clin Proc 49:636–641, 1974
130. Sutherland JM, Glueck HI, Gleser G: Hemorrhagic disease of the newborn: Breast feeding as a necessary factor in the pathogenesis. Am J Dis Child 113:524–533, 1967
131. Thaler E, Balzar E, Kopsa H, Pinggera W: Acquired Antithrombin III deficiency patients with glomerular proteinuria. Haemostasis 7:257–272, 1978
132. Thiagarajan P, Shapiro SS, De Marco L: A monoclonal IgM gamma coagulation inhibitor with phospholipid specificity: Mechanism of a lupus anticoagulant. J Clin Invest 66:397–405, 1980
133. Thomas DP, Ream J, Stuart RK: Platelet aggregation in patients with Laennec's cirrhosis of the liver. N Engl J Med 276:1344–1348, 1967

134. Thompson AR, Harker LA: Manual of Hemostasis and Thrombosis, 3rd ed, p 117. Philadelphia, FA Davis, 1983

135. Tracy PB, Peterson JM, Nesheim MB et al: Interaction of coagulation factor V and factor Va with platelets. J Biol Chem 254:10354, 1979

136. Tytgat GN, Collen D, Verstraete M: Metabolism of fibrinogen in cirrhosis of the liver. J Clin Invest 50:1690–1701, 1971

137. Vaziri ND, Branson HE, Ness R: Changes of coagulation factors IX, VIII, VII, X and V in nephrotic syndrome. Am J Med Sci 280:167–171, 1980

138. Verstraete M, Vermylen C, Vermylen J et al: Excessive consumption of blood coagulation components as cause of hemorrhagic diathesis. Am J Med 38:899–908, 1965

139. Von Felten A, Straub W, Frick PG: Dysfibrinogenemia in a patient with primary hepatoma: First observation of an abnormality of fibrin monomer aggregation. N Engl J Med 280:405–409, 1969

140. Webster WP, Mandel SR, Strike LE et al: Factor VIII synthesis: Hepatic and renal allografts in swine with von Willebrand's disease. Am J Physiol 230:1342–1348, 1976

141. Webster WP, Zukowski CF, Hutchins P et al: Plasma factor VIII synthesis and control as revealed by canine organ transplantation. Am J Physiol 22:1147–1154, 1971

142. Weiss AE, Cederbaum AI: Diagnosis and treatment of intravascular coagulation. Am Fam Physician 8:110–119, 1973

143. Weiss AE, Easterling WE, Odom MH et al: Defibrination syndrome after intra-amniotic infusion of hypertonic saline. Am J Obstet Gynecol 113:868–874, 1972

144. Whaun JM, Oski FA: Experience with disseminated intravascular coagulation in a children's hospital. Can Med Assoc J 18:963–967, 1972

145. Yatzidis H, Richet G: Activite de certaines proteines de la coagulation dans le plasma et les urines au cours du syndrome nephrotique. Rev Fr Etud Clin Biol 2:717, 1957

146. Zarrabi MH, Zucker S, Miller F et al: Immunologic and coagulation disorders in chlorpromazine-treated patients. Ann Intern Med 91:194–199, 1979

147. Zetterval O, Nilsson IM: Acquired von Willebrand's disease caused by a monoclonal antibody. Acta Med Scand 204:521–528, 1978

148. Zimmerman TS, Ruggeri ZM: Von Willebrand's disease. Clin Haematol 12:175–200, 1983

149. Zipursky A, deSa D, Hsu E et al: Clinical and laboratory diagnosis of hemostatic disorders in newborn infants. Am J Pediatr Hematol Oncol 1:217–226, 1979

Platelet Production and Structure   7

George A. Fritsma

CASE STUDY

A 38-year-old white woman came to the emergency room with multiple bruises on her limbs and trunk. She had no history of physical trauma, recent infection, chills, fever, malaise, or anorexia. She had first noticed the presence of bruises on her body upon arising in the morning about 3 days prior to seeking medical attention and said that their number had increased daily without any sign of trauma. There was no known family history of hemorrhage or easy bruising. Upon questioning the patient recalled incidents of epistaxis and menorrhagia. She was gravida 2, para 2 but not currently pregnant.

The patient was 5 feet, 5 inches tall, weighed 132 pounds, was pale, and had a blood pressure of 116/74, a pulse of 74, 15 respirations per minute, and a temperature of 98.5°F. She was in no acute distress. Lymph nodes were not enlarged, lungs were clear, and spleen and liver were normal in size. Neurologic examination was unremarkable. Purpura and petechiae were noted on the arms, legs, and trunk. There was no evidence of an active infection.

Initial Laboratory Data

CBC
    Hemoglobin 10.8 g/dl
    Hematocrit 32.7%
    RBCs 3.7 × 10⁶/μl

MCV 88 fl
MCH 29.2 pg
MCHC 30.3%
WBCs $9.2 \times 10^3/\mu l$
   Seg. neutrophils 67%
   Bands 3%
   Lymphocytes 24%
   Monocytes 4%
   Eosinophils 2%
   Platelets $12,000/\mu l$
Coagulation parameters
   PT 11.6 sec.
   APTT 41.3 sec.
   Bleeding time 11.5 min.
Urinalysis
   2+ occult blood
Chemistry screen: All within normal limits except
   Serum iron 37 μg/dl
   TIBC 480 μg/dl

The patient was admitted, and a bone marrow aspiration was performed to determine the reason for the low platelet count. All parameters were normal except for an increase in the number of megakaryocytes. Megakaryocyte morphology was normal. The patient was placed on a course of prednisone therapy, and after 6 days the platelet count went up to 40,000 and the bleeding time dropped to 6 minutes. Immunologic testing revealed the presence of anti-Pl^{A1} autoantibody.

Significant laboratory findings included the platelet count, bleeding time, and evidence of a mild normocytic/normochromic anemia. The possibility of acute leukemia is ruled out by the white count and the normal bone marrow parameters. Thrombocytopenia may be caused by diminished platelet production associated with aplastic anemia, leukemia, drug administration, or tumor replacement of myelogenous tissue. In diminished platelet production the characteristic marrow pattern includes diminished numbers of megakaryocytes. Platelet destruction is often caused by immune phenomena that include antibody attachment and reticuloendothelial clearance of platelets. The bone marrow is normal except for a responsive increase in megakaryocyte number. In chronic platelet destruction the morphology of the megakaryocytes is normal.

This patient was diagnosed as having chronic immune thrombocytopenic purpura (ITP), also termed *idiopathic thrombocytopenic purpura.* This is an autoimmune disease caused by the presence of autoantibodies specific for platelets. It most often attacks women of child bearing age. The mild normocytic-normochromic anemia, when present, is due to chronic blood loss and accompanying mild iron deficiency. Corticosteroids are used to control antibody production. Treatment with platelet concentrate is ineffective because of the immune reaction.

After 7 days the patient was released. Prednisone therapy was continued, and she was instructed to have regular platelet counts performed.

The *thrombocyte,* or *platelet,* is a 2- to 4-micrometer (μm) cytoplasmic fragment that circulates in the peripheral blood and participates in hemostasis both directly and through the intrinsic mechanism of coagulation. When the peripheral platelet count is low, clot formation is delayed and inadequate. Although normal platelets interact physically and biochemically with the coagulation mechanism at several points of the intrinsic and common pathways, platelets are usually called elements of *primary hemostasis* because their activity is most often associated with contact activation.

Platelets are called "cells" in this text and most texts, but they are actually cell fragments that, like mature erythrocytes, lack nuclei. Unlike erythrocytes, platelets are cytoplasmic fragments of much larger bone marrow cells, the *megakaryocytes.* Megakaryocytes mature and differentiate within the bone marrow along with other *myeloid* cells and upon maturity release portions of their cytoplasm to the peripheral blood. The nature and control of megakaryocyte maturation are similar to the maturation process of other cell lines.

Following release from the bone marrow, platelets remain viable for an average of 10 days. Although platelets appear uncomplicated in light microscopy, their ultrastructure is complex, changing with age and activation. The number and distribution of platelets in the peripheral blood are closely controlled, and when platelets reach the end of their life span, their destruction follows a carefully prescribed process.

This chapter describes the *myelogenous* source of platelets and shows how they are released from the bone marrow to the peripheral blood under the control of humoral messengers. The appearance of the platelet in the stained peripheral blood smear and in transmission electron microscopy (TEM) is described in detail. The structural elements of the platelet are described in relation to platelet function, which is examined in detail in Chapter 8.

HISTORY

Julius Bizzozero first described the megakaryocyte in 1882, identifying it and the *osteoclast* as the two largest cells in the bone marrow.[1] Megakaryocytes reach 150 μm in diameter and contain a single, multilobulated nucleus, a feature that distinguishes them from the multinucleate osteoclasts. Osteoclasts are *syncytial* macrophages lying adjacent to the *osseous trabeculae* that constitute bone. Osteoclasts are nonmyelogenous marrow cells that break down calcified bone and release ionic calcium into the plasma (Fig. 7-1).[11]

The first written description of circulating platelets as formed elements appeared in 1842 (see Chap. 1), but Bizzozero was the first researcher to recognize their adhesive properties and role in coagulation.[1] In 1906 J. Homer Wright published a paper that provided an important insight into the morphologic link between megakaryocytes and platelets.[14] Examining peripheral blood smears stained with "improved Romanowski stain" (later named Wright stain), he described an intracytoplasmic blue hyaline matrix that surrounds central violet granules in both megakaryocytes and circulating platelets. The additional observation that both platelets and megakaryocytes form pseudopods caused Wright to theorize a structural and functional relationship. His precocious conclusions were largely ignored until the electron microscope was applied to the study of blood cells, mostly in the late 1940s and early 1950s.

Much of the information on the ultrastructure of megakaryocytes and platelets in

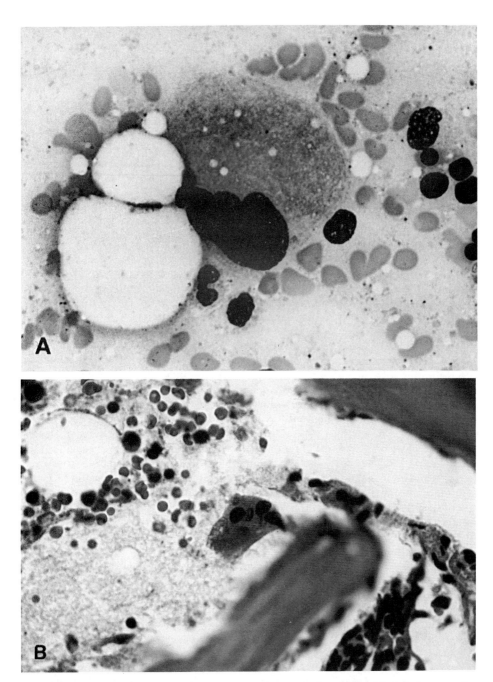

FIG. 7-1. (A) Photomicrograph of a bone marrow smear megakaryocyte with abundant granular cytoplasm and multilobulated nucleus (Wright stain, original magnification ×450, 15% reduction). (B) Photomicrograph of an osteoclast with multiple nuclei (hematoxylin eosin stain, original magnification ×450, 15% reduction).

the remainder of this chapter is based on a series of reviews published in the 1960s, notably that of J. F. David-Ferreira.[2]

ORIGIN OF MEGAKARYOCYTES

Stem Cell Mechanisms

The megakaryocyte is similar to other myeloid cells in having an undifferentiated *hematopoietic stem cell* precursor. A stem cell is capable of differentiating into one of several separate and distinct cell lines while simultaneously maintaining itself through *asymmetric mitosis*. This means that when cell division occurs, one daughter cell remains *pluripotential,* while the other, responding to a variety of partially studied environmental stimuli, enters a pathway of differentiation.

Control of Megakaryocyte Production

The hematopoietic stem cell can differentiate into myelocytic, erythrocytic, and mega-karyocytic cell lines. Recruitment to a cell line in each case depends on the presence of a plasma-soluble or *humoral* messenger protein, termed a *poietin*. For example, *erythro-poietin,* a secretion of the *juxtaglomerular apparatus* of the nephron, induces prolifera-tion of erythrocyte precursors by attaching to a recognition protein on the membrane of the stem cell. The plasma level of erythropoietin varies with tissue oxygen saturation measured by specialized kidney cells. Thus the kidney provides the link between oxy-gen saturation level of body cells and erythrocytic proliferation.

Another humoral substance, *thrombopoietin,* induces stem cell differentiation into megakaryocytes. In a 1961 experiment, plasma from platelet-depleted or *thrombo-cytopenic* rabbits was purified and given to normal mice.[10] The mice developed a transient *thrombocytosis*. In 1968 this experiment was repeated, but selenomethion-ine-75 (^{75}Se) was added to the thrombocytopenic rabbit plasma and injected into the normal mice. The ^{75}Se radioisotope is incorporated into newly formed DNA, so when it was detected in the nuclei of mouse marrow megakaryocytes a few hours after adminis-tration, the conclusion was reached that new megakaryocytes were being formed in response to the humoral substance. Thrombopoietin is known to be a glycoprotein, but its amino acid structure has not been characterized because thrombopoietin is difficult to separate from plasma in a form pure enough for biochemical characterization. The structure of thrombopoietin could be similar to erythropoietin, but the function is separate.[3] The site of production is not clear, but laboratory animal nephrectomy exper-iments suggest that the kidney is the primary site and that the liver and spleen are probable secondary sites.[9]

Thrombopoietin is not the only regulatory substance affecting megakaryocyte re-cruitment. Recent investigations suggest that a second substance, *megakaryocyte col-ony stimulating factor (Meg-CSF)* plays a role. Meg-CSF production depends solely on the mass of bone marrow megakaryocytes and is inversely proportional to their num-ber. Meg-CSF recruits stem cells for megakaryocytic differentiation but does not influ-ence growth or proliferation of committed megakaryocytes. "Ancillary" bone marrow cells — macrophages or lymphocytes — may be the source of Meg-CSF, and decreases in megakaryocyte mass somehow stimulate production of Meg-CSF by these cells. The current model for megakaryocyte proliferation postulates that Meg-CSF induces differentiation of the hematopoietic stem cell to the progenitor stage, while thrombopoietin regulates the number of mitotic divisions, the size, and the cytoplasmic content of the maturing megakaryocyte. Where the influence of Meg-CSF leaves off and thrombopoietin begins, and how the two regulators influence each other are questions that await resolution (Fig. 7-2). The mechanism by which thrombopoietin and Meg-CSF levels respond to platelet availability and megakaryocyte mass, respectively, is also unknown, as is whether the thrombopoietin response is to circulating platelets or to their total mass. A bone marrow smear from an animal with acute thrombocytopenia has a normal number of megakaryocytes but an increase in average size and DNA content. In chronic thrombocytopenia, size and DNA content are normal, but the number of megakaryocytes is increased.

The structural cells of the bony matrix influence megakaryocytopoiesis. Hematopoietic stem cells proliferate near osteoblasts, or *stromal* cells, the cells that both produce and compose the bony matrix.[13] In one experiment an animal is subjected to hematopoietic stress. Increases of granulopoietic cells are localized in the bone mar-

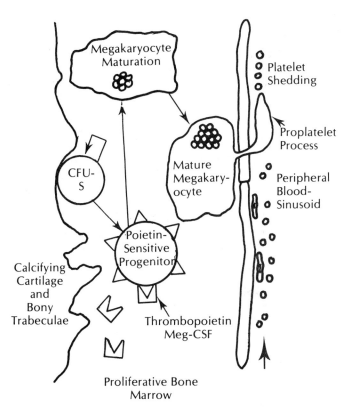

FIG. 7-2. Recruitment of the megakaryocyte from the colony-forming units (CFUs) in the proliferative bone marrow. Thrombopoietin, Meg-CSF, and the presence of bony matrix combine to impart poietin sensitivity and initiate megakaryocytic differentiation. Early maturation of the megakaryoblast and promegakaryocyte proceeds in quiescent bone marrow areas. The megakaryocyte migrates to the margin of the sinusoid to initiate the shedding process.

row, while erythropoiesis proceeds in the spleen. In another experiment, when marrow stem cells are injected into the spleen of irradiated mice, erythroid elements grow in the red pulp, granulocytic colonies form along the trabeculae, and megakaryocytic cells grow beneath the capsule. This localization implies a structural cell–proliferative cell relationship. In culture, hematopoietic cells seem to possess increased proliferative capacity when grown together with stromal cells. These experiments demonstrate that communication between structural elements and hematopoietic cells seems to promote both growth and differentiation. After the stem cell has undergone asymmetric mitosis, the daughter cell becomes sensitive to the influence of the poietin, and differentiation proceeds. The change in sensitivity is related to membrane receptor changes and may be influenced by stromal cells. Megakaryocyte growth now occurs in relatively quiet areas of the bone marrow until maturity, when the cells move to the margin of the *sinusoid.*

DIFFERENTIATION OF MEGAKARYOCYTES

Endomitosis

Light microscopic examinations of Wright-stained bone marrow smear preparations do not reveal the youngest cells committed to the megakaryocyte lineage. The megakaryocytic elements that are recognized by their size and distinct nuclear lobulation have already undergone the early stages of *endomitosis* and contain increased DNA concentrations. Endomitosis is the process of nuclear division without formation of separate daughter cells. It is unique to megakaryocytes in the human bone marrow (Fig. 7-3).[8]

The earliest stage, or *megakaryocytic progenitor,* is a daughter cell formed after the first hematopoietic stem cell mitotic division that is committed to the megakaryocyte cell line by the action of thrombopoietin. In cell culture, megakaryocytic progenitors, usually referred to as *colony-forming units (CFU-Meg)* may, with appropriate nutrients, proliferate into mature megakaryocytes. Megakaryocyte progenitor cells are presumed to contain only the normal, or 2N, level of DNA and cannot be distinguished morphologically from stem cells or other committed progenitor cells.[6]

Early endomitosis proceeds without production of cytoplasm; consequently, the youngest megakaryocytic cells are morphologically indistinguishable from other small

Megakaryocytic Endomitosis

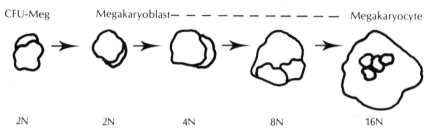

CFU-Meg   Megakaryoblast— — — — — — — — — — —   Megakaryocyte

2N   2N   4N   8N   16N

FIG. 7-3. Megakaryocytic endomitosis. Cytoplasmic growth appears at the 4N or 8N stage. Mitosis ends soon after, reaching 16N, 32N, or 64N. Cytoplasmic volume is related to the ploidy. *CFU-Meg,* colony-forming unit megakaryocyte.

bone marrow cells. Studies on human bone marrow have shown that these young cells produce surface membrane *markers* similar to those detected on circulating platelets. *Liganded* antisera — that is, specific antibodies chemically bound to measurable substances such as radioisotopes, fluorescent dyes, or enzymes — are employed in immunologic techniques to identify young megakaryocytic markers. Immune labeling is used to detect these cells in both light microscopic and TEM techniques and demonstrates them to be morphologically similar to small lymphocytes.

In the megakaryocytic progenitor stage, duplication of nuclear material proceeds to the 4N or 8N level, whereupon cytoplasmic changes render the cell morphologically distinguishable from other bone marrow elements. Mitosis does not occur beyond the progenitor stage; instead, the nucleus increases in size and lobulation. There is no proportional relationship between the amount of DNA present and the degree of nuclear lobulation, but there is a relationship between DNA concentration and cytoplasmic volume. When the 4N or 8N stage is reached, the now morphologically distinguishable cell is referred to as a *megakaryoblast.* Endomitosis continues as the cell grows; endomitosis stops at 16, 32, or 64N, somewhere in the middle of the promegakaryocyte stage.

Maturation

In most classification systems based on light microscopic examination of Wright-stained bone marrow smear preparations, three stages of megakaryocytes are identified: *stage I,* or *megakaryoblast; stage II,* or *promegakaryocyte;* and *stage III,* or *megakaryocyte* (Fig. 7-4). Stage I is the smallest and least differentiated, measures 15 μm to 50 μm in diameter, is round, and contains an unlobulated nucleus that occupies the majority of the cell. The cytoplasm is basophilic. On TEM the nucleus is shown to contain a high percentage of active euchromatin and relatively little nuclear condensation. The active

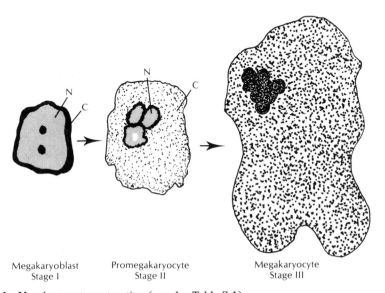

|Megakaryoblast|Promegakaryocyte|Megakaryocyte|
|Stage I|Stage II|Stage III|

FIG. 7-4. Megakaryocyte maturation (see also Table 7-1).

cytoplasm is characterized by the presence of *rough endoplasmic reticulum* (RER), characteristic of a protein-producing cell, an active *Golgi apparatus,* and *mitochondria,* but no granules. Review Table 7-1 for a summary of the stage characteristics.

Stage II megakaryocytes are also termed *promegakaryocytes* or *maturing megakaryocytes.* These are larger than megakaryoblasts, measuring 20 μm to 80 μm, irregular in shape, and with abundant cytoplasm. The nucleus is always lobulated and demonstrates greater peripheral chromatin condensation. The cytoplasm at this stage still contains plenty of RER, but the Golgi apparatus is now surrounded by *lysosomes*— small vesicles containing a variety of lytic enzymes whose hemostatic purpose is somewhat vague.

Also evident in stage II is the early development of the *demarcation membrane system (DMS).* A plasma membrane is generated throughout the cytoplasm in this stage, eventually resulting in full compartmentalization. There is both invagination and internal proliferation of the membrane structure, which will eventually result in the formation of individual platelets.

Stage III megakaryocytes are the most abundant megakaryocytic elements in the bone marrow, constituting some 85% of all megakaryocytes observed in smears from normal donors. These cells are huge, many up to 150 μm in diameter, and are best observed using 100× or low-power magnification. The nuclear material is distributed into many closely apposed lobules resembling a stack of coins or a bunch of balloons. The cytoplasm is abundant and is azurophilic because of the presence of the DMS and *granules.* Ultrastructural studies reveal that the DMS has now extended throughout the cytoplasm and that the nuclear chromatin is mostly condensed into *heterochromatin.*

TABLE 7-1
Megakaryocyte Maturation

Characteristic	Megakaryoblast	Promegakaryocyte	Megakaryocyte
Shape	Round to oval	Irregular	Irregular
Size	15–50 μm in diameter	20–80 μm at widest dimension	Up to 150 μm at widest dimension
N/C ratio	5 : 1	1 : 1	Mostly cytoplasm
Nucleus	Round to oval; chromatin dispersed and light staining; nucleoli present	Lobulated; chromatin condensed near periphery and medium staining; nucleoli are vestigial.	Highly lobulated, like a stack of coins or a bunch of balloons; chromatin is clumped.
Cytoplasm	Basophilic; clear Golgi apparatus area; deep blue stain due to presence of RER; mitochondria	Lightly granular due to presence of lysosomes; demarcation system	Highly granular due to lysosomes, alpha granules, and dense bodies; demarcation system is complete; margin is rough, undefined; pseudopodia may be present due to thrombosthenin.

Two other types of cytoplasmic granules are added during stage III. These are *dense bodies,* containing ionic calcium, serotonin, and ADP, and *alpha granules,* which contain a variety of procoagulant glycoproteins similar or identical to plasma procoagulants. Multiplicity of cytoplasmic granules gives the azure staining quality to the megakaryocyte. Also visible is a marginal zone rich in *actin* and *myosin.* These microfilamentous molecules, collectively termed *actomyosin,* are identical to the molecules that constitute the *myofilaments* of skeletal muscle and through their contractile property provide for locomotion and reorganization of the cell. *Thrombosthenin* is another term for actomyosin when found in megakaryocytes or platelets. Within the megakaryocyte–platelet system, the terms *actomyosin* and *thrombosthenin* are used synonymously.

In scanning of the bone marrow for cell classifications, all megakaryocytic stages combined make up from 0.1% to 0.5% of all myelocytic elements.

Megakaryocyte Fragmentation and Platelet Dispersal

Platelet dispersal from the bone marrow follows a well-defined process. Mature megakaryocytes migrate to a point near the wall or endothelial lining of the bone marrow *sinusoids* (see Fig. 7-3). Sinusoids are specialized capillaries with enlarged lumina and *fenestrations,* or "windows," penetrating the endothelial lining cells. The megakaryocyte extends a teardrop-shaped pseudopod or *proplatelet process* through a fenestration or a gap between endothelial cells and into the lumen, where peripheral blood passes rapidly (Fig. 7-5). The processes lengthen, bead, and disperse into peripheral blood as platelets.

The residual "naked nucleus" is soon phagocytosed by bone marrow macrophages. The time required for the entire maturation and release process is 3 days in the rat or rabbit but 4 to 5 days in the human.[13]

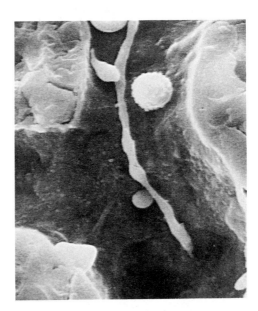

FIG. 7-5. Scanning electron photomicrograph of a proplatelet process. (DeBruyn PH: Structural substrates of bone marrow function. Semin Hematol 18:179–183, 1981)

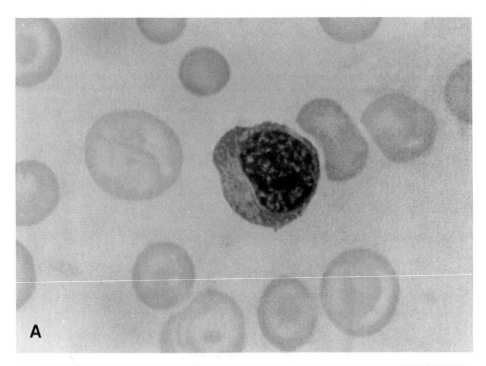

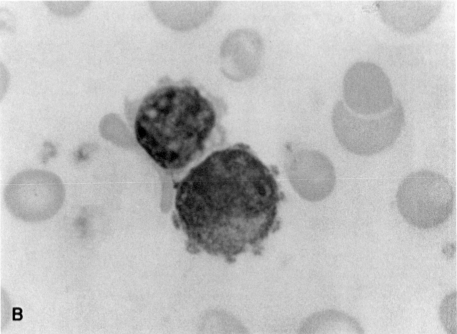

FIG. 7-6. *(A)* Photomicrograph of a peripheral blood circulating micromegakaryocyte in essential thrombocythemia (Wright stain, original magnification ×1000). *(B)* Photomicrograph of two circulating micromegakaryocytes with cytoplasmic tags in essential thrombocythemia (Wright stain, original magnification ×1000).

Although most platelets are produced in the bone marrow, any quiet site within the body where megakaryocytic progenitors can collect and where a structure is present to support the release mechanism may serve as an alternative. The lungs, for example, retain megakaryocytes and produce about 10% of circulating platelets. Small megakaryocytes, often termed *micromegakaryocytes* (Fig. 7-6), pass routinely through the peripheral blood from the bone marrow to the lungs and other peripheral sites and may on rare occasions be detected during routine smear examination. These cells closely resemble small circulating lymphocytes and may be misidentified unless attention is drawn to the distinguishing morphologic feature of the "naked nucleus." The presence of micromegakaryocytes in peripheral blood is uncommon and is most likely an indication of a *myeloproliferative disorder.*

PLATELET STRUCTURE

Wright Stain Morphology

In Wright-stained peripheral blood smears, platelets appear as discoid or *lentiform* (bean-shaped) cytoplasmic fragments with a mean of 2.5 μm in diameter or longest dimension (Fig. 7-7, A). The range of normal size is wide: 1.5 μm to 6.5 μm. Most platelets fall in the range of 1.5 μm to 3.5 μm, but a minor population of larger cells with a mean diameter of 5 μm is also present. The wide range of size is a function of the random way in which platelets fragment during production. There is some evidence that large platelets are young cells that have most recently dispersed from megakaryocytes, while small platelets are older.[8] In disorders such as ITP, in which platelet life span is significantly shortened, large cells predominate in the peripheral smear. The larger platelets possess greater metabolic activity than smaller cells, one reason why a patient with ITP may manifest no symptoms of hemorrhage in the face of remarkably low platelet counts.

Physiologically normal large platelets must be distinguished from *giant platelets* (Fig. 7-8, B), which are as large as or larger than nearby erythrocytes. Their presence, like the presence of micromegakaryocytes in peripheral blood, may indicate a myeloproliferative disorder such as *chronic myelocytic leukemia* or *essential thrombocythemia.* Giant platelets are not seen in the smears of hematologically normal persons and are associated with abnormal or uncontrolled maturation.

The cytoplasm of Wright-stained platelets is purple-blue and translucent, and a few granules may be faintly visible under light microscopy (see Fig. 7-7, A). The granules are often centrally located and surrounded by relatively clear cytoplasm. Wright referred to these regions as the *granulomere* and the *hyalomere,* placing some significance on their distribution. Regionalization is probably caused by the activation and slight contraction of platelets that occurs when they contact the glass slide. The margin may often be irregular, with several spinous processes (Fig. 7-8), also a property of glass contact.

Ultrastructure

TEM studies reveal platelets to be exceptionally complex (Fig. 7-9), lentiform in overall shape, and smooth-margined. The margin is punctured by multiple pores that are the

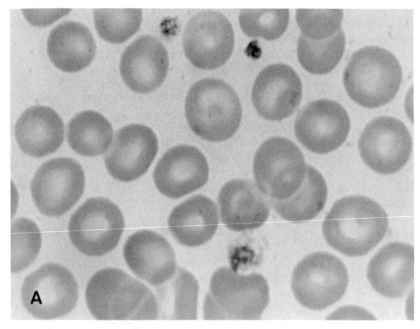

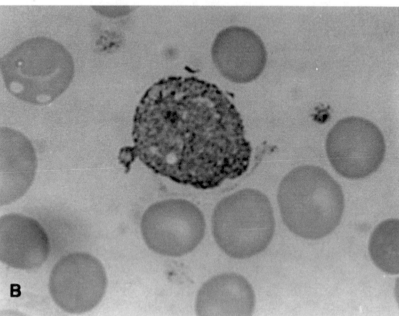

FIG. 7-7. *(A)* Photomicrograph of a normal peripheral blood smear with small and large platelets (Wright stain, original magnification × 1000). *(B)* Photomicrograph of a giant platelet in a peripheral blood smear in essential thrombocythemia (Wright stain, original magnification × 1000).

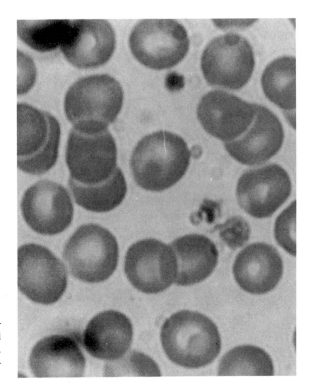

FIG. 7-8. Photomicrograph of circulating platelets in peripheral blood. Note the spinous processes. (Wright stain, original magnification ×1000)

mouths of the *open canalicular system (OCS)*, also known as the *surface connecting system (SCS)*. No other human cells are so porous.

The platelet may be subdivided into three zones: the *peripheral zone*, the *membranous zone*, and the *organelle zone* (Fig. 7-10). The contents of each of these zones are as follows:

Peripheral zone
    Platelet membrane
    Exterior coat, or *glycocalyx*
    Thrombosthenin-rich submembrane
    Circumferential microtubules
Membranous zone
    Open canalicular system
    Dense tubular system
Organelle zone
    Mitochondria
    Dense bodies
    Alpha granules
    Lysosomes
    Glycogen particles

Each of these zones is considered in turn.

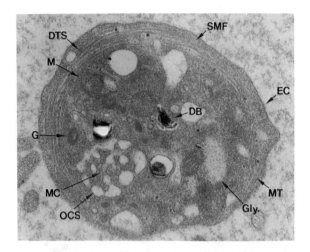

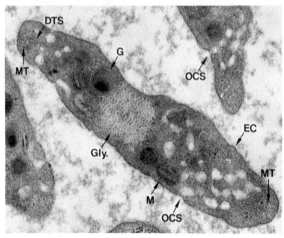

FIG. 7-9. Transmission electron photomicrographs of circulating platelets in flat *(top)* and longitudinal *(bottom)* section. *DTS*, dense tubular system; *SMF*, submembrane filaments; *EC*, exterior coat, or glycocalyx; *DB*, dense body; *MT*, microtubules; *Gly.*, glycogen particle; *OCS*, open canalicular system (surface-connecting); *MC*, membrane complex; *G*, alpha granule; *M*, mitochondria (38% reduction); White JG, Gerrard JM: Interaction of microtubules and microfilaments in platelet contractile physiology. Meth Achiev Exp Pathol 9:1–39, 1979)

Peripheral Zone

The platelet membrane, like the membranes of most human body cells, is composed of two layers of phospholipids (Fig. 7-11). A typical phospholipid molecule, phosphatidylinositol, is demonstrated in Figure 7-12. Phospholipids are composed of a three-carbon triglyceride-derived backbone where the carbon linked to the phosphoric acid (phosphate) radical is designated carbon 3. Carbon 1 is usually ester-bound to a saturated fatty acid, and carbon 2 to an unsaturated fatty acid. The phosphate portion of the phospholipid molecule, which is ionized and carries a charge, is called the *polar head group.* Because of the charge the polar head group has affinity for water molecules and is consequently termed *hydrophilic.* The fatty acid portion of the molecule is neutral in charge and tends to be insoluble in water; therefore it is termed *hydrophobic.* In a typical human cellular membrane, phospholipid molecules form a bilayer, with the polar head groups oriented toward both the aqueous plasma surrounding the cell and the internal cytoplasm; the fatty acid or *acyl* "tails" orient themselves toward each other (see Fig. 7-11). This results in the typical *trilaminar* appearance of the *fluid*

Platelet Ultrastructure

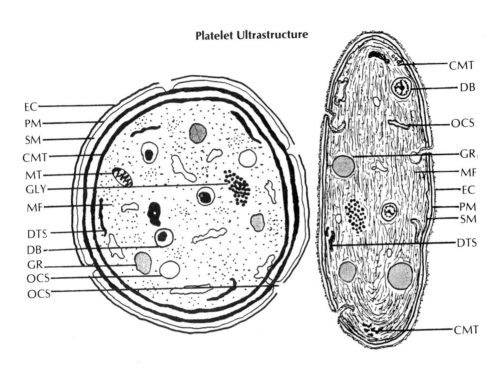

Key:
- PM: Platelet Membrane
- EC: Exterior Coat or Glycocalyx
- SM: Sub-membrane Microfilaments (Thrombosthenin)
- CMT: Circumferential Microtubules
- OCS: Open Canalicular System (Surface-connecting)
- DTS: Dense Tubular System
- MT: Mitochondria
- DB: Dense Body
- GR: Granule (Alpha Granule or Lysosome)
- GLY: Glyogen Particle
- MF: Microfilament (Thrombosthenin)

FIG. 7-10. Diagram of platelet ultrastructure. (Fritsma GA, Engelmann G, Yousof M: A review of platelet function and Testing. Am J Med Technol 47:723–729, 1981)

mosaic membrane model. The distribution of phospholipids is asymmetric because some species of the molecule are found in higher concentrations in the inner leaflet than in the outer leaflet.

Distributed throughout the phospholipid bilayer are globular integral membranous proteins. By weight, membrane proteins make up about half the membrane mass.[8] These proteins extend partly through or transfix the lipid bilayer and may extend laterally from the membrane for some distance. The proteins that extend from the inner leaflet often attach to cytoplasmic proteins, while those that are located at the outer leaflet bear carbohydrate molecules and are termed *glycoproteins*. Integral membrane

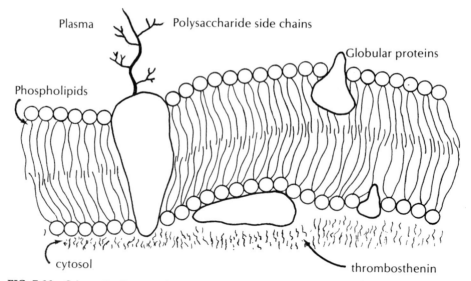

Plasma   Polysaccharide side chains

Globular proteins

Phospholipids

cytosol   thrombosthenin

FIG. 7-11. Schematic diagram of the phospholipid bilayer of a plasma membrane. The hydrophilic heads *(circles)* are directed toward the plasma and cytoplasm; the hydrophobic tails are directed inward. Proteins are embedded within or floating on the surface. Polysaccharide sidechains rise above the surface. Thrombosthenin is concentrated just under the surface.

proteins drift freely in lateral directions, provided that they are not immobilized through attachment to cytoplasmic proteins. However, their depth in the lipid bilayer is fixed, dictated by the secondary structure of the proteins. An abundance of sialic acid (neuraminic acid) provides a negative surface charge.

Five functional groups of integral membrane proteins have been described: *pumps, channels, receptors, enzymes, and structural proteins.* A given protein may serve more than one of these purposes. For example, a protein may be both structural and a receptor. Pumps effect active transport of ions across the membrane, channels allow for passage of small molecules, and receptors are usually glycoproteins that provide a recognition mechanism and localized binding of various activating substances. En-

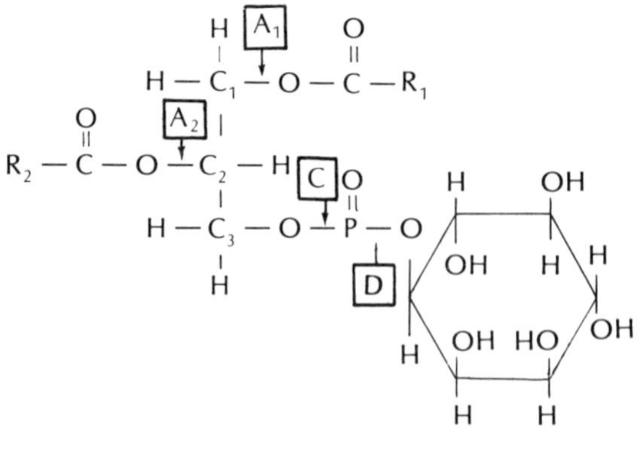

FIG. 7-12. Phosphatidylinositol (PI) is one of the membrane phospholipids. In platelets it is often concentrated on the inner leaflet of the bilayer. The ester bonds may be hydrolyzed by a variety of phospholipases *(letters in squares).* R_1 is a saturated fatty acid. R_2 is unsaturated; in PI it is often arachidonic acid. (Fritsma GA, Engelmann G, Yousof M: Control mechanisms in platelet activation. Am J Med Technol 47:813–817, 1981)

zymes may catalyze a variety of localized reactions. For example, a phospholipase serves to release unsaturated fatty acid from the number 2 carbon of the phospholipid backbone. Structural proteins may connect with the internal cytoskeleton. Glycoproteins that extend from the outer leaflet are often antigenic. Some of these glycoproteins share immunologic identity with glycoproteins of erythrocytes and leukocytes, while others are found only on platelets. Because of their antigenicity, surface glycoproteins may become involved in autoimmune reactions such as ITP.

Membrane phospholipids are important to the function of the platelet. When platelet receptor glycoproteins encounter certain specific chemical stimuli, termed activators or *agonists*, membrane-bound phospholipases catalyze the release of unsaturated fatty acids from the number 2 carbon of the phospholipid backbone.[7] These 20-carbon fatty acids are converted into *prostaglandins, thromboxanes*, and *prostacyclins*, all of which serve as intracellular messengers, directing the reorganization of the cell. In addition, phospholipid fragments of the membrane serve as sites of prothrombin activation by binding Factors V_a and X_a and by serving as a site for each of the serine protease reactions of the coagulation pathway (see Chap. 8).

The glycocalyx or exterior coat is composed of the polysaccharide side-chains of integral membrane glycoproteins plus an accumulation of additional proteins that are similar to plasma proteins and are of either plasma or platelet origin. Although all circulating blood cells tend to accumulate plasma materials on their surfaces, the glycocalyx of the platelet is unusually thick: 150 Å to 200 Å. Plasma coagulation factors predominate: fibrinogen, prothrombin, and Factors VII, IX, and X have been eluted from the surface of washed platelets. The canals of the OCS are inward extensions of the coated plasma membrane that expand the surface area and volume of the glycocalyx.

Components of the glycocalyx are essential to platelet function. Surface glycoproteins have been separated by electrophoresis into five fractions commonly designated by Roman numerals I through V. Fraction I contains a receptor protein that provides a binding site for plasma procoagulant Factor VIII/von Willebrand factor (vWF), essential to platelet adhesion. Fractions IIb and IIIa form a combined site that binds fibrinogen, necessary for aggregation (see Chap. 8). Fraction V contains a thrombin substrate. The procoagulants of the glycocalyx participate in plasma coagulation, which proceeds in part directly on the platelet surface.

Thrombosthenin microfilaments are dispersed throughout platelet cytoplasm. They are more heavily concentrated just within the plasma membrane, where they articulate with proteins of the inner leaflet.[5] All microfilaments are randomly arranged in the resting cell but become reoriented in parallel bundles upon activation as they participate in shape change. During activation they are found in higher concentrations in pseudopodic processes with the parallel arrangement still intact. Some microfilaments remain distributed throughout the cytoplasm.

Mature platelets also possess microtubules. Microtubules are hollow, nonbranching cylinders that are 22 nm in diameter and many micrometers in length and are straight, curved, or spirally wound. They are composed of *tubulin* protein dimers that polymerize to form the wall of the microtubule (Fig. 7-13). Tubulin dissociates in the presence of certain drugs such as vincristine or colchicine or at refrigerator temperature. In nucleated body cells that engage in mitosis, microtubules form the spindle fibers that direct chromatid separation during anaphase. In platelets the microtubules are assembled in an equatorial pattern referred to as the circumferential band of microtubules (CMT).

In a transmission electron photomicrograph of a platelet viewed through its short-

Tubulin
Dimers

Microtubule

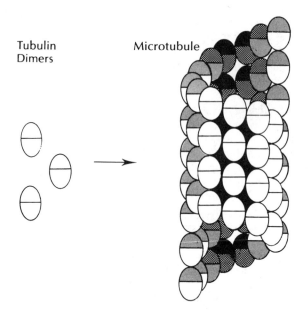

FIG. 7-13. Tubulin dimers condense to form microtubules. The tubule is a hollow bundle of 13 filaments, each made from stacked molecules of protein.

est axis (as it presents its widest face), the CMT is visible around the entire periphery. When viewed in longitudinal section, cross sections of the CMT are visible at two sites (see Fig. 7-9). The CMT appears to be a single helical microtubule that preserves the discoid or lentiform shape of the resting, circulating platelet.[11] CMTs cannot be demonstrated in newly formed platelets, nor are they visible when platelets have been exposed to refrigerator temperatures for brief periods. Chilled platelets lose their discoid shape but regain it when rewarmed to 37°C as the microtubules reform.[12] The CMT articulates with many of the microfilaments concentrated near the inner membrane layer. Together these structures form the platelet cytoskeleton that maintains its resting shape.

When the platelet becomes activated during adhesion or aggregation, a process known as reorganization results in redistribution of the organelles toward the center of the cell (see Chap. 8). This reaction accounts for the appearance of the granulomere and hyalomere seen in light microscopic preparations and is essential to the secretion of granular contents. At first glance, it would seem that reorganization is directed by the CMT; however, the tubulin molecule is noncontractile. Associated platelet microfilaments deliver the contractile force, while the CMT provides control and orientation of the reorganization process. At the time of reorganization the CMT disappears, reappearing in dispersion throughout the contractile cell and concentrated in pseudopodic fragments that may lend some structural rigidity. The centrally located organelles are now surrounded by a dense band of microfilaments rich in thrombosthenin.

Some authors group microfilaments, microtubules, and the aqueous cytoplasm into a separate "sol-gel" zone.

Membranous Zone
The platelet is the only blood cell that possesses an OCS, a patent internal extension of the plasma membrane twisting through the cell and giving it its vacuolar appearance in

cross section. There are no specialized contents. The material contained within the canaliculi is the same as that which constitutes the glycocalyx of the peripheral zone; spongelike, the platelet is capable of transporting a large mass of exterior coat material.

Platelets are secretory cells. Most cells secrete when vesicles fuse with the plasma membrane, releasing their contents to the surface. Platelet granules move toward the center during reorganization, requiring a separate mechanism to convey their contents to the outside. The OCS has been shown to connect with granules and to communicate with the outside, providing a route for secretion. Granules are squeezed during shape change, and their contents pass through the OCS to the outside.

The OCS is also essential to platelet activation early in the contractile process. When agonists are bound at the plasma membrane, the OCS conveys chemical messages inward, much as the tubules of the T-system in skeletal muscle conduct free calcium. The chemical information introduced by the OCS is processed in adjacent structures.

The dense tubular system (DTS) is one such structure. The DTS is a membranous condensation of smooth endoplasmic reticulum (SER) of the developing megakaryocyte and is analogous in origin and function to the *sarcoplasmic reticulum* of skeletal muscle. In all parts of the cell the DTS is apposed to the OCS. The DTS is the primary site for sequestration of internally functional calcium; release of this calcium is essential to cell activation. Adenyl cyclase, the enzyme that converts adenosine triphosphate (ATP) to cyclic adenosine monophosphate (cAMP), is located in the DTS. The cAMP promotes uptake of free calcium into the DTS, preventing platelet activation. Several of the enzymes associated with formation of the prostaglandins and thromboxanes (*cyclooxygenase, thromboxane synthetase*) are also present in the DTS at physiologically active concentrations. So are some of the phospholipases that catalyze release of the unsaturated fatty acids from the second carbon position of the phospholipid molecule.

The response to an activation stimulus, therefore, is transmitted to the DTS via the OCS, resulting in release of free calcium. The free calcium then initiates contraction of thrombosthenin microfilaments, controlling platelet reorganization. A full treatment of this rather complex activation process is given in Chapter 8.

Organelle Zone

Like other cells, platelets have mitochondria and glycogen granules. They do not have nuclei and do not possess protein synthesizing organelles such as RER or a Golgi apparatus. Three types of storage organelles are present: lysosomes, alpha granules, and dense bodies.[4] Lysosomes resemble the primary or azurophil granules in human blood granulocytes and contain microbiocidal enzymes, neutral proteinases, and acid hydrolases (see Contents of Platelet Granules). The proportions of contents vary from granule to granule; some are rich in peroxidase, some in acid β-galactosidase, and some in acid β-glycerophosphatase. Lysosomes respond to activating substances to secrete their enzymes, but their role in the hemostatic mechanism still requires definition. Secretion of contents requires a stronger stimulus than the secretion of materials from dense bodies and alpha granules. Furthermore, separate types of stimuli result in a variety of lysosomal release reactions. Definition of subpopulations among lysosomes may help to demonstrate their purpose.

In standard osmium TEM preparations, lysosomes and alpha granules are indistinguishable. Both are round to elongated and osmiophilic, with moderate electron density, thus appearing to be uniformly filled with a homogeneous dark gray substance. A few may have a slightly granular appearance or a central zone more dense than the rest

CONTENTS OF PLATELET GRANULES

DENSE BODIES

ATP
ADP
Ca^{2+}
Serotonin

ALPHA GRANULES

Fibrinogen
Factor V
Fibronectin
Albumin
Kallikrein
Glycoprotein G
α_2-Antiplasmin
Thrombospondin
Platelet factor 4
β-Thromboglobulin
Platelet-derived growth factor

LYSOSOMES

β-Hexosaminidase
β-Galactosidase
β-Glucuronidase
α-Arabinosidase
β-Glycerophosphatase
Aryl-sulfatase

of the material, simulating a "bull's eye."[7] Some morphologists conclude that alpha granules are larger than lysosomes and that the "bull's-eye" is not seen in lysosomes.

Alpha granules store at least 20 proteins that participate in hemostatic reactions. Most are homologous to plasma proteins, although they are probably of platelet origin. Five coagulation cofactors (vWF, fibrinogen, Factor V, high-molecular-weight kininogen, and fibronectin) and four plasma protease inhibitors (α_1-antitrypsin, α_2-macroglobulin, C1-esterase inhibitor, and α_2-antiplasmin) have been localized to the alpha granule. Platelet-specific proteins such as platelet factor 4, β-thromboglobulin, platelet-derived growth factor, and thrombospondin are known to be present. These four are important for their physiologic roles and may also be employed as laboratory markers for platelet activation, since they are not found in other blood cells. Additional factors are believed to be present in the alpha granule, and at least one, Factor XIII, is cytosolic.

Dense bodies are distinguishable from the other storage organelles in TEM preparations. They are smaller than alpha granules, and more electron-dense. Frequently the very dense material does not fill the entire space surrounded by membrane, leaving clear areas called lacunae. This appearance is an artifact of preparation and has no physiologic significance. Dense bodies contain serotonin, ATP, ADP, ionic calcium, and pyrophosphate. These substances are secreted during platelet activation and participate in the recruitment and activation of neighboring platelets and in modifying surrounding vasculature. In "storage pool disease," platelets have fewer dense bodies. Patients with this disorder have a mild hemorrhagic tendency, and their platelets do not aggregate normally. See Chapter 10 for a full description.

PLATELET KINETICS AND LIFE SPAN

Normal human marrow contains about 6×10^6 megakaryocytes per kilogram of body weight, and each megakaryocyte may produce thousands of platelets. In fact, megakaryocytes produce about 35,000 platelets per microliter of blood per day, a rate that may be increased six to eight times under stress, such as occurs in acute thrombocytopenia. Two thirds of the total body volume of platelets resides within the circulation, but one third is sequestered within the red pulp of the spleen. How the spleen promotes pooling is unknown, but it appears that platelets tend to adhere to the surfaces of splenic sinusoids. In splenomegaly vast numbers of platelets become sequestered, sometimes up to 90% of the total circulating platelet mass. In splenectomized persons, nearly 100% of platelets are retained within the circulation.

Platelets may be labeled with ^{51}Cr or ^{111}In, both of which bind firmly and have little effect on clearance. Experiments using these labeled preparations have demonstrated that the mean life span in humans averages 6.9 to 9.9 days, with a turnover rate of 10% per day. In conditions of platelet destruction such as immune thrombocytopenia, the life span may be shortened to less than 1 day, and bone marrow production fails to compensate.

Although platelets are often destroyed in peripheral vessels during functional activities, most destruction occurs in the bone marrow, spleen, and liver. Studies show that clearance of radiolabeled platelets in the circulation is linear, indicating that cell destruction is based on senescence. The physiological mechanism that detects platelet age is unknown but may rely on changes caused by the repeated involvement of platelets in minor hemostatic activities. When life span is shortened, as in ITP, thrombotic thrombocytopenic purpura, and hemolytic–uremic syndrome, the clearance curve is more nearly exponential, indicating that the pathologic destructive mechanism is blind to platelet age.

CONCLUSIONS

What were originally perceived as insignificant blood fragments turn out to be active participants in hemostasis and a part of a complex system. Platelet production in the bone marrow, under the control of a humoral mechanism, is responsive to physiologic and pathologic demands. Platelet structure is designed to provide for ongoing homeostasis. Each portion of the cell contributes to the physiological maintenance and repair of the circulatory system and may extend to participation in inflammatory systems.

Chapter 8 demonstrates how the structure of platelets relates to their function.

REFERENCES

1. Bizzozero J: Über einen neuen Formbestandtheil des Blutes und die rolle bei der Thrombose und der Blutgerinning. Virchows Arch [A] 90:261, 1882
2. David-Ferreira JF: The blood platelet: Electron microscopic studies. In Bourne GH, Danielli JH (eds): International Review of Cytology. New York, Academic Press, 1964
3. Evatt BL, Levin J, Algazy KM: Partial purification of thrombopoietin from the plasma of thrombocytopenic rabbits. Blood 54:377–388, 1979
4. Fukami MH, Salganicoff L: Human platelet storage organelles: A review. Thromb Haemost 38:963–970, 1977
5. Gerrard JM, White JG: The structure and function of platelets with emphasis on their contractile nature. Pathobiol Annu 6:31–59, 1979
6. Gewirtz AM: Human megakaryocytopoiesis. Semin Hematol 23:27–42, 1986
7. Holmsen H: Platelet metabolism and activation. Semin Hematol 22:219–240, 1985
8. Long MW: Current concepts in the development and regulation of the bone marrow megakaryocyte. J Med Technol 1:681–686, 1984
9. McDonald TP, Andrews RB, Clift R, Gottsell M: Characterization of a thrombocytopoietic-stimulating factor from kidney cell culture medium. Exp Hematol 9:288, 1981
10. Odell TT Jr, McDonald TP, Detweiler TC: Stimulation of platelet production by serum of platelet-depleted rats. Proc Soc Exp Biol Med 108:146–149, 1961
11. Ross MH, Reith EJ: Histology: A Text and Atlas. Philadelphia, JB Lippincott, 1985
12. White JG, Gerrard JM: Interaction of microtubules and microfilaments in platelet contractile physiology. Methods Achiev Exp Pathol 9:1–39, 1979
13. Williams WJ, Beutler E, Erslev AJ, Lichtman MA: Hematology, 3rd ed. New York, McGraw-Hill, 1983
14. Wright JH: The origin and nature of blood plates. Boston Med Surg J 154:643–645, 1906

Platelet Physiology

8

Larry D. Brace

CASE STUDY* A 26-year-old woman was seen for treatment of a life-long mild bleeding problem. Other members of her family had exhibited a similar bleeding disorder. Her platelet count was normal, but the results of a bleeding time were prolonged. Blood was drawn for platelet aggregation studies. Platelet aggregation in response to arachidonic acid was completely absent. In addition, her platelets were unresponsive to addition of U46619 (a thromboxane A_2 mimetic). Epinephrine addition to platelet-rich plasma (PRP) caused primary aggregation only. Addition of ADP in a concentration sufficient to cause primary and secondary aggregation in normal PRP induced shape change and primary aggregation, but only minimal secondary aggregation. Collagen addition to her PRP caused shape change, but only a minimal aggregation response. In addition, the release reaction (evaluated by lumiaggregometry) was defective, demonstrating reduced ATP (and therefore ADP and serotonin) release. In contrast, thrombin addition caused normal platelet aggregation and secretion, and her platelets agglutinated normally in response to ristocetin addition. In an attempt to further evaluate the unresponsiveness of this patient's platelets to arachidonic acid or U46619 addition, mixing experiments were performed. Arachidonic acid was added to PRP obtained from a normal donor. The aggregated platelets

* Adapted from Wu KK, Le Breton GC, Tai H-H, Chen Y-C: Abnormal platelet response to thromboxane A_2. J Clin Invest 67:1801–1804, 1981

were removed by centrifugation, and the supernate plasma was mixed with another normal donor's PRP and PRP from the patient under study. Addition of the supernate plasma caused aggregation of the normal donor's PRP, but not the patient's PRP. The ability of the patient's platelets to generate thromboxane A_2 (TXA_2) in response to arachidonic acid addition was measured by a radioimmunoassay (RIA) technique and found to be normal.

Prostacyclin (PGI_2) is the most potent known inhibitor of platelet activation. PGI_2 interacts with a specific receptor on the platelet surface, resulting in adenylate cyclase activation. Adenylate cyclase activation causes ATP conversion to cyclic adenosine monophosphate (cAMP), resulting in increased intracellular cAMP, measurable by cAMP assay. In normal platelets, this PGI_2-induced increase in cAMP can be inhibited by addition of the thromboxane mimetic U46619. However, when U46619 and PGI_2 were added to this patient's platelets, the increase in intracellular cAMP was not inhibited.

Discussion

The results presented above indicate defective secondary aggregation, an impaired release reaction, and failure of platelets to respond to arachidonic acid addition. The primary release disorders of platelets may be due to an abnormality of one or more of the enzymes involved in arachidonic acid metabolism, leading to reduced TXA_2 formation (the so-called aspirinlike defects). Alternatively, the platelet dense granules may fail to accumulate and/or store ADP, ATP, and serotonin and therefore do not have sufficient quantities of these compounds to release (storage pool deficiency). The disorder observed in this patient was due to a different mechanism, since her platelets formed normal quantities of TXA_2, and thrombin caused her platelets to aggregate and release normally. Her disorder appeared to be due to a defect in platelet responsiveness to TXA_2. Three lines of evidence support this conclusion. First, her platelets failed to respond to preformed TXA_2 in the mixing experiments. Second, platelet aggregation in response to U46619, which acts directly at the TXA_2 receptor, was not observed. Finally, U46619 failed to suppress the cAMP elevation caused by addition of PGI_2 to her platelets.

Conclusions

The bleeding disorder in this patient is probably due to a membrane abnormality in the patient's platelets, most likely a specific TXA_2 receptor abnormality.

Human blood platelets, when activated, undergo a complex series of morphologic and biochemical changes known as *shape change, aggregation,* and *secretion* (release) of the contents of their internal storage organelles. In addition, the platelet surface undergoes biochemical changes that confer the physical property known as "adhesion." The ability of platelets to adhere to a nonendothelial surface, aggregate, and secrete is a major component of the overall hemostatic mechanism. A defect in any of these platelet functions almost always leads to a bleeding disorder. The severity of the bleeding disorder depends on the severity and type of the platelet function abnormality.

In addition to platelet–platelet and platelet–vessel wall interactions, platelets and platelet products interact in the chemical coagulation sequence to promote clotting and limit blood loss following blood vessel damage. Conceptually, the hemostatic mechanism can be thought of as a triangle, the sides of which consist of the chemical coagulation sequence, platelets, and the vascular endothelium. When these three components are in balance, normal hemostasis is maintained, while a defect in any one of these components may lead to a bleeding or thrombotic disorder.

The purposes of this chapter are (1) to examine the physical and biochemical events involved in platelet activation and (2) to discuss the interaction of platelets and platelet products with the coagulation mechanism and the vascular endothelium. This discussion should lead to a better understanding of the intricacies of and interactions between the components of the hemostatic mechanism and should aid the reader to better understand the pathophysiology of bleeding problems encountered in the platelet disorders discussed in Chapter 10.

PLATELET ACTIVATION FUNCTIONS

Adhesion

Adhesion may be defined as the ability of platelets to attach to *nonendothelial* surfaces but not to one another. The intact vascular endothelium is a continuous nonthrombogenic surface to which platelets normally will not adhere. However, when the endothelium is disrupted as in vascular injury, subendothelial structures (particularly collagen) are exposed, and platelets adhere to the nonendothelial surfaces. Adhesion is the first response of platelets to vascular injury. The degree to which platelets respond to vessel injury is determined by the extent of the injury. For example, if a blood vessel is markedly dilated, the junctions between adjacent endothelial cells may separate. Platelets adhering to the edges of separated endothelial cells may be sufficient to bridge the gap between the endothelial cells. These adherent platelets will usually remain morphologically normal and may detach at a later time and reenter the circulating blood. Platelets that adhere to the exposed basement membrane generally undergo degranulation (the release reaction) and may attract additional platelets to completely cover the basement membrane. Platelets that undergo the release reaction do not reenter the circulation.

If, on the other hand, damage is sufficiently severe to breach the vessel wall, platelets will adhere to the exposed subendothelial surfaces within seconds. These adhering platelets rapidly undergo the release reaction. Over the next few minutes, additional platelets from blood flowing out of the wound adhere to the platelets already attached (aggregate). These platelets also undergo release, and the process is repeated until a *hemostatic plug* large enough to occlude the damaged site is formed. Thus, the formation of a definable clot occurs within a few minutes of vessel damage.

While the physical events involved in platelet adhesion are well documented, the biochemical events are less well defined. *Collagen* is a major component of the connective tissue that constitutes the vessel wall and supports the vascular endothelium. Exposed collagen fibrils are the major attachment site for platelet adhesion. A plasma protein, *von Willebrand factor* (vWF), is also required for normal platelet adhesion and is essential for the formation of a normal platelet thrombus.

vWF is a glycoprotein synthesized in endothelial cells and megakaryocytes.[158] This protein is present in circulating blood, is deposited in the subendothelial matrix by endothelial cells, and is also stored within the platelet alpha granules[57,185,212] (see Chap. 2 for a discussion of vWF structure and function). The subendothelial vWF binding site appears to be located on collagen; adsorption and binding are optimal in the presence of large vWF multimers and fibrillar collagen.[160]

For normal platelet adhesion to occur, vWF must bind to both the platelet surface and collagen. While the site on vWF that binds to the platelet surface has not been clearly defined, it is most likely different from the vWF binding site for collagen.[175] The vWF binding site on the platelet is generally considered to be *glycoprotein Ib (GP Ib)*[135] (see discussion of membrane glycoproteins in Chap. 7). Evidence that GP Ib is the binding site for vWF has come primarily from the study of platelets congenitally deficient in GP Ib *(Bernard-Soulier syndrome)*. Bernard-Soulier syndrome results in failure of platelets to bind vWF, defective adhesion of platelets, and a resultant bleeding disorder.

Ruggeri and associates have demonstrated that vWF will also bind to a site related to the *GP IIb–IIIa* complex when platelets are activated by thrombin or ADP.[156] However, this binding may not be physiologically relevant, since the GP IIb–IIIa complex is the platelet binding site for fibrinogen. Fibrinogen is present in far greater quantities than vWF, and fibrinogen effectively competes with vWF for binding to GP IIb–IIIa.[144,146,164] Therefore, when platelets are activated, almost all of the GP IIb–IIIa binding sites will bind fibrinogen rather than vWF.

While plasma vWF does not normally bind to the circulating quiescent platelet, binding to platelets can be observed under certain circumstances. vWF is rich in sialic acid and therefore has a relatively strong negative charge. Platelets also have a negatively charged surface; thus electrostatic repulsion appears to inhibit the binding of vWF.[158] If the negative charge on either platelets or vWF is reduced, binding of vWF to platelets is enhanced.[47] *Ristocetin* (an antibiotic with a positive charge) has been widely used *in vitro* to study the interaction of vWF with platelets. Ristocetin has the ability to cause platelet *agglutination* in the presence of normal vWF (ristocetin cofactor activity).[203] The ability of ristocetin to agglutinate platelets has been shown to reside in its positive charge. It is this positive charge of ristocetin that is thought to decrease the negative charge on the platelet surface to facilitate the binding of vWF.[38,165] The electrostatic repulsion between the platelet surface and vWF may be important in preventing unwarranted interactions in the circulation.[158]

In addition to the presence of vWF in the subendothelium and circulating blood, the alpha granules of platelets also contain a significant amount of vWF. This storage pool represents about 20% of the total circulating vWF and is composed primarily of the larger-molecular-weight multimers that are more hemostatically active.[113,157,212] However, this pool of vWF is not available for the initial adhesion of platelets. Alpha granule vWF is released only during secretion (release reaction), an activation process subsequent to adhesion.

The interaction between platelets, vWF, and the subendothelium is shown diagrammatically in Figure 8-1. When subendothelial structures are exposed, high-molecular-weight multimers of vWF are adsorbed from the blood by collagen. The adsorbed vWF supplements the collagen-bound vWF produced by endothelial cells and becomes available for attachment to platelet GP Ib. The importance of plasma vWF in this process is demonstrated by the fact that both normal plasma vWF and subendothelial bound vWF are necessary for optimal adhesion to occur.[136,182] Less than optimal adhesion is observed when plasma vWF is deficient.

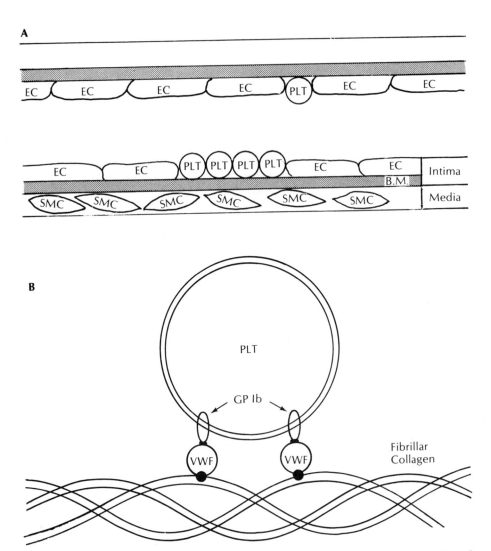

FIG. 8-1. Platelet adherence to subendothelial structures. (*A*) Drawing of a cross section through a small artery showing platelet adherence to the basement membrane. The intima is composed of the endothelial cell monolayer and the basement membrane. The basement membrane contains fibrillar collagen and vWF secreted by endothelial cells. The media contains primarily smooth muscle cells and connective tissue. (*B*) Enlarged drawing of platelet attachment to the basement membrane demonstrating vWF binding to fibrillar collagen and binding of platelet GP Ib to vWF. Note that vWF has separate binding sites for collagen and GP Ib. *PLT*, platelet; *EC*, endothelial cell; *SMC*, smooth muscle cell; *B.M.*, basement membrane; *vWF*, high-molecular-weight von Willebrand multimers; *GP Ib*, platelet membrane glycoprotein Ib.

The importance of platelet adhesion in the maintenance of normal hemostasis is illustrated by the observation that patients with vWF abnormalities or patients with a deficiency in platelet membrane GP Ib have bleeding disorders (see Chap. 10).

Two laboratory procedures can be used to test the ability of platelets to limit blood loss following vascular injury. The *tourniquet test* is used to induce vascular dilatation and minor endothelial damage. If platelets do not adhere properly to the damage sites, red blood cells will escape from the vessels, producing numerous petechiae on the surface of the skin. The *bleeding time test,* primarily a test of platelet function *in vivo,* measures the time required for bleeding to stop after a small incision is made on the volar surface of the forearm. If platelet function is normal, bleeding will stop within a specified period (depending on the technique used), whereas abnormal platelet function usually results in a prolonged bleeding time. These tests are described in more detail in Chapter 9.

An *in vitro* laboratory procedure can also be used to test platelet adhesion. In this test, blood is collected by a two-syringe technique. The blood in the first syringe is added to EDTA anticoagulant and used for a platelet count. The blood in the second syringe is then passed through a glass-bead column at a constant flow rate. As the blood exits the glass-bead column, it is collected in EDTA anticoagulant and used for a second platelet count. A platelet adhesion defect is detected when most of the platelets fail to adhere to the glass beads. Abnormal results are obtained from blood of patients with vWF abnormalities and platelet GP Ib deficiency. This test is described in more detail in Chapter 9.

Shape Change

Shape change is generally regarded to be the most sensitive index of platelet activation. Under normal conditions, platelets circulate in the blood as ovoid disks, approximately 2 μm to 4 μm in diameter. Exposure of platelets to any of a variety of platelet stimulators (agonists) leads to a change from ovoid disks to spheres with pseudopodia. If the stimulus is sufficiently strong, the platelets aggregate (stick to one another) and secrete the contents of their internal storage organelles.

The precise events involved in the platelet shape change process are not fully elucidated. However, it has been proposed that the state of reactivity of the platelet is governed by the availability of ionic, cytosolic calcium. In this connection, Brace and colleagues and others have shown that many agonists (e.g., ADP, thrombin, thromboxane A_2, prostaglandin H_2, collagen) promote internal redistribution of calcium from membrane-bound stores (such as the dense tubular system [DTS] or internal plasma membrane) into the cytoplasm.[24-26,106,139] This free cytosolic calcium then becomes available for platelet activation processes such as platelet shape change. Epinephrine appears to be an exception, in that the interaction of epinephrine with its receptor on the platelet surface appears to open a calcium channel, allowing calcium to enter the cell.[138] When the calcium entering the cell reaches a sufficient level, additional calcium from internal stores appears to be released. This process has been termed "calcium-stimulated calcium release." For reasons that are not clear, epinephrine does not cause platelet shape change.

The discoid shape of unstimulated platelets is maintained by a circumferential band of microtubules immediately beneath the plasma membrane[207] (Fig. 8-2, *A*; see also Fig. 7-10). There is a transient disassembly of microtubules during shape change, but they reassemble in the pseudopods where they seem to provide some structural support. The dissolution of the circumferential microtubules is triggered by rising cytosolic calcium levels.

In 1959, Bettex-Galland and Luscher extracted the protein thrombosthenin from platelets; this protein constitutes about 15% of the platelet cellular protein.[16,17] Further studies have revealed that thrombosthenin is identical to naturally occurring muscle protein, actomyosin. High cytosolic calcium levels promote contraction, while decreased calcium levels inhibit contraction, similar to actomyosin function in smooth muscle cells.[1,77] Electron microscopic studies of activated platelets have revealed that during shape change the randomly dispersed organelles become centralized and encircled by a web of microfilaments (Fig. 8-2, *B*). It was once thought that the circumferential microtubules simply contracted to centralize the internal organelles. It is now known that during activation, the band of microfilaments that centralizes the internal organelles is a separate structure composed primarily of actomyosin.

In summary, the events involved in shape change include calcium-triggered dissolution of circumferential microtubules with loss of the ovoid disk shape. The microtubules reassemble in the pseudopods during the transformation from ovoid disks to spheres with pseudopods. During shape change, the increased cytoplasmic calcium levels lead to the formation of a contractile gel of microfilaments of actomyosin. These microfilaments contract around the randomly dispersed organelles, forcing the organelles to the center of the cell. The exact function of the contractile microfilaments and centralization of the granules is not known with certainty. However, centralization of the granules is probably involved in secretion (a subsequent activation process), during which the contents of the storage organelles are extruded into the exterior of the platelet. If the activation stimulus is strong and cytoplasmic calcium levels rise to sufficiently high levels, aggregation and secretion will ensue. If the stimulus is insufficient to cause aggregation, however, the shape change process will reverse itself, and the platelets will resume the ovoid disk shape.

Aggregation

Platelet aggregation may be defined as the process during which platelets stick to one another (cohesion). Aggregation is an energy-dependent process requiring ATP derived primarily from glycolysis, but also to some extent from oxidative phosphorylation in the mitochondria. Glucose is the primary fuel used for energy production, although fructose, mannose, and galactose can be utilized—albeit with much less efficiency.[81] Experiments have shown that when oxidative phosphorylation in mitochondria is blocked, the ATP derived from glycolysis alone is sufficient to support the energy requirements of aggregation.[81]

The process of platelet activation is initiated when an *agonist* interacts with a specific receptor on the platelet surface. The mode of action and the internal events stimulated by each of the platelet agonists will be discussed in a later section of this chapter. In this section, the discussion of aggregation will be limited to the events that occur on the external surface of the platelet and that mediate platelet–platelet interaction. In this connection, fibrinogen and external calcium are required for the aggregation process.[121] Although plasma fibrinogen is sufficient for aggregation, experiments have shown that platelets contain a store of fibrinogen that can be released and, under certain circumstances, can support aggregation in the absence of plasma fibrinogen.[80,183]

The interaction of an agonist with its receptor and the subsequent internal events

(Text continues on p 238.)

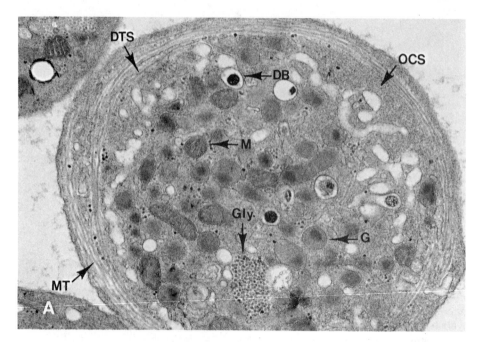

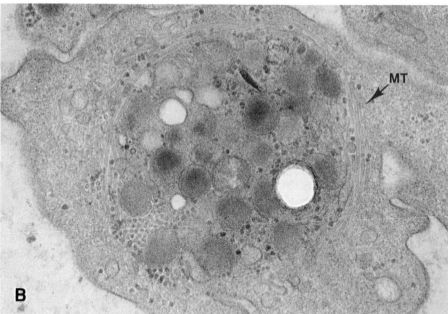

FIG. 8-2. Transmission electron micrographs of thin sections of platelets in various stages of activity. *(A)* A normal resting discoid human platelet cut in the equatorial plane. A circumferential band of microtubules *(MT)* supporting the lentiform appearance lies just under the surface. Many granules *(G)*, occasional mitochondria *(M)*, a few dense bodies *(DB)*, and masses of glycogen particles *(Gly.)* fill the cytoplasm. Elements of two channel systems, the open canalicular system *(OCS)*, communicating with the cell surface, and the dense tubular system *(DTS)*, derived from rough endoplasmic reticulum of the parent megakaryocyte, are randomly dispersed in the cytoplasmic matrix. (Original magnification ×25,000) *(B)* A shape-changed platelet from a sample of PRP stirred with the calcium ionophore A23187. The cell has lost its discoid form, become an irregular sphere, and developed pseudopods. Organelles are concentrated in the cell center and are enclosed within a tight-fitting ring of microtubules and microfilaments *(MT)*. The physical transformation stimulated by aggregating agents resembles a process of internal contraction. (Original magnification ×43,000)

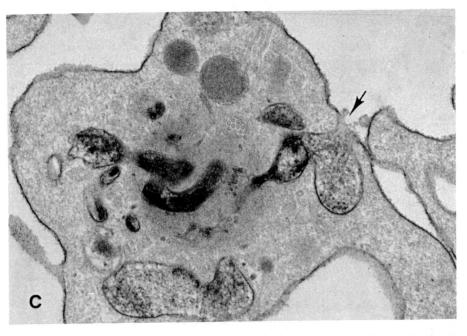

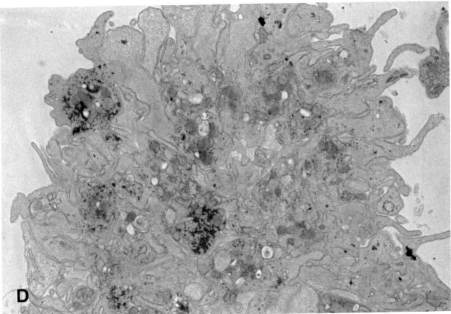

FIG. 8-2 *(Continued)*. *(C)* An activated platelet in the process of secretion. This cell was stirred with thrombin and then fixed in solutions containing tannic acid. Tannic acid combines with granule products and deposits osmic acid as an electron-dense stain. Communication between granules and channels of the OCS and the cell surface *(arrow)* is clearly delineated. (Original magnification ×43,000) *(D)* Platelet aggregate formation. A segment of de-endothelialized rabbit aorta was exposed to human blood in a flow chamber. A large platelet aggregate, also referred to as a platelet thrombus, has formed on the exposed subendothelium. The aggregate is identical in appearance to those that develop in samples of PRP stirred with potent aggregating agents *in vitro*. (Original magnification ×8000) *DB*, dense body; *DTS*, dense tubular system; *G*, granules; *Gly.*, glycogen; *M*, mitochondria; *MT*, microtubules; *OCS*, open canalicular system. (Transmission electron micrographs courtesy of Dr. James G. White, Regents' Professor and Associate Dean for Research, Departments of Laboratory Medicine and Pathology, and Pediatrics, University of Minnesota)

bring about specific changes on the membrane surface. In particular, the fibrinogen binding site becomes exposed, and fibrinogen is bound to the platelet membrane. The fibrinogen binding site has been shown to be the GP IIb–IIIa complex.[12,64] In the unstimulated platelet, GP II and GP III exist as separate proteins. However, when cytoplasmic calcium levels rise, the GP IIb–IIIa complex is formed in an *intracellular* calcium-dependent process, and fibrinogen is bound to the platelet surface.[55,56,134,143] Fibrinogen binding to GP IIb–IIIa leads to the *extracellular* calcium-dependent formation of fibrinogen/fibrin bridges between adjacent platelets and the formation of a platelet aggregate. Fibrinogen appears to have two platelet binding sites: a low-affinity site on the alpha chain and a high-affinity site on the gamma chain.[78,100,142] The precise arrangement of the fibrinogen/fibrin-calcium bridges between platelets has not been determined at this time, and other proteins such as fibronectin and thrombospondin, which bind to the GP IIb–IIIa complex, may be involved.[63,146]

The importance of fibrinogen, calcium, and the GP IIb–IIIa complex in the formation of platelet aggregates can be illustrated in the following examples. If blood is collected in EDTA rather than citrate, platelet aggregation will not occur. This is because EDTA binds calcium with high affinity, and calcium will not be available for the aggregation process. Although citrate complexes calcium, the affinity is not as high; consequently, sufficient free calcium remains to support aggregation. If platelets are isolated in a medium free of fibrinogen and under conditions in which platelet fibrinogen will not be secreted, platelets will not aggregate in response to the usual platelet-aggregating agents. Finally, if monoclonal antibodies directed against the platelet GP IIb–IIIa complex are added, the fibrinogen receptor will not be available for fibrinogen binding, and aggregation will not occur.[11,39,52] This finding is supported in that platelets deficient in GP IIb and GP IIIa (Glanzmann's thrombasthenia) will not aggregate in response to platelet aggregating agents.

Depending on the agonist or the concentration of agonist used, aggregation may proceed in two waves or phases, usually called primary and secondary aggregation. During the primary phase of platelet aggregation, small aggregates of platelets form. If small concentrations of agonist are used (*e.g.*, low concentrations of ADP), secondary aggregation may not occur, and the aggregates will begin to dissociate. After a time, nearly all of the aggregates will resolve into individual platelets. Therefore, primary aggregation is said to be reversible. If slightly higher concentrations of the agonist are used, primary aggregation will occur, followed by a variable lag time and then secondary aggregation (Fig. 8-2, *C*). The onset of secondary aggregation also marks the beginning of secretion (see below). In fact, secondary aggregation is dependent on the products released during secretion, particularly the ADP released from dense bodies. In turn, secretion is dependent on the formation of thromboxane inside the platelet except when thrombin is used as the platelet aggregating agent. If the thromboxane pathway is blocked by aspirin or other cyclooxygenase inhibitors (*in vivo* or *in vitro*), secondary aggregation will be inhibited, and only primary aggregation will be observed. If even higher concentrations of the agonist are used, a single wave of aggregation that combines primary and secondary aggregation may be observed. Whether a single wave or discernible primary and secondary waves of aggregation are observed is dependent on the agonist used. Some agonists, such as epinephrine, are absolutely dependent on secretion for secondary aggregation. If the thromboxane pathway is inhibited, epinephrine will induce only primary aggregation no matter how high the concentration used.

Although secondary aggregation is often considered irreversible, recent experiments have shown that secondary aggregation can be reversed. Addition of the potent platelet inhibitor PGI$_2$ or the thromboxane receptor antagonist 13-azaprostanoic acid (13-APA) to PRP can reverse platelet aggregation even after the onset of secondary aggregation.[108,140] This reversal of aggregation by PGI$_2$ and 13-APA is time dependent. Several minutes after the onset of secondary aggregation, addition of even high concentrations of PGI$_2$ will not cause reversal of aggregation. The inability to reverse aggregation after several minutes has elapsed is probably due to time-dependent stabilization of the platelet–platelet bridges, a process not affected by prostacyclin.

Secretion (Release Reaction)

Secretion (the release reaction) marks the final phase of platelet activation, and, as discussed above, is the cause of secondary aggregation. Secretion is the process whereby platelets release the contents of internal storage organelles. When the internal ionic calcium concentration reaches a sufficient level, secretion begins. Although the precise details of secretion are not known, the process appears to involve fusion of the storage granule membranes with the plasma membrane and release of the granule contents to the exterior of the platelet (exocytosis). The platelet granule membranes are not released but become part of the platelet cytoplasmic membrane.[81] Secretion induced by most agonists involves the formation of thromboxane, which elevates the cytosolic calcium concentration to a level adequate for secretion. Thrombin is an exception. It can induce secretion independent of the formation of thromboxane. Therefore, thrombin can be considered to be a *direct* secretagogue (*i.e.,* can cause secretion independent of aggregation).

Secretion proceeds in stages, primarily dependent on the cytosolic concentration of calcium, although other messengers may be involved. The contents of the dense granules are secreted first, followed by the contents of alpha granules. Finally, the lysosomal contents are secreted (Table 8-1).[81]

Human platelet dense bodies (dense granules) contain macromolecular complexes of calcium, ADP, ATP, and serotonin in very high concentrations. Because of the high metal ion (calcium) content, these granules appear electron dense in transmission electron micrographs, a feature from which the term *dense bodies* was derived.[81] When released to the exterior of the platelet, these products become available in very high local concentrations to promote additional platelet aggregation. As noted earlier, the released ADP is responsible for secondary aggregation and is a potent platelet activating agent. The released calcium may also promote platelet aggregation, since calcium is required for the fibrinogen/fibrin bridges between platelets. The released serotonin (5-HT) has several functions. Serotonin by itself is a weak platelet activating agent, but it promotes the activation of platelets by other agonists such as ADP.[46] In addition, serotonin is a powerful vasoconstrictor and reduces blood flow through the damaged vessel. It is also a potent stimulator of smooth muscle PGI$_2$ production and potentiates the ability of platelet-derived growth factor (PDGF) to stimulate prostacyclin production by smooth muscle cells.[41]

The function of released ATP is uncertain. The addition of high concentrations of ATP *in vitro* actually inhibits the platelet activating effects of ADP. However, the amount of ATP released during secretion is not adequate to inhibit ADP. Therefore, the overall effect of dense granule release is to promote vasoconstriction and additional platelet aggregation, thus limiting blood loss during vascular injury.

Secretion from dense bodies can be measured simultaneously with platelet aggre-

TABLE 8-1
Characteristics of Human Platelet Storage Granules

Granule	Contents	Function(s)
Dense granules	ADP	Platelet activation
	ATP	?
	Serotonin	Platelet activation, vasoconstriction, promotion of PGI_2 production by endothelial cells
	Phosphate	?
	Calcium	Platelet aggregation
	Guanine nucleotides	?
Alpha granules	Fibrinogen	Platelet aggregation, thrombus formation
	vWF	Platelet adhesion to collagen
	Plasminogen	Clot lysis
	High-molecular-weight kininogen	Contact activation
	Fibronectin	?
	α_2-Antiplasmin	Plasmin inhibition
	Factor V	Clot formation
	Albumin	?
	C1 esterase inhibitor	Complement inhibition
	Platelet factor 4	Heparin neutralization, inflammation, chemotactic for fibroblasts, hypersensitivity reactions, inhibition of contact activation
	β-Thromboglobulin	Heparin binding, chemotactic for fibroblasts
	Platelet basic protein	Platelet factor 4 and β-thromboglobulin precursor mitogen
	PDGF	Chemotactic for polymorphonuclear leukocytes and monocytes, promotion of lipid metabolism
	Thrombosponsin	Platelet aggregation, heparin binding (?)
Lysosomes	α-Arabinosidase	?
	Aryl-sulfatase	?
	β-Galactosidase	?
	β-Glucuronidase	?
	β-Glycerophosphatase	?
	β-Hexosaminidase	?

gation in the laboratory with the aid of an instrument called the lumiaggregometer[53] (see Chap. 9). This measurement relies on the cosecretion of ATP with ADP, calcium, and serotonin from dense granules. Luciferin-luciferase (a firefly tail extract) is added to the PRP, and an agonist is added. ATP released from dense bodies interacts with the luciferin-luciferase. This interaction results in luminescence, which can be detected by the instrument. The amount of luminescence is proportional to the amount of ATP (and thus calcium, serotonin, and ADP) released. This measurement is useful in examining the ability of a platelet activating agent to cause secretion or in assessing dense granule storage pool deficiency.

Like dense bodies, the contents of alpha granules are released by exocytosis from activated platelets. The alpha granule membranes appear to fuse with the membranes of the surface-connected canalicular system. This membrane fusion leads to surface expression of alpha granule membrane proteins (GP IIb and GPIIIa) and some alpha granule proteins such as high-molecular-weight kininogen and platelet fibrinogen.[64,65,183] Approximately 20 different proteins have been demonstrated in isolated alpha granules.[65] These proteins can be divided into two groups: those consisting of proteins that are similar or identical to (homologues of) plasma proteins, and those that are platelet specific. The homologues of plasma proteins include albumin, fibrinogen, vWF, plasminogen, high-molecular-weight kininogen, C1 esterase inhibitor, fibronectin, α_2-antiplasmin, coagulation Factor V, and two components of the complement system.[33,45,58,66,85,86,98,101,162,163,190,213] The function of these proteins will not be discussed here, with the exception of fibrinogen. The production of platelet alpha granule fibrinogen appears to be under different genetic control than plasma fibrinogen.[54,59] Fibrinogen isolated from alpha granules of platelets from patients with congenital plasma dysfibrinogenemia does not contain the same defect as the plasma fibrinogen of these same patients. The alpha granule fibrinogen is normal in both structure and function.[93,181]

Four platelet-specific proteins have been well characterized: platelet factor 4 (PF$_4$), β-thromboglobulin (βTG), PDGF, and thrombospondin. Thrombospondin, a major alpha granule protein, is not truly a platelet-specific protein, since endothelial cells also appear to produce thrombospondin.[86,132] The function of thrombospondin and the other platelet-specific proteins is discussed in the following sections.

PLATELET FACTOR 4. The PF$_4$ monomer contains 70 amino acids and has a molecular weight of 7800 daltons.[49,79,131,181,199] It probably exists *in vivo* as a tetramer and is secreted from alpha granules in a complex with a high-molecular-weight proteoglycan (protein and polysaccharide) carrier.[7,130] PF$_4$ has unusually high affinity for heparin. When the PF$_4$–proteoglycan carrier complex is exposed to heparin, the carrier (proteoglycan) is released, and PF$_4$ binds heparin, neutralizing its anticoagulant activity.

The best-characterized function of PF$_4$ is its heparin-neutralizing activity. However, PF$_4$ appears to have several other functions whose physiologic relevance has yet to be established. PF$_4$ is chemotactic for neutrophils and monocytes and may be responsible for the role of platelets in mediating inflammatory reactions.[50] PF$_4$ can stimulate histamine release by basophils and therefore may be implicated in hypersensitivity reactions.[29] Since PF$_4$ also has chemotactic activity for fibroblasts, a role in wound healing has been suggested.[166] In addition, PF$_4$ appears to inhibit the contact activation system of the coagulation mechanism.[200,202] Finally, a high-affinity PF$_4$ binding site on platelets has been demonstrated. PF$_4$ binding at this site results in increased sensitivity to other aggregating agents and thus appears to promote platelet aggregation.[86]

β-THROMBOGLOBULIN. The βTG protein has a molecular weight of approximately 8800 daltons and an amino acid sequence very similar to that of PF$_4$.[9] Like PF$_4$, βTG probably exists as a tetramer and binds heparin with heparin neutralizing activity.[128,129] However, in comparison with PF$_4$, βTG has a low affinity for heparin, and its physiological significance in heparin neutralization is uncertain. βTG has been shown to have potent chemotactic activity for fibroblasts and therefore may play an important role in vessel wound healing.[166]

During attempts to isolate βTG, another protein, called platelet basic protein (PBP), has been isolated.[141] This protein appears to be a precursor of both βTG and PF$_4$.[86]

PLATELET-DERIVED GROWTH FACTOR. PDGF appears to consist of two distinct polypeptide chains, but the precise amino acid sequence has not been determined.[95,150] As indicated by its name, PDGF stimulates the growth of other cells (*i.e.*, has mitogenic activity). Receptors for PDGF have been identified on a variety of cell types including vascular smooth muscle cells and skin fibroblasts.[20,89,211] When PDGF interacts with its receptor, cellular DNA synthesis is stimulated and cell proliferation is promoted.[184] Thus, when a blood vessel is damaged and platelets are activated, PDGF is liberated during secretion, smooth muscle growth is stimulated, and wound healing is promoted.

PDGF has also been implicated in the pathologic process of atherosclerosis.[155] Ross and colleagues have speculated that the development of atherosclerosis involves wound repair, but without the normal control mechanisms, leading to thickening of the vessel wall intima.[154,155] In addition to stimulating smooth muscle growth, PDGF also appears to promote accumulation of lipid, a component of atherosclerotic plaques. PDGF also has chemotactic activity for monocytes and neutrophils, smooth muscle cells, and fibroblasts.[14,51,71,92,167] These properties of PDGF make an attractive working model of atherosclerotic plaque development.

THROMBOSPONDIN. The protein thrombospondin received its name because it was first isolated from thrombin-stimulated platelets.[103,105,120] Thrombospondin is a multimeric protein with a molecular weight of approximately 410,000 to 420,000 daltons and a subunit weight of 130,000 to 145,000 daltons. It appears to be a calcium-binding protein that is cleaved by proteolytic enzymes (such as thrombin or trypsin) with the release of an NH$_2$-terminal polypeptide that contains a heparin binding site.[37,103,104] Thrombospondin released from alpha granules binds to specific receptors on the platelet surface that appear to be surface-expressed fibrinogen. Gartner and co-workers have suggested that thrombospondin plays a role in platelet aggregation.[60] An interaction between thrombospondin and fibrinogen has been demonstrated, as has crosslinking between released thrombospondin and surface-bound fibronectin and collagen. These observations suggest that the interactions among these three proteins are important in platelet aggregation and adhesion. As noted previously, thrombospondin is not a true platelet-specific protein, since it is also produced by human endothelial cells.[132]

There is currently a great deal of interest in platelet secretion products, particularly in the measurement of the platelet-specific proteins. Radioimmunoassays have been developed for measurement of PF$_4$ and βTG and have been used to detect *in vivo* platelet activation (see Chap. 9). Such measurements may become important as clues to ongoing thromboembolic disorders and as indicators of therapeutic success.

Platelets also contain lysosomal granules. Lysosomal granule contents are released by exocytosis during secretion. These granules resemble small alpha granules but are usually round and in electron micrographs do not have the eccentric zone of osmophilic material typical of alpha granules.[85] They contain a wide variety of typical lysosomal enzymes (see Table 8-1). Only a portion of the lysosomal granule contents are released even during maximal secretion, and not all agonists are capable of causing maximal lysosomal release.[2,82]

The function of platelet lysosomes is not well understood. Platelets do not function in bacterial killing, the usual function of lysosomes. The secreted enzymes may play a role in viscous metamorphosis or resolution of the platelet plug formed at the site of vascular damage, but no direct evidence for these functions exists.

BIOCHEMISTRY OF PLATELET ACTIVATION

Production and Function of Thromboxane

Only small amounts of free ionic calcium are present in the cytosol of the quiescent platelet; free calcium in the cytosol is estimated to be 10^{-7} M. Whenever platelets become activated, cytosolic calcium levels rise. Where does this calcium come from? Available evidence indicates that there are at least two pools of intracellular calcium. The DTS in the platelet is known to accumulate calcium in high concentration and can release this calcium upon appropriate stimulation.[61,97,159] Another pool of calcium is thought to be associated with the cytoplasmic surface of the plasma membrane, perhaps bound to polyphosphatidylinositol.

As discussed in Chapter 7, phosphatidylinositol (PI) is a component of the platelet membrane and is located preferentially on the inner surface of the plasma membrane. Some of the PI is enzymatically converted to diphosphatidylinositol (DPI) and triphosphatidlyinositol (TPI) (phosphatidylinositol-4'-monophosphate and phosphatidylinositol-4',5'-bisphosphate, respectively). PI constitutes about 4% of the total membrane phospholipids, while the polyphosphatidylinositols (DPI and TPI) constitute about 1%.[112] The unique structure of TPI, with its two closely spaced phosphate groups at the 4 and 5 positions of inositol (Fig. 8-3), represents a potential binding site for ionic calcium.[123] In addition, the fatty acid esterified to the number 2 position of the phosphoinositides is almost exclusively arachidonic acid. These properties of phosphoinositides (*i.e.*, the preferential location on the inner leaflet of the membrane, the potential

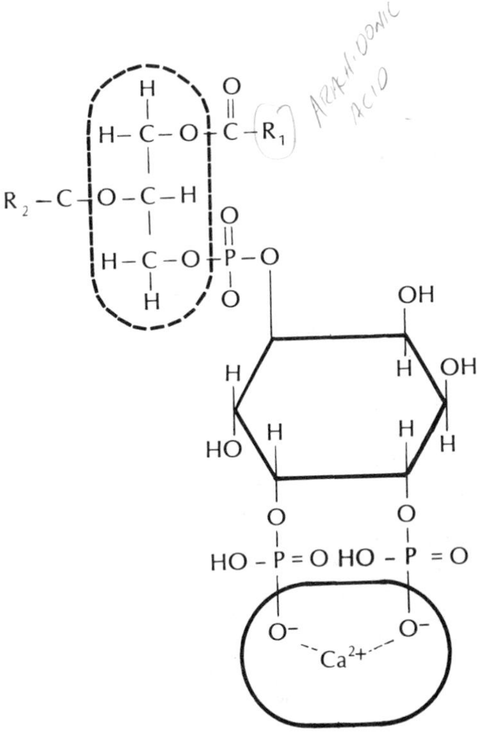

FIG. 8-3. Structure of TPI. The glycerol backbone is enclosed in the broken line. The potential calcium binding region is enclosed by the solid line. R_1, a saturated fatty acid; R_2, an unsaturated fatty acid, usually arachidonic acid.

ability to bind calcium, and the high content of arachidonic acid) make it an attractive target for membrane signaling during platelet activation.

Interaction of an agonist with its receptor on the platelet surface leads to rapid turnover of the phosphatidylinositides and calcium mobilization from membrane-bound stores into the cytoplasm. The rapid turnover and resynthesis of the polyphosphatidylinositols has been referred to as the PPI cycle or PPI response (Fig. 8-4).[123] TPI is hydrolyzed to a diglyceride (DG) and inositol triphosphate. The DG can be cycled back to PI (and ultimately TPI) or further degraded (see below). The DG is cycled back to PI in two steps: it is phosphorylated at the 3 position to form phosphatidic acid, and subsequently an inositol molecule is attached to yield PI.

At the same time that the PPI cycle begins, the PI cycle is also initiated.[148] In this cycle PI is converted to DG by phospholipase C (PLC), and DG is recycled to PI as in the PPI cycle (see Fig. 8-4). Unlike the PPI cycle, the PI cycle appears to *require* calcium, since the enzyme responsible for breakdown of PI to DG (PLC) is dependent on calcium for activity.[18,153] Thus it may be that TPI turnover releases sufficient calcium to activate PLC and initiate the PI cycle. It should be noted, however, that no direct evidence for the linkage of these two cycles is currently available.

Recently, another mechanism for calcium release and initiation of the PI cycle has

PI and PPI Cycles

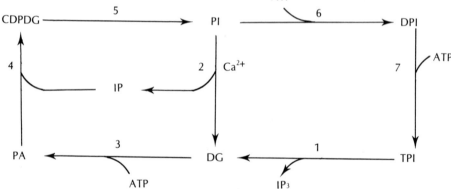

FIG. 8-4. The PI (phosphatidylinositol) and PPI (polyphosphatidylinositol) cycles. The numbers indicate the enzymes in the PI and PPI cycles and are listed below. TPI is acted upon by a TPI-specific phosphodiesterase to yield diacylglycerol (DG) and inositol triphosphate (IP_3). PI is acted upon by the calcium-requiring PI-specific phospholipase C (PLC) to yield DG and inositol phosphate (IP). DG is phosphorylated by DG kinase in a reaction requiring ATP to form phosphatidic acid (PA). PA is converted by diglyceride cytidyltransferase to cytidine diphosphate diacylglycerol (CDPDG). CDPDG is converted to PI by diacylglycerol inositol transferase. PI can be converted to DPI by PI kinase and ATP. DPI is converted to TPI by DPI kinase and ATP. The cycle on the left is known as the PI cycle, the cycle on the right the TPI cycle. PI, phosphatidylinositol; DPI, phosphatidylinositiol 4-bisphosphate; TPI, phosphatidylinositol 4 5-bisphosphate; DG, diacylglycerol; PA, phosphatidic acid; CDPDG, cytidine diphosphate diacylglycerol; IP, inositol phosphate; IP_3, inositol triphosphate; 1, TPI-specific phosphodiesterase; 2, PI-specific phosphodiesterase (PLC); 3, diacylglycerol kinase; 4, diacylglycerol cytidyl transferase; 5, diacylglycerol inositol transferase; 6, PI kinase; 7, DPI kinase.

been proposed. Reaction of an agonist with its receptor on the surface of the platelet causes activation of DG kinase, which acts on preformed DG (known to exist in small quantities in the membrane) to form phosphatidic acid. (PA; Fig. 8-5). PA is proposed to cause calcium mobilization, which activates PLC. Hydrolysis of PI by activated PLC initiates the PI cycle, with subsequent formation of DG and more PA.[84] The mechanism

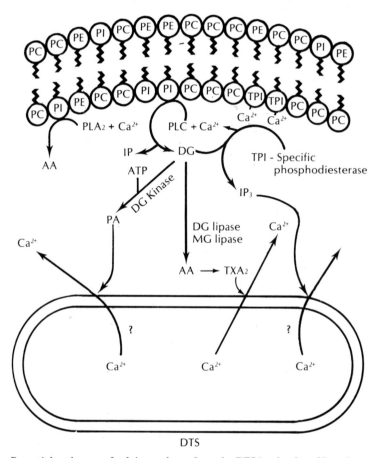

FIG. 8-5. Potential pathways of calcium release from the DTS in platelets. Note the asymmetric distribution of phospholipids in the membrane, with preferential concentration of the PIs on the inner leaflet and phosphatidylethanolamine *(PE)* on the outer leaflet. TPI breakdown releases inositol triphosphate *(IP3)* DG, and perhaps calcium. IP_3 may be a messenger for release of calcium from the DTS. PLA_2 in the presence of calcium hydrolyzes PI to release AA. PLC in the presence of calcium hydrolyzes PI to yield IP and DG. DG is metabolized by DG and MG lipases to yield AA. AA is converted to thromboxane A_2 *(TXA2)* by enzymes of the DTS membrane, and TXA_2 causes calcium release from the DTS. Alternatively, DG can be phosphorylated to PA. PA has been proposed as a messenger for calcium release from the DTS. *PC*, phosphatidylcholine; *PE*, phosphatidylethanolamine; *PI*, phosphatidylinositol; *TPI*, phosphatidylinositol 4,5-bisphosphate; *PLC*, phospholipase C; PLA_2, phospholipase A_2; *IP*, inositol phosphate; IP_3, inositol triphosphate; *AA*, arachidonic acid; TXA_2, thromboxane A_2; *DTS*, dense tubular system; *PA*, phosphatidic acid; *DG lipase*, diacylglycerol lipase; *MG lipase*, monoacylglycerol lipase; *DG*, diacylglycerol (diglyceride); *?*, release of calcium from the DTS by this agent has not been proved.

by which PA causes calcium mobilization is proposed to be that of an ionophore (*i.e.*, an agent capable of transporting ions across biologic membranes) for calcium. However, this proposed property of PA has never been demonstrated in intact platelets.

More recently, it has been suggested that TPI breakdown to DG and inositol triphosphate is critical to platelet activation. Berridge and Irvine have proposed that the lipid-soluble DG activates protein kinase C, while water-soluble inositol triphosphate is the messenger for release of internal calcium (see Fig. 8-5).[15] Protein kinase C causes the phosphorylation of myosin light chain kinase, a reaction that is necessary for actomyosin contraction.[133] Protein kinase C activation requires calcium and is greatly amplified by DG. It is not known whether inositol triphosphate acts as a calcium carrier or interacts with a receptor to cause calcium release.

Thus, initiation of the PI and PPI cycles by interaction of platelet activating agents with their receptors on the platelet surface causes the release or production of several agents that may participate as internal messengers for platelet activation. Specifically, these are calcium and arachidonic acid (AA) release, and DG, PA, and inositol triphosphate formation. The relative contribution of each of these agents to platelet activation has not been determined.

Concurrent with the activities of the PI and PPI cycles is the liberation of AA. As discussed above, DG can be enzymatically recycled to PI. However, platelets also contain DG and monoglyceride lipases.[147] Acting in concert, these two enzymes are capable of reducing DG to glycerol and two free fatty acids, one of which is AA (Fig. 8-6). It is not clear at this point which of the two enzymes is responsible for arachidonic acid release. The DG lipase may act directly at the 2 position of DG to directly release AA. Alternatively, it may act at the 1 position to yield a monoglyceride (MG) upon which MG lipase acts to liberate AA. Another possibility is that AA is released by both mechanisms.

An alternate mechanism of AA release involves the enzyme phospholipase A_2 (PLA_2). This enzyme acts directly at the 2 position of PI to release AA, and, like PLC, PLA_2 is calcium dependent (see Fig. 8-6).[48] However, kinetic studies of the activity of PLA_2 suggest that release of AA by PLA_2 is too slow to account for the rate of appearance of free AA during platelet activation.[133,186] Therefore, the physiologic role of PLA_2 in AA release is not known with certainty.

AA, once released, may be re-esterified into phospholipids (see above) or further metabolized in the platelet by the heme-containing enzyme cyclooxygenase (Fig. 8-7). Platelets are active in resynthesizing phospholipids and can use glycerol as the starting material. Current evidence indicates that the great majority of fatty acids released are re-esterified into phospholipids without further metabolism. However, cyclooxygenase (CO) converts some of the released AA (a 20-carbon fatty acid) to the cyclic endoperoxide prostaglandin G_2 (PGG_2). PGG_2 is rapidly converted by the enzyme peroxidase to another cyclic endoperoxide, prostaglandin H_2 (PGH_2). PGH_2 is acted on by the enzyme thromboxane synthase to form TXA_2, the most potent platelet activating agent known[74,75] (see Fig. 8-7). TXA_2 interacts with a specific receptor in the platelet to cause further calcium release and platelet activation (including the release reaction). TXA_2 has a very short half-life (probably less than 1 minute) and spontaneously degrades to a stable metabolic thromboxane end-product, thromboxane B_2 (TXB_2). Antibodies against TXB_2 have been developed, so TXB_2 can now be measured by an RIA technique. Although under normal conditions almost all of the PGH_2 formed is converted to TXA_2, it should be noted that PGH_2 is itself a powerful platelet activator that, like TXA_2, causes internal calcium mobilization.[24-26]

In close proximity to the inner surface of the plasma membrane is a membraneous

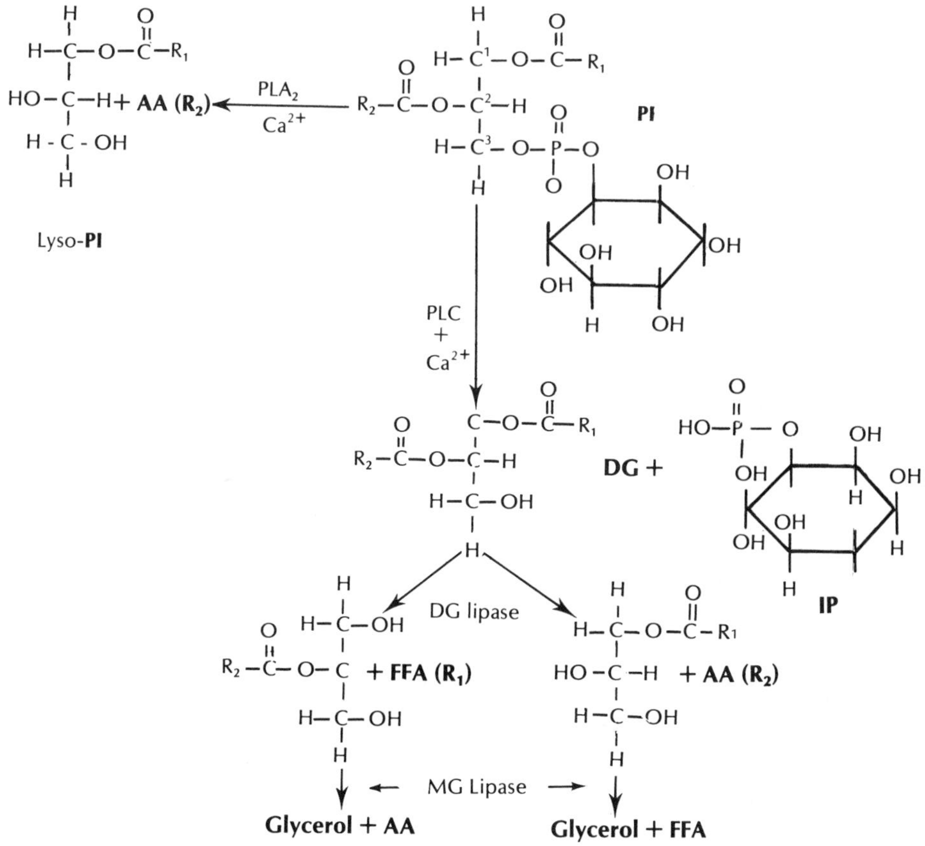

FIG. 8-6. Mechanisms of arachidonic acid release from PI. Arachidonic acid *(AA)* can be directly released from PI by the action of calcium-requiring phospholipase A$_2$ *(PLA$_2$)* to yield lyso-phosphatidylinositol *(lyso-PI)* and AA. Alternatively, PI is broken down to diacylglycerol *(DG)* and inositol phosphate *(IP)* by the calcium-requiring PLC. DG is further catabolized by DG lipase to a monoglyceride *(MG)* and a free fatty acid *(FFA)* or an MG and an AA. The monoglyceride is acted upon by MG lipase to form glycerol and AA or glycerol and an FFA. *PLA$_2$*, phospholipase A$_2$; *PI*, phosphatidylinositol; *lyso-PI*, lyso-phosphatidylinositol; *PLC*, phospholipase C; *DG*, diacylglycerol; *IP*, inositol phosphate; *DG lipase*, diacylglycerol lipase; *R$_1$*, saturated fatty acid; *R$_2$*, arachidonic acid; *AA*, arachidonic acid; *FFA*, free fatty acid; *MG lipase*, monoacylglycerol lipase.

structure known as the dense tubular system, or DTS (see Figs. 7-12 and 8-2, *A*). TXA$_2$ (and PGH$_2$) can cause release of calcium from the DTS, and the enzymes responsible for the metabolism of AA to thromboxane (*i.e.,* CO and thromboxane synthase) are localized on the membranes of the DTS.[31,62,159] Thus, thromboxane is formed on the DTS membranes, calcium is released from the DTS, and the cytosolic calcium levels rise (see Fig. 8-5). This rise in cytosolic calcium supports additional platelet activation processes such as actomyosin contraction, secretion, and so forth. Because the DTS is close to the plasma membrane (from which AA is released), AA can be efficiently transformed to TXA$_2$ by the enzymes of the DTS membranes. While it is logical to suppose

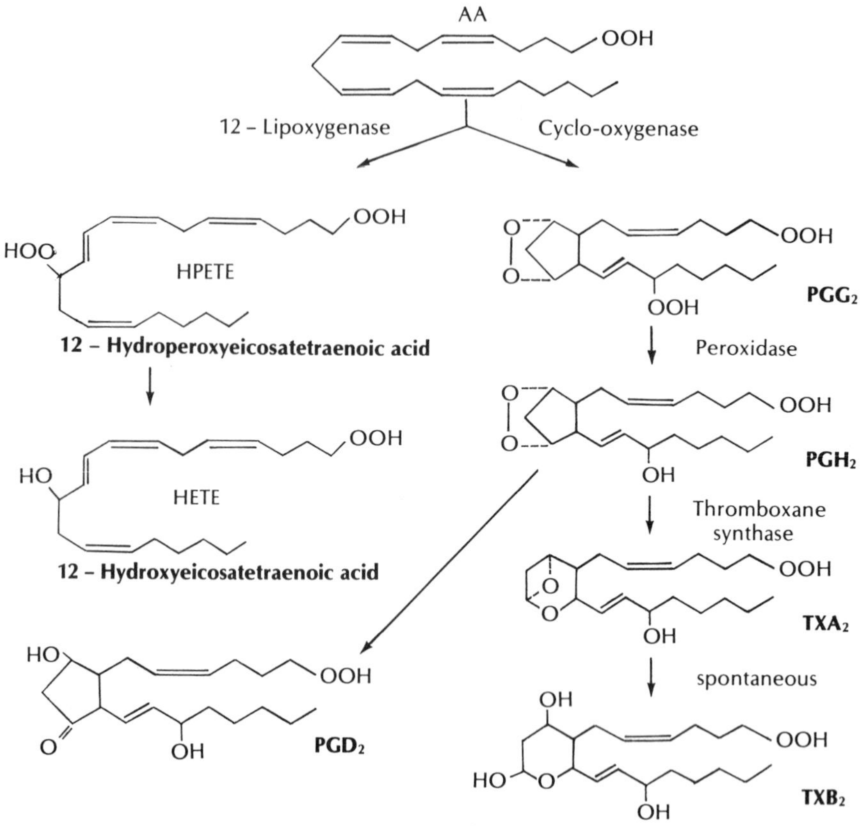

FIG. 8-7. Pathways of AA metabolism in the platelet. PGG_2, prostaglandin G_2; PGH_2, prostaglandin H_2; PGD_2, prostaglandin D_2; TXA_2, thromboxane A_2; TXB_2, thromboxane B_2.

that the thromboxane receptor is located on the DTS, this has not been proved. However, Lim and colleagues have recently presented evidence for isolation of the thromboxane receptor from platelet membranes, and the location of the thromboxane receptor in platelets should be identified in the near future.[111] In addition to the ability to release calcium, the DTS can also actively accumulate calcium.[159] The ability of the DTS to actively accumulate and release calcium provides an attractive analogy to the sarcoplasmic reticulum of muscle.

Because AA metabolism has a central role in platelet activation, numerous drugs that inhibit various steps in the thromboxane pathway have been developed. These drugs are used in an attempt to regulate platelet reactivity. Examples of these drugs include indomethacin and aspirin (which inhibit the CO) and thromboxane synthase inhibitors (which inhibit the conversion of PGH_2 to TXA_2). However, total blockade of thromboxane production *in vivo* does not generally lead to bleeding, probably because only one pathway of platelet activation is inhibited. In fact, the observation that severely thrombocytopenic patients have hemorrhagic problems while patients on aspirin do not is testament to the ability of platelets to be activated through pathways other than thromboxane. The following section examines the role of other platelet agonists in platelet activation.

Agonists of Platelet Activation

Arachidonic Acid

AA (see Fig. 8-7) can be added directly to platelet suspensions as either the free acid or the sodium salt. This exogenous AA is rapidly taken up by the platelets, and, in essence, the need for release of AA from membrane phospholipids is bypassed. The absorbed AA is then available to platelet CO and is rapidly converted to TXA_2 (see Figs. 8-7 and 8-8), a potent platelet activator. When AA is added to intact functional platelets, a single wave of platelet aggregation is observed. This is because TXA_2 induces platelets to aggregate by first causing platelets to secrete ADP from dense granules. Thus, in the case of TXA_2, secretion and aggregation occur almost simultaneously. If platelet CO is inhibited, AA-induced aggregation and secretion will not occur, and only shape change will be observed. Thus, AA is a useful tool in the clinical laboratory to assess the function of the thromboxane pathway in platelets.

ADP

The structure of ADP is shown in Figure 8-9. The outer surface of the platelet membrane contains specific ADP receptors.[19,115] These ADP receptors are coupled to the enzyme adenylate cyclase located on the inner surface of the plasma membrane (see Fig. 8-8). Adenylate cyclase is responsible for converting ATP to cAMP (see Fig. 8-8). Increased cellular cAMP levels lead to a decrease in free calcium in the cytoplasm, which inhibits platelet activation. Owen and Le Breton have proposed that calcium is pumped from the cytoplasm into a storage site, perhaps the DTS, by a cAMP-driven cation pump[139] (see Fig. 8-8). The ADP receptor is coupled to adenylate cyclase through an inhibitory subunit. When ADP interacts with the receptor, adenylate cyclase is actually inhibited (*i.e.,* negative coupling). This ADP-induced inhibition of adenylate cyclase prevents an increase in cellular cAMP levels and therefore inhibits the mechanism responsible for *lowering* the cytosolic calcium level. In addition, when ADP reacts with the receptor, calcium is mobilized from intracellular stores, thus raising the cytosolic calcium level.[107] Thus the mechanism for lowering the concentration of cytoplasmic calcium (*i.e.,* production of cAMP) is inhibited while calcium is released from an internal pool. The release of calcium from a storage pool and inhibition of adenylate cyclase lead to an elevated cytoplasmic calcium concentration. The high cytosolic calcium concentration also inhibits adenylate cyclase, which in turn further inhibits cAMP production. In the intact platelet the released calcium is used to initiate the internal activation mechanisms discussed in the preceding section.

When the ability of ADP to activate platelets is tested *in vitro* by platelet aggregometry, a concentration of ADP that causes biphasic platelet aggregation — that is, primary and secondary aggregation — can be found. The secondary aggregation is caused by the release of ADP during secretion and is dependent on the formation of thromboxane. If the CO is inhibited and the same concentration of ADP is used, only primary aggregation will be observed. If, however, much higher concentrations of ADP are used, a monophasic aggregation curve will be obtained. This is because the ADP normally supplied by secretion (responsible for secondary aggregation) has, in essence, been replaced by the added ADP. Thus, nearly the same degree of platelet aggregation can be obtained through the use of ADP in CO-inhibited platelets, but much higher concentra-

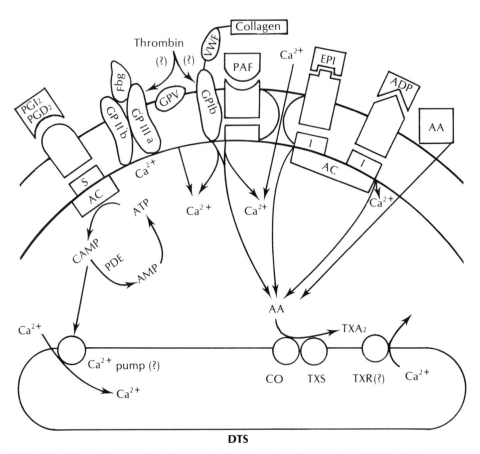

FIG. 8-8. Effects of receptor binding on the platelet surface. Interaction of ADP with its receptor causes coupling of adenylate cyclase *(AC)* to its inhibitory subunit *(I)* and inhibition of AC enzyme activity. Concurrently, calcium is released from an internal store, and AA is released from membrane phospholipids. When epinephrine *(EPI)* binds to the α_2 receptor, AC becomes coupled to its inhibitory subunit. In addition, a calcium channel appears to be opened, allowing calcium to enter the cell. The rising intracellular calcium concentration triggers AA release from membrane phospholipids. The binding of platelet activating factor (PAF) to its receptor also appears to open a calcium channel, perhaps the same channel as epinephrine, allowing calcium to enter the cell. In addition, calcium appears to be released from an internal store, and AA is released from membrane phospholipids. The interaction of thrombin with its receptor (GP Ib and/or GP V) causes calcium release from an internal store and AA release from membrane phospholipids. However, the ability of thrombin to activate platelets is not dependent on AA release. Collagen binding to GP Ib in the presence of vWF also causes calcium and AA release. The GP IIb–IIIa complex is the fibrinogen *(Fbg)* receptor. However, platelets must be activated by an agonist in order for fibrinogen to bind. The ability of GPIIb–IIIa to bind Fbg may depend on elevated cytosolic calcium concentration. Binding of the inhibitory prostaglandins (PGI$_2$, PGD$_2$) to receptors couples AC to the stimulatory subunit, activating AC. In its activated state, AC rapidly converts ATP to cAMP. cAMP appears to stimulate a calcium sequestering mechanism on the DTS (a calcium pump), causing cytosolic calcium to enter the DTS and leading to reduced cytosolic calcium concentration. It should be noted that reduced cytosolic calcium concentration is stimulatory for AC, while elevated cytosolic calcium is inhibitory to AC. cAMP is broken down to AMP by the action of a phosphodiesterase

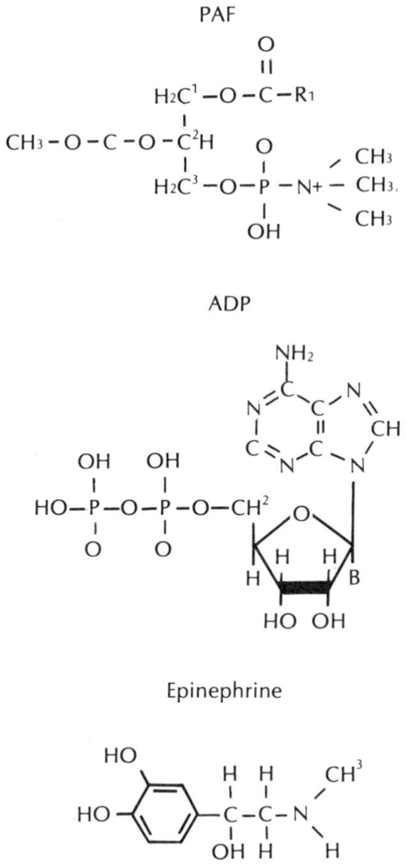

PAF

$$O$$
$$||$$
$$H_2C^1-O-C-R_1$$
$$|$$
$$CH_3-O-C-O-C^2H \quad O$$
$$| \quad | \quad \nearrow CH_3$$
$$H_2C^3-O-P-N^+-CH_3.$$
$$| \quad \searrow CH_3$$
$$OH$$

ADP

$$NH_2$$

$$OH \quad OH$$
$$| \quad |$$
$$HO-P-O-P-O-CH^2$$
$$| \quad |$$
$$O \quad O$$

$$HO \quad OH$$

Epinephrine

$$HO$$
$$HO \quad \quad H \quad H \quad CH^3$$
$$| \quad | \quad \nearrow$$
$$C-C-N$$
$$| \quad | \quad \searrow$$
$$OH \quad H \quad H$$

FIG. 8-9. Chemical structures of platelet-activating factor *(PAF)*, ADP, and epinephrine.

tions of ADP are required than when untreated platelets are used. If only a high concentration of ADP is used in the clinical laboratory to evaluate platelet reactivity, the ability of platelets to secrete ADP cannot be assessed.

Two other adenosine phosphate compounds, ATP and AMP, will also bind to the ADP receptor. Both AMP and ATP are actually antagonists of ADP-induced platelet activation and can reverse ADP-induced platelet aggregation.[19] When ATP or AMP is

(PDE). AMP can be rephosphorylated to ATP. Exogenously added AA does not interact with a cytoplasmic membrane receptor but is absorbed by the platelet. AA (either absorbed or released from membrane phospholipids) is rapidly converted to TXA_2 by the action of CO and thromboxane synthase *(TXS)* located on the DTS membranes. TXA_2 causes calcium release from the DTS, perhaps by binding to a thromboxane receptor *(TXR)* on the DTS. *AA*, arachidonic acid; *EPI*, epinephrine; *PAF*, platelet activating factor; *vWF*, von Willebrand factor; *GP*, glycoprotein; *FBG*, fibrinogen; *PGI_2*, prostaglandin I_2; *PGD_2*, prostaglandin D_2; *AC*, adenylate cyclase; *S*, stimulatory subunit of AC; *I*, inhibitory subunit of AC; *cAMP*, cyclic AMP; *PDE*, cAMP phosphodiesterase; *CO*, cyclooxygenase; *TXS*, thromboxane synthase; *TXR*, thromboxane receptor; *TXA_2*, thromboxane A_2, *(?)*, not yet proven.

bound to the receptor, no activation occurs, and ADP binding to the receptor is inhibited (*i.e.,* they are competitive inhibitors). However, high concentrations of ATP and AMP are required. The ability to reverse platelet aggregation is useful in experimental evaluation of platelet activation mechanisms, but is probably of minor physiological importance.

In addition to the adenine nucleotides contained in dense bodies, the platelet cytosol contains a metabolically active pool of adenine nucleotides (ATP, ADP, and AMP) that is used primarily to provide energy to the cell. This metabolic pool of adenine nucleotides is not released during secretion and therefore is not available to enhance platelet activation processes by interacting with the platelet ADP receptors.[83]

Epinephrine

The structure of epinephrine is shown in Figure 8-9. In the human, at least three different receptors for epinephrine are known: α_1, α_2, and β. The platelet surface contains only α_2 receptors, which, like ADP receptors, are negatively coupled to adenylate cyclase (see Fig. 8-8). Epinephrine is an unusual agonist. When epinephrine interacts with the α_2 receptor on platelets, shape change does not occur. The mechanism of action of epinephrine appears to involve a calcium channel, presumably in close proximity or attached to the α_2 receptor (see Fig. 8-8). When epinephrine binds to the receptor, adenylate cyclase is inhibited, and the calcium channel opens, allowing calcium to cross the membrane and enter the cytoplasm. However, epinephrine does not appear to directly cause calcium mobilization from an intracellular store, like ADP.[138] Eventually, cytoplasmic calcium reaches a level sufficient to trigger internal platelet activation, leading to thromboxane formation and secretion. The ability of epinephrine to cause platelet activation is absolutely dependent on extracellular calcium. When extracellular calcium is chelated by addition of EDTA, no epinephrine-induced platelet activation is observed. Platelet activation induced by epinephrine addition can also be inhibited by the α_2 receptor blocking agent phentolamine or the calcium channel blocker verapamil.[138] For epinephrine to cause secondary aggregation and secretion, thromboxane must be formed. Unlike ADP, thromboxane-dependent secondary aggregation and secretion cannot be bypassed by adding higher concentrations of epinephrine. If platelet CO is inhibited, epinephrine will induce only primary aggregation, no matter how much epinephrine is added.

When platelet activation is assessed by platelet aggregometry, epinephrine causes biphasic (primary and secondary) aggregation. However, there are several exceptions in which epinephrine will induce only primary aggregation: (1) inhibition of the platelet CO, (2) platelet storage pool deficiency in which the pool of releasable ADP in the dense granules is too small to trigger secondary aggregation, and (3) a deficiency in one of the enzymes responsible for thromboxane production. In these cases only primary aggregation (10%–20% aggregation) is observed. In addition, epinephrine fails to induce aggregation (either primary or secondary) when added to platelets of patients with thrombasthenia.

Collagen

Collagen is the component of the subendothelium to which platelets adhere, in an interaction requiring vWF. This interaction among platelets, vWF, and collagen (see Fig. 8-8) is also capable of causing platelet aggregation, providing a laboratory marker to assess platelet function. As with epinephrine, collagen-induced platelet aggregation is dependent on an intact thromboxane pathway; inhibition of this pathway results in impaired collagen-induced aggregation. Collagen-induced aggregation is always accompanied by a lag time (lag phase) of variable length dependent on the concentration of collagen added and platelet reactivity. During the lag phase, shape change may be observed. Shape change is followed by platelet aggregation in a monophasic wave dependent on thromboxane formation and subsequent secretion. The interaction of collagen with platelets slowly releases calcium from an intracellular storage pool, resulting in shape change. Aggregation and secretion begin when the intracellular concentration becomes adequate to activate the phospholipases, resulting in AA release from membrane phospholipids and thromboxane formation.

The collagen preparations used in *in vitro* laboratory testing of platelet function vary considerably in quality, depending on the source and method of preparation. Several genetically distinct types of collagen have been identified. Types I, III, IV, and V are found in the vessel media and adventitia and surrounding connective tissues.[117] Types IV and V are also found in the subendothelium. Collagen types I and III are more potent platelet activators than IV and V, which may partially explain why vessel injuries that penetrate the subendothelium result in a greater hemostatic response than those that do not.[8,206] However, the ability to bind vWF and activate platelets depends more on the *structure* of the collagen than the collagen type. In this regard, fibrillar collagen is a much better platelet activating agent than collagen monomers. Therefore, one is cautioned to "know your collagen" when assessing platelet function.

Thrombin

The serine protease thrombin is a potent platelet aggregating agent that does not depend on the thromboxane pathway for its activity. Thrombin is capable of directly causing secretion (*i.e.*, it is a direct secretagogue). Thrombin is also extremely potent in elevating platelet cytosolic calcium concentration, a property probably responsible for the ability of thrombin to cause aggregation and secretion.

The interaction of thrombin and the platelet membrane that leads to platelet activation has not been clarified (see Fig. 8-8). It is known that thrombin binds to the membrane glycoprotein GP Ib (which also appears to be the vWF binding site). Therefore, GP Ib has been proposed as the functional thrombin binding site.[122,135] On the other hand, thrombin has the ability to hydrolyze GP V. Thus GP V has also been proposed as the functional thrombin binding site.[27] The observation that platelets obtained from patients with Bernard-Soulier syndrome (which are congenitally deficient in GP Ib) aggregate when thrombin is added indicates that binding of thrombin to GP Ib is not necessary for platelet activation, supporting the notion that GP V is the functional receptor for thrombin. However, membrane glycoprotein analysis of platelets from patients with Bernard-Soulier syndrome reveals that these platelets are devoid of GP V as well as GP Ib.[35] It is therefore difficult to reconcile the ability of thrombin to activate platelets that apparently lack GP Ib and GP V. In this regard Brendt and Phillips have shown that GP V is a surface (peripheral) protein and is only loosely bound to the platelet surface.[28] Because it is loosely bound to the platelet surface, GP V may be lost from platelets of patients with Bernard-Soulier syndrome during the rigorous procedures necessary for identification of platelet glycoproteins. However, GP V *would* be present on platelets in plasma. Therefore, GP V is available on the surface of platelets in PRP obtained from patients with Bernard-Soulier syndrome, but lost during isolation of these same platelets for glycoprotein analysis.[180] However, GP V is *not* lost from normal platelets during isolation procedures for glycoprotein analysis. Solum has hypothesized that GP Ib in some way stabilizes GP V on the membrane of normal platelets and therefore is not lost during glycoprotein analysis.[180] This theory has not yet been proven, and the functional receptor for thrombin remains an open question. Even if one accepts that cleavage of GP V by thrombin causes platelet activation, it is not clear how cleavage of this peripheral protein transmits the signal for platelet activation to the interior of the platelet. Therefore, research into the mechanism of thrombin-induced platelet activation remains an area of active experimentation and interest.

For several reasons, thrombin is infrequently used in the clinical laboratory to assess platelet reactivity. First, thrombin is somewhat difficult to use, since the concentrations that cause platelet aggregation are close to those causing coagulation of the plasma. More importantly, because of its action as a direct secretagogue, thrombin almost always causes platelet aggregation. Therefore, not much information is gained by using thrombin to assess platelet function. However, one potential use of thrombin *depends* on its direct secretory capability. Thrombin can be added to platelets suspected of having storage pool deficiency, and the amount of ATP released can be quantified with the lumiaggregometer. Thus, thrombin can be used to separate storage pool deficiency from aspirinlike defects of the thromboxane pathway in platelets.

Platelet-Activating Factor (PAF)

In the early 1970s, Benveniste and associates observed that exposure of platelets to antigen-sensitized rabbit leukocytes caused platelet aggregation and release.[13] This "platelet-activating factor" was shown to be released from the leukocytes and was subsequently identified as a choline-containing phospholipid with an unusual structure.[34,114] PAF has an acetyl group attached at the 2 position by an *ether* linkage. Most phospholipids have a fatty acid attached at the 2 position of the phospholipid by an *ester* linkage (see Fig. 8-9). The structure of PAF has been identified as acetyl glyceryl ether phosphorylcholine (1-0-alkyl-2-acetyl-*sn*-glycero-3-phosphocholine), or AGEPC, as it is sometimes called.[76] The acetyl group attached by an ether linkage makes PAF unique among phospholipids and appears to account for its numerous activities. These activities range from platelet activation to participation in acute allergic and inflammatory reactions and anaphylaxis. The discussion here will be confined to its role in platelet activation.

The platelet membrane appears to contain specific receptors for PAF, which is a potent platelet activator.[161] Investigations are currently under way to elucidate the events that follow binding of PAF to this receptor (see Fig. 8-8). In this regard PAF appears to share features of epinephrine-induced platelet aggregation. Lee and colleagues have provided evidence that PAF stimulates an influx of calcium across the platelet membrane (as does epinephrine) and suggested that PAF functions as a calcium ionophore.[110] However, Serhan and colleagues were unable to demonstrate that PAF has calcium ionophoretic activity.[168] PAF-induced influx of calcium can be inhibited by blocking the platelet α receptors; blockade of α receptors also inhibits epinephrine-induced calcium influx[110] (see Fig. 8-7). In addition, PAF seems to share a feature of other platelet agonists (such as ADP) in that binding to its receptor initiates the PI and PPI cycles. Calcium in turn is mobilized from an internal storage pool, and arachidonic acid is released from membrane phospholipids.[102,110,170,173] Of additional interest is the recent observation by Alam and co-workers that, under certain circumstances, platelets are themselves capable of making PAF.[3] Thus it may be that PAF formation by platelets reinforces the platelet activating effects of the primary agonist and the thromboxane that is subsequently formed.

PAF is not currently used in the clinical laboratory to assess platelet reactivity.

However, PAF remains of great clinical interest because it is produced and released by other cells that interact with platelets. For example, rabbits whose leukocytes have been sensitized to a specific antigen respond to an intravenous antigenic challenge by producing PAF.[145] PAF causes *in vivo* platelet activation and histamine release from the rabbit leukocytes and is chemotactic for neutrophils. Consequently, these animals develop an anaphylactic reaction concurrently with thrombocytopenia and neutropenia.[145] These and many additional experiments indicate that PAF plays a role in both normal and pathologic platelet activation processes.

Ristocetin

Ristocetin was initially developed as a broad-spectrum antibiotic. However, ristocetin cannot be used as a therapeutic agent because it causes *in vivo* platelet agglutination and thrombocytopenia. Ristocetin induces the binding of vWF to GP Ib (a property termed *ristocetin cofactor activity*), resulting in platelet agglutination (see section on adhesion for a discussion of ristocetin-induced vWF binding). It is necessary to emphasize that ristocetin promotes *agglutination*, not aggregation. Even formaldehyde-fixed platelets are agglutinated by ristocetin, though they are metabolically inert and cannot be aggregated by any platelet aggregating agent.[4,116] Ristocetin-induced platelet agglutination requires the presence of vWF, particularly the high-molecular-weight multimers. Therefore, platelets from most patients with von Willebrand disease do not agglutinate normally when ristocetin is added to PRP from these patients. Thus, while it is not a useful antimicrobial agent, ristocetin can be used as a diagnostic reagent in the hemostasis laboratory. Bernard-Soulier syndrome (congenital deficiency of GP Ib) and von Willebrand disease are the only known conditions in which ristocetin-induced agglutination is abnormal (see Chap. 9).

Other Agents

In addition to the major platelet agonists discussed above, a wide variety of other agents are known to cause platelet aggregation. Examples include antigen–antibody complexes, certain bacterial endotoxins, some antibiotics, and serotonin (although a very weak agonist by itself). Even heparin, a major therapeutic and prophylactic anticoagulant, has been shown to activate platelets *in vivo* and *in vitro* in some patients, paradoxically resulting in arterial and venous thrombosis and thromboembolism.[10,21–23]

The mechanism of action of the platelet aggregating agents has been determined primarily *in vitro* by adding a single agent and then examining the physical and biochemical events that follow. It should be kept in mind that platelet activation *in vivo* is an entirely different phenomenon. *In vivo*, platelets are usually exposed simultaneously to a variety of platelet activating agents. For example, when a blood vessel is severely damaged, platelets are exposed not only to collagen but also to thrombin (formed by activation of the coagulation cascade), ADP and serotonin (released from dense granules), epinephrine (from the circulating blood), and perhaps PAF (produced by leukocytes or even platelets themselves). Thus, numerous platelet activation pathways are almost simultaneously stimulated and reinforce one another. Experiments have shown that small concentrations of two aggregating agents that by themselves produce only minor platelet activation produce major platelet aggregation when added together. Thus, platelet activating agents tend to potentiate the effects of one another (*i.e.,* their effects become more than additive). Potentiation is physiologically relevant, since platelets *in vivo* are not exposed to the high concentrations of activating agents that are used to cause platelet activation *in vitro*. In addition, two of the agents formed or released during *in vivo* platelet activation (TXA_2 and serotonin) are powerful vasocon-strictors and also aid in limiting blood loss following vascular injury.

Inhibitors of Platelet Activation

While platelets are a necessary element in the repair process for injured blood vessels, the repair process itself may lead to important pathologic events. For example, forma-tion of a platelet plug at a site of vascular damage may lead to changes in arterial blood flow because of mechanical obstruction or *vasospasm,* and may be the cause of certain types of angina. Also, release of fibrin – platelet *emboli* may be responsible for some cases of transient ischemic attacks or for initiating sudden fatal cardiac arrhythmias. Acute thrombotic occlusions involving platelets can precipitate *transmural* myocardial infarction, strokes, and cessation of blood flow through bypass graphs or shunts.[172] In addition, it is now known that the release of growth factors from stimulated platelets plays an important role in the development of atherosclerosis. Atherosclerosis may be the single most important cause of chronic vascular disease in man.[172] Because plate-lets are involved in such a wide variety of pathologic processes, a great interest in drugs that modulate platelet reactivity has evolved. In particular, interest has centered on the potential prophylactic and therapeutic benefit of drugs in preventing and halting patho-logic processes involving platelets. In the following section, two major approaches to altering platelet reactivity (inhibition of the thromboxane pathway and elevation of intracellular cAMP), and the drugs used to accomplish this, will be examined.

Inhibition of the Thromboxane Pathway

Inhibition of the thromboxane pathway in platelets is an attractive approach to modula-tion of platelet reactivity because of thromboxane's central role in platelet activation. In addition, inhibition of the thromboxane pathway does not reduce the ability of platelets to adhere to the subendothelium or totally eliminate the ability of platelets to respond to other agonists. The objective of thromboxane pathway inhibition is to reduce reactivity, particularly platelet aggregability, without eliminating the capacity of platelets to re-spond to major vessel damage. Three classes of drugs have been used to inhibit the thromboxane pathway: CO inhibitors, thromboxane synthase inhibitors, and throm-boxane receptor blocking agents. The latter two groups remain experimental at this time.

CYCLOOXYGENASE INHIBITORS. *Aspirin.* The anti-inflammatory, analgesic (pain-relieving) and antipyretic (fever-reducing) effects of acetylsalicylic acid (aspirin) were known long before its mechanism of action was discovered. Aspirin is an irreversible inhibitor of platelet CO, preventing the conversion of AA to cyclic endoperoxides and thromboxane.[179,194] As will be discussed later, aspirin also inhibits endothelial cell CO. Acetylsalicylic acid donates its acetyl group to (acetylates) CO, forming salicylic acid and irreversibly acetylated CO (Fig. 8-10). After acetylation, CO is incapable of convert-ing AA to the cyclic endoperoxide PGG_2, a thromboxane precursor. Since platelets can not synthesize CO, the thromboxane pathway is inhibited for the life of the platelet. Megakaryocytes, however, *do* synthesize CO, and newly released platelets will contain the active enzyme. Over a period of approximately 10 days (the half-life of platelets in the circulation), normal reactivity to arachidonic acid is recovered as old platelets are removed and replaced by platelets containing active CO.

Indomethacin and sulindac have actions similar to those of aspirin and are given to patients for their anti-inflammatory and analgesic – antipyretic properties. However,

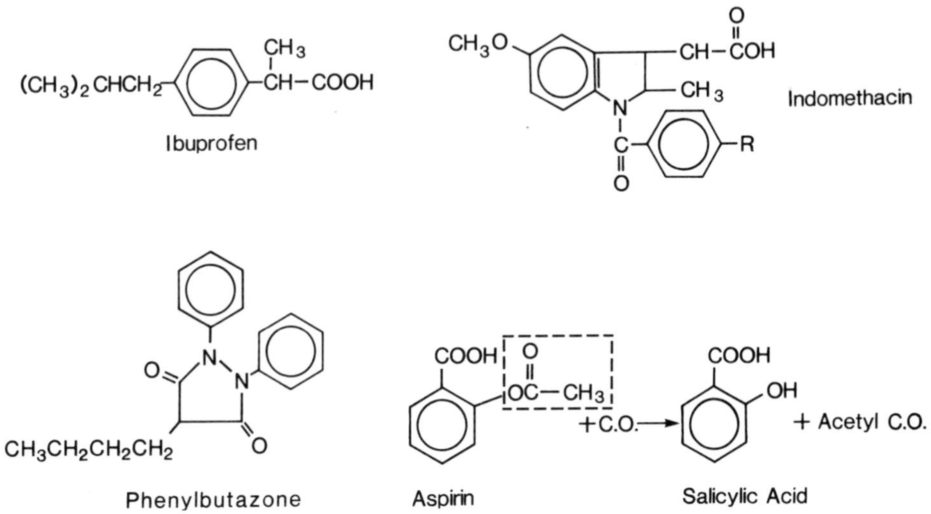

FIG. 8-10. Chemical structures of several common CO inhibitors. The acetyl group of aspirin is enclosed by the broken line. This acetyl group is transferred to CO, yielding the inactive metabolite salicylic acid and irreversibly inactivated CO.

unlike aspirin, sulindac and indomethacin are competitive inhibitors and do not permanently inhibit platelet CO. Therefore, platelets recover their ability to metabolize AA within 1 to 2 days after discontinuation of drug intake. Indomethacin (Indocin; see Fig. 8-10) and sulindac are used primarily to treat rheumatoid arthritis and have a few other selected applications. Their use is limited because of toxic side-effects.

Pyrazolone derivatives (phenylbutazone and sulfinpyrazone). Phenylbutazone (see Fig. 8-10) is the most commonly used pyrazolone derivative. It inhibits CO and therefore has anti-inflammatory, antipyretic, and analgesic properties. In addition, phenylbutazone promotes the renal excretion of uric acid (*i.e.*, it is uricosuric). Because of this combination of properties, phenylbutazone can be used in the treatment of acute gout as well as rheumatoid arthritis and allied disorders. Because it has toxic side-effects, phenylbutazone is used only when other agents are not effective.

Recent attention has focused on the sulfoxide derivative sulfinpyrazone (Anturane). The most active property of this agent is its uricosuric effect. However, sulfinpyrazone also prolongs the survival of platelets in patients with various thromboembolic disorders and is known to inhibit a number of platelet functions including the release reaction, adherence to subendothelium, and synthesis of prostaglandins. The effectiveness of sulfinpyrazone as an antithrombotic and prophylactic agent is currently being evaluated in a number of large clinical studies.[5,6,171]

Propionic acid derivatives, a relatively new group of aspirinlike agents, are rapidly gaining wide acceptance as effective anti-inflammatory, antipyretic, and analgesic drugs. Ibuprofen (Motrin, Advil; see Fig. 8-10) is the most widely used drug of this group and has recently been approved for nonprescription use. Although these agents are as effective as aspirin, indomethacin, or phenylbutazone, they are usually better tolerated and therefore may offer significant advantages for the patient. Naproxen and fenoprofen are agents of this group that are approved for use in the US by prescription only. Two additional propionic acid derivatives, flurbiprofen and ketoprofen, have not yet been approved for use in the US.

Other CO inhibitors. In addition to the drugs discussed above, a variety of less commonly used CO inhibitors are available for clinical use, including the fenamic acid derivatives (mefanamic acid) and tolmetin.

The list of CO inhibitors described above is by no means complete. However, since ingestion of these agents will affect the outcome of platelet aggregation testing in the clinical laboratory, the most commonly used agents have been discussed. One should keep in mind that more than 200 nonprescription preparations contain aspirin. In addition, numerous nonprescription compounds containing ibuprofen are now available. When platelet aggregation studies are ordered, it is necessary to get an *accurate history of drug intake to correctly interpret the results of platelet function studies.*

AGENTS THAT AFFECT INTRACELLULAR cAMP. *Prostacyclin* (PGI_2; Fig. 8-11), synthesized by vascular endothelial cells from AA, is the most potent known inhibitor of platelet aggregation and activation. Endothelial cells contain CO, which converts AA, released from membrane phospholipids, to PGH_2. PGH_2 is then converted to PGI_2 by the enzyme prostacyclin synthase. PGI_2 is released into the circulation by endothelial cells through an unknown mechanism. In the circulation, PGI_2 has a half-life of approximately 1 minute and is rapidly degraded to a stable metabolic end-product, 6-keto-$PGF_{1\alpha}$. Antibodies specific for 6-keto-$PGF_{1\alpha}$ have been produced in animals, and an RIA technique for the measurement of 6-keto-$PGF_{1\alpha}$ has been developed. The short half-life

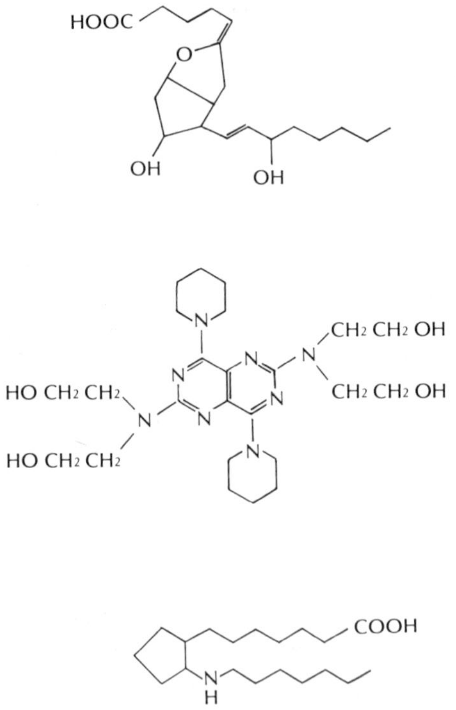

Prostacyclin

Dipyridamole

13 - Azaprostanoic Acid

FIG. 8-11. Chemical structures of the platelet inhibitors PGI_2 dipyridamole, and 13-APA.

of PGI_2 suggests that it must act at or near the site of production. In addition to platelet effects, PGI_2 has direct effects on blood vessels. PGI_2 is a powerful vasodilator, a property opposite that of TXA_2.

Platelet membranes contain a receptor for PGI_2 that is coupled to adenylate cyclase through a stimulatory subunit. When PGI_2 reacts with its receptor on the platelet surface, adenylate cyclase is activated and rapidly converts intracellular ATP to cAMP (see Fig. 8-8). When intracellular cAMP concentration rises, free cytosolic calcium is shifted to a membrane-bound form, resulting in a decrease in free cytoplasmic calcium concentration.[24,26,139]

Platelet activating agents have exactly the opposite effect on cytosolic free calcium concentration. Since PGI_2 and platelet activating agents affect cytosolic free calcium in opposite directions, addition of PGI_2 should inhibit the effects of a platelet activating agent. In fact, if a platelet activating agent that increases cytosolic calcium concentration is added to platelets pretreated with PGI_2 platelet activation is inhibited.[26] If PGI_2 is added shortly after the platelet activating agent, platelet activation will be reversed.[24] Owen and Le Breton have suggested that cAMP activates a calcium "pump" on the DTS (see Fig. 8-8), leading to an increased calcium concentration within the DTS and a decreased calcium concentration in the cytosol.[97,139] Hack and colleagues have recently provided support for this concept.[73] They found a Ca^{2+}-ATPase on DTS membranes that is associated with the ability of the DTS to sequester calcium. A calcium pump on the DTS may be one mechanism by which the platelet is able to control the level of cytosolic calcium and thus its state of reactivity.

Because PGI_2 has a short half-life, the effect on platelets is transient. When the PGI_2 concentration declines to a level that no longer stimulates the adenylate cyclase, the intracellular cAMP level begins to fall. Platelets contain an enzyme that rapidly degrades cAMP to AMP, cAMP phosphodiesterase. Unless there is continued cAMP production, cAMP phosphodiesterase rapidly returns the cAMP concentration to its basal level, and inhibition of platelet activation is removed.

The therapeutic and prophylactic effect of aspirin and aspirinlike drugs in the prevention of postoperative thromboembolism, reinfarction, and so forth has been evaluated in a number of large clinical trials. The discovery that endothelial cell CO is also inhibited by aspirin and aspirinlike drugs may explain why these agents have not provided the therapeutic benefit that was expected. In addition to preventing the proaggregatory production of thromboxane, the ability of vascular endothelium to synthesize PGI_2 is also inhibited by aspirin and aspirinlike drugs. In retrospect, the doses of CO inhibitors used in clinical trials were higher than that required to inhibit platelet CO. As a result, additional studies to find a dose of these agents that inhibits platelet function while producing minimal effects on vascular PGI_2 production are in progress. Unlike platelets, the vascular endothelium is capable of synthesizing new CO, and after a small dose of aspirin, the capacity to produce PGI_2 is regenerated within a few hours. Thus, the protective effect of PGI_2 again becomes available while thromboxane production by platelets remains inhibited. Whether or not periodic, low-dose aspirin therapy will be more effective than high doses remains to be proven.

The clinical use of PGI_2 has remained experimental for several reasons. First, the short half-life of PGI_2 necessitates the use of fairly large quantities to achieve the desired effect, making use of PGI_2 prohibitively expensive. Perhaps more importantly, the potent vasodilating effect of PGI_2 causes a sharp, undesirable drop in blood pressure. These limitations have led to the synthesis of several prostacyclin analogues in an attempt to find an agent that has a longer half-life, is less expensive, and does not have the adverse effects on blood pressure. Unfortunately, all of the prostacyclin analogues tested so far have caused a reduction in blood pressure.

   Dipyridamole (Persantine) (see Fig. 8-11) is a vasoactive drug that inhibits the enzyme responsible for cAMP breakdown, cAMP phosphodiesterase. This drug by itself produces little, if any, effect on platelets. Dipyridamole-treated platelets aggregate normally in response to platelet activating agents. However, dipyridamole potentiates the effects of agents that stimulate cAMP production by preventing breakdown of cAMP. Thus, when phosphodiesterase is inhibited and cAMP production is stimulated, cytosolic cAMP levels remain high even after the stimulus for cAMP production is removed. As a result, platelet aggregation is inhibited. Dipyridamole is usually used in combination with other platelet inhibitors.[32,169]

   THROMBOXANE SYNTHASE INHIBITORS.   Inhibition of thromboxane synthase is a relatively new approach to modulation of platelet reactivity. Several agents are available for experimental use, but none have been approved for clinical use. These agents block the conversion of PGH_2 to TXA_2 but do not always inhibit platelet aggregation. The inability of thromboxane synthase inhibitors to inhibit platelet aggregation is probably due to the ability of PGH_2 to interact with the thromboxane receptor and cause platelet aggregation. Smith and colleagues have hypothesized that the reason these agents inhibit platelet aggregation in some cases but not others is that PGH_2 metabolism is shunted to PGD_2 production[70,176,178] (see Fig. 8-7). They have shown that PGH_2 can be enzymatically and nonenzymatically converted to PGD_2, and PGD_2 stimulates cAMP production in platelets[176,177] (see Fig. 8-8). It is possible that in those instances in which thromboxane synthase inhibitors block platelet aggregation, PGH_2 is more efficiently converted to PGD_2. Whether thromboxane synthase inhibitors will prove to be effective antiplatelet agents is not known.

   THROMBOXANE RECEPTOR ANTAGONISTS.   Thromboxane receptor antagonists are the newest line of drugs developed to inhibit platelet activation. Most of these agents are analogues of prostaglandins or prostaglandin precursors, such as 13-APA (13-azaprostanoic acid[91,109] (see Fig. 8-11). They bind to the thromboxane receptor and competitively inhibit the binding of PGH_2 and TXA_2 but do not inhibit formation of the cyclic endoperoxides or thromboxane. When platelets treated with a thromboxane receptor antagonist are stimulated, normal amounts of TXA_2 and PGH_2 are formed. However, TXA_2 and PGH_2 production does not affect platelets, since the site at which they must react to cause platelet activation is blocked. *In vitro*, these agents are effective in inhibiting platelet aggregation caused by thromboxane production. Several of these agents are currently being evaluated in animal studies, but it is too early to draw any conclusions about their efficacy *in vivo*. Like thromboxane synthase inhibitors, thromboxane receptor antagonists have not been approved for clinical use.

PLATELET INTERACTIONS

Under normal conditions the vascular endothelium forms a continuous, or near continuous, inner lining of blood vessels to which platelets do not adhere (*i.e.*, it is a nonthrombogenic surface). However, when the endothelium is disrupted, platelets interact with components of the vessel wall and coagulation mechanism, with several important consequences. The role of platelets in halting blood loss has already been discussed and will not be addressed here. Instead, the discussion will now focus on the interaction of platelets with the coagulation mechanism and various cells of the vessel wall and the effects produced by these interactions.

Platelet – Endothelial Cell Interaction

Perhaps the most important property of endothelial cells is their capacity to synthesize PGI_2. PGI_2 inhibits platelet function, thus *preventing* interactions between platelets and endothelial cells.[127,205] The pro-aggregatory effects of thromboxane formed by platelets can be viewed as being countered by the inhibitory actions of PGI_2 produced by endothelial cells. Therefore, PGI_2 production contributes to the nonthrombogenic property of endothelial cells. Even activated platelets do not directly interact with intact endothelial cells.

Under certain circumstances, activated platelets can influence PGI_2 production by endothelial cells. When platelet AA metabolism is inhibited, endothelial cells are capable of using thromboxane precursors generated by activated platelets to make PGI_2—the so-called "steal hypotheses."[127] The ability of endothelial cells to steal prostaglandin intermediates for PGI_2 production makes the concept of thromboxane synthase inhibitors as potential therapeutic and prophylactic agents very attractive. However, it is not clear whether the "steal" process plays an important physiological role.

It is interesting to note that most agents that stimulate platelet activation also stimulate PGI_2 production by endothelial cells.[87,204] In this regard, endothelial cells near the site of vascular damage are exposed to platelet activating agents and produce more PGI_2 than endothelial cells farther away from the damage site (Fig. 8-12, A). Increased PGI_2 production by endothelial cells near site of damage is probably an important physiological event, since it serves to inhibit platelet function and limit thrombus extension beyond the site of damage.

Platelet – Smooth Muscle Cell Interaction

Platelets that are exposed to subendothelial structures become activated and undergo secretion. One of the released proteins, platelet-derived growth factor or PDGF, has powerful effects on the underlying smooth muscle cells and plays a role in normal wound healing. PDGF is a chemotactic factor for smooth muscle cells, causing migration of these cells from the media to the intima at the site of injury (see Fig. 8-12, A). In addition, PDGF is also a powerful mitogen, stimulating the *proliferation* of both smooth muscle cells in the media and fibroblasts in the underlying supporting tissues (see discussion of PDGF above). Proliferation of smooth muscle cells is necessary for repair of the vessel wall; fibroblast proliferation is necessary for repair of tissues underlying the vasculature. At the cellular level, PDGF promotes DNA synthesis, increased amino acid transport into the cells, increased protein and cholesterol synthesis, increased lipid metabolism, and an increase in receptors for low-density lipoproteins, events associated with cell growth.[72,137,184,208]

At least initially, the lumen of the repaired vessel is slightly narrowed because of subendothelial proliferation of smooth muscle cells (Fig. 8-12, B). With time, the lumen size may be restored, or the constriction may remain. Almost paradoxically, the process of repair may participate in the development of atherosclerotic plaque deposition. Repeated damage and repair at the same site may lead to permanent narrowing of the vessel lumen because of smooth muscle proliferation. Also, because PDGF stimu-

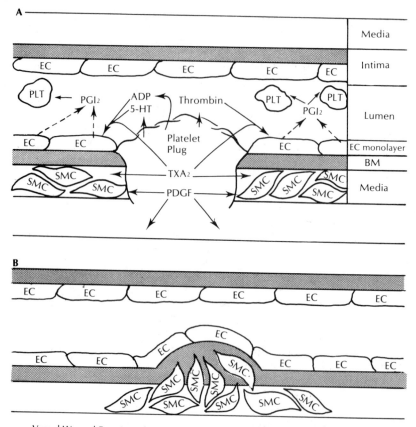

Vessel Wound Repair with Intimal Thickening and Narrowing of Vessel Lumen

FIG. 8-12. *(A)* Drawing of a transverse section through a small artery showing the effects of products released from a platelet plug. ADP, serotonin (5-HT), thrombin, and TXA_2 promote PGI_2 formation and release from endothelial cells near the site of vessel damage. The released PGI_2 inhibits platelet function and limits extension of the thrombus. Serotonin and TXA_2 stimulate smooth muscle contraction in the vessel media and are powerful vasoconstrictors. In addition, serotonin stimulates PGI_2 production by smooth muscle cells and potentiates the ability of PDGF to stimulate smooth muscle PGI_2 production. PDGF is a powerful mitogen for smooth muscle cells and fibroblasts and stimulates their growth. PDGF also promotes the production of PGI_2 by smooth muscle cells. *(B)* Drawing of a transverse section through a small artery after wound healing. Note the thickening of the vessel intima and media due to smooth muscle cell proliferation and slight narrowing of the vessel lumen. *EC*, endothelial cell; *BM*, basement membrane (composed primarily of collagen); *SMC*, smooth muscle cell; *PLT*, platelet; *5-HT*, serotonin; *TXA_2*, thromboxane A_2; *PGI_2*, prostacyclin (prostaglandin, I_2); *PDGF*, platelet-derived growth factor.

lates lipid metabolism and cholesterol synthesis, lipid tends to be deposited at the site of repair.[154] Hyperlipoproteinemic persons appear to deposit relatively more lipid at these sites, which may partially explain their higher incidence of atherosclerotic vascular disease.

In addition to the effects of PDGF on smooth muscle cells, PDGF is also chemotactic for monocytes and neutrophils. The attraction of monocytes to damage sites may aid in repair of the vessel, since monocytes and macrophages also produce a growth factor that stimulates smooth muscle growth. Finally, endothelial cells also participate in the healing process by producing a growth factor (EGF) that stimulates smooth muscle proliferation.

Two other products released from activated platelets, TXA_2 and serotonin (5-HT), have direct effects on smooth muscle cells. They cause smooth muscle cell proliferation and therefore are powerful vasoconstrictors (see Fig. 8-12, *A*). Vasoconstriction helps limit blood loss from a damaged vessel.

Though platelets do not appear to significantly affect endothelial cell growth, it is necessary to briefly discuss endothelial growth to complete the picture of vessel wall repair. Endothelial cell growth is controlled by a process called contact inhibition. In a normal blood vessel, endothelial cells form a continuous monolayer on the inside of the vessel. Whenever that layer is disrupted, contact inhibition of growth is removed. Endothelial cells no longer in contact with one another begin to proliferate until the monolayer is reestablished. Thus, endothelial regrowth is stimulated by the process that initially caused disruption of the endothelium.

Platelet Interactions With the Coagulation Mechanism

The observation that the platelet glycocalyx contains high concentrations of numerous coagulation proteins and that platelets contain forms of several plasma proteins points to one of the roles of platelets in promoting coagulation: they serve to concentrate coagulation proteins at the site of vascular damage and thus promote hemostasis (see Chap. 7). In addition, the platelet surface itself plays a critical role in activation of certain of the coagulation proteins.

Platelet Factor 3

The concept of platelet factor 3 (PF_3) is an old one derived from *in vitro* testing and the realization that platelets (or at least platelet products) have a necessary role in the activation of the coagulation mechanism. PF_3 was later identified as a phospholipid component of the platelet membrane, and assays for "PF_3 availability" were developed. The realization that phospholipids could substitute for platelets and platelet membranes gave rise to the activated partial thromboplastin reagents, which contain a contact activator (such as ellagic acid) and a platelet substitute. Many textbooks still use illustrations of the coagulation mechanism showing interaction sites for PF_3. We have chosen to replace the term *PF_3* with the more descriptive phrase *platelet-derived phospholipid.*

The Role of Platelets in Contact Activation

Factor XII (the inactive or zymogen form) undergoes a conformational change when exposed to a negatively charged surface such as subendothelial structures or activated platelets. The conformational change makes Factor XII more susceptible to proteolytic cleavage by plasma kallikrein and other proteases.[68,152] The conformationally changed zymogen also has slight enzymatic activity that may be sufficient to initiate the coagulation cascade by cleaving prekallikrein to kallikrein or by converting surface-bound Factor XII to XII_a[36,210] (Fig. 8-13). The activated form of Factor XII (XII_a) is primarily generated through limited proteolytic cleavage by kallikrein, and the active component is released into the fluid phase.[151] Factor XII_a is an active enzyme capable of the cleavage and activation of prekallikrein and Factor XI. Prekallikrein is associated with high-molecular-weight kininogen (HMWK) in plasma, and this complex binds to the platelet

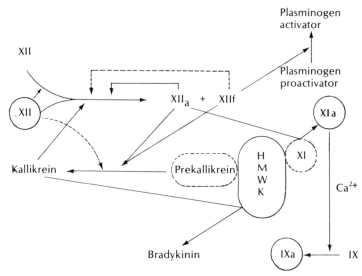

FIG. 8-13. Contact activation mechanisms. High-molecular-weight kininogen *(HMWK)* binds to a negatively charged surface and binds prekallikrein and Factor XI. Factor XII bound to a negatively charged surface undergoes conformational change and becomes capable of cleaving prekallikrein to kallikrein. Kallikrein has two major enzymatic activities: (1) it converts Factor XII to its most active form, XII_a and XII fragments (XII_f), and (2) it cleaves HMWK to release the vasoactive peptide bradykinin. Factors XII_a and to some extent XII_f are also capable of converting Factor XII to XII_a and XII_f (positive feedback amplification). In addition, Factors XII_a and XII_f actively convert prekallikrein to kallikrein to reinforce the cycle of Factor XII activation. Factor XII_a also converts Factor XI (bound to HMWK) to XI_a, and XI_a then binds to the negatively charged surface. Bound Factor XI_a actively converts Factor IX to IX_a, and IX_a then binds to the negatively charged surface. Finally, Factor XII_f promotes the conversion of plasminogen proactivator to plasminogen activator. Factors enclosed by solid lines are bound to negatively charged surfaces (e.g., the platelet surface). Factors enclosed by the broken lines are bound to HMWK. Solid arrows indicate major pathways. Broken arrows indicate minor pathways. *XII,* Factor XII; *XII_a,* activated Factor XII; *XII_f,* Factor XII fragments; *XI,* Factor XI; *XI_a,* activated Factor XI; *IX,* Factor IX; *IX_a,* activated factor IX.

surface.[119] In addition to binding prekallikrein, HMWK also binds Factor XI.[189] Thus, the necessary elements for contact activation are concentrated on the platelet surface or subendothelial structures bound to HMWK[209] (see Fig. 8-13).

Factor XII (activated by conformational change or proteolysis) can cleave prekallikrein to kallikrein. The active enzyme, kallikrein, can remain bound on the surface or be released to the plasma. Bound and free kallikrein is capable of converting additional Factor XII to XII_a.[36,174,210] The free kallikrein, a serine protease, utilizes surface-bound Factor XII as a substrate to form XII_a and Factor XII fragments $(XII_f;$ see Fig. 8-13). Autodigestion of Factor XII_a (by Factor XII_a) also produces Factor XII_f. Factor XII fragments can catalyze the conversion of Factor XII to XII_a but are much more efficient in converting prekallikrein to kallikrein and plasminogen proactivator to plasminogen activator.[151] Plasminogen activator converts plasminogen to the active enzyme, plasmin. Once formed, plasmin can activate Factor XII in the same manner as kallikrein.[30] These interactions between kallikrein and Factor XII form a positive feedback loop to reinforce the production of both XII_a and kallikrein and promote contact activation (see Fig. 8-13). The proteolytic activation of Factor XII and prekallikrein is further enhanced if the platelets are activated.[198,201]

Once formed, Factor XII_a acts on Factor XI bound to HMWK to form Factor XI_a and cleavage products (see Fig. 8-13). Factor XI_a remains bound to the activated platelet surface at specific sites, where it is protected from inactivation by plasma proteinase inhibitors.[198] Factor XII_a and XII fragments are also capable of activating Factor VII and therefore may promote coagulation via the extrinsic system.[99,149,198] In addition to activating Factor XII, kallikrein also rapidly cleaves surface-bound and free HMWK, yielding the vasoactive peptide bradykinin (see Fig. 8-13). Bradykinin promotes vasoconstriction and also affects endothelial cell PGI_2 and TXA_2 production.[42,87] While platelets play a role in *promoting* contact activation, studies suggest that PF_4 secreted from platelets later in the hemostatic process can produce negative feedback effects by *inhibiting* contact activation (*i.e.,* inhibiting plasma prekallikrein activation).[200,202]

The observation that persons deficient in Factor XII (Hageman factor) do not have a bleeding diathesis *may* be explained by the observation that *activated* platelets seem to proteolytically activate Factor XI independent of Factor XII. Activation of Factor XI by this mechanism is dependent on kallikrein, enhanced by HMWK, and requires the binding of Factor XI to specific receptors on the surface of activated platelets.[67,198] The precise details of Factor XI activation by this pathway are not known. It is interesting to note that people with Factor XII deficiency do not have a bleeding abnormality but are prone to thromboembolic problems. Mr. Hageman (in whom the deficiency was initially described) and several others with Factor XII deficiency died of complications associated with thromboembolism. It is speculated that their thromboembolic problems are associated with the inability to convert plasminogen proactivator to plasminogen activator due to the Factor XII deficiency. As a result, their ability ro resolve thrombi would be compromised.

Factor XI_a bound to the platelet surface acts on Factor IX to produce the active cleavage product IX_a in a reaction requiring calcium (see Fig. 8-13). Factor XI_a binds to the platelet surface via its amino-terminal γ-carboxyl groups and is protected from inactivation by plasma proteinase inhibitors.[195] The physiologic substrate for Factor IX_a is Factor X.[94]

The Role of Platelets in Factor X Activation

The physiologic activation of Factor X by IX_a occurs on the platelet surface. Factor IX_a, Factor VIII, and Factor X bind to the platelet surface at adjacent sites (Fig. 8-14). Although Factor IX_a and X bind via their γ-carboxyl groups, Factor VIII is bound noncovalently. Factor VIII serves as a cofactor for Factor X activation, and its function as a cofactor is enhanced by thrombin modification.[88,188] Although Factor IX_a can activate Factor X in the absence of Factor VIII, the reaction proceeds 300,000-fold faster in the presence of thrombin-modified Factor VIII (VIII_m or VIII_a).[90] The Factor X_a formed on the platelet surface remains attached, and this environment protects it from inactivation by plasma proteinase inhibitors.[125,187,197]

In contrast to Factor X activation via the intrinsic system, platelets do not appear to play a role in the activation of Factor X by the extrinsic system.[197] In the extrinsic pathway, Factor X is rapidly converted to X_a in a reaction requiring Factor VII_a, calcium, and a tissue factor (tissue extract, or "juice"). It is also important to recognize that Factor VII_a, calcium, and tissue factor can also activate Factor IX, but not as efficiently as Factor XI_a in the intrinsic pathway.[196,214]

The Role of Platelets in Prothrombin Activation

In the presence of calcium, Factor X_a binds specifically and reversibly to high-affinity receptors on the platelet, and binding of Factor X_a closely correlates with prothrombin

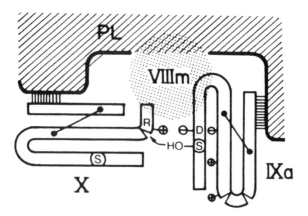

FIG. 8-14. Intrinsic Factor X activation. Factors IX_a and X are bound to the phospholipid surface (*PL, crosshatched area*) by calcium bridges through their γ-carboxyglutamic acid residues (Gla). Factor VII, having been modified by thrombin (*VIIIm; stippled circle*) binds nonionically to the phospholipid surface and serves as the cofactor in the activation by an as yet undefined mechanism. The steps of catalysis established for tryptic-like cleavage involve binding of substrate (Factor X) with an Arg *(R)* group ionically attaching to an Asp *(D)* residue in the bottom of the binding pocket near the active-center Ser *(S)* of the enzyme (Factor IX_a). The active-center Ser forms an unstable acyl intermediate that is hydrolyzed, cleaving the Arg–Ile peptide bond to generate Factor X_a. *PL*, platelet; *small lines connecting Factors X and IX_a to the platelet surface*, Gla residues near the amino terminus; *circled S*, active serine site of the enzyme; *D*, aspartic acid residue; *R*, arginine residue; *X*, Factor X; *IX_a*, activated Factor IX; *VIII_m*, thrombin-modified Factor VIII; *solid lines between filled circles*, disulfide bridges. (Thompson AR, Harker LA: Manual of Hemostasis and Thrombosis. Philadelphia, FA Davis, 1983)

activation.[43,96,124,126] The high-affinity receptor for Factor X_a is activated Factor V (V_a).[125,191] Factor V is modified by thrombin to its active form, and thus the active form of Factor V is also known as V_m. The terms V_a and V_m are used interchangeably. Factors V and V_m bind to the platelet surface, although the binding sites are different; both bind to low-affinity sites, but only V_m binds to high-affinity sites.[193] Thrombin-modified Factor V (V_m) binds to its surface receptor and to Factor X_a in a 1-to-1 complex.[191] The platelet surface appears to contain at least 2500 binding sites for Factor V_m. The binding of some activated factors to the platelet surface occurs more rapidly on, or is facilitated by, activated platelets. However, Factor V_m and X_a binding does not appear to be facilitated by platelet activation and will occur at nearly the same rate in the presence of a phospholipid substitute.[118]

In the presence of calcium, prothrombin (bound to the platelet surface or a phospholipid substitute) is rapidly converted to thrombin by the bound V_m–X_a complex (Fig. 8-15). A phospholipid environment is required for efficient conversion of prothrombin to thrombin. The rate of conversion of prothrombin to thrombin is about 300,000-fold greater when Factor X_a is bound to V_m and platelet phospholipid than when Factor X_a is not bound.[118] The thrombin formed in this reaction is released into the plasma, where it enzymatically converts fibrinogen to fibrin.

As indicated in Chapter 2, activated protein C is capable of degrading Factor V. However, activation of Factor V to V_m and its binding to platelets are required.[40,44,192] Apparently, activated protein C cannot degrade unbound Factor V or V_m. In addition,

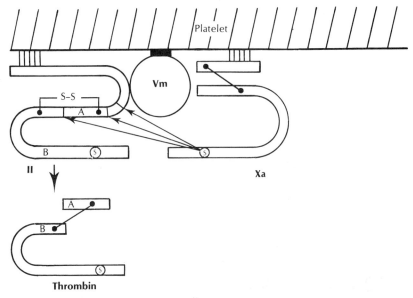

FIG. 8-15. Prothrombin activation. Thrombin-modified Factor V (V_m) binds with high affinity to sites on the platelet surface. Bound V_m is the high-affinity receptor for Factor X_a. Factor X_a bound to V_m and the platelet surface (or a phospholipid substitute) rapidly converts prothrombin (also bound to the platelet surface or a phospholipid substitute) to thrombin in the presence of calcium. Cleavage of prothrombin by Factor X_a occurs at three sites on the prothrombin molecule. The active enzyme, thrombin, and a cleavage peptide are released into the plasma. The A and B chains of thrombin are held together by a disulfide bond. The small lines connecting Factors II and X_a to the platelet surface represent the Gla residues near the amino terminus. *A,* A chain of thrombin; *B,* B chain of thrombin; *circled S,* active serine sites of the enzymes; V_m, thrombin-modified Factor V; *II,* Factor II (prothrombin), X_a, activated Factor X.

binding of Factor X_a to Factor V_m appears to protect platelet-bound Factor V_m from proteolytic degradation by activated protein C.[44,192] Activated protein C also degrades Factor VIII_m. Inactivation of Factors V_m and VIII_m by activated protein C is physiologically important, as illustrated by the observation that patients deficient in protein C have thromboembolic disease.[69]

In summary, platelets play an important role in promoting clot formation. The platelet glycocalyx contains several coagulation proteins, and additional coagulation proteins can be released from platelet granules during secretion. In addition, the platelet surface possesses high-affinity receptors for certain coagulation proteins, including receptors for the Factor XI_a – HMWK complex, the prekallikrein – HMWK complex, Factor XI_a, the Factor X_a – V_a complex, and prothrombin. As a result, platelets promote the activation of prekallikrein, Factors XII, XI, IX, and X, and prothrombin. Finally, binding to the platelet surface also appears to protect certain activated coagulation proteins from inactivation by plasma proteinases. Because platelets adhere to sites of vascular damage and become activated, platelets can be viewed as a means of localizing coagulation reactions to the sites of blood vessel injury, thus promoting hemostasis.

REFERENCES

1. Adelstein RS, Conti MA: The characterization of contractile proteins from platelets and fibroblasts. Cold Spring Harbor Symp Quant Biol 37:599–605, 1972
2. Akkerman JWN, Holmsen H: Interrelationship between platelet responses: Studies on the burst in proton liberation, lactate production and oxygen uptake during platelet aggregation and Ca^{2+} secretion. Blood 57:956–966, 1981
3. Alam I, Smith JB, Silver MJ: Human and rabbit platelets form platelet-activating factor in response to calcium ionophore. Thromb Res 30:71–79, 1983
4. Allain JP, Cooper HA, Wagner RH et al: Platelets fixed with paraformaldehyde: A new reagent for assay of von Willebrand factor and platelet aggregating factor. J Lab Clin Med 85:318–328, 1975
5. Anturane Reinfaction Italian Study Group: Sulfinpyrazone in postmyocardial infarction. Lancet 1:237–242, 1982
6. The Anturane Reinfarction Trial Research Group: Sulfinpyrazone in the prevention of sudden death after myocardial infarction. N Engl J Med 302:250–256, 1980
7. Barber AJ, Kaser-Glanzmann R, Jakabova M et al: Characterization of chondroitin sulfate proteoglycan carrier for heparin-neutralizing activity (PF_4) released from human blood platelets. Biochim Biophys Acta 286:312–329, 1972
8. Barnes MJ, Bailey AJ, Gordon JL, MacIntyre DE: Platelet aggregation by basement-associated collagens. Thromb Res 18:375–388, 1980
9. Begg BS, Pepper DS, Chesterman CN et al: Complete covalent structure of human beta-thromboglobulin. Biochemistry 17:1739–1744, 1978
10. Bell WR, Royall RM: Heparin-associated thrombocytopenia: A comparison of three heparin preparations. N Engl J Med 303:902–907, 1980
11. Bennett JS, Hoxie JA, Leitman SF et al: Inhibition of fibrinogen binding to stimulated human platelets by a monoclonal antibody. Proc Natl Acad Sci USA 80:2417–2421, 1983
12. Bennett JS, Vilaire G, Cines DB: Identification of the fibrinogen receptor on human platelets by photoaffinity labeling. J Biol Chem 257:8048–8054, 1982
13. Benveniste J, Henson PM, Cochrane CG: Leukocyte-dependent histamine release from rabbit platelets: The role of IgE, basophils and a platelet-activating factor. J Exp Med 136:1356–1377, 1972
14. Bernstein LR, Antoniades HN, Zetter BR: Migration of cultured vascular cells in response to plasma and platelet-derived growth factors. J Cell Sci 56:71–82, 1982
15. Berridge MJ, Irvine RF: Inositol triphosphate, a novel second messenger in cellular signal transduction. Nature 312:315–321, 1984
16. Bettex-Galland M, Luscher EF: Extraction of an actomyosin-like protein from human thrombocytes. Nature 184:276–277, 1959
17. Bettex-Galland M, Luscher EF: Thrombosthenin: A contractile protein from thrombocytes: Its extraction from human blood platelets and some of its properties. Biochim Biophys Acta 49:536–547, 1963
18. Billah MM, Lapetina EG, Cautrecasas P: Phosphatidylinositol-specific phospholipase-C of platelets: Association with 1,2-diacylglycerol-kinase and inhibition by cyclic-AMP. Biochem Biophys Res Commun 90:92–98, 1979
19. Born GVR: Aggregation of blood platelets by adenosine diphosphate and its reversal. Nature 194:927–929, 1962
20. Bowen-Pope DF, Ross R: Platelet-derived growth factor. II. Specific binding to cultured cells. J Biol Chem 257:5161–5171, 1982
21. Brace LD, Fareed J: An objective assessment of the interaction of heparin and its fractions with human platelets. Semin Thromb Hemost 11:190–198, 1985
22. Brace LD, Fareed J: Heparin-induced platelet aggregation is inhibited by antagonists of the thromboxane pathway. Thromb Res 39:533–539, 1985
23. Brace LD, Fareed J: Biochemical and pharmacological studies on the interaction of PK 10169 and its subfractions with human platelets. Haemostasis 16:93–105, 1986

24. Brace LD, Venton DL, Le Breton GC: Reversal of thromboxane A_2/prostaglandin H_2 and ADP-induced calcium release in intact platelets. Am J Physiol 249(Heart Circ Physiol 18):H8–H13, 1985

25. Brace LD, Venton DL, Le Breton GC: Prostaglandin H_2 causes calcium mobilization in intact human platelets. In Bailey JM (ed): Prostaglandins, Leukotrienes, and Lipoxins, pp 333–344. New York, Plenum, 1985

26. Brace LD, Venton DL, Le Breton GC: Thromboxane A_2/prostaglandin H_2 mobilizes calcium in human blood platelets. Am J Physiol 249(Heart Circ Physiol 18):H1–H7, 1985

27. Brendt MC, Phillips DR: Interaction of thrombin with platelets: Purification of the thrombin substrate. Ann NY Acad Sci 370:87–95, 1981

28. Brendt MC, Phillips DR: Purification and preliminary physicochemical characterization of human platelet membrane glycoprotein V. J Biol Chem 256:59–65, 1981

29. Brindley LL, Sweet JM, Goetzl EJ: Stimulation of histamine release from human basophils by human platelet factor 4. J Clin Invest 72:1218–1223, 1983

30. Burrowes CE, Morat HZ, Soltay MJ: The kinin system of human plasma. VI. The action of plasmin. Proc Soc Exp Biol Med 138:959–966, 1971

31. Carey F, Menashi S, Crawford N: Localization of cyclo-oxygenase and thromboxane synthetase in human platelet intracellular membranes. Biochem J 204:847–851, 1982

32. Chesebro JH, Fuster V, Elveback LR et al: Effect of dypyridamole and aspirin on late vein-graft patency after coronary bypass operations. N Engl J Med 310:209–214, 1984

33. Chesney CM, Pifer D, Colman RW: Subcellular localization and secretion of factor V from human platelets. Proc Natl Acad Sci USA 78:5180–5184, 1981

34. Clark PO, Hanahan DJ, Pinckard RN: Physical and chemical properties of platelet-activating factor obtained from human neutrophils and monocytes and rabbit neutrophils and basophils. Biochim Biophys Acta 628:69–75, 1980

35. Clemetson KJ, McGregor JL, James E et al: Characterization of the platelet membrane glycoprotein abnormalities in Bernard-Soulier syndrome and comparison with normal by surface-labeling techniques and high-resolution two-dimensional gel electrophoresis. J Clin Invest 70:304–311, 1982

36. Cochrane CG, Griffin JH: Molecular assembly in the contact phase of the Hageman factor system. Am J Med 67:657–664, 1979

37. Coligan JE, Slayter HS: Structure of thrombospondin. J Biol Chem 259:3944–3948, 1984

38. Coller BS, Gralnick HR: Studies on the mechanism of ristocetin-induced platelet agglutination: Effects of structural modification of ristocetin and vancomycin. J Clin Invest 60:302–312, 1977

39. Coller BS, Peerschke EI, Scudder LE et al: A murine monoclonal antibody that completely blocks the binding of fibrinogen to platelets produces a thrombasthenic like state in normal platelets and binds GP IIb and/or GP IIIa. J Clin Invest 72:325–338, 1983

40. Comp PC, Esmon CT: Activated protein C inhibits platelet prothrombin-converting activity. Blood 54:1271–1281, 1979

41. Coughlin SR, Moskowitz MA, Antoniades HN, Levine L: Serotonin receptor-mediated stimulation of bovine smooth muscle cell prostacyclin synthesis and its modulation by platelet-derived growth factor. Proc Natl Acad Sci USA 78:7134–7138, 1981

42. Crutchley DJ, Ryan JW, Ryan US et al: Bradykinin-induced release of prostacyclin and thromboxanes from bovine pulmonary artery endothelial cells. Biochim Biophys Acta 751:99–107, 1983

43. Dahlback B, Stenflo J: Binding of bovine coagulation factor Xa to platelets. Biochemistry 17:4939–4945, 1978

44. Dahlback B, Stenflo J: Inhibitory effect of activated protein C on activation of prothrombin by platelet-bound factor Xa. Eur J Biochem 107:331–335, 1980

45. Davey MG, Luscher EF: Release reactions of human platelets induced by thrombin and other agents. Biochim Biophys Acta 165:490–506, 1968

46. De Clerck F, Van Gorp L: Induction of circulating platelet aggregates by release of endogenous 5-hydroxytryptamine in the rat (abstr #82). Thromb Haemost 46:29, 1981

47. De Marco L, Shapiro SS: Properties of human asialo-Factor VIII: A ristocetin-independent platelet-aggregating agent. J Clin Invest 168:321–328, 1981
48. Derksen A, Cohen P: Patterns of fatty acid release from endogenous substrates by human platelet homogenates and membranes. J Biol Chem 250:9342–9347, 1975
49. Deuel TF, Keim PS, Farmer M et al: Platelet factor 4: Complete amino acid sequence. Proc Natl Acad Sci USA 74:2256–2258, 1977
50. Deuel TF, Senior RM, Chang D et al: Platelet factor 4 is chemotactic for neutrophils and monocytes. Proc Natl Acad Sci USA 78:4584–4587, 1981
51. Deuel TF, Senior RM, Huang JS et al: Chemotaxis of monocytes and neutrophils to platelet-derived growth factor. J Clin Invest 69:1046–1049, 1982
52. DiMinno G, Thiagarajan P, Perussia B et al: Exposure of platelet fibrinogen binding sites by collagen, arachidonic acid, and ADP: Inhibition by a monoclonal antibody to the GP IIb–IIIa complex. Blood 61:140–148, 1983
53. Feinman RD, Lubowsky I, Charo I, Zabinski MP: The lumiaggregometer: A new instrument for simultaneous measurement of secretion and aggregation. J Lab Clin Med 90:125–129, 1977
54. Francis CW, Nachman RL, Marder VJ: Plasma and platelet fibrinogen differ in chain content. Thromb Haemost 51:84–88, 1984
55. Fujimoto T, Ohara S, Hawiger J: Thrombin induced exposure and prostaglandin induced inhibition of receptors for F VIII/vWF on human platelets. J Clin Invest 69:1212–1222, 1982
56. Fujimura K, Phillips DR: Calcium cation regulation of GP IIb–IIIa complex formation in platelet cell membranes. J Biol Chem 258:10247–10252, 1983
57. Fulcher CA, Zimmerman TS: Characterization of the human Factor VIII procoagulant protein with a heterologous precipitating antibody. Proc Natl Acad Sci USA 79:1648–1652, 1982
58. Ganguly P: Studies on platelet proteins. III. The identity of platelet and serum albumins. Biochim Biophys Acta 188:78–88, 1969
59. Ganguly P: Isolation and some properties of fibrinogen from human blood platelets. J Biol Chem 247:1809–1816, 1972
60. Gartner TK, Gerrard JM, White TF et al: Fibrinogen is the receptor for the endogenous lectin of human platelets. Nature 289:688–690, 1981
61. Gerrard JM, Butler AM, Graff G et al: Prostaglandin endoperoxides promote calcium release from a platelet membrane fraction in vitro. Prostaglandins Med 1:373–385, 1978
62. Gerrard JM, White JG, Rao GHR, Townsend D: Localization of platelet prostaglandin production in the platelet dense tubular system. Am J Pathol 83:283–298, 1976
63. Ginsberg MH, Wolff R, Marguerie G et al: Thrombospondin binding to thrombin-stimulated platelets: Evidence for a common protein binding mechanism. Clin Res 32:308A, 1984
64. Gogstad GO, Brosstak F, Krutnes MB et al: Fibrinogen-binding properties of the human platelet glycoprotein IIb–IIIa complex: A study using crossed-radioimmunoelectrophoresis. Blood 60:663–671, 1982
65. Gogstad GO, Hagen I, Kormso R et al: Evidence for release of soluble, but not membrane-integrated proteins from human platelet alpha granules. Biochim Biophys Acta 670:150–152, 1981
66. Gogstad GO, Stormorken H, Solum NO: Platelet alpha-2-antiplasmin is located in the platelet alpha granules. Thromb Res 31:387–390, 1983
67. Greengard JS, Ersdal E, Griffin JH: Binding of purified high molecular weight kininogen, factor XI and factor XIa to washed human platelets (abstr). Blood 62:256, 1983
68. Griffin JH: Role of surface in surface-dependent activation of Hageman factor (blood coagulation factor XII). Proc Natl Acad Sci USA 75:1998–2002, 1978
69. Griffin JH, Evatt B, Zimmerman JS et al: Deficiency of protein C in congenital thrombocytic disease. J Clin Invest 68:1370–1373, 1981
70. Grimm LJ, Knapp DR, Senator D, Halushka PV: Inhibition of platelet thromboxane synthesis by 7-(1-imidazolyl)heptanoic acid: Dissociation from inhibition of aggregation. Thromb Res 24:307–317, 1981

71. Grotendorst GR, Seppa HEJ, Kleinman HK et al: Attachment of smooth muscle cells to collagen and their migration towards platelet-derived growth factor. Proc Natl Acad Sci USA 76:3669–3672, 1981

72. Habenicht AJR, Glomset JA, Ross R: Relation of cholesterol and mevalonic acid to the cell cycle in smooth muscle and Swiss 3T3 cells stimulated to divide by platelet-derived growth factor. J Biol Chem 256:12329–12335, 1981

73. Hack N, Croset M, Crawford N: Studies on the bivalent-cation-activated ATPase activities of highly purified human platelet surface and intracellular membranes. Biochem J 233:661–668, 1986

74. Hamberg M, Svensson J, Samuelsson B: Thromboxanes: A new group of biologically active compounds derived from prostaglandin endoperoxides. Proc Natl Acad Sci USA 72:2294–2298, 1975

75. Hamberg M, Svensson J, Wakabayshi T, Samuelsson B: Isolation and structure of two prostaglandin endoperoxides that cause platelet aggregation. Proc Natl Acad Sci USA 71:345–349, 1974

76. Hanahan DJ, Demopoulos CA, Liehr J, Pinckard RN: Identification of platelet-activating factor isolated from rabbit basophils as acetyl glyceryl ether phosphorylcholine. J Biol Chem 255:5514–5516, 1980

77. Hathaway DR, Adelstein RS: Human platelet myosin light chain kinase requires the calcium-binding protein calmodulin for activity. Proc Natl Acad Sci USA 76:1653–1657, 1979

78. Hawiger J, Timmons S, Kloczewiak M et al: Gamma and alpha chains of human fibrinogen possess sites reactive with human platelet receptors. Proc Natl Acad Sci USA 79:2068–2071, 1982

79. Hermodson M, Schmer G, Kurachi K: Isolation, characterization and primary amino acid sequence of human platelet factor 4. J Biol Chem 252:6276–6279, 1977

80. Holme R, Sixma JJ, Murer EH et al: Demonstration of platelet fibrinogen secretion via the surface connecting system. Thromb Res 3:347–356, 1973

81. Holmsen H: Platelet metabolism and activation. Semin Hematol 22:219–240, 1985

82. Holmsen H, Day HJ: The selectivity of the thrombin-induced platelet release reaction: Subcellular localization of released and retained substances. J Lab Clin Med 75:840–855, 1970

83. Holmsen H, Day HJ, Setkowsky C: Secretory mechanisms: Behavior of adenine nucleotides during platelet release reaction induced by adenosine diphosphate and adrenaline. Biochem J 129:67–82, 1972

84. Holmsen H, Kaplan KL, Dangelmaier DA: Differential energy requirements for platelet responses: A simultaneous study of dense granule, alpha-granule and acid hydrolase secretion, arachidonate liberation, phosphatidylinositol turnover and phosphatidate formation. Biochem J 208:9–18, 1982

85. Holt JC, Niewiarowski S: Secretion of plasminogen by washed human platelets (abstr). Circulation 62:342, 1980

86. Holt JC, Niewiarowski S: Biochemistry of alpha granule proteins. Semin Hematol 22:151–163, 1985

87. Hong SL: Effect of bradykinin and thrombin on prostacyclin synthesis in endothelial cells from calf and pig aorta and human umbilical cord vein. Thromb Res 18:787–795, 1980

88. Hoyer LW, Trabold NC: The effect of thrombin on human factor VIII. J Lab Clin Med 97:50–64, 1981

89. Huang JS, Huang SS, Kennedy B et al: Platelet-derived growth factor: Specific binding to target cells. J Biol Chem 257:8130–8136, 1982

90. Hultin MB: Role of human factor VIII in factor X activation. J Clin Invest 69:950–958, 1982

91. Hung SC, Ghali NI, Venton DL, Le Breton GC: Specific binding of the thromboxane antagonist 13-azaprostanoic acid to human platelet membranes. Biochim Biophys Acta 728:171–178, 1983

92. Ihnatowycz IO, Winocour PD, Moore S: A platelet-derived factor chemotactic for rabbit arterial smooth muscle cells in culture. Artery 9:316–327, 1981

93. Jandrot-Perus M, Mossesson MW, Denninger MH et al: Studies of platelet fibrinogen from a

subject with congenital plasma fibrinogen abnormality (Fibrinogen Paris I). Blood 54:1109–1116, 1977

94. Jesty J, Spencer AK, Nemerson Y: The mechanism of action of factor X: Kinetic control of alternative pathways leading to the formation of activated factor X. J Biol Chem 49:5614–5622, 1974

95. Johnsson A, Heldin CH, Westermark B et al: Platelet-derived growth factor: Identification of constituent polypeptide chains. Biochem Biophys Res Commun 104:66–74, 1982

96. Kane WH, Lindout MJ, Jackson CW et al: Factor Va–dependent binding of factor Xa to human platelets. J Biol Chem 255:1170–1174, 1980

97. Kaser-Glanzman R, Jakabova M, George JN, Luscher EF: Stimulation of calcium uptake in platelet membrane vesicles by adenosine 3′,5′-cyclic monophosphate and protein kinase. Biochim Biophys Acta 566:429–440, 1977

98. Keenan JP, Solum NO: Quantitative studies on the release of platelet fibrinogen by thrombin. Br J Haematol 23:461–466, 1972

99. Kisiel W, Fujikawa K, Davie EW: Activation of bovine factor VII (proconvertin) by factor XIIa (activated Hageman factor). Biochemistry 16:4189–4193, 1979

100. Kloczewiak M, Timmons S, Hawiger J: Localization of a site interacting with human platelet receptors on the carboxy-terminal segment of the human fibrinogen gamma chain. Biochem Biophys Res Commun 107:181–187, 1982

101. Koutts J, Walsh PN, Plow EF et al: Active release of human Factor VIII–related antigen by adenosine diphosphate, collagen and thrombin. J Clin Invest 62:1255–1263, 1978

102. Lapetina EG: Platelet-activating factor stimulates the phosphatidylinositol cycle. Appearance of phosphatidic acid is associated with the release of serotonin in horse platelets. J Biol Chem 257:7314–7317, 1982

103. Lawler JW, Chao FC, Cohen CM: Evidence for calcium-sensitive structure in platelet thrombospondin: Isolation and partial characterization of thrombospondin in the presence of calcium. J Biol Chem 257:12257–12265, 1982

104. Lawler JW, Slayter HS: The release of heparin-binding peptides from platelet thrombospondin by proteolytic action of thrombin, plasmin and trypsin. Thromb Res 22:267–279, 1981

105. Lawler JW, Slayter HS, Coligan JE: Isolation and characterization of a high molecular weight glycoprotein from human platelets. J Biol Chem 253:8609–8616, 1978

106. Le Breton GC, Dinerstein RJ, Roth LJ, Feinberg H: Direct evidence for intracellular divalent cation distribution associated with platelet shape change. Biochem Biophys Res Commun 71:362–370, 1976

107. Le Breton GC, Feinberg H: ADP-induced changes in intraplatelet Ca^{++} ion concentration. Pharmacologist 16:699, 1974

108. Le Breton GC, Venton DL: Thromboxane A$_2$ receptor antagonism selectively reverses platelet aggregation. In Samuelsson B, Ramwell PW, Paoletti R, (eds): Advances in Prostaglandin and Thromboxane Research, pp 497–503. New York, Raven Press, 1980

109. Le Breton GC, Venton DL, Enke SE, Halushka PV: 13-Azaprostanoic acid: A specific antagonist of the human blood platelet thromboxane/endoperoxide receptor. Proc Natl Acad Sci USA 76:4097–4101, 1979

110. Lee TC, Malone B, Blank ML et al: 1-Alkyl-2-acetyl-sn-glycero-3-phosphocholine (platelet activating factor) stimulates calcium influx in rabbit platelets. Biochem Biophys Res Commun 102:1261–1268, 1981

111. Lim CT, Kattelman EJ, Arora Sk et al: Partial purification and identification of thromboxane A$_2$/prostaglandin H$_2$ receptor protein in human platelets (abstr #1117). Fed Proc 45(3):346, 1986

112. Lloyd JV, Nishizawa EE, Mustard JF: Effect of ADP-induced shape change on incorporation of ^{32}P into platelet phosphatidic acid and mono-, di- and triphosphatidyl inositol. Br J Haematol 25:77–99, 1973

113. Lopex-Fernandez MF, Ginsberg MH, Ruggeri ZM et al: Multimeric structure of platelet Factor VIII/von Willebrand factor: The presence of larger multimers and their reassociation with thrombin stimulated platelets. Blood 60:1132–1138, 1982

114. Lynch JM, Lotner GZ, Betz SJ, Henson PM: The release of platelet activating factor by stimulated rabbit neutrophils. J Immunol 123:1219–1226, 1979
115. MacFarlane DE, Mills DCB: The effects of ATP on platelets: Evidence against the central role of released ADP in primary aggregation. Blood 46:309–320, 1975
116. MacFarlane DE, Stibbe J, Kirby EP et al: A method for assaying von Willebrand Factor (ristocetin cofactor). Thromb Diath Haemorrh 34:306–308, 1975
117. Madri JA, Dreyer B, Pitlick FA, Furthmayr H: The collagenous components of the subendothelium: Correlation of structure and function. Lab Invest 43:303–315, 1980
118. Majerus PW, Miletich JP, Kane WH et al: The formation of thrombin on the platelet surface. In Mann KG, Taylor FB Jr (eds): The Regulation of Coagulation, pp 215–233. New York, Elsevier/North-Holland, 1980
119. Mandle R, Colman RW, Kaplan AP: Identification of prekallikrein and high molecular weight kininogen as a complex in human plasma. Proc Natl Acad Sci USA 11:4179–4183, 1976
120. Margossian SS, Lawler JW, Slayter HS: Physical characterization of platelet thrombospondin. J Biol Chem 256:7495–7500, 1981
121. Marguerie GA, Plow EF: Interaction of fibrinogen with its platelet receptor: Kinetics and effect of pH and temperature. Biochemistry 20:1074–1080, 1981
122. McGregor JL,Brochier J, Wild F et al: Monoclonal antibodies against platelet membrane glycoproteins: Characterization and effect on platelet function. Eur J Biochem 131:427–436, 1983
123. Michell RH: Is phosphatidylinositol really out of the calcium gate? Nature 296:492–493, 1982
124. Miletich JP, Jackson CM, Majerus PW: Interaction of coagulation factor Xa with human platelets. Proc Natl Acad Sci USA 74:4033–4036, 1977
125. Miletich JP, Jackson CM, Majerus PW: Properties of the factor Xa binding site on human platelets. J Biol Chem 253:6908–6916, 1978
126. Miletich JP, Majerus DW, Majerus PW: Patients with congenital factor V deficiency have decreased factor Xa binding sites on their platelets. J Clin Invest 62:824–831, 1978
127. Moncada S, Vane JR: Arachidonic acid metabolites and the interactions between platelet and blood-vessel walls. N Engl J Med 300:1142–1147, 1979
128. Moore S, Pepper DS: Identification and characterization of a platelet specific release product: Beta-thromboglobulin. In Gordon JL (ed): Platelets in Biology and Pathology, pp 293–311. Amsterdam, Elsevier Biomedical Press, 1976
129. Moore S, Pepper DS, Cash JD: The isolation and characterization of a platelet-specific beta-globulin and the detection of anti-urokinase and anti-plasmin released from thrombin-aggregated washed human platelets. Biochim Biophys Acta 379:360–369, 1975
130. Moore S, Pepper DS, Cash JD: Platelet antiheparin activity: The isolation and characterization of platelet factor 4 released from thrombin-aggregated washed human platelets and its dissociation into subunits and the isolation of membrane-bound antiheparin activity. Biochim Biophys Acta 379:370–384, 1975
131. Morgan FJ, Begg GS, Chesterman CN: Complete covalent structure of human platelet factor 4. Thromb Haemost 42:1652–1660, 1979
132. Mosher DF, Doyle MJ, Jaffe EA: Synthesis and secretion of thrombospondin by cultured human endothelial cells. J Cell Biol 93:343–348, 1982
133. Murer EH: The role of platelet calcium. Semin Hematol 22:313–323, 1985
134. Nachman RL, Leung LLK: Complex formation of platelet membrane glycoprotein IIb and IIIa with fibrinogen. J Clin Invest 69:263–269, 1982
135. Okumura T, Jamieson GA: Platelet glycocalicin: A single receptor for platelet aggregation induced by thrombin or ristocetin. Thromb Res 8:701–706, 1976
136. Olson JD, Moake JL, Collins MF et al: Adhesion of human platelets to purified solid-phase von Willebrand factor: Studies of normal and Bernard-Soulier platelets. Thromb Res 32:115–122, 1983
137. Owen AJ, Geyer RP, Antoniades HN: Human platelet-derived growth factor stimulates amino

acid transport and protein synthesis by human diploid fibroblasts in plasma-free media. Proc Natl Acad Sci USA 79:3203–3207, 1982

138. Owen NE, Feinberg H, Le Breton GC: Epinephrine induces calcium uptake in human blood platelets. Am J Physiol 239:H483–H488, 1980

139. Owen NE, Le Breton GC: Ca^{2+} mobilization in blood platelets as visualized by chlortetracy-cline fluorescence. Am J Physiol 241(Heart Circ Physiol 10): H613–H619, 1981

140. Parise LV, Venton DL, Le Breton GC: Prostacyclin potentiates 13-azaprostanoic acid–induced platelet deaggregation. Thromb Res 28:721–730, 1982

141. Paul D, Niewiarowski S, Varma KG et al: Human platelet basic protein associated with anti-heparin and mitogenic activities: Purification and partial characterization. Proc Natl Acad Sci USA 77:5914–5918, 1980

142. Peerschke EIB, Galanakis DK: Binding of fibrinogen to ADP-treated platelets. Comparison of plasma fibrinogen fractions and plasmic fibrinogen derivatives. J Lab Clin Med 101:453–460, 1983

143. Phillips DR, Baughan AK: Fibrinogen binding to human platelet plasma membranes: Identification of two steps requiring divalent cations. J Biol Chem 258:10240–10246, 1983

144. Pietu G, Cherel G, Marguerie G et al: Inhibition of von Willebrand factor–platelet interaction by fibrinogen. Nature 308:648–649, 1984

145. Pinckard RN: Platelet-activating factor. Hospital Practice 18(11):67–76, 1983

146. Plow EF, Srouji AH, Meyer D et al: Evidence that three adhesive proteins interact with a common recognition site on activated platelets. J Biol Chem 259:5388–5391, 1984

147. Prescott SM, Majerus PW: Characterization of 1,2-diacylglycerol hydrolysis in human plate-lets. J Biol Chem 258:764–769, 1983

148. Putney JW: Recent hypotheses regarding the phosphatidyl inositol effect. Life Sci 29:183–194, 1981

149. Radcliffe R, Bagdasarian A, Colman R, Nemerson Y: Activation of bovine factor VII by Hage-man factor fragments. Blood 50:611–617, 1977

150. Raines EW, Ross R: Platelet-derived growth factor. I. High yield purification and evidence for multiple forms. J Biol Chem 257:5154–5160, 1982

151. Revak SD, Cochrane CG: The relationship of structure and function in human Hageman factor: The association of enzymatic and binding activities with separate regions of the molecule. J Clin Invest 57:852–860, 1976

152. Revak SD, Cochrane CG, Griffin JH: The binding and cleavage characteristics of human Hageman factor during contact activation. J Clin Invest 59:1167–1175, 1977

153. Rittenhouse-Simmons S: Production of diglyceride from phosphatidylinositol in activated human platelets. J Clin Invest 63:580–587, 1979

154. Ross R: The arterial wall and atherosclerosis. Annu Rev Med 30:1–15, 1979

155. Ross R, Glomset J: The pathogenesis of atherosclerosis. N Engl J Med 295:420–425, 1976

156. Ruggeri ZM, De Marco L, Gatti L et al: Platelets have more than one binding site for von Willebrand Factor. J Clin Invest 72:1–12, 1983

157. Ruggeri ZM, Mannucci PM, Federici AB et al: Multimeric composition of factor VIII/von Willebrand factor following administration of DDAVP: Implications for pathophysiology and therapy of von Willebrand's disease subtypes. Blood 59:1272–1278, 1982

158. Ruggeri ZM, Zimmerman TS: Platelets and von Willebrand disease. Semin Hematol 22:203–218, 1985

159. Rybicki JP, Venton DL, Le Breton GC: The thromboxane antagonist, 13-azaprostanoic acid, inhibits arachidonic acid–induced Ca^{2+} release from isolated platelet membrane vesicles. Biochim Biophys Acta 751:66–73, 1983

160. Santoro SA: Adsorption of von Willebrand factor/factor VIII by the genetically distinct inter-stitial collagens. Thromb Res 21:689–693, 1981

161. Satouchi K, Pinckard RN, McManus LM, Hanahan DJ: Modification of the polar head group of acetyl glyceryl ether phosphorylcholine and subsequent effects upon platelet activation. J Biol Chem 256:4425–4432, 1981

162. Schmaier AH, Smith PM, Colman RW: Platelet C1 inhibitor: A secreted alpha granule subcellular protein. J Clin Invest 75:242–250, 1985

163. Schmaier AH, Zuckerberg A, Silverman C et al: High molecular weight kininogen: A secreted platelet protein. J Clin Invest 71:1477–1489, 1983

164. Schullek J, Jordan J, Montgomery RR: Interaction of von Willebrand Factor with human platelets in the plasma milieu. J Clin Invest 73:421–428, 1984

165. Seaman GVF: Electrochemical features of platelet interactions. Thromb Res 8 (Suppl II): 235–246, 1976

166. Senior RM, Griffin GL, Huang JS et al: Chemotactic activity of platelet alpha granule proteins for fibroblasts. J Cell Biol 96:382–385, 1983

167. Seppa H, Grotendorst G, Seppa S et al: Platelet-derived growth factor is chemotactic for fibroblasts. J Cell Biol 92:584–588, 1982

168. Serhan C, Anderson P, Goodman E et al: Phosphatidate and oxidized fatty acids are calcium ionophores: Studies employing arsenazo III in liposomes. J. Biol Chem 256:2736–2741, 1981

169. Sharma GVRK, Khuri SF, Josa M et al: The effect of antiplatelet therapy on saphenous vein coronary artery bypass patency. Circulation (II) 68:218–221, 1983

170. Shaw JO, Klusick SJ, Hanahan DJ: Activation of rabbit platelet phospholipase and thromboxane synthesis by 1-0-hexadecyl/octadecyl-2-acetyl-sn-glyceryl-3-phosphorylcholine (platelet activating factor). Biochim Biophys Acta 663:222–229, 1981

171. Sherry S: The anturane reinfarction trial. Circulation 62(Suppl V):218–221, 1980

172. Sherry S: Clinical aspects of antiplatelet therapy. Semin Hematol 22:125–134, 1985

173. Shukla SD, Hanahan DJ: AGEPC (platelet activating factor) induced stimulation of rabbit platelets: Effects on phosphatidylinositol, di- and tri-phosphoinositides and phosphatidic acid metabolism. Biochem Biophys Res Commun 106:697–703, 1982

174. Silverberg M, Thompson R, Miller G, Kaplan AP: Initiation of the intrinsic coagulation pathway: Autoactivatability of human Hageman factor and mechanisms by which the light chain derived from HMW-kininogen functions as a co-factor in the activation of prekallikrein, factor XI, and Hageman factor. In Mann KG, Taylor FB Jr. (eds): The Regulation of Coagulation, pp 531–541. New York, Elsevier/North-Holland, 1980

175. Sixma JJ, Sakariassen KS, Stel HV et al: Functional domains of von Willebrand factor: Recognition of discrete tryptic fragments by monoclonal antibodies that inhibit interaction of von Willebrand factor with platelets and with collagen. J Clin Invest 74:736–744, 1984

176. Smith JB: Effect of thromboxane synthetase inhibitors on platelet function: Enhancement by inhibition of phosphodiesterase. Thromb Res 28:477–485, 1982

177. Smith JB, Ingerman CM, Silver MJ: Prostaglandin D_2 inhibits the aggregation of human platelets. Thromb Res 5:291–299, 1974

178. Smith JB, Ingerman CM, Silver MJ: Formation of prostaglandin D_2 during endoperoxide-induced platelet aggregation. Thromb Res 9:413–418, 1976

179. Smith JB, Willis AL: Aspirin selectively inhibits prostaglandin production in human platelets. Nature New Biol 231:235–237, 1971

180. Solum NO: Platelet membrane proteins. Semin Hematol 22:289–302, 1985

181. Soria J, Soria C, Samama M et al: Human platelet fibrinogen: A protein different from plasma fibrinogen. Pathol Biol (Paris) 24 (Suppl): 15–17, 1976

182. Stel HV, Sakariassen KS, de Groot PG et al: vonWillebrand factor in the vessel wall mediates platelet adherence. Blood 65:85–90, 1985

183. Stenberg PE, Shuman MA, Levine SP et al: Redistribution of alpha granules and their contents in thrombin-stimulated platelets. J Cell Biol 98:748–760, 1984

184. Stiles CD, Capone GT, Scher CD et al: Dual control of cell growth by somatomedins and platelet-derived growth factor. Proc Natl Acad Sci USA 76:1279–1283, 1979

185. Sussman II, Rand JH: Subendothelial deposition of von Willebrand's factor requires the presence of endothelial cells. J Lab Clin Med 100:526–532, 1982

186. Sutherland CA, Amin D: Relative activities of rat and dog platelet phospholipase A_2 and diglyceride lipase. J Biol Chem 257:14006–14010, 1982

187. Teitel JM, Sosenberg RD: Protection of factor Xa from neutralization by the heparin–antithrombin complex. J Clin Invest 71:1383–1391, 1983

188. Thompson AR, Harker LA: Coagulation. In Thompson AR, Harker LA (eds): Manual of Hemostasis and Thrombosis, 3rd ed, pp 21–33. Philadelphia, FA Davis, 1984

189. Thompson E, Mandle R, Kaplan AP: Association of factor XI and high molecular weight kininogen in human plasma. J Clin Invest 60:1376–1379, 1977

190. Tracy PB, Eide LC, Bowie EJW et al: Radioimmunoassay of Factor V in human plasma and platelets. Blood 60:59–63, 1982

191. Tracy PB, Nesheim ME, Mann KG: Coordinate binding of factor Va and factor Xa to the unstimulated platelet. J Biol Chem 256:743–751, 1981

192. Tracy PB, Nesheim ME, Mann KG: Proteolytic alterations of factor Va bound to platelets. J Biol Chem 258:7264–7267, 1983

193. Tracy PB, Peterson JM, Nesheim ME et al: Interaction of coagulation factor V and factor Va with platelets. J Biol Chem 254:10354–10361, 1979

194. Vane JR: Inhibition of prostaglandin synthesis as a mechanism of action for aspirin-like drugs. Nature New Biol 231:232–235, 1971

195. Walsh PN: The effects of collagen and kaolin on the intrinsic coagulant activity of platelets: Evidence for an alternative pathway in intrinsic coagulation not requiring factor XII. Br J Haematol 22:393–405, 1972

196. Walsh PN: Platelet-mediated coagulant protein interactions in hemostasis. Semin Hematol 22:178–186, 1985

197. Walsh PN, Biggs R: The role of platelets in intrinsic factor Xa formation. Br J Haematol 22:743–760, 1972

198. Walsh PN, Griffin JH: Contributions of human platelets to the proteolytic activation of blood coagulation factors XII and XI. Blood 57:106–118, 1981

199. Walz DA, Wu VY, de Lamo R et al: Primary structure of human platelet factor 4. Thromb Res 11:893–898, 1977

200. Weerasinghe KM, Scully MF, Kakkar VV: A platelet derived inhibitor of plasma prekallikrein activation. Thromb Res 32:519–529, 1983

201. Weerasinghe KM, Scully MF, Kakkar VV: The effect of collagen mediated platelet release on plasma prekallikrein activation. Thromb Haemost 51:37–41, 1984

202. Weerasinghe KM, Scully MF, Kakkar VV: Inhibition of the cerebroside sulphate (sulfatide)–induced contact activation reactions by platelet factor four. Thromb Res 33:625–631, 1984

203. Weiss HJ, Hoyer LW, Rickles FR et al: Quantitative assay of plasma factor deficient in von Willebrand's disease that is necessary for platelet aggregation: Relationship to factor VIII procoagulant activity and antigen content. J Clin Invest 52:2708–2716, 1973

204. Weksler BB, Ley CW, Jaffe EA: Stimulation of endothelial cell prostacyclin production by thrombin, trypsin, and the ionophore A23187. J Clin Invest 62:923–930, 1978

205. Weksler BB, Marcus AJ, Jaffe EA: Synthesis of prostaglandin I_2 (prostacyclin) by cultured human and bovine endothelial cells. Proc Natl Acad Sci USA 74:3922–3926, 1977

206. Wester J, Sixma JJ, Geuze JJ, Heijnes HFG: Morphology of the hemostatic plug in human skin wounds: Transformation of the plug. Lab Invest 41:182–192, 1979

207. White JG: Platelet microtubules and microfilaments: Effect of cytochalasin B on structure and function. In Caen JP (ed): Platelet Aggregation, pp 15–52. Paris, Masson et Cie, 1971

208. White LD, Cornicelli JA: Platelet-derived growth factor stimulates low density lipoprotein receptor activity in cultured human fibroblasts. Proc Natl Acad Sci USA 77:5962–5966, 1980

209. Wiggins RC, Bouma BN, Cochrane CG, Griffin JH: Role of high molecular weight kininogen in surface-binding and activation of coagulation factor XI and prekallikrein (Hageman factor, contact activation, frbrinolysis). Proc Natl Acad Sci USA 74:4636–4640, 1977

210. Wiggins RC, Cochrane CG: The autoactivation of rabbit Hageman factor. J Exp Med 150:1122–1133, 1979

211. Williams LT, Tremble P, Antoniades HN: Platelet derived growth factor binds specifically to receptors on vascular smooth muscle cells and the binding becomes non-dissociable. Proc Natl Acad Sci USA 79:5867–5870, 1982

212. Zucker MB, Broekman MJ, Kaplan KL: Factor VIII – related antigen in human blood platelets: Localization and release by thrombin and collagen. J Lab Clin Med 94:675–682, 1979
213. Zucker MB, Mosesson MW, Broekman MJ et al: Release of fibronectin (cold-insoluble globulin) from alpha granules induced by thrombin and collagen; lack of requirement for plasma fibronectin in ADP-induced platelet aggregation. Blood 54:8–12, 1979
214. Zur M, Nemerson Y: Kinetics of factor IX activation via the extrinsic pathway: Dependence of Km on tissue factor. J Biol Chem 225:5703–5707, 1980

Tests of Platelet Number and Function   9

George A. Fritsma

A healthy 22-year-old white woman came to the hematology clinic in no apparent distress. She indicated that she was a medical technology student who had just completed several coagulation laboratory exercises. During one laboratory exercise a classmate performed a bleeding time test on her, and the result was 19 minutes. Because this result was well above the normal limit, her instructor recommended that she request a coagulation workup.

The patient indicated that she had no history of easy bruising, and she recalled no episodes of menorrhagia, epistaxis, or hemorrhage after dental surgery. She had been healthy for 6 months prior to the bleeding time test, had never been pregnant, and was not pregnant at this time. There was no family history of hemorrhage. She had not taken aspirin for at least 1 week prior to the day of the bleeding time test.

The patient was 5 feet, 2 inches tall, weighed 114 pounds, and had a blood pressure of 120/82, a pulse of 68, 13 respirations per minute, and a normal temperature. No petechiae or purpura were noted on legs, arms, or trunk. Spleen and liver were normal, and there was no evidence of lymphadenopathy.

The patient was instructed to avoid all medication for 10 days and report to the laboratory for a routine coagulation screen and CBC. Results are shown here.

Laboratory Data

CBC
   Hemoglobin 13.4 g/dl
   Hematocrit 41.1%
   RBC $4.2 \times 10^6/\mu l$
   WBC $7.3 \times 10^3/\mu l$
   Platelets 310,000/μl
PT 11.2 sec.
APTT 29.4 sec.
TT 14 sec. (control, 16 sec.)
Bleeding time 13 min.

After a second office visit, platelet aggregometry was ordered. The results were as follows:

AGONIST	TRACING
ADP (10^{-6}M)	Primary aggregation followed by return to baseline
Epinephrine	Primary aggregation followed by return to baseline
Collagen	No aggregation
Thrombin	No aggregation
Ristocetin	Full (80%) agglutination

These findings imply that the patient has a mild storage pool disorder. The significant results include bleeding time and platelet aggregometry with ADP, epinephrine, collagen, and thrombin. All other laboratory results were within normal limits.

A prolonged bleeding time result may imply either an abnormality affecting the integrity of the vasculature or a platelet abnormality. Since the platelet count was normal and there was no apparent bruising, an abnormality of platelet function was suspected. This was confirmed by the aggregometry tracings. Primary aggregation followed by platelet disaggregation indicates that the platelets do not secrete internal agonists upon extrinsic challenge. Inadequate secretion may be caused by storage pool disorder or a disorder of platelet activation (aspirinlike syndrome). In storage pool disorder the platelet dense bodies are poorly developed, with low concentrations of ADP, calcium, and serotonin. In aspirinlike syndrome, platelet enzymes responsible for activation, like cyclooxygenase or prostaglandin synthase, are congenitally deficient. In either case, secondary aggregation cannot proceed because there is no release of internal aggregating agents. Aggregometry with thrombin as the agonist helps distinguish between the two situations. Thrombin bypasses the requirement for prostaglandin production and causes direct secretion of platelet organelle contents. The lack of response to thrombin in this case implies storage pool disorder.

There was a discrepancy between the bleeding time determined by the student and the later laboratory bleeding time, although both were elevated. This could be explained by faulty technique in the first case. The bleeding time test is difficult to control and may be prolonged by the use of an uncontrolled skin puncture or excessive forearm blood pressure. Another possibility is that although the patient reported no aspirin ingestion, several patent medicines contain salicylates without including the term *aspirin* in their name. She may have taken one of these. Salicylate is a nonsteroidal anti-inflammatory drug that irreversibly acetylates platelet cyclooxygenase to prevent activation. Nonsteroidal anti-inflammatory drugs will affect the bleeding in any event, but especially in mild storage pool disorder.

Because the patient was experiencing no hemorrhagic symptoms, the disorder was presumed to be mild, and she was encouraged to resume her normal activities with the precaution that she eliminate the use of aspirin or aspirin products. If she later requires major surgery, a full coagulation panel should be included in the preliminary laboratory workup.

Tests for evaluation of platelets include *platelet counts* and *platelet function tests.* Platelet counts are reliable and have become routine procedures in automated hematology laboratories. The combination of platelet counting and bone marrow megakaryocyte estimation yields extensive information about platelet production and consumption, and about the risks of hemorrhage and thrombosis. Computation of *mean platelet volume (MPV)* adds to the clinical understanding of platelet kinetics.

Clinical tests of platelet function are generally less reliable than the time-tested platelet count. The most commonly applied test, and one that has enjoyed a comeback since 1977, is the *bleeding time (BT)* test.[17] This simple procedure may be used to detect functional platelet abnormalities even when the count is normal or increased. Unfortunately the BT is sometimes prolonged in the presence of vascular rather than platelet abnormalities, so interpretation demands scrupulous attention to technique and a knowledge of the clinical condition of the patient.

Platelet aggregometry and *platelet retention* tests are commonly applied *in vitro* qualitative or semiquantitative assays of platelet function that require specially designed laboratory instruments. These results are subject to technologists' interpretation. The retention test was developed by E. W. Salzman in 1963, when it was called the test of platelet *adhesiveness.*[23] The retention procedure has enjoyed limited acceptance in clinical laboratories because it is difficult to perform reliably. Although also technically demanding, aggregometry has become popular in the clinical laboratory and is performed often.[4]

Immunoassay of the plasma concentration of platelet-specific secretions such as *platelet factor 4* or *β-thromboglobulin* is the newest type of test for platelet activation. Immunoassays are technically less demanding than aggregometry and are easily adapted for routine use, but their results are not easy to interpret clinically. Immunologic tests are described in detail in Chapter 12.

These tests and a few others of limited application, such as *capillary fragility, antiplatelet antibody,* and *platelet immune complexes,* make up the entire spectrum of platelet physiology tests. The purpose of this chapter is to identify each clinically useful laboratory test of platelet number and function. The principle of each test protocol is reviewed to demonstrate where it fits in the overall hemostatic scheme. The clinical significance and interpretation of each procedure using normal values are also described in detail.

SPECIMEN COLLECTION

Chapter 3 provides a full discussion of whole blood collection techniques for platelet testing. Blood collected for platelet counts is treated as a sample collected for a complete blood count (CBC). A solution of tripotassium *ethylenediamine tetraacetic acid (EDTA; Sequestrene, Versene)* is the recommended anticoagulant. EDTA is provided in commercial evacuated glass tubes, and is effective both as a preservative and as an anticoagulant when the sample is well mixed immediately after collection. Commercially available vacuum tubes containing EDTA are identified with a lavender stopper. The samples may be held for up to 5 hours at room temperature after collection or up to 24 hours at 4°C without significant change in the platelet count. If the platelet count is to be performed at the same time as a CBC, however, the test should be completed within 4 hours of specimen collection. Furthermore, a stained peripheral blood smear from the EDTA tube for platelet count estimation must be made within 2 hours of collection to avoid anticoagulant-induced distortion of cell morphology.[8] EDTA tubes may not be used for collection of samples for platelet function tests both because the calcium chelating effect of the EDTA causes *in vitro* suppression of platelet activity, and the glass tube surface tends to induce platelet activation.

There is a bizarre, but not uncommon, consequence of EDTA blood sample collection called *platelet satellitism*, or *platelet–neutrophil adherence* (Fig. 9-1). On the blood smear, platelets encircle polymorphonuclear neutrophils, and the platelet count is falsely decreased, sometimes to below the normal range.[21] This phenomenon is seen only in EDTA samples; when smears are made from samples drawn in potassium sodium oxalate, sodium citrate, or heparin, satellitism is not seen. Platelet satellitism is not related to functional abnormalities of the blood, drug usage, or the clinical condition of the patient, and appears to be an *in vitro* phenomenon caused by some ill-defined

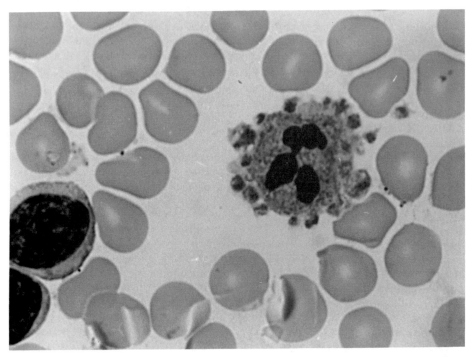

FIG. 9-1. Photomicrograph of platelet–neutrophil adherence on a peripheral blood smear from an EDTA whole blood specimen (satellitism) (Wright stain, original magnification ×1000).

autoimmune activity. Platelet satellitism must always be reported when detected because it causes *spurious thrombocytopenia* and may be involved in some as yet unspecified clinical abnormality.[18]

Samples collected for platelet function studies, such as those that are collected for plasma coagulation factor quantitation, require special preparation and handling. The two-syringe technique (described in Chap. 3) must be employed, and the blood sample may come into contact only with plastic, not glass. A buffered solution of 0.109M (3.2%) or 0.129M (3.8%) sodium citrate is placed in the second syringe prior to collection in sufficient volume to ensure that the final ratio of anticoagulant solution to whole blood–anticoagulant mixture is 1:10. The venipuncture must be made without trauma, and as soon as the blood is drawn into the anticoagulated syringe, the sample must be gently and thoroughly mixed. Commercially prepared evacuated glass tubes with blue stoppers, designed for collection of plasma samples for routine coagulation testing, may not be used for tests of platelet function.

PHYSICAL EXAMINATION

Detection of a bleeding disorder begins with a careful history and physical examination. Since a hemorrhagic tendency is not always apparent, it is essential to obtain details of the bleeding history of the patient and the patient's relatives. *Petechiae,* hemorrhages into the skin or mucous membrane of less than 3 mm in diameter; *ecchymoses,* hemorrhages greater than 3 mm; and *purpura;* generalized skin and mucous membrane hemorrhages, are the more common physical signs of platelet or vascular disorders. Minor cuts may result in prolonged bleeding. Gastrointestinal bleeding and prolonged or excessive bleeding after surgery are sometimes seen in thrombocytopenia.[25]

Hemophilia and coagulation disorders, by contrast, usually have widespread bleeding episodes: bleeding from the urinary and gastrointestinal tract, into joints, and into the peritoneum. Though the symptoms of hemophilia seem more profound, platelet and coagulation disorders may both become life-threatening.

CAPILLARY FRAGILITY

The signs of hemorrhagic blood vessel disorders resemble those of platelet disorders. For this reason, tests of capillary fragility, described here, are performed to rule out capillary disease when a platelet disorder is suspected.

Tourniquet Test

Because many hemostatically normal people exhibit a tendency to bruise easily, tests of capillary fragility are rarely conclusive. To perform the tourniquet test, developed about 1910 by two German physicians, Theodor Rumpel and Stockbridge Carl Leed, a blood pressure cuff is placed around the patient's arm and inflated to a pressure between the *systolic* and *diastolic* levels of the patient's blood pressure. After 5 minutes the cuff is deflated. Several minutes later, the arm is examined for subcutaneous petechiae just distal to where the cuff had been placed. More than five petechiae per 3-cm-diameter circle may indicate a blood vessel disorder. See Chapter 1 for a discussion of the causes of vascular disorders.

Capillary Fragility Test

In the capillary fragility test a negative-pressure device called a *petechiometer* is used instead of the tourniquet (Fig. 9-2). The suction cup is applied to the volar surface of the forearm for 1 to 2 minutes, then released. After several minutes the cup is removed, and the area of skin underneath is examined for subcutaneous petechiae. When 1 or more petechiae appear, the test is considered to be positive for capillary fragility. This approach is more comfortable for the patient and may be repeated several times for increased accuracy.

Neither the tourniquet test nor the petechiometer test is completely reliable, since many normal persons exhibit positive test results. The technologist and phlebotomist should be aware, however, that the appearance of numerous petechiae during the employment of a tourniquet for routine venipuncture may be significant and should be reported to the attending physician as an indication that further studies are warranted.

PLATELET COUNTING AND SIZING

Clinical Purpose of the Platelet Count

The reference interval for peripheral blood platelet counts for adult men and women is 150 to 440×10^3 cells per microliter of whole blood.[24] *Thrombocytopenia*, defined as a count below $150 \times 10^3/\mu l$, may be the result of a variety of disorders that are characterized by a pathologic increase in the consumption of platelets or diminished platelet production. *Immune (idiophathic) thrombocytopenic purpura (ITP), neonatal isoim-*

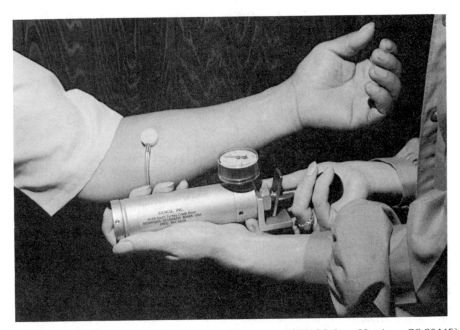

FIG. 9-2. The SIENCO DP-647 petechiometer. (Courtesy of SIENCO, Inc., Morrison, CO 80465)

mune *thrombocytopenia, posttransfusion purpura, thrombotic thrombocytopenic pur-pura (TTP)*, and *disseminated intravascular coagulation (DIC)* are disorders in which the platelet life span is significantly shortened and in which platelet consumption is not replenished by marrow production. Thrombocytopenias in which diminished platelet production is the primary cause include *Bernard-Soulier syndrome (BSS)*, *aplastic anemia*, and the *acute lymphocytic* and *acute nonlymphocytic leukemias*. Chapter 10 reviews these diseases. Thrombocytopenia is also an expected side-effect of cancer chemotherapy.

Platelet counts are performed routinely in all laboratories, usually to detect throm-bocytopenia. Profound thrombocytopenia is a common cause of hemorrhage and may be a medical emergency. Most physicians choose to initiate platelet concentrate therapy by administering 4 to 6 random-donor units when the count drops to below 20 $\times$ $10^3/\mu l$.[12] The decision is influenced by the clinical condition of the patient, evidence of hemorrhage, and whether the fall in count is abrupt or gradual. The number of platelets in a single unit of platelet concentrate is sufficient to increase the platelet count of a healthy person by about 10 $\times$ $10^3/\mu l$.[12] The effect of platelet concentrate in a patient with bleeding, fever, or increased platelet destruction is variably diminished. The im-portance of the platelet count in a thrombocytopenic patient experiencing hemorrhage is underscored by the number of times it is ordered as an emergency or "stat" procedure.

An elevated platelet count is termed *thrombocytosis* or *thrombocythemia*. Throm-bocytosis is often present in infection, in inflammation, and after surgery.[22] In these conditions thrombocytosis may be thought of as an acute-phase reaction secondary to the condition. The platelet count will fall to the normal range after symptoms are resolved. Thrombocytosis may also be associated with nonhematologic malignancy. During inflammation, platelet counts between 500 and 800 $\times$ $10^3/\mu l$ are regularly observed and seldom warrant medical intervention.

Primary thrombocytosis is rare and usually indicates a myeloproliferative disorder such as *essential thrombocythemia*. In this case platelet counts often reach levels higher than 1000 $\times$ $10^3/\mu l$, creating a remarkably cluttered blood smear (Fig. 9-3). The clinical consequences of these extreme counts are variable and may not be injurious, but the underlying condition is a cause for concern.

Manual Platelet Count

Platelet counts are performed manually in most clinical laboratories despite the avail-ability of platelet counting instruments. Manual counting is necessary to calibrate instruments or to analyze samples with exceptionally high or low platelet counts that are beyond the range of instrument accuracy, or in cases when instruments are unavail-able.

Direct visual examination using phase-contrast microscopy is the most reliable manual approach to platelet counting. Brecher and Cronkite developed this method in 1950.[6] Capillary or venous blood (collected in EDTA) is diluted in a 1.1% solution of ammonium oxalate with a specially designed pipette. Ammonium oxalate hemolyzes the red cells while leaving platelets and white cells intact. The suspension is placed in the chamber of a special *hemocytometer* designed for phase-contrast microscopy that has standard *Neubauer* rulings (Fig. 9-4). Once the suspension is added, the hemocy-tomer is placed on the microscope stage and examined by the technologist to distin-guish between platelets and other objects. The platelets located within a defined area

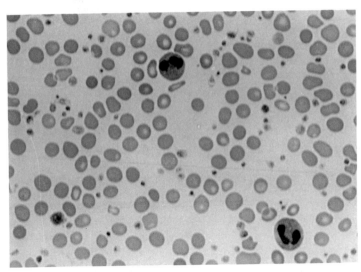

FIG. 9-3. Photomicrograph of the peripheral blood smear from a patient with essential thrombocythemia, in which the platelet count is greater than $1000 \times 10^3/\mu l$ (Wright stain, original magnification $\times 450$).

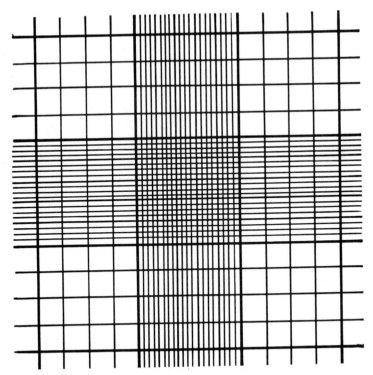

FIG. 9-4. Counting area of a standard Neubauer hemocytometer. The 25 small squares in the center square millimeter are used for the platelet count (approximately $100\times$ actual size).

are counted, and a computation is used to convert the raw value to platelets $\times 10^3/\mu l$. Results are compared to the reference interval.

The coefficient of variation for repeated performances of phase-contrast platelet counts is 11% under ideal conditions, and 16% under standard laboratory conditions.[7] (See Chapter 3 for a definition of coefficient of variation.) In some laboratories an ordinary light microscope is substituted for the phase instrument, raising the coefficient of variation to as high as 20% to 25%. Blood collection techniques also affect count reliability. Capillary blood samples will yield consistently lower counts with greater variation because platelets tend to adhere to the edges of the collection wound. Venous blood samples must be well mixed at the time of collection to prevent *in vitro* platelet aggregation and plasma coagulation. Since no method is available for calibration or control of manual platelet counts, accuracy depends on the exercise of careful technique.

When the phase-contrast platelet count is used to calibrate automated counting instruments, accuracy may be ensured when the calibration sample is averaged from quadruplicate counts performed by two technologists.

Automated Platelet Count Using Platelet-Rich Plasma

Automated platelet counts may be performed using either well-mixed whole blood or platelet-rich plasma (PRP). In either approach, results that fall in the range of $50 \times 10^3/\mu l$ to $500 \times 10^3/\mu l$ are more reliable when determined automatically than manually. Instrument counts are made on a greater number of particles than manual counts. Consequently, the coefficient of variation for automated counts may be as small as 4%, whereas the best achievable for the Brecher-Cronkite phase microscope manual count is 11%. Most instruments also contain circuitry that distinguishes between platelets and small nonbiologic particles, eliminating the need for visual recognition and differentiation of debris from platelets.

The PRP technique begins with an aliquot of whole blood for which the hematocrit has previously been determined. The blood is mixed carefully, placed in a plastic capillary tube, and allowed to stand in a position between 10° and 30° from vertical for 30 to 90 minutes, permitting the erythrocytes to settle. Specialized centrifugation may replace sedimentation, providing PRP in 5 to 10 minutes. Centrifugation is superior to sedimentation because it is more rapid and because leukocytes that remain in the PRP of sedimented samples tend to cause falsely lowered counts. Since the centrifugation time and centrifugal force must be carefully controlled, specially designed centrifuges are used. The Coulter Thrombo-fuge (Coulter Electronics, Hialeah, FL 33010) is one example of a centrifuge designed for PRP preparation.[9]

A measured volume (3.33 μl or 6.66 μl) of PRP is suspended in 10 ml or 20 ml of an electrolyte solution such as Isoton (Coulter) or Hematall (Fisher Diagnostics, Orangeburg, NY 10962) to achieve a 1:3030 dilution. The suspension is then placed on the sample stand of a particle-counting instrument such as a Coulter ZBI. When the instrument cycle is started, the suspension passes through a 70-μm orifice through which is passing a small electrical current. Each time a particle passes through the orifice, an increase in impedance to the current flow produces an electronic "pulse" or "spike." Each spike is measured electronically and recorded. The number of electronic pulses is proportional to the number of particles that pass through the orifice.

After several seconds, a numerical result corresponding to the number of pulses in 100 μl of platelet suspension appears on the face of the instrument. This number is used to compute platelets per microliter of whole blood using a Platelet Calculator, a device that is supplied with the platelet counting kit. This calculator provides a whole blood result based on the previously determined hematocrit and compensates both for platelet-free plasma trapped within the sedimented erythrocytes and for particle coincidence.

PRP results become unreliable if the numerical display value on the counting instrument is below 1000 or above 30,000. Hematocrit values below 20 or above 50 result in loss of linearity. In these cases, manual counts are performed instead of automated counts.

Since platelets are small, with an MPV of 7.5 to 10.5 femtoliters (fl), platelet counts are easily affected by the presence of debris or microcytic erythrocytes in PRP dilutions. Figure 9-5 demonstrates the relationship between debris, platelet, and erythrocyte size distributions. When the platelet count is low, pulses generated by particles of debris cause a significant elevation. When microcytes are present, as in iron-deficiency anemia or thalassemia, red cells are counted as platelets. These phenomena may be managed by manipulating the threshold controls of the instrument. The lower threshold may be set to coincide with the valley between debris and platelets, appropriately termed the *lower valley*. The upper threshold may be similarly set at the level of the *upper valley* between platelets and red cells (see Fig. 9-5). The upper and lower valley levels will differ for each patient sample. However, standard PRP-based platelet counting instruments provide no means for displaying or analyzing the valleys and have fixed threshold settings. These instruments tend to give falsely elevated platelet counts in cases of microcytosis or when there is an artifactual increase in the size and average volume of debris. The presence of debris causes unacceptable false elevation of a low platelet count.

An electronic analyzer that displays a frequency distribution histogram of particle size may be connected to the platelet counter. This device produces a graph similar to the one shown in Figure 9-5 that displays the upper and lower valleys. The Coulter Channelyzer is such a device. Platelets are passed through the aperture until a fre-

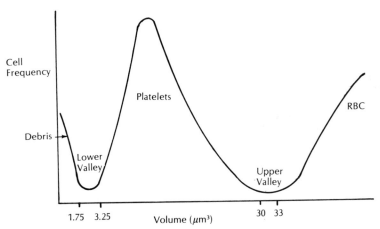

FIG. 9-5. Cell volume frequency distribution histogram demonstrating the range of normal platelet volume and the valleys separating platelets from debris (*lower*) and erythrocytes (*upper*).

quency distribution graph is produced (usually 10,000 particles are sufficient). The graph is examined, and the particle volumes at the level of the valleys are computed. Threshold settings on the instrument are changed to coincide with the valleys, and the count is initiated. The Channelyzer tracing serves as a qualitative expression of platelet sample volume and was used routinely for this purpose until the incorporation of MPV measurements on multiparametric instruments. See the subsequent section on platelet size analysis for further details about MPV.

Automated Platelet Counts Using Whole Blood

Another type of automated platelet counter uses a whole blood specimen instead of PRP. One example is the ULTRA-FLO 100 Platelet Counter (Clay-Adams Co., Parsippanny, NJ 07054), an instrument marketed in the 1980s that employs the principle of *hydrodynamic focusing*. A 1:910 suspension of whole blood in buffered saline is directed through a 60-μm orifice surrounded by a stream of isotonic "sheath fluid" (Fig. 9-6). An electrical current passes through the orifice with the cells so that an electronic pulse will be generated each time a particle passes the orifice. Platelets yield pulses in an amplitude range equivalent to their size, between 3.25 μm^3 and 33 μm^3, while erythrocytes give pulses proportional to their volume, greater than 33 μm^3. Electronic "channels" permit discrimination between platelet and erythrocyte pulses so that they are counted separately. Hydrodynamic focusing provides a sensitivity to particle size not achievable by other means. To perform a platelet count on the ULTRA-FLO 100 the erythrocyte count is first determined by another technique. The erythrocyte count is then dialed by thumbwheel into the display on the front of the instrument, the diluted

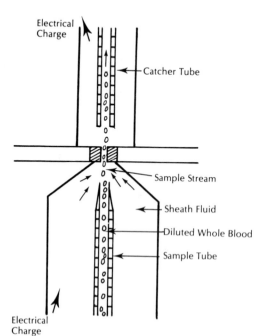

Electrical
Charge

Catcher Tube

Sample Stream

Sheath Fluid

Diluted Whole Blood

Sample Tube

Electrical
Charge

FIG. 9-6. Hydrodynamic focusing: the focused aperture tube.

sample of whole blood is inserted onto the sample tube, and the count is initiated. When the instrument counts a number of erythrocytes proportional to the dialed-in value, the cycle ends and the platelet count is displayed on the face of the instrument. The displayed count is actually based on the ratio between platelet pulses and erythrocyte pulses. In this approach the accuracy of the platelet count depends only on the accuracy of the erythrocyte count and not on the accuracy of the dilution prepared for counting.

The particle size counting thresholds for the ULTRA-FLO 100 are preset and cannot be changed to reflect movement of upper and lower valleys. However, special circuits monitor the levels of pulses in the range of 1.75 μm^3 to 3.25 μm^3 (lower valley) and 30 μm^3 to 33 μm^3 (upper valley). When the pulse count exceeds preset limits in each range, panel alarms are triggered to indicate that the count is suspect. When there is an upper valley alarm, the operator may switch to a *MICRO* mode, in which counting proceeds at between 3.25 μm^3 and 30 μm^3 volume. When there is a lower valley alarm, the operator must remove the sample and perform a manual platelet count or use the PRP method with a Channelyzer.

Most multiparameter hematologic instruments provide a platelet count as a routine part of the complete blood count. Whole blood samples are introduced directly into the instrument, which makes appropriate dilutions internally. The erythrocyte:platelet ratio is determined, and the threshold setting "floats" electronically to the upper and lower valley locations to provide accurate counts. As in all instrumental analyses, the accuracy of counts between 50 and 500 $\times$ $10^3/\mu l$ is acceptable, while low and high counts must still be performed by hand.

For procedural protocols for automated platelet counting devices, the reader is referred to the technical manuals that accompany the platelet counters.

Platelet Size Analysis: The Clinical Use of the MPV

The MPV is the arithmetic mean cell volume for a sample platelet population. Though the concept of MPV has existed for many years, practical clinical assessment of platelet size has been limited to semiquantitative notations based on smear examination and to visual inspection of Channelyzer-generated platelet size distribution curves (platelet histograms). Most multiparametric hematology instruments now automatically analyze the platelet population and present a platelet histogram. Figure 9-7 shows a platelet histogram from normal human blood. Note that the distribution is "log-normal," meaning that the curve tails off gradually to the right. The instrument analyzes the generated histogram to determine whether it is log-normal and then computes the platelet count and the MPV by integration. If the curve does not fit the expected distribution, the instrument count and MPV cannot be accurately computed and are not displayed. When this happens, the platelet count must be performed manually and the MPV report deleted.

There is no single range of normals for the MPV. When the platelet count is 150 $\times$ $10^3/\mu l$, the MPV reference interval is approximately 9 fl to 12 fl, but at a count of 400 $\times$ 10^3, the range drops to 7.5 fl to 10 fl.[2] The inverse relationship of normal platelet count to normal MPV is demonstrated in the nomogram developed by Bessman (Fig. 9-8). The MPV may rise to above the normal limit in a variety of diseases in which increased platelet destruction is evident such as in ITP or DIC. This is an "appropriate" elevation that reflects bone marrow regeneration of platelets. Under these conditions the MPV is associated with a diminished platelet count and an increase in the number of bone

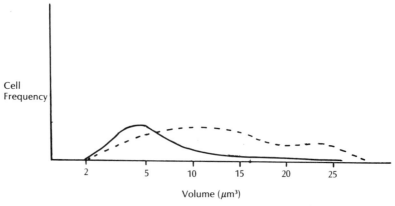

FIG. 9-7. Platelet volume frequency distribution histogram comparing a normal distribution *(solid line)* and a population of large platelets *(broken line).*

marrow megakaryocytes.[1] ITP patients recovering from thrombocytopenic episodes demonstrate decreasing MPVs as their platelet counts rise.

Patients with thrombocytopenia and *decreased* MPVs suffer from the hypoproliferation of marrow elements found in aplastic anemia, megaloblastic anemia, or anticancer chemotherapy and may have a poorer prognosis than patients with thrombocytopenia and high MPVs. Cancer chemotherapy induces a diminished MPV concurrent with thrombocytopenia, but as bone marrow regenerates, the MPV will rise before the platelet count. Failure of the MPV to rise in such instances suggests continuing bone marrow suppression. Thrombocytopenia secondary to hypersplenism is associated

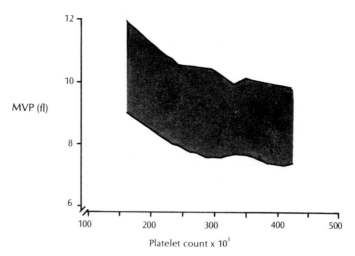

FIG. 9-8. Nomogram representing the reference range of MPV at various platelet counts. (Bessman JD, Williams LJ, Gilmer PR Jr: The inverse relation of platelet size and count in normal subjects, and an artifact of other particles. Am J Clin Pathol 76:289–293, 1981)

with a reduced MPV, perhaps because there is preferential sequestration of the larger platelets.

In most cases of secondary thrombocytosis, a low MPV is expected. However, in essential thrombocythemia the MPV usually falls in the normal range. In essential thrombocythemia the platelet histogram is not log-normal but bimodal because of the presence of a population of large platelets (see Fig. 9-7). The MPV remains normal when this population is small, but may rise when the large cells constitute a significant proportion of the population.

Quality Control for Platelet Counts

Two types of commercial platelet control suspensions are available: preserved normal human platelets and synthetics. Human platelet controls are harvested from PRP and suspended in a solution of plasma with glutaraldehyde (a membrane crosslinking agent), surface-active agents to prevent activation, formalin, and other stabilizers. Synthetic controls are composed of polystyrene particles suspended in sodium azide solution.[20] Human platelet suspensions provide the expected range of platelet volumes but have a short shelf life and may be altered by preservatives. Synthetics are inert but do not reflect the size distributions of fresh platelets. Low- and normal-range controls are incorporated in routine runs of platelet counts and are compared to predetermined action limits as described in Chapter 3. Controls are not used to calibrate platelet counting instruments; instead, calibration is performed by manually counting the platelets of fresh whole blood from a normal donor.

Whole blood controls with platelet components are available for multiparametric instruments. In most cases these are preserved human whole blood materials, although some incorporate nonhuman components such as mammalian platelets, avian erythrocytes that simulate leukocytes, and human erythrocytes. Some of these materials now provide MPV values.

Platelet Estimation From Blood Smears

All platelet counts must be confirmed by examination of the monolayer portion of a properly stained blood smear. Five to eight monolayer fields are scanned with a 100X (oil-immersion) objective, and the number of platelets per field is counted and averaged. In a patient with a normal erythrocyte count, an average of 8 to 20 platelets per high-power field is normal.[8] The average is multiplied by 20,000 and the product compared to the visual or instrumental count. If the two figures do not agree within 20%, the blood smear should be examined for the presence of platelet clumps, giant platelets, platelet adhesion to polymorphonuclear neutrophils, microcytes, or erythrocytic fragments (Fig. 9-9). The instrument count and estimate must be repeated, and if a discrepancy still exists, the cause must be determined. Giant platelets, clumping, and adherence can cause spuriously low platelet counts, while the presence of microcytes and schizocytes will elevate the count.

In laboratories where there is no instrumentation for routine platelet counting, platelet estimates must be reported. The following terms are used:

Fewer than 8 platelets/1000X field: Platelets decreased
8 to 20 platelets/1000 X field: Platelets adequate
More than 20 platelets/1000X field: Platelets increased

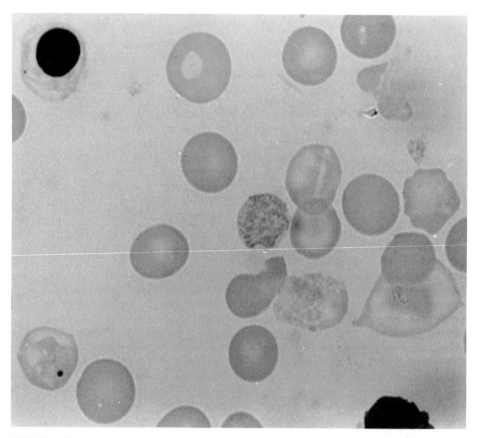

FIG. 9-9. Photomicrograph demonstrating microcytes and platelets in the peripheral blood smear of a patient with iron-deficiency anemia (Wright stain, original magnification ×1000).

Because platelet distribution depends on erythrocyte concentration, when the erythrocyte count is not within the normal range, platelet estimation from the smear is unreliable.

THE BLEEDING TIME TEST

An injury to a capillary bed exposes subendothelial collagen fibrils. Circulating platelets adhere to the collagen and aggregate to form a hemostatic platelet plug. The adequacy of both the adhesion and aggregation components of platelet function may be assessed by making a small, controlled puncture wound and measuring the duration of bleeding. Early approaches to BT tests were nonstandard, and critical nonplatelet variables such as skin thickness, intracapillary pressure, and size and depth of the wound were sources of profound variation. The earliest attempt at standardization was made by Duke in 1912.[11] The Duke BT was performed with a standard lancet to prick the earlobe and required blotting the wound every 30 seconds with filter paper. Duke's approach was used until the mid-1970s but was difficult to standardize because wound depth in the earlobe was hard to control.

The Ivy BT was described in 1941.[17] In this approach a blood pressure cuff is placed around the upper arm and inflated to 40 mm Hg. A site on the volar surface of the forearm near the antecubital crease is selected and prepared, then punctured with a lancet. The wound is blotted with filter paper every 30 seconds. The skin thickness in this area varies only slightly from one person to another; thus, the bleeding BT is better standardized, provided that the area is free of superficial blood vessels, rashes, hair, and scar tissue. The only variables that remain are the size and depth of the wound.

In 1977 the Simplate Bleeding Time Device (Organon Teknika, Parsipanny, NJ 07054) was introduced. This is a spring-loaded lancet that produces a uniform incision 5 mm long and 1 mm deep. The Simplate is designed to be used in the Ivy BT method to eliminate variation in wound size. The blood pressure cuff is placed around the upper arm and inflated to 40 mm Hg. A site is selected and cleansed with alcohol and allowed to air dry. The Simplate is placed firmly on the site and triggered. The wound is blotted every 30 seconds with filter paper, taking care that the paper does not contact the wound. Blotting continues at the same interval until bleeding stops, and the time is recorded.

The normal range for the Ivy BT using the Simplate is 2 to 9 minutes. The time is prolonged in thrombocytopenia, hereditary and acquired platelet dysfunctions, von Willebrand disease, afibrinogenemia, severe hypofibrinogenemia, and some vascular bleeding disorders. A single dose of aspirin will cause a small but significant prolongation of the BT in about 50% of normal persons. Many other drugs may affect results. Surgicutt (International Technidyne Corporation, Edison, NJ 08817) is another, more recently introduced incision-making instrument.

The Ivy method with the Simplate or Surgicutt device is the simplest and most common screening test for platelet dysfunction and is always applied before other more elaborate tests are performed. The Mielke Template method, in which three parallel incisions are made 1 mm deep and 9 mm long guided by a template, is a further modification. This method is more reproducible and sensitive but tends to leave noticeable scars. The Simplate and Surgicutt methods may also leave scars, but these are minimized by the application of a pressure dressing upon completion.

PLATELET AGGREGOMETRY

When a wound forms and subendothelial collagen fibrils are exposed, platelets adhere to the injured surface. The adhesion of additional platelets to the first layer of platelets is called aggregation. During aggregation, platelets release calcium, ADP, and serotonin to recruit more platelets and promote further aggregation. The *in vitro* measurement of platelet aggregation is useful for detection of congenital and acquired platelet dysfunctions resulting in hemorrhage and in some circumstances may be used to test for the risk of thrombosis. The laboratory test for aggregation is called aggregometry.[5]

Specimen Preparation

Aggregometry is performed with PRP and platelet-poor plasma (PPP). A sample of whole blood is collected in sodium citrate by the two-syringe technique (see Chap. 3). PRP is prepared by taking a portion of the whole blood sample and centrifuging for 10 minutes at a relative centrifugal force (RCF) of 200g. The plasma is removed and stored in a covered vial at ambient temperatures. The remaining whole blood is centrifuged again, this time at 1000g for 15 minutes, resulting in a supernate of PPP. The PPP is removed from the red cells, placed in a covered vial, and stored at ambient temperatures.

Operation of the Platelet Aggregometer

Aggregometry is performed in an aggregation meter, a specialized photometer with a stirring device that maintains PRP in an even suspension in its sample cuvet (Fig. 9-10). PRP is adjusted to a count of about 300×10^3 platelets per microliter by mixing with PPP. This mixture is placed in a cuvet equipped with a clean plasticized stir bar that turns at 800 to 1200 RPM, keeping the platelets in suspension. The cuvet with the PRP is warmed to 37°C and maintained at this temperature throughout the aggregometry procedure. White incident light is directed toward the sample cuvet. Transmitted light, the intensity of which varies in proportion to the level of aggregation in the plasma, is continuously monitored and recorded on the strip chart (Fig. 9-11). First, PPP is placed in a cuvet and moved to the cuvet well. The operator sets the pen at full deflection or the equivalent of 100% light transmission. The PPP is now replaced by a second cuvet containing 0.45 ml of PRP, and the pen moves downward, reflecting the diminished transmission of light. As the PRP is stirred, the pen stabilizes at a point near 0% transmission. This is called the baseline. After a brief period, 20 µl of an aggregating agent or *agonist* is mixed with the PRP. In 60 to 90 seconds the platelets change in shape from discoid to spherical with pseudopods. Small aggregates form, more light passes through the PRP, and the pen begins to move towads 100% light transmission. The ensuing aggregation reaction is continuously recorded for about 15 minutes.

In normal PRP the pen tracing may take one of three paths depending on the type and concentration of agonist (Fig. 9-12). If there is a strong stimulus, the pen deflects rapidly towards 100% transmission, resulting in a smooth *monophasic* arc leveling off at between 60% and 80% (see Chap. 8 for a complete description of physiologic events during aggregation). The platelets will not disaggregate, and the pen will remain at this level as long as the instrument is allowed to run. A moderate stimulus results in a *biphasic* curve. The pen deflects rapidly to a point about halfway between baseline and

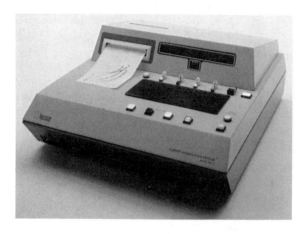

FIG. 9-10. Platelet Aggregation Profiler (Courtesy of Bio/Data, Hatboro, PA 19040).

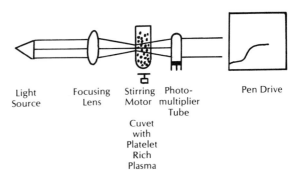

Light Source   Focusing Lens   Stirring Motor   Photo-multiplier Tube   Pen Drive

Cuvet with Platelet Rich Plasma

FIG. 9-11. Aggregometer light path: platelet suspension in the cuvet.

full aggregation, pauses for several seconds, then continues to record events until full aggregation is reached. The first deflection is the primary curve, the latter is secondary, and the two curves are separated by a plateau. The primary curve records the direct response of platelets to the agonist: shape change and the formation of small aggregates. The secondary curve reflects complete aggregation following release of intrinsic ADP. The contents of the organelles are secreted during the latter portion of primary aggregation and during the plateau phase, causing complete aggregation. In the third case, when agonist stimulus is low, *primary aggregation* may be followed by *disaggregation*. The partially aggregated platelets do not secrete granule contents. Instead, they resume their original discoid shape, and the pen returns to the baseline after 1 to 2 minutes.

Because the PRP is being stirred, the motion of the platelets causes the pen to oscillate slightly throughout the aggregation process. The oscillations broaden as aggregate size increases, and they become pronounced when the irreversible stage is reached. Thus a typical aggregometry tracing is somewhat jagged.

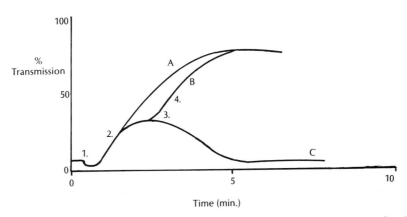

FIG. 9-12. Platelet aggregometry tracings. *A,* monophasic curve; *B,* biphasic curve; *C,* primary aggregation followed by disaggregation; *1,* addition of agonist; *2,* primary wave; *3,* plateau; *4,* secondary wave.

Commonly Employed Agonists

The agonists most often used in clinical aggregometry are ADP, epinephrine, collagen, arachidonic acid (AA), and ristocetin. The applications for each of these are discussed in turn.

ADP at a concentration of about 1×10^{-6}M induces a biphasic curve. The exact concentration required to give a biphasic curve is determined by the individual laboratory and varies with each plasma sample, depending on the pH, the presence of biochemical inhibitors, and the temperature. When the concentration of ADP is low, primary aggregation occurs, followed by disaggregation; when the concentration of ADP is high, the curve is monophasic. The normal response of 0.45 ml plasma to 20 μl of ADP at optimal concentration is a biphasic curve that reaches 60% to 80% of full deflection. Patients with *thrombocytopathies* such as *aspirinlike disorder*, in which prostaglandin synthesis is diminished, or *storage pool deficiency*, in which granule contents are inadequate, generate primary aggregation followed by disaggregation. In *Glanzmann's thrombasthenia* there is no response to ADP (refer to Chap. 10 for details of these diseases).

Epinephrine is prepared from a 1:1000 solution of adrenaline chloride (Parke-Davis, Detroit, MI 48232). Epinephrine produces a biphasic curve at a concentration of 1.16×10^{-5}M when 20 μl are used in about 0.45 ml PRP. The resulting aggregometry tracings are the same as expected when ADP is used as the agonist, and the responses to thrombocytopathies and thrombasthenia are similar to those induced by ADP. ADP and epinephrine aggregometry are used to confirm each other.

Collagen is difficult to prepare, so most laboratories purchase lyophilized type IV fibrillar collagen preparation, the type of collagen that is most abundant in the basement membrane of the tunica intima of vessels. Aggregometry with collagen is the most analogous to *in vivo* platelet activation. There is no primary wave of aggregation. When 20 μl of the agonist is added to 0.45 ml PRP, a brief lag phase follows, during which the pen may deflect to a point below the baseline, indicating loss of transmission of light due to shape change. Within 30 to 60 seconds, secondary aggregation begins, and a monophasic curve develops, reaching 60% to 80% transmission. Thrombocytopathy and thrombasthenia will result in complete inhibition of the collagen-induced curve.

Arachidonic acid is used infrequently to assess the viability of the thromboxane pathway of platelets. Undiluted AA is added to PRP to induce a monophasic aggregometry curve with virtually no lag phase. Abnormalities in the thromboxane pathway such as "aspirinlike syndrome" result in complete suppression of the curve.

Nonsteroidal anti-inflammatory agents such as aspirin suppress secretion of ADP and cause a thrombocytopathic pattern of primary aggregation followed by disaggregation.[13] Abnormal aggregation patterns occur in the presence of dipyridamole, certain antidepressant drugs, and fibrin or fibrinogen degradation products. Conditions such as uremia and dysproteinemia may also affect aggregation. The patient is instructed to avoid all drugs for 1 week before blood is collected for aggregometry, and particularly to avoid the anti-inflammatories. If the patient has taken aspirin, time and dosage are recorded and subsequently noted with the results.

Ristocetin, developed as an antibiotic in the late 1950s, was shown in laboratory trials to cause thrombocytopenia in animals and was never placed on the therapeutic market. It is still available as a reagent and may be purchased from Pacific Hemostasis Laboratories (Los Angeles, CA 90034). Although the platelet test is usually referred to as *ristocetin aggregation*, the drug actually induces platelet *agglutination* by reducing the repulsion effect of negative platelet plasma membrane charges, similar to antisera-induced formation of red cell aggregates in immunohematologic reactions. There is no shape change, no expenditure of energy, and no secretion in ristocetin-induced reactions. For ristocetin aggregation to proceed, von Willebrand factor (vWF; ristocetin cofactor) must be present, and the platelets must possess an intact surface membrane, including the vWF receptor site glycoprotein Ib (GP Ib).

Ristocetin induces a monophasic aggregation curve in normal PRP. Patients with all subtypes of von Willebrand disease except type IIb exhibit a loss of the ristocetin reaction, although all other agonists produce normal aggregation curves. Addition of exogenous vWF will restore the ristocetin aggregation reaction, confirming the diagnosis. In patients with *BSS (Bernard-Soulier syndrome)* a congenital change in the phospholipid membrane includes loss of the GP Ib receptor site. The diminished or absent ristocetin reaction is not corrected by addition of vWF. Absence of ristocetin aggregation that is corrected by the addition of vWF indicates von Willebrand disease, while the lack of correction indicates BSS.

Any discussion of von Willebrand disease must indicate the variation in laboratory results both from one patient to another, and from time to time in the same patient (see Chap. 5). Under the best of conditions the test for the ristocetin cofactor is diagnostic in about 70% of cases, and it is nondiagnostic in type IIB von Willebrand disease. A given patient may have a normal result one time and demonstrate loss of ristocetin aggregation at another time. It is necessary to perform a panel of procedures including BT, Factor VIII activity (FVIII:C) assay, and Factor VIII–related antigen (FVIIIR:AG) assay to confirm the diagnosis suggested by the ristocetin aggregation results. Confirmation is made by a clinical trial of Factor VIII therapy in which either the prolonged BT is directly corrected or the rise in Factor VIII clotting activity is delayed.

One refinement of ristocetin aggregometry is the substitution of formalin-fixed normal reagent platelets for patient's platelets, which results in a proportional relationship between the level of vWF and the aggregometry response of the reagent platelets. Comparison of the aggregation results of patient's plasma to the results of standard dilutions of normal plasma permits quantitation of the vWF level.

Summary

A typical clinical platelet aggregometry battery includes the use of the agonists ADP, collagen, epinephrine, and ristocetin. AA and thrombin may be added. A pattern of suppressed aggregation in ADP and epinephrine with a normal response in ristocetin indicates a thrombocytopathy, thrombasthenia, or drug-related effect. Further differentiation may be gained by examining the shape of the curve. Primary aggregation followed by disaggregation indicates thrombocytopathy; a complete loss of aggregation may mean thrombasthenia. Normal aggregation in ADP and epinephrine with loss of ristocetin aggregation indicates von Willebrand disease or BSS. These may be distinguished by addition of exogenous vWF, which corrects the aggregometry in von Willebrand disease but not in BSS.

LUMIAGGREGOMETRY

The *lumiaggregometer* may be used to simultaneously measure platelet aggregation and secretion.[14] This instrument, available from Chrono-log Corporation (Havertown,

PA 19083), records both light transmission through PRP and emission of chemiluminescence generated by ATP in the presence of "firefly extract" (Chronolume, Chrono-
log Corporation).[10] The procedure for lumiaggregometry differs little from conventional aggregometry but simplifies the diagnosis of platelet dysfunction.[16] Although
ADP is the active aggregation-inducing secretion, ATP is released at the same time as
ADP from platelet organelles. The concentrations of released ATP and ADP are in a
constant ratio, so measurement of ATP serves to diagnose platelet release or storage
defects even though ADP is the active material.

To perform lumiaggregometry, count-adjusted PRP (0.45 ml) is placed in a cuvet
and firefly extract is added. An agonist is then added, and the PRP is monitored simultaneously for aggregation and secretion. The first agonist used is always *thrombin*, which
induces full aggregation and release independent of the prostaglandin pathway, as
described in Chapter 8. Luminescence induced by thrombin is measured, recorded, and
compared with the luminescence produced by other agonists. Normal secretion induced by ADP, epinephrine, collagen, or AA produces luminescence at about 50% of
that resulting from thrombin stimulation. Figure 9-13 depicts simultaneous aggregation and secretion responses of PRP to epinephrine. In lumiaggregometry, aggregation
curves are monophasic, but detection of the release reaction does not rely on demonstration of the secondary curve as is required in conventional aggregometry, since ATP-gen-
erated luminescence serves as the release indicator.

In Glanzmann's thrombasthenia both aggregation and secretion responses are lost.
In storage pool disorder, collagen, ADP, or epinephrine induces a diminished aggregation and diminished ATP release, while AA induces normal aggregation with diminished ATP release (Fig. 9-14). The response to AA agonist differs from the response to
ADP and epinephrine because AA supplies an adequate external source of prostaglandin substrate. In aspirinlike syndrome, a defect in cyclooxygenase or prostaglandin
synthetase activity results in absence of AA-induced aggregation because no prostaglandins are produced in spite of the adequate substrate supply (see Fig. 9-14). The
effect of aspirin ingestion is the same. For lumiaggregometry techniques, refer to the
technical manuals supplied by the instrument manufacturer.

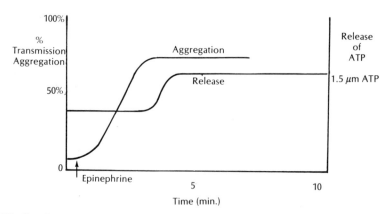

FIG. 9-13. Lumiaggregometry tracings showing simultaneous aggregation and release.

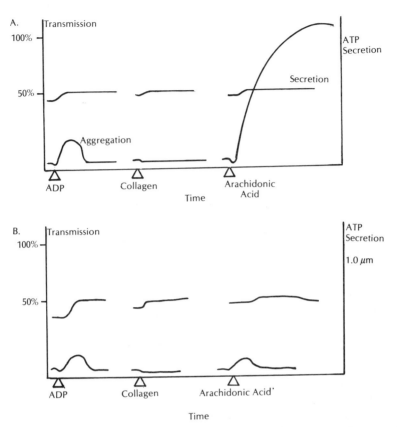

FIG. 9-14. Lumiaggregometry. (*A*) Aggregation and secretion responses to three agonists in storage pool disorder. (*B*) Responses to the same agonists in aspirinlike syndrome.

PLATELET RETENTION

The platelet retention test measures the decrease in platelet count that occurs when fresh whole blood is allowed to contact a foreign surface for a specified period. The earliest retention procedure was devised by Borchgrevink in 1960.[3] In the Borchgrevink method, whole blood is collected from a capillary puncture immediately after and again several minutes after the wound was made. Platelet counts are performed on both samples. The difference between the two counts is believed to represent a measure of platelet adhesion to the exposed collagen fibrils of the wound.

The Salzman technique employs nonsiliconized glass beads as the foreign surface.[23] Whole blood is collected by venipuncture with the two-syringe technique and a scalp-vein "butterfly" infusion set. The first 2 ml of whole blood are collected in a syringe, the syringe is removed from the infusion set, and the blood is placed in a tube containing 0.02 ml of 15% K_3EDTA and mixed. The end of the infusion set is then attached to the free end of a nonsiliconized glass bead filter column (Pacific Hemostatis Laboratories, Inc., Los Angeles, CA 90034). A syringe is attached to the other end of the column, and another 2 ml of whole blood is withdrawn. Withdrawal of the syringe plunger must be at a constant rate and is usually performed on a Harvard Infusion-Withdrawal Apparatus (Harvard Apparatus, Inc., Dover, MA 02030). The pump withdraws blood at a constant rate through the column. The sample in the second syringe is placed in a second tube of anticoagulant, and platelet counts are performed on both samples. Duplicate samples for both the preglass and glass phases are usually drawn.

The results are determined using this calculation:

$$\text{Percent retention} = \frac{P - Pg}{P} \times 100$$

Where P = the platelet count without glass bead retention

Pg = the platelet count after glass bead retention

Normal retention ranges from 31% to 83%. Levels below 25% indicate inadequate platelet retention, often seen in von Willebrand disease. Reproducible results depend on the constant flow of the whole blood, the regularity of the glass beads used, and the length of the column.

Originally the platelet retention test was believed to be a measure of platelet adhesion. Review Chapter 8, Platelet Physiology, for the distinction between platelet adhesion and aggregation. It is now clear that retention of platelets on glass beads is equally dependent on both adhesion and aggregation, and that the platelet retention test is confirmatory for aggregometry results without adding additional information. A method for platelet retention is provided in Williams, Appendix 43.[25]

MEASUREMENT OF PLATELET SECRETIONS

Availability of Platelet Phospholipid (Platelet Factor 3)

During platelet activation, plasma membrane phospholipid particles are released and become involved in plasma coagulation. There are two steps in the coagulation mechanism in which platelet phospholipid is necessary: conversion of Factor X to X_a by the complex of intrinsic Factors VIII and IX_a, and conversion of prothrombin to thrombin by the complex of Factors V and X_a (Fig. 9-15), reviewed in Chapter 2. Phospholipids from other sources, such as nearby tissue, may also contribute to the reaction; however, when the source is platelets, the phospholipid has traditionally been called platelet factor 3 (PF_3). In cases of thrombocytopenia or thrombocytopathy with diminished platelet activation, inadequate levels of platelet phospholipid are generated, resulting in incomplete coagulation. One measure of platelet phospholipid availability is the *prothrombin consumption (serum prothrombin)* test, a clot-based assay that measures the level of available prothrombin in a serum sample after coagulation is complete.

Ten milliliters of blood are drawn by the two-syringe technique, and the blood is dispensed into a clean siliconized glass or plastic tube without anticoagulant. The sample is placed at 37°C for 2 hours, and the supernatant serum is collected. A prothrombin time is performed on the serum by employing a prothrombin reagent enriched with fibrinogen and Factor V (Simplastin-A, Organon Teknika, Parsippany, NJ 07054).

Any time interval from addition of reagent to clot formation greater than 25 seconds is normal for the prothrombin consumption time test. A result under 20 seconds

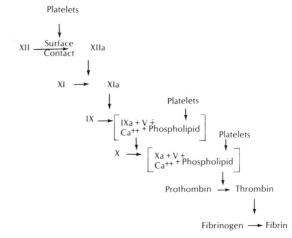

FIG. 9-15. Platelets contribute to the coagulation mechanism at three or more points. (Modified from Fritsma GA, Engelmann G, Yousof M: A review of platelet function and testing. Am J Med Technol 47:723–727, 1981)

indicates the presence of unconsumed prothrombin in the serum sample. This may be the result of inadequate platelet phospholipid or the absence of one of the intrinsic clotting Factors VIII, IX, XI, or XII. An activated partial thromboplastin time (APTT) is performed on a plasma sample from the same patient. If the result of the APTT test is normal, intrinsic factors are present at functional levels. If the APTT is normal, a shortened prothrombin consumption time indicates an inadequate level of platelet phospholipid. Since it is unlikely that a primary disorder of platelet phospholipid availability exists, abnormal results more likely indicate inadequate platelet activation, one result of which is diminished phospholipid release.

Platelet-Specific Secretions

Platelets store, produce, and secrete a variety of proteins, most of which are analogues of plasma proteins, such as vWF, fibrinogen, and plasma Factor V (see Chap. 7). Certain low-molecular-weight proteins produced and stored by platelets are absent from other systems; for example, platelet factor 4 (PF_4), β-thromboglobulin (βTG), platelet-derived growth factor (PDGF), and thrombospondin. The properties of these materials are described in Chapter 8. Because of their platelet specificity, measurement of these proteins may provide clinical information about platelet activation that cannot be gained from aggregometry or retention studies. Immunologic measurement of PF_4 and βTG has been perfected, and radioimmunoassay or enzyme immunoassay kits are available. A review of available kits and the principle of their activity is provided in Chapter 12.

Elevation of platelet-specific proteins in serum may indicate conditions of spontaneous platelet activation *in vivo*. Increases have been detected in patients following myocardial infarction, in those with coronary artery disease, and in those with other conditions related to thrombotic risk. The value of these procedures depends on whole blood collection techniques that minimize *in vitro* platelet activation. The presence of relatively high concentrations of PF_4 and βTG in platelet alpha granules means that activation after sample collection will yield extreme increases in the concentrations of these materials.

No clinical significance has been associated with diminished levels of βTG or PF$_4$ in serum or plasma. Measurement of the release of these platelet-specific proteins during aggregometry does not contribute to the diagnosis of storage pool disorders.

MISCELLANEOUS PLATELET PROCEDURES

Platelet Survival

Platelet life span is measured through the use of *in vivo* labeling of platelets with radioisotopes that bind securely without themselves changing platelet survival. Isotopes used routinely for survival determination include ^{32}P-diisopropylfluorophosphate, ^{75}Se-methionine, ^{35}S, ^{111}In-indium oxide, ^{14}C-serotonin, and ^{51}Cr-chromate. Labels are administered by injection, and serial samples are withdrawn to determine levels of radioactivity in whole blood or PRP. Normal survival by these methods is 8 to 12 days. In autoimmune thrombocytopenic purpura the mean survival time is less than 1 day.

Circulating Platelet Antibodies

There are a variety of platelet surface membrane antigens, some of which, like Pl^{A1}, are platelet specific. In ITP, circulating autoantibodies or alloantibodies attach to the platelet-specific antigen and induce phagocytosis by cells of the mononuclear–phagocyte system. In some cases, complement-mediated direct destruction of antibody-coated platelets occurs. These antibodies may be detected either directly on the surface of the patient's platelets or indirectly in patient serum through application of solid-phase enzyme immunoassay techniques.[15]

In the direct technique, PRP from the patient is adjusted to a count of $25 \times 10^3/\mu l$, then placed in cuvets for several hours. The platelets coat the walls of the cuvets. The plasma is washed from the coated cuvets, and enzyme-conjugated anti–human IgG is added. A positive result indicates that the platelets were bound by immunoglobulin.

In the indirect technique, pools of O Rh-negative PRP are collected and allowed to coat cuvets. Test serum is then placed in the coated cuvets, and the antibody, if present, is allowed to react with the platelet membranes. After washing, the antibody is detected with enzyme-conjugated anti–human IgG. Serial dilution techniques may be used to quantitate the results.

Clot Retraction

When normal whole blood is allowed to clot in a glass tube, the clot will retract from the walls of the tube after a few hours, leaving clear serum visible around the clot. Clot retraction depends on normal platelet function, intact thrombosthenin, and the presence of magnesium, ATP, and pyruvate kinase. In thrombocytopenia or platelet function disorders, clot retraction is poor or absent. In the past, quantitative clot retraction procedures were devised to test for platelet function. These procedures have been supplanted by aggregometry, retention, and measures of platelet release. It is nevertheless important for the trained technologist to observe the clotting properties of routine blood samples to detect possible clinical abnormalities of platelets.

REFERENCES

1. Bessman JD: The relation of megakaryocyte ploidy to platelet volume. Am J Hematol 16:161–170, 1984
2. Bessman JD, Williams LJ, Gilmer PR: The inverse relation of platelet size and count in normal subjects, and an artifact of other particles. AM J Clin Pathol 76:289–293, 1981
3. Borchgrevink CF: A method for measuring platelet adhesiveness *in vivo*. Acta Med Scand 168:157, 1960
4. Born GVR: Aggregation of blood platelets by adenosine diphosphate and its reversal. Nature 194:927, 1962
5. Born GVR: Quantitative investigation into the aggregation of blood platelets. J Physiol (Paris) 16:68, 1962
6. Brecher G, Cronkite MP: Morphology and enumeration of human blood platelets. J Appl Physiol 3:365–377, 1950
7. Brecher G, Schneidermann M, Cronkite EP: The reproducibility and constancy of the platelet count. Am J Clin Pathol 23:15–26, 1953
8. Brown BA: Hematology: Principles and Procedures, 4th ed. Philadelphia, Lea & Febiger, 1984
9. Bull BS, Schneiderman MA, Brecher G: Platelet counts with the Coulter counter. Am J Clin Pathol 44:678–688, 1965
10. Detwiler TC, Feinman RJ: Kinetics of the thrombin-induced release of adenosine triphosphate by platelets: Comparison with release of calcium. Biochemistry 12:2462–2468, 1973
11. Duke WW: The pathogenesis of purpura haemorrhagica with especial reference to the part played by the blood platelets. Arch Intern Med 10:445, 1912
12. Eisenstaedt R: Blood component therapy in the treatment of platelet disorders. Semin Hematol 23:1–7, 1986
13. Ens GE: Hemostasis. Part III. Platelet function testing and hereditary and acquired disorders of platelet function. Am J Med Technol 48:119–127, 1982
14. Feinman RD, Lubowsky J, Caro IF et al: The lumi-aggregometer: A new instrument for simultaneous measurement of secretion and aggregation. J Lab Clin Med 90:125–129, 1977
15. Finley PR, Fletcher C: Laboratory tests in immune thrombocytopenia. J Med Technol 1:709–715, 1984
16. Ingerman-Wojenski CM: Simultaneous measurement of platelet aggregation and the release reaction in platelet-rich plasma and in whole blood. J Med Technol 1:697–701, 1984
17. Ivy AC, Nelson D, Bucher G: The standardization of certain factors in the cutaneous "venostasis" bleeding time technique. J Lab Clin Med 26:1812, 1941
18. Kjeldsberg CR, Swanson J: Platelet satellitism. Blood 43:831–836, 1974
19. Kumar R, Ansell JE, Canoso RT, Deykin D: Clinical trial of a new bleeding device. Am J Clin Pathol 70:642, 1978
20. Lott JA, Hartzell RK, Longberry J: Synthetic materials for platelet quality control. Am J Med Technol 49:43–48, 1983
21. McAlee PS, Edelman RJ: Platelet–neutrophil adherence. Lab Med 19:147–148, 1979
22. Robbins G, Barnard DL: Thrombocytosis and microthrombocytosis: A clinical evaluation of 372 cases. Acta Haemat 70:175–182, 1983
23. Salzman EW: Measurement of platelet adhesiveness: A simple *in vitro* technique demonstrating an abnormality in von Willebrand's disease. J Lab Clin Med 62:724, 1963
24. Thompson AR, Harker LA: Manual of Hemostasis and Thrombosis, 3rd ed. Philadelphia, FA Davis, 1983
25. Williams WJ, Beutler E, Erslev AJ, Lichtman MA: Hematology, 3rd ed. New York, McGraw-Hill, 1983

Platelet Disorders 10

Gerald L. Davis
George A. Fritsma

CASE STUDY

A 32-year-old white man was brought to the emergency room after a series of seizures over a period of several hours. He reported that he had been well until about 4 days prior to this episode, when he had begun to experience episodic fevers. The fever was highest in the evening hours and near normal in mornings. During the time his history was taken, the patient experienced another seizure.

Examination revealed a well-developed white male, weight 175 pounds, 22 respirations per minute, pulse 95, temperature 101.4°F, and blood pressure 112/72. He was in mild distress except during seizures, pale, sweating, and complaining of malaise. There were several unexplained bruises on his extremities and trunk. Examination of head, eyes, ears, nose, and throat revealed no infection, nor was there any evidence of an infected wound. Heart and bowel sounds were normal, and the abdomen was not distended. He experienced no pain upon palpation of the abdomen.

Dilantin was administered to control convulsions, and the patient was admitted for observation. Initial laboratory orders included a complete blood count, coagulation workup, and urinalysis. Results were as follows:

CBC
Hemoglobin 9.8 g/dl
Hematocrit 31.2%
Erythrocytes $3.7 \times 10^6/\mu l$
MCV 84.5 fl

MCH 26.5 pg
MCHC 31.8%
Leukocytes 9800/μl
  Bands 3%
  Neutrophils 67%
  Lymphocytes 21%
  Eosinophils 3%
  Monocytes 6%
Platelets 32 $\times$ 10^3/μl
Morphology: Moderate microcytes, few spherocytes, few schistocytes
Coagulation tests
  PT 12.3 sec. (control 11.6)
  APTT 34.5 sec. (control 32.1)
  TT 18.5 sec. (control 21.2)
  BT 14 min. (normal range 3 – 7.5)
Urinalysis
  Appearance: Hazy, brown
  Hemoglobin 2+
  Red cells 4 – 7 per hpf
  White cells 2 – 5 per hpf
  All other parameters: Within normal limits

Seizure activity was stabilized after 24 hours, but the patient began to experience epistaxis, increased bruising, and oozing of blood from the gums. The fever remained above 100°F after repeated measures. After 2 days, gastric bleeding was noted, and an epigastric tube was inserted to suction the blood. At this time laboratory parameters were repeated. The significant changes are as follows:

CBC:
  Hemoglobin 7.2 g/dl
  Hematocrit 22.3%
  Erythrocytes 2.90 $\times$ 10^6/μl
  Morphology: Marked schistocytosis, microcytosis, spherocytosis
  Platelets 11 $\times$ 10^3/μl
Coagulation parameters: Within normal limits

The disorder was diagnosed as thrombotic thrombocytopenic purpura (TTP). TTP is a bleeding disorder characterized by low platelet count, microangiopathic anemia, fever, and neurologic imbalance. Uremia may develop. TTP is caused by activation of platelets in the microvasculature for reasons that are not especially clear. The anemia is hemolytic, caused by the presence of microthrombi deposited in capillaries that result in rupture of erythrocytes.

The patient was first treated with platelet transfusions. These slowed the hemorrhage briefly; however, after a few hours the platelet count had dropped to the previous level. A biopsy of the kidney revealed deposition of microthrombi in blood vessels. A plasma exchange was carried out by plasmapheresis, followed by prednisone therapy. Hemorrhage slowed and stopped. After 7 days the platelet count returned to 52 $\times$ 10^3, and the hemoglobin went up to 9.5 g/dl. The reticulocyte count at 7 days was 8.9%. The patient continued to improve on prednisone therapy and was sent home on day 14.

Hemorrhagic and thrombotic diseases result from derangement of one of the four hemostatic components: platelets, blood vessels, coagulation, and fibrinolysis (see Chap. 1). Because platelets play a central role in primary hemostasis, the most common hemorrhagic hemostatic abnormalities involve platelets alone or in combination with the other systems. Adhesion to foreign surfaces, aggregation, secretion, and formation of a hemostatic plug require intact platelets that react with vascular lining and coagulation factors. When platelets are functionally disturbed or in short supply, the initial stages of hemostasis are diminished or lost.

The circulation is a sealed fluid system and obeys certain hydraulic principles. As a result, blood flowing through the smallest vessels, the capillaries, produces the highest *shear* force. Platelets encounter difficulty in adhering to capillary walls because of the forces that oppose adhesion. Consequently, clinical symptoms of platelet disorders are mainly associated with small vessel or mucosal bleeding. Classic symptoms include petechiae, ecchymosis, *epistaxis* (nosebleed), and prolonged bleeding from small wounds. Purpura, menorrhagia, renal hemorrhage, and gastrointestinal hemorrhage are present in more severe platelet disorders. Hemorrhagic disorders caused by changes in vascular integrity demonstrate similar symptoms, but coagulation deficiencies such as the hemophilias are more often associated with internal bleeding into joints and body cavities such as the peritoneum.

Platelet, vessel, and coagulation abnormalities also result in increased clotting or thrombotic disorders. The mechanisms whereby platelets promote clotting are poorly understood, although research is proceeding in the area of platelet–vessel wall interactions and atherosclerosis. In this chapter, thrombotic disorders involving platelets are mentioned in relation to only a few conditions, such as essential thrombocythemia, in which the correlation is clear. Chapter 11 provides a complete discussion of thromboembolic disorders and hypercoagulation syndromes.

Platelet disorders are divided into two categories: abnormal count or diminished function (thrombocytopathy). Platelets must be present in adequate numbers to support normal hemostasis. The usual reference interval for the adult human platelet count (PLC) is 150 to 400×10^3 platelets per microliter of whole blood (see Chap. 9). A PLC above the reference interval is termed *thrombocytosis* or *thrombocythemia*, while a count below 150×10^3 cells per microliter is thrombocytopenia. A clinical distinction is made between PLCs of 50 to $150 \times 10^3/\mu l$, which are classified as mild thrombocytopenia, and counts below 50×10^3, which are described as severe. PLC disorders may be hereditary, congenital, or acquired, as demonstrated in Table 10-1.

Platelet functional disorders are called thrombocytopathies. Often a platelet disorder is first suspected by an alert technologist, performing a venipuncture, who perceives the appearance of petechiae upon application of the tourniquet. In many cases, petechiae and ecchymoses are visible on the skin of a patient with a normal PLC, indicating a possible thrombocytopathy. A test for platelet function, such as bleeding time (BT) or platelet aggregometry, is then necessary (Chap. 9). The reference interval for an Ivy BT with a standard puncture device such as the Simplate (Organon Teknika, Parsipanny, NJ 07054) is 2.75 to 8 minutes.[9] The combination of a prolonged BT and normal PLC establishes the presumption of a thrombocytopathy. Aggregometry test

TABLE 10-1
Nomenclature of the Thrombocytopenias

Type	Megakaryocytic Hypoplasia	Ineffective Thrombopoiesis	Increased Destruction
Hereditary	Thrombopoietin deficiency Fanconi's anemia Thrombocytopenia with absent radii	May-Hegglin anomaly Bernard-Soulier syndrome Wiskott-Aldrich syndrome	
Congenital	Congenital leukemia Neonatal rubella Maternal drug ingestion		Hemolytic disease of the newborn Preeclampsia Infection Drug sensitivity
Acquired nonimmune	Aplastic anemia Drugs, other chemicals Radiation Viruses Marrow infiltration Carcinoma Leukemia Multiple myeloma Lymphoma Myelofibrosis Tuberculosis Paroxysmal nocturnal hemoglobinuria Systemic lupus erythematosus	Vitamin B_{12} and folate deficiency Erythroleukemia Leukemia Iron-deficiency anemia	Thrombotic thrombocytopenic purpura Disseminated intravascular coagulation Hemolytic–uremic syndrome Thrombin-related Transfusions Infections Hypersplenism Hemorrhage Extracorporeal perfusion
Acquired immune			Acute immune (idiopathic) thrombocytopenic purpura Chronic immune (idiopathic) thrombocytopenic purpura Neonatal thrombocytopenic purpura Drug-induced thrombocytopenic purpura Posttransfusion purpura

(Courtesy of Donna M. Corriveau)

CONGENITAL PLATELET FUNCTION DEFECTS

Disorders of platelet adhesion
  von Willebrand disease
  Bernard-Soulier syndrome
Disorders of primary platelet aggregation
  Glanzmann's thrombasthenia
  Afibrinogenemia
Disorders of platelet secretion
  Storage pool deficiency
  Aspirinlike defects

results are employed to confirm this diagnosis, classify the disorder, and suggest appropriate treatment.

Thrombocytopathies, like PLC disorders, are inherited or acquired. *Bernard-Soulier syndrome, Glanzmann's thrombasthenia, aspirinlike syndrome, and storage pool disorder* are hereditary thrombocytopathies. Storage pool disorders are common; the others are rare. Acquired disorders include platelet reactions to drugs, especially the nonsteroidal anti-inflammatory agents (NSAIAs), and *disseminated intravascular coagulation (DIC)*. Some thrombocytopathies result from intrinsic pathologic lesions of the platelets, some from extrinsic conditions. The classification of the thrombocytopathies is given under Congenital Platelet Function Defects.

Several conditions are a result of a combination of thrombocytopathy with PLC disorders. Bernard-Soulier syndrome is an inherited hemorrhagic thrombocytopenia with impaired platelet function. Essential thrombocythemia is an acquired myeloproliferative disorder with extremely high PLCs and diminished platelet activity. In most cases of thrombocytopenia, ingestion of NSAIAs has a profound effect on platelet function, modifying the results of the BT and causing the appearance of petechiae.

The PLC and BT are the most informative and commonly employed screens of the platelet component of hemostasis. The PLC is a routine screen used to detect quantitative disorders. Modern platelet counting equipment also generates a measure of platelet volume known as mean platelet volume (MPV). The BT is sensitive to quantitative and qualitative disorders as well as vascular abnormalities (see Chap. 9). In persons with normal vascular and platelet function, BT results are inversely proportional to the PLC in the range below 100×10^3 per microliter (Fig. 10-1). Because of this relationship, many investigators suggest that the BT is redundant to the PLC and therefore valueless in the patient with severe thrombocytopenia (count below $50 \times 10^3/\mu l$). Others argue that some patients with young, "hyperactive" platelets have a normal BT even with a very low PLC ($30 \times 10^3/\mu l$). This combination is accompanied by an elevated MPV. In addition to the BT, MPV, and PLC, platelet aggregometry, measurement of platelet secretions, platelet retention, and morphologic examination are used to detect and define platelet abnormalities.

The emphasis of this chapter is on etiology (cause), pathophysiology (mechanism), clinical manifestations, and laboratory diagnosis of PLC disorders and thrombo-

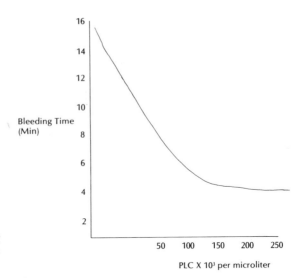

16
14
12
10

Bleeding Time
(Min)   8

6

4

2

50   100   150   200   250

PLC X 10³ per microliter

FIG. 10-1. Inverse relationship of PLC and BT when the PLC is below 100×10^3 cells per microliter.

cytopathies. Each disorder in Table 10-1 and under Congenital Platelet Function Defects is discussed in turn, beginning with thrombocytopenia, then thrombocytosis, and concluding with thrombocytopathy.

THROMBOCYTOPENIA

Thrombocytopenia is characteristic of the most common platelet disorders, and laboratory diagnosis of thrombocytopenia is based on the PLC and MPV and the appearance and number of megakaryocytes in a bone marrow smear preparation. The clinical laboratory technologist has a particular responsibility to accurately and rapidly determine the existence of thrombocytopenia and to notify the attending physician. Severe thrombocytopenia (PLC below 50×10^3 cells per microliter) is often a medical emergency that requires swift and appropriate treatment such as administration of platelet concentrate. Analysis of clinical manifestations alone is inadequate to determine the cause.

Thrombocytopenia is the result of inherited, congenital, or acquired lesions. Whatever the cause, there are three mechanisms responsible for thrombocytopenia: *megakaryocytic hypoplasia* (diminished or suppressed megakaryocytopoiesis, also called *amegakaryocytic thrombocytopenia*), *ineffective thrombocytopoiesis,* and *increased sequestration and destruction of platelets* (Fig. 10-2). In megakaryocytic hypoplasia, the number of megakaryocytes in the bone marrow is decreased.[3] In a normal Wright-stained crush or wedge preparation of bone marrow material, one observes one to three megakaryocytes per $100 \times$ magnification, "low-power" microscope field (Fig. 10-3). Diminished bone marrow megakaryocyte numbers and peripheral blood thrombocytopenia suggests the presumption of megakaryocytic hypoplasia. MPV is in the normal

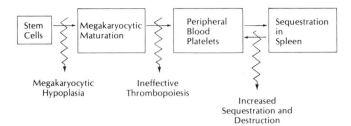

FIG. 10-2. Schematic diagram of platelet kinetics, indicating the sites of lesions for megakaryocytic hypoplasia, ineffective thrombopoiesis, and increased sequestration and destruction (courtesy of Donna Corriveau).

range for a low PLC (9–12 femtoliters [fl]) or slightly decreased (approximately 8 fl), depending on the specific disorder, so the expected observed diameter of stained peripheral blood smear platelets is 2 µm or less. The Bessman nomogram (see Fig. 9-8) demonstrates the relationship of MPV to PLC. The life span of platelets in all forms of megakaryocytic hypoplasia, measured by radioactive phosphate (DFP^{32}) or chromium (^{51}Cr) is normal, that is, approximately 9.5 days.[6]

In ineffective thrombocytopoiesis, megakaryocyte maturation and dispersion of platelets into the circulation are defective but unsuppressed. The majority of megakaryocytes possess ultrastructural flaws and fail to mature to the point of platelet dispersion. These abnormal megakaryocytes are destroyed by macrophages in the bone mar-

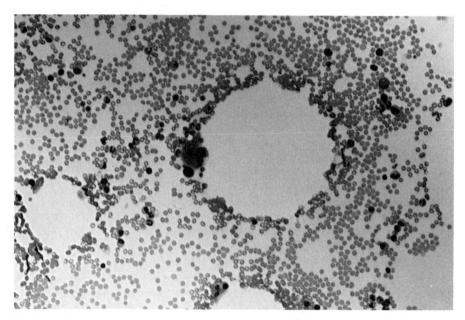

FIG. 10-3. Photomicrograph of megakaryocytes in a normal bone marrow smear (Wright stain, original magnification ×100).

row. Marrow estimates reach 14 or more megakaryocytes per low-power field, and their appearance is marked by nuclear abnormalities like chromatin fragmentation, hypo-lobulation, or chromatin bridging. Sometimes megakaryocytes develop to the point of platelet dispersion, but platelets are destroyed as they are freed from the surrounding cytoplasm. For those platelets that reach the peripheral blood, life span is normal, and the MPV is between 9 fl and 12 fl.

Thrombocytopenia caused by increased sequestration and destruction of platelets results in hyperproliferation of megakaryocytes. The bone marrow examination reveals increased numbers of megakaryocytes without the nuclear anomalies seen in ineffective thrombocytopoiesis. The platelet life span is reduced; in immune (idiopathic) thrombocytopenic purpura (ITP), for example, platelets survive less than 4 days. The MPV exceeds 12 fl in most cases of platelet destruction because the only platelets in the circulation are newly dispersed. Young, newly dispersed platelets are larger ($4-6$ μm) and functionally more active than platelets that have been in the circulation for several days. The peripheral blood PLC is low (often in the range of 50×10^3 or less), and platelets have an average diameter of 4 μm to 6 μm.

Thrombocytopenia Caused by Megakaryocytic Hypoplasia

Hereditary forms of megakaryocytic hypoplasia (amegakaryocytic thrombocytopenia) include *thrombopoietin deficiency, Fanconi's anemia,* and *thrombocytopenia with absence of radii (TAR).*

Thrombopoietin Deficiency

Thrombopoietin is a plasma hormone, produced by either macrophages or the kidney, that acts on marrow progenitor cells to increase the number, rate of maturation, size, and ploidy of megakaryocytes (Chap. 7). A decrease in the platelet pool causes an increase in thrombopoietin activity and increased thrombocytopoiesis. Thrombocytopenia resulting from thrombopoietin deficiency has been reported in a few cases when fresh normal plasma transfusions appear to trigger maturation of previously arrested megakaryoblasts and an increase in the peripheral blood PLC in patients whose thrombocytopenia was not accompanied by other hematologic changes.[20] Investigators presumed that the plasma provided the trigger that caused the production of thrombopoietin. Arguments against a thrombopoietin-deficient mechanism for thrombocytopenia cite the established ability of erythropoietin to stimulate megakaryocytopoiesis. Nevertheless, the strength of the evidence presented in the literature gives credence to the concept of thrombopoietin deficiency.[3] In the laboratory the presence of diminished bone marrow megakaryocytes in otherwise normal myelogenous tissue suggests this diagnosis.

Fanconi's Anemia and Thrombocytopenia With Absence of Radii

Fanconi's anemia *(constitutional infantile panmyelopathy, infantile aplastic anemia)* and TAR syndrome are examples of hereditary megakaryocytic hypoplasia. Both appear to be inherited as autosomal-recessive traits, although some argue that they are induced during fetal development and should be considered congenital. The pancytopenia (hypoplasia in all cell lines) of Fanconi's anemia develops slowly over a period of months or years, becoming symptomatic between 18 months and 10 years. In TAR, thrombocytopenia is apparent at birth and is fatal during the first year of life in more than 90% of cases. Another difference between the two disorders is that the megakaryocytic hypoplasia of TAR is seldom accompanied by a decrease in the granulocytic and erythrocytic cell lines.

Both Fanconi's anemia and TAR are accompanied by various malformations such as skin pigmentation; hypoplasia of the spleen, kidney, or heart; microcephaly; and bilateral absence of radii or thumbs. Patients have cardiac insufficiency and mental and sexual retardation. Laboratory features include thrombocytopenia and absence of megakaryocytes, and in Fanconi's the usual markers for anemia and granulocytopenia such as diminished erythrocyte count and neutrophil count. In TAR, organelle contents are diminished or absent, resulting in a storage pool deficiency with abnormal aggregometry results. A description of storage pool deficiencies is given later in this chapter.

Congenital Megakaryocytic Hypoplasia
Congenital megakaryocytic hypoplasia is common in infants infected prenatally with cytomegalovirus or rubella, or infants whose mothers ingested thiazide diuretics. Thiazides appear to have a direct toxic effect on the fetal bone marrow. Congenital leukemia may first present as megakaryocytic hypoplasia. TAR and Fanconi's anemia are often classified as congenital disorders.

Acquired Megakaryocytic Hypoplasia
Acquired megakaryocytic hypoplasia is part of the aplastic anemia syndrome. Aplastic anemia is a pancytopenia prevalent in age groups below 20 and over 60. This condition produces weakness and pallor due to decreased erythropoiesis, infection due to decreased granulopoiesis, and hemorrhage due to decreased thrombocytopoiesis. Epistaxis and menorrhagia are early hemorrhagic symptoms, followed by purpura. The prognosis depends on the severity of the pancytopenia. In aplastic anemia, hemorrhage and infections are the most common cause of death. In at least 50% of cases of aplastic anemia the cause is unknown, but in the remainder of cases the cause is exposure to a drug, some other chemical, or ionizing radiation. Chloramphenicol, thiazide diuretics, estrogen and penicillin are four of the more than 80 drugs that have been identified as etiologic agents of aplastic anemia. Benzene and benzene derivatives are industrial and environmental chemicals implicated regularly. Radiation therapy and myelosuppressive drugs that acetylate nucleic acids like cytosine arabinoside, employed therapeutically in the treatment of solid tumors, leukemia, and lymphomas, eventually become the cause of aplastic anemia or acute leukemia in approximately 1% of those treated. Acute aplastic crises secondary to viral infection, hemolytic anemias, and autoimmune disorders also present with hemorrhagic symptoms.

Laboratory manifestations include all the findings associated with normocytic/normochromic anemia and granulocytopenia, as well as thrombocytopenia. Coagulation tests are normal except for the BT, which is prolonged, and the capillary fragility test, results of which are positive. The bone marrow is fatty, with scattered pockets of hematopoietic cells.

Thrombocytopenia With Ethanol Ingestion
Ethanol ingestion causes thrombocytopenia, but the cause of the observed effects of alcohol on megakaryocyte development is not known. This type of thrombocytopenia is

most often associated with the "binge" drinker. Megakaryocytopenia occurs after 5 to 10 days of whiskey ingestion even when folic acid is administered simultaneously. In the most severe cases the PLC drops to $10 \times 10^3/\mu l$, but bleeding is rarely a problem. When ethanol is discontinued, rebound thrombocytosis occurs, with PLCs greater than $600 \times 10^3/\mu l$ for several weeks.

Marrow Replacement
Marrow replacement of myelogenous tissue by tumor cells results in megakaryocytic hypoplasia. In acute leukemia, blastic cells create a tumor load in the bone marrow that crowds out all normal elements, causing thrombocytopenia and anemia. Although thrombocytopenia is most prevalent in acute lymphocytic leukemia, it is routinely identified in acute nonlymphocytic leukemia. The chronic DIC that accompanies acute promyelocytic leukemia contributes to thrombocytopenia in that disorder. DIC is initiated by the release of procoagulant material from leukemic promyelocytes during chemotherapy. *Metastatic carcinoma, plasma cell myeloma, Hodgkin's disease, and non-Hodgkin's lymphoma* are other neoplasms that replace normal marrow elements. *Myelofibrosis, miliary tuberculosis, and Gaucher's disease* are nonmalignant disorders that cause megakaryocytic hypoplasia through marrow replacement. Gaucher's disease is a lipid metabolism disorder in which marrow crowding of megakaryocytes is compounded by splenic sequestration and phagocytosis of platelets.

In leukemia the bone marrow and peripheral blood are filled with the malignant clones of cells. The task of the hematology laboratory is to identify these cells while routinely recording the PLC to monitor and document the effects of supportive therapy. In other conditions that cause marrow replacement, peripheral blood smears demonstrate immature erythrocytes and neutrophils. This indicates the presence of *extramedullary hematopoiesis*, which is the proliferation of myelogenous tissue in nonmarrow spaces of the spleen, liver, and lungs (Fig. 10-4). PLCs are diminished, and platelet morphology may be bizarre: giant platelets (platelets that are larger than nearby erythrocytes), agranular platelets, and platelets with abnormal or crystallized granules are seen (Fig. 10-5).

Thrombocytopenia Caused by Ineffective Thrombocytopoiesis

In ineffective thrombocytopoiesis the number of megakaryocytes in the bone marrow is normal to increased, but maturation of megakaryocytes and dispersion of platelets into the circulation are suppressed. Conditions that disrupt the maturation of the megakaryocyte or dispersion of platelets result in ineffective thrombocytopoiesis. In ineffective thrombocytopoiesis up to 90% of thrombocytopoietic elements, including megakaryocytes or newly produced platelets, are destroyed before platelets are dispersed. Except in Wiskott-Aldrich syndrome, the platelets that survive the destructive mechanism and are dispersed have a normal life span. Bone marrow examination reveals an increased number of megakaryocytes in both thrombocytopenia due to ineffective thrombocytopoiesis and thrombocytopenia due to increased sequestration and destruction, so determination of platelet life span by radioactive tagging is frequently the only laboratory method available to distinguish these disorders.

The distinction between causes of thrombocytopenia affects treatment decisions. Thrombocytopenia caused by ineffective thrombocytopoiesis is often treated with

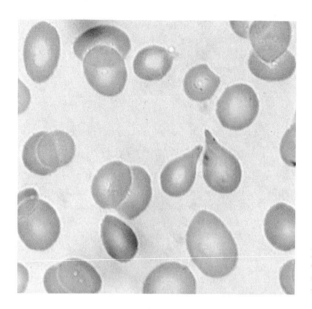

FIG. 10-4. Photomicrograph of peripheral blood cells seen in extramedullary hematopoiesis (Wright stain, original magnification × 1000).

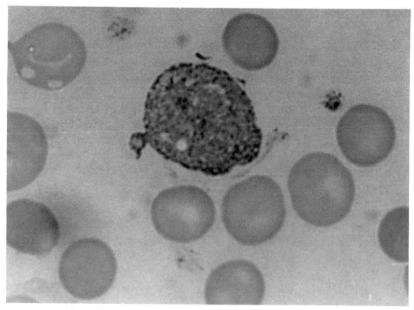

FIG. 10-5. Photomicrograph of a giant platelet in acute nonlymphocytic leukemia (Wright stain, original magnification × 1000).

platelet concentrate. Platelet concentrate is useless in the treatment of most cases of thrombocytopenia in which increased sequestration and destruction is the mechanism.

Hereditary Forms

Hereditary forms of ineffective thrombopoiesis include *May-Hegglin anomaly, Bernard-Soulier syndrome, and Wiskott-Aldrich syndrome.*

   MAY-HEGGLIN ANOMALY AND BERNARD-SOULIER SYNDROME. May-Hegglin anomaly and Bernard-Soulier syndrome are thrombocytopenias demonstrating giant platelets in the peripheral blood smear (Fig. 10-6). A giant platelet is one that is larger than nearby

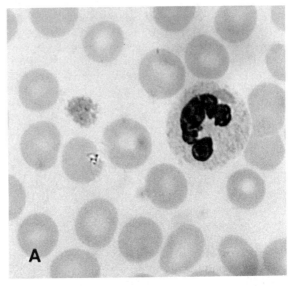

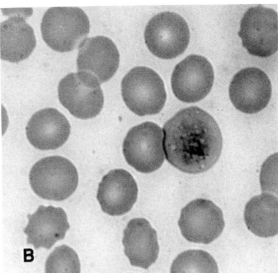

FIG. 10-6. *(A)* Photomicrograph of a peripheral blood platelet and neutrophil with a Döhle body in May-Hegglin anomaly (Wright stain, original magnification ×1000). *(B)* Photomicrograph of a large grayish platelet typical of Bernard-Soulier syndrome (Wright stain, original magnification ×1000).

erythrocytes and that displays some structural abnormalities such as hypogranularity. Giant platelets differ markedly from the large young platelets of thrombocytopenia due to increased sequestration and destruction, which have an MPV of 12 fl or more, are 4 μm to 6 μm in diameter, and are normal in structure. MPV levels for giant platelets have not been established.

May-Hegglin is an autosomal-dominant anomaly with neutrophils with cytoplasmic *Döhle bodies* and giant platelets. Döhle bodies are blue-staining inclusions located near the plasma or nuclear membrane. Ultrastructural studies have shown that Döhle bodies are cytoplasmic areas packed with dense fibrils of messenger RNA.[5] No such structural abnormality is evident in the platelets or megakaryocytes of persons with May-Hegglin anomaly, but about one third have mild asymptomatic thrombocytopenia. Hemorrhage is rare, in spite of thrombocytopenia.

Bernard-Soulier syndrome is an autosomal-recessive trait characterized by both thrombocytopenia and platelet inability to adhere to foreign surfaces. In Bernard-Soulier syndrome, Döhle bodies are normally not present in neutrophils. The presence or absence of Döhle bodies is an important criterion for separating May-Hegglin anomaly from Bernard-Soulier syndrome. Platelet aggregometry employing the agonist ristocetin is routinely used to diagnose Bernard-Soulier syndrome, so a full discussion of this disorder is deferred to the section on qualitative platelet disorders.

WISKOTT-ALDRICH SYNDROME. Wiskott-Aldrich syndrome is a sex-linked immunodeficiency disease characterized by eczema, thrombocytopenia, and recurrent infections in young boys. A dual mechanism accounts for the thrombocytopenia: ineffective thrombocytopoiesis and increased sequestration and destruction. Ineffective thrombocytopoiesis is the major component; the platelet life span is not sufficiently shortened to account for the degree of thrombocytopenia observed.[23] Bone marrow megakaryocytes are normal to increased in number, with ultrastructural abnormalities that contribute to premature platelet destruction.

Wiskott-Aldrich platelets are structurally abnormal. Diminished levels of adenine nucleotides are reflected in the lack of dense bodies observed in transmission electron microscopy. Furthermore, there is diminished aerobic metabolism and consequently fewer mitochondria. Although some support an autoimmune mechanism, most evidence shows that the shortened life span of Wiskott-Aldrich platelets is a result of the diminished metabolism, and that the spleen removes these defective platelets earlier than normal platelets in reponse to their intrinsic defect. Normal platelets achieve a normal life span when infused into a Wiskott-Aldrich patient. The platelets of this disorder have defective aggregometry patterns with a lack of a secondary wave of aggregation following administration of the agonists ADP, epinephrine, or collagen. The response to thrombin is normal. The aggregation curve in Wiskott-Aldrich syndrome is typical of a storage pool deficiency.

Wiskott-Aldrich platelets are referred to as microplatelets because the MPV is routinely below 8 fl. By contrast, in ITP the shortened platelet life span is accompanied by an MPV of 12 fl. or higher. Wiskott-Aldrich syndrome is often fatal owing to repeated debilitating infections. The mortality in this syndrome is more a result of immunodeficiency than the platelet abnormality. The most successful treatment for the thrombocytopenia is splenectomy, which exposes the immunodeficient patient to the risk of infection but corrects the shortened platelet life span. Bone marrow transplantation has been attempted with some success.

Acquired Forms

Acquired forms of ineffective thrombocytopoiesis include *megaloblastic anemia, erythroleukemia (Di Guglielmo's syndrome), and myelodysplasia.*

MEGALOBLASTIC ANEMIA. Megaloblastic anemia is caused by vitamin B_{12} or folate deficiency and is characterized by morphologic abnormalities and hypercellularity of the red and white cell precursors in a bone marrow smear. Abnormalities include asynchrony of maturation, uneven hemoglobinization of erythroblasts, hypersegmentation of mature granulocyte nuclei, and nuclear breakdown, or karyorrhexis. Megakaryocytes appear normal, although some reports indicate hypersegmentation of nuclei. In the peripheral blood thrombocytopenia is mild; erythrocytes are macrocytic, with MCVs above 100 fl; and neutrophils are hypersegmented. Platelet production is only about 10% of the expected value, based on anticipated megakaryocyte pool and platelet life span. In rare situations the thrombocytopenia is severe, and hemorrhage becomes the initial complaint of the patient, especially in aspirin ingestion. Within 5 to 10 days of the initiation of vitamin therapy, the platelet count returns to normal.

ERYTHROLEUKEMIA. Erythroleukemia is an acute nonlymphocytic leukemia caused by uncontrolled proliferation of erythrocytic precursors. While marrow replacement becomes a factor in the late stages, thrombocytopenia is mostly due to the combination of megakaryocytic hypoplasia and ineffective thrombocytopoiesis. Bone marrow megakaryocytes are decreased or absent. Platelet transfusions are required for the patient's survival, but survival is determined more by the progression of the disease overall than by platelet function or number.

MYELODYSPLASIA. *Myelodysplasia* is the general name for a group of hematologic disorders that are associated with increased and abnormal hematopoiesis with a cytopenia of one or more cell lines. Typically the patient is a man of 45 years or older. Myelodysplasia is characterized by a mild macro-ovalocytic anemia (hemoglobin approximately 10 g/dl), morphologic aberrations of granulocytes *(Pelgeroid neutrophils)*, and megaloblastic maturation patterns in myelogenous tissue. The anemia is refractory to vitamin B_{12} or folate treatment, and because of the propensity of these patients to develop acute nonlymphocytic leukemia, myelodysplasia is also referred to as *preleukemia. Refractory anemia, sideroblastic anemia,* and *chronic myelomonocytic leukemia* are examples of myelodysplasia. In myelodysplasia, ineffective thrombocytopoiesis results in mild thrombocytopenia that occasionally accounts for hemorrhagic symptoms. One form of myelodysplasia that has megakaryocytic hypolobulation and elevated PLCs is called *5q — syndrome* for its cytogenetic abnormality. Discussion of 5q — syndrome properly fits in the section on thrombocytoses.

Thrombocytopenia Caused by Increased Platelet Sequestration and Destruction

Nonimmune

A rapid fall in the PLC with no apparent hemorrhage to account for the loss of platelets suggests increased sequestration and destruction of platelets with shortened platelet life span. Megakaryocytic proliferation and platelet production is increased to as much as eight times normal in response to platelet consumption, provided that the marrow is otherwise normal. In some patients the PLC stabilizes at near normal because the rate of production reaches the rate of loss. This condition is referred to as a *compensated thrombocytolytic response,* and platelet life span is still shortened. The peripheral blood percentage of young, recently dispersed, platelets is increased. These platelets have greater functional ability and a higher MPV than mature platelets. The diameter of young platelets on a stained peripheral blood smear averages 4 μm to 6 μm.

The mechanism for excess removal of platelets from the circulation is either sequestration by the spleen and liver or destruction in these organs plus other tissues. Except in the case of excess sequestration due to splenomegaly, the division between sequestration and destruction is artificial because both mechanisms operate in every condition. The pathophysiologic trigger of sequestration and destruction is immune or nonimmune mediated. This section is a consideration of nonimmune-mediated thrombocytopenia caused by increased platelet sequestration and destruction. This classification includes the acquired disorders *TTP, hemolytic–uremic syndrome (HUS), and DIC.*

TTP, HUS, and DIC are thrombocytopenias that present with *microangiopathic hemolytic anemia.* In microangiopathic hemolytic anemia the stained blood smear reveals schistocytes, microcytes, helmet cells, dacryocytes, and decreased platelets. This morphologic pattern reflects fragmentation of red cells and trapping of platelets as they pass intravascular fibrin strands or damaged vascular lining. Mechanical disruption of erythrocytes and platelets is also reflected in diminished results of life span studies.

General differences among TTP, HUS, and DIC are given in Table 10-2. Briefly the major differences are age, mechanism, and treatment. TTP is prevalent in adult females, HUS in young people, and DIC in all age groups. TTP is caused by some plasma component that is altered in infusion or exchange of fresh plasma. HUS is secondary to renal disease with proteinuria, hematuria, and azotemia (elevated blood urea nitrogen). Often blood urea nitrogen (BUN) levels exceed 100 mg/dl. Renal dialysis is effective in the treatment of HUS. Renal disease is sometimes seen in TTP but is not as severe. In DIC platelet consumption is associated with thrombin generation and fibrin formation. Heparin is administered to arrest coagulation, thus reducing platelet consumption and hemolysis.

THROMBOTIC THROMBOCYTOPENIC PURPURA. The thrombocytopenia of TTP, like that of ITP, results from increased platelet consumption and decreased platelet life span. In ITP, immunoglobulin-coated platelets are removed by mononuclear phagocytic cells of the spleen and liver, but in TTP platelets are destroyed intravascularly as a consequence of thrombus formation and aggregation in arterioles, venules, and capillaries throughout the body. It is important that one not confuse ITP with TTP, since treatment approaches differ considerably: TTP is treated with platelet concentrate and

TABLE 10-2

Characteristics of the Various Forms of Nonimmune Platelet Consumption

Characteristic	HUS	TTP	DIC
Age	Childhood	Adulthood (women)	All
Mechanism	Uremia	Plasma component	Secondary to inflammation
Treatment	Dialysis	Plasmapheresis	Heparin

plasma exchange, and ITP is treated by immunosuppression. TTP is more dangerous; the mortality rate exceeded 90% until plasma exchange therapy dropped it to 20%.

TTP was first described by E. Moschcowitz in 1924, and it is sometimes referred to as Moschcowitz' syndrome.[12] Incidence is 1/1,000,000 per year, with a predilection for 30- to 40-year-old women. The ratio of affected females to males overall is 3:2. TTP produces a "diagnostic triad" of hemorrhage, microangiopathic hemolytic anemia, and neurologic changes such as confusion, lack of coordination, or convulsions. Other symptoms include fever and renal disease, and some authors include these in a "diagnostic pentad." Histologic examination reveals multiple dispersed microvascular thrombi containing fibrin and platelets, presumed to be the cause of the diagnostic symptoms.

The etiology of TTP is unknown. It occurs with infections, surgery, injury, penicillin therapy, influenza vaccination, *Bartonella* bacteremia, rheumatoid arthritis, systemic lupus erythematosus, hyperacute rejection of renal allografts, and pregnancy. These conditions have in common a tendency to damage vascular endothelium. It should be noted that immune-complex formation also causes damage to the endothelium. Newer evidence suggests that TTP is due to the deficiency of an unknown plasma factor that is required for synthesis of prostacyclin (PGI_2) by endothelium. Experimental exposure of rat aortic rings to normal plasma stimulates PGI_2 production from endothelial cells. In contrast, PGI_2 synthesis is absent following exposure of rat aortic rings to plasma collected from a patient during a TTP episode, but stimulated by her postexchange plasma.

Evidence has also been presented that suggests that normal plasma contains a factor that inhibits platelet *agglutination*. TTP plasma causes or permits *in vitro* platelet agglutination unless first mixed with normal plasma. The ability of TTP plasma to induce agglutination may require the presence of large platelet membrane binding Factor VIII: von Willebrand factor (vWF) multimers (see Chap. 5) like those synthesized by cultured human endothelial cells. Such multimers were demonstrated in four patients with chronic relapsing TTP. During periods of relapse the levels of VIII: vWF multimers were reduced. TTP patients may lack a depolymerase that reduces the size of endothelial cell–produced multimers. Plasma transfusions provide the depolymerase in this experimental model.[7]

The multiplicity of theories suggests that several pathologic mechanisms may combine to create the TTP syndrome, or that TTP may be a group of similar disorders.

Laboratory findings in TTP include severe thrombocytopenia, with PLC results less than 10×10^3 platelets per microliter. Reflective of the hemolytic process, lactate dehydrogenase (LDH) activity levels and unconjugated bilirubin levels are markedly increased. The LDH level is usually above 1000 U/liter when a technique with a reference interval of 225 U to 450 U/liter of whole blood is used, and may reach as high as 10,000 U/liter. Erythrocyte isoenzymes of LDH — LD1 and LD2 — are present. The LDH level correlates with the severity of the disorder and is the most sensitive indicator of recovery and relapse. Bilirubin, a product of hemoglobin catabolism, is usually increased, and the fraction present is unconjugated bilirubin, a finding consistent with intravascular hemolysis. Anemia is severe, and hemoglobin levels are below 10 g/dl, in some cases as low as 7 g/dl of whole blood. The blood smear reveals decreased platelets, schistocytes, and marked polychromasia. The polychromasia is reflective of the marked reticulocytosis, which ranges from 2% to 20% but may be greater than 50%.

Neurologic symptoms include transient or fluctuating headache, vertigo, abnormal speech, confusion, loss of memory, and coma. Mild fever, between 100°F and 102°F, although not a presenting symptom, develops in more than 95% of patients in the course of the illness. Renal complications are reflected in elevated BUN and creatinine levels. The BUN may go as high as 80 mg/dl of whole blood (reference interval less than 20 mg/dl) but seldom exceeds that level. Creatinine levels may go as high as 3 mg/dl (top limit of normal 1.5 mg/dl). Renal abnormalities are less severe than in HUS.

Symptoms of TTP are similar to many symptoms of DIC. This has lead many authors and researchers to speculate that the two disorders arise from a single pathophysiologic mechanism, but there is no evidence to support a role for DIC in the pathophysiology of TTP. Patients with TTP have normal prothrombin time and activated partial thromboplastin time results, and normal levels of fibrinogen, Factor V, and Factor VIII. Fibrinogen survival time is normal. The severe intravascular hemolysis of TTP occasionally triggers DIC.

In summary, TTP is a complex and dangerous syndrome. The cause of the syndrome is unknown, but evidence supports the deficiency of some plasma factor still under investigation that is supplied in normal plasma. Typical laboratory findings in TTP include decreased platelets, decreased hemoglobin, reticulocytosis, schistocytes, and elevated BUN, creatinine, LDH, and bilirubin. The prothrombin time, activated partial thromboplastin time, and fibrinogen levels are all normal in TTP.

HEMOLYTIC-UREMIC SYNDROME. Clinically, HUS resembles TTP except that it predominates in children less than 4 years old and is self-limiting. It is often a sequel to an acute viral infection, and it affects males and females equally. The childhood form of HUS has a mortality rate of 33%, the adult form 61%. Physical symptoms include purpura, pallor, drowsiness, hepatosplenomegaly, hypertension, and renal failure. The cardinal signs of HUS are hemolytic anemia, renal failure, and thrombocytopenia. The anemia is typical of a hemolytic process, with a hemoglobin less than 10 g/dl, an elevated reticulocyte count, and the presence of schistocytes in the peripheral blood. The leukocyte count is elevated. Renal failure is reflected in elevated BUN and creatinine levels and the presence of red cells, protein, and casts in urinary sediment. Thrombocytopenia is mild to moderate.

In HUS, platelet consumption occurs primarily in the kidney. Thrombocytopenia in HUS may be caused by infection-induced immune-complex formation, formation of platelet microaggregates in the kidneys, or kidney vasculature-induced platelet sequestration or injury. Histologic sections showing fibrin strands in the kidney, hepatosplenomegaly, and shortened platelet life span are evidence for kidney-induced platelet injury; however, experiments using radioactive platelets from platelet-rich plasma have not confirmed significant platelet sequestration by the kidney. There is some indication of genetic predisposition.

Patients with HUS are treated with renal dialysis. As uremic symptoms disappear, the PLC returns to normal. The adult version of HUS responds favorably to heparin therapy and administration of NSAIAs.

DISSEMINATED INTRAVASCULAR COAGULATION. In DIC (see Chap. 6) thrombocytopenia is associated with diminished Factors V and VIII and fibrinogen, caused by *in vivo* thrombin generation. In acute DIC platelet consumption is rapid, and the resultant thrombocytopenia is severe. In chronic DIC compensatory thrombocytopoiesis results in moderately low to normal platelet count.

GIANT HEMANGIOMA. *Giant hemangioma* is a congenital benign vascular tumor that causes thrombocytopenia and pathologic thrombin generation in the newborn. Platelets are sequestered and destroyed within the tumor, and if the tumor is large, severe thrombocytopenia, hypofibrinogenemia, and purpura develop. Fragmentation of red cells is an expected finding in the stained smear. Treatment includes the use of corticosteroids, radiation therapy, and surgical excision, although in most cases the tumor spontaneously regresses.

In vivo platelet activation is characteristic of the nonimmune thrombocytopenias TTP, HUS, and DIC. The platelet release measurement techniques for platelet factor 4 and β-thromboglobulin are elevated (see Chap. 12).

Immune

Immune mechanisms account for the second group of thrombocytopenias caused by increased sequestration and destruction. *Autoimmune* thrombocytopenias are disorders in which immunoglobulins against platelet membrane self-antigens develop: *acute or chronic ITP, drug-induced thrombocytopenia,* and thrombocytopenia secondary to other autoimmune disorders such as *systemic lupus erythematosus (SLE). Alloimmune (isoimmune)* thrombocytopenias include *neonatal thrombocytopenia,* in which fetal platelets are destroyed by maternal immunoglobulins, and *posttransfusion purpura.* The pathophysiology of these thrombocytopenias begins with platelet binding of antiplatelet IgG, immune complexes, or complement, causing sequestration and clearance by cells of the mononuclear phagocyte system in the spleen and liver.

CHRONIC IMMUNE (IDIOPATHIC) THROMBOCYTOPENIC PURPURA. Chronic ITP (CITP) begins with an insidious onset of easy bruising, petechiae formation, and menorrhagia.[6] Demographic analysis indicates that adults between 20 and 50, with a female preponderance of $3:1$ or $4:1$, contract CITP. The typical patient is a woman of childbearing age. Untreated CITP is eventually fatal; remissions are rare, although the course of the illness extends from several months to several years and varies from mild to severe. Several modes of successful treatment are available, and the mortality rate for treated CITP is less than 0.5%

CITP is also referred to as "idiopathic" thrombocytopenic purpura, although the current trend is to let the "I" stand for immune. Idiopathic means unknown, indicating that little is known about the etiology of CITP autoimmunity. The term *immune* describes the pathophysiology of CITP but fails to distinguish it from thrombocytopenia secondary to clinically distinct autoimmune conditions like SLE or rheumatoid arthritis (RA). Consequently, many clinicians prefer *idiopathic* to *immune* when describing CITP. In common clinical usage the terms are synonymous. The term *idiopathic* is not appropriate in cases of acute ITP (AITP), in which the etiology of the thrombocytopenia is clear.

Evidence for a humoral mechanism was initially suggested by the occurrence of transient thrombocytopenia in neonates born of mothers with CITP and confirmed later by the administration of CITP plasma to normal volunteers.[10] The agent is a platelet-associated IgG (PAIgG) immunoglobulin of autoimmune origin (Fig. 10-7). The PAIgG antibody is measurable in plasma and on platelet membranes by immunologic methods and is shown to bind platelets in at least 90% of cases of CITP. While a minuscule concentration of PAIgG coats platelets in normal persons, just as small amounts of erythrocyte-coating immunoglobulins are always present on normal red cells, CITP patients have much larger concentrations. The plasma PAIgG titer is inversely related to the PLC but does not predict the severity of clinical symptoms, which are mitigated by the appearance of young, metabolically competent platelets in the peripheral blood. The spleen is a major site for synthesis of PAIgG.[10]

PAIgG binds membranes of platelets in typical reactions involving the Fab terminus of the immunoglobulin and antigenic structures of the membrane (see Fig. 10-7).

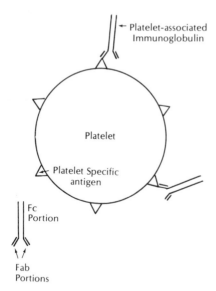

FIG. 10-7. Diagram of an autoimmune reaction between PAIgG and platelets.

The specificity of this reaction is undetermined, although the antigen Pl^{A1} is proposed in several cases. Removal of coated platelets is mediated by Fc receptors on the membranes of mononuclear phagocytes that recognize and attach the bound immunoglobulin. The rate of removal of PAIgG-coated platelets is decreased by immune blocking of cellular Fc receptors. Studies with ^{51}Cr-labeled platelets demonstrate that phagocytic clearance occurs in the spleen when symptoms are mild, and in both spleen and liver as the symptoms become severe. Platelet life span is decreased in proportion to PLC (Fig. 10-8). PAIgG attaches to megakaryocytes and in some patients suppresses thrombocytopoiesis, but in most cases the shortened platelet life span is partially compensated for by increased marrow platelet production. This is reflected in the increased numbers of megakaryocytes seen in examination of stained bone marrow smears.

Splenectomy results in remission in at least 50% of cases of CITP. The PLC returns to normal, and so do the platelet life span and levels of PAIgG activity. Some reports indicate that diminished immunoglobulin activity is a result of the dilution of young platelets with old in the circulation after splenectomy. These experiments indicate that less antibody is bound by the older cells than the younger. The diminished PAIgG level also indicates the role of splenic immunogenic tissue in producing the immunoglobulin. In another 30% of cases, splenectomy results in incomplete remission.

Clinical and laboratory diagnosis of CITP requires exclusion of sepsis, DIC, or drug sensitivity. Upon initial presentation of CITP, the PLC may range from 5 to 75×10^3 cells per microliter. Anemia is sometimes present if blood loss has occurred. Bleeding time is prolonged, results of the capillary fragility test are positive because of the thrombocytopenia, and the MPV is above 12 fl. Results of the antihuman globulin (direct Coombs) test are sometimes positive when autoimmune hemolytic anemia is present. Alkaline phosphatase activity is elevated. Prothrombin time and activated partial thromboplastin time test results are normal.

Stained peripheral blood smears in CITP confirm the decreased PLC. All the platelets are large, with a diameter between 4 μm and 6 μm, but their morphology and granularity are normal. In a few cases, bizarre or fragmented platelets are seen with

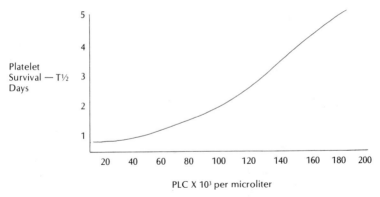

FIG. 10-8. Relationship between PLC and platelet survival in CITP.

condensed or crystallized granules. The large platelets of CITP do not resemble the giant platelets of May-Hegglin anomaly, Bernard-Soulier syndrome, or myeloproliferative disorders. Giant platelets are morphologically abnormal and larger than erythrocytes. Bone marrow megakaryocytes are increased in number but normal in appearance.

Several immunologic methods are available for detection and measurement of PAIgG; however, lack of specificity, complex methodology, and the presence of biologic false-positives have made them difficult to interpret. Consequently, measurement of PAIgG has remained a research activity. The amount of surface IgG plus the amount of IgG found in the interior of the platelet are termed *total IgG* in solubilization experiments. Total IgG exceeds surface-bound IgG by about five times. Following solubilization of platelet-rich plasma, total IgG is measured by radial immunodiffusion, immunoelectrophoresis, or nephelometry. The result is a semiquantitative estimate of PAIgG. This measurement is not specific for CITP because autoimmune conditions resulting in secondary thrombocytopenia such as SLE demonstrate increased levels of PAIgG.

When the PLC goes below 50×10^3 cells per microliter, corticosteroid treatment is initiated. Prednisone is assumed to suppress the phagocytic activity of macrophages, inhibit splenic sequestration and phagocytosis of antibody-coated platelets, and improve capillary structural integrity. If corticosteroid therapy is ineffective, splenectomy is necessary. Splenectomy results in complete remission in at least 50% of patients, and another 30% experience an elevation of the platelet count sufficient to eliminate the need for further therapy.[13] In 20% of cases, splenectomy does not induce remission, and corticosteroids are continued. Further therapy includes the use of vincristine, cyclophosphamide, and azathioprine.

NEONATAL THROMBOCYTOPENIA OF CITP. When CITP is present during pregnancy, *neonatal thrombocytopenia* is a possibility. While some authors refer to this disorder as *autoimmune neonatal thrombocytopenia,* the mechanism is alloimmune from the standpoint that the mother's PAIgG crosses the placental barrier and coats fetal platelets. The immunoincompetent fetus does not synthesize PAIgG. During pregnancy, exposure of fetal platelets to immunoglobulin is best assessed with a measure of maternal IgG antiplatelet antibody and not maternal platelet count. The major risk to the fetus is intracranial hemorrhage during vaginal delivery. If the mother's PLC is below $100 \times 10^3/\mu l$, or if during the early stage of delivery the fetal PLC, performed on blood collected from a scalp vein, is below 50×10^3, the baby is delivered by cesarean section.

Neonatal thrombocytopenia is self-limiting, and in most newborns the platelet count returns to normal after 3 to 4 weeks, depending on the rate of clearance of maternal PAIgG. During this period the PLC is performed regularly and may be severely diminished, although serious bleeding occurs only rarely. Even if no symptoms of neonatal thrombocytopenia exist, PLCs of newborns of mothers with CITP are checked repeatedly during the first 2 months of life.

ACUTE IMMUNE THROMBOCYTOPENIC PURPURA. AITP is a common disease of childhood, with a predilection for children between ages 2 and 6. AITP affects males and females equally and occasionally occurs in adults. In nearly 80% of cases the onset is 1 to 3 weeks after an acute viral illness such as an upper respiratory infection. Like viral illnesses, peak incidence of AITP is in the winter and sping. Sudden onset of petechiae, ecchymoses, and purpura in otherwise healthy children is usually the first indication of AITP. Epistaxis, hematuria, and gastrointestinal hemorrhage are other presenting symptoms. Thrombocytopenia is profound; counts below $20 \times 10^3/\mu l$ are common, but mortality is less than 1%. Intracranial hemorrhage is the most dangerous outcome of the thrombocytopenia.

Thrombocytopenia lasts 3 days to 6 months and may recur after remission. Occasionally in older girls, AITP moderates but remains as CITP. Laboratory findings are limited to the PLC, bleeding time, and anemia associated with hemorrhage.

The cause of AITP is not established, although association with viral illness implies formation of *immune complexes*. An immune complex is the particle formed when an immunoglobulin reacts with a soluble antigen such as a circulating virus. Immune complexes may circulate, then become deposited on the platelet surface. The reaction with the platelet is apparently nonspecific, and the platelet is an "innocent bystander" that is cleared by the mononuclear phagocyte system. Table 10-3 is a comparison of CITP and AITP.

TABLE 10-3
Characteristics of Acute Versus Chronic ITP

Characteristic	Acute	Chronic
Duration	<6 months	Months to years
Onset of bleeding	Sudden	Gradual
Population	2–6 years	20–50 years
Sexual predilection	None	Female to male ratio of 3 : 1 or 4 : 1
Seasonal pattern	Higher incidence in winter and spring	None
Predisposing factors	Majority experienced viral illness.	None
Platelet count on admission	$<20 \times 10^3/\mu l$	$30-80 \times 10^3/\mu l$
Platelet life span	Shortened	Shortened
Spontaneous remission	90% of patients	Uncommon
Therapy	Good response to corticosteroids; splenectomy is rare.	Corticosteroids may be helpful; splenectomy is common.

(Courtesy of Donna M. Corriveau)

DRUG-INDUCED IMMUNE THROMBOCYTOPENIA. Certain drugs suppress bone marrow activity and cause pancytopenia, as described earlier in this chapter. In *drug-induced thrombocytopenia* resulting from increased platelet consumption, bone marrow mega-karyocyte numbers are normal or increased, but platelet survival is markedly de-creased. Drugs that have caused immune thrombocytopenia are listed in Table 10-4. Clinical symptoms are those of acute thrombocytopenia that disappears after with-drawal of the drug.

Quinine and *quinidine* derivatives mediate thrombocytopenia through an immune mechanism similar to the mechanism that mediates AITP. The quinidine derivative is a *hapten* (a substance that elicits an immune response when bound to carrier protein but reacts with preformed specific antibody in the absence of the protein) that binds to a plasma carrier protein. The drug–protein complex elicits a quinine-specific alloim-mune antibody response that on reexposure binds the drug alone. The drug–antibody complex now binds to a high-affinity membrane site; in the case of quinidine the site appears to be the glycoprotein Ib (GP Ib) receptor, the same receptor that interacts with ristocetin and vWF. Platelets from patients with Bernard-Soulier syndrome lack GP Ib and do not bind the drug–antibody complex. The complex recruits complement, which binds to the platelet surface. The presence of the immune complex and complement results in platelet clearance by the mononuclear phagocyte system. Note that "tonic water" contains quinine and may be the cause of drug-induced thrombocytopenia. The patient must be questioned not only about drug ingestion, but also the consumption of tonic-containing beverages like the popular "gin and tonic." Withdrawal of the drug results in rapid remission of thrombocytopenia, but the reaction recurs if the drug is readministered.

The other drugs listed in Table 10-4 cause thrombocytopenia through immune-complex formation, as described for quinine/quinidine. Quinine/quinidine is the only drug that has been shown to participate in a reaction that fixes complement. Although the time-honored *complement fixation* technique may be used to determine the speci-ficity of the quinine/quinidine-specific immunoglobulins, it does not work for other drugs and is technically demanding and time consuming. In most clinical situations the drug that causes thrombocytopenia is easy to implicate without a laboratory test,

TABLE 10-4
Common Drugs Causing Immune Thrombocytopenia

Class	Examples	No. of Cases
Analgesics	Aspirin, acetaminophin, phenylbutazone	31
Antibacterials	Sulfonamides, rifampicin, para-aminosalicy-late, ampicillin, cephalothin	54
Alkaloids	Quinidine, quinine	100
Sedatives, anticonvul-sants	Allylisopropylacetylurea, diphenylhydantoin, carbamazepine	45
Sulfonamide derivatives	Chlorthalidone, furosemide, chlorpropamide	35
Miscellaneous	Arsenical antiluetics, chloroquine, chlorothia-zide, gold salts, insecticides	153

so the laboratory contribution is limited to performance of the PLC and platelet morphology.

Heparin is implicated in an immune-mediated thrombocytopenia that is associated with arterial thrombosis.[2] Patients treated with heparin for thromboembolic disorders occasionally develop thrombosis associated with a high degree of morbidity and mortality. In many cases the limb with arterial occlusions develops gangrene, and amputation is necessary. The difficulty with *heparin-induced thrombocytopenia* is that the clinician is bound to use additional heparin in response to the symptoms, leading to further platelet activation and increased thrombus formation. A heparin-dependent antiplatelet antibody mediates immune-complex formation, deposition on platelets, and aggregates of platelets.

SLE is an autoimmune disorder that occasionally presents with a clinical picture similar to CITP, underscoring the need for careful differential diagnosis. Platelet destruction may begin at any point in the course of SLE as well, and antiplatelet antibodies have been identified. Corticosteroid therapy and splenectomy produce remissions in SLE with about the same frequency as in CITP.

ALLOIMMUNE DISORDERS. *Alloimmune disorders* include *neonatal thrombocytopenia* and *posttransfusion purpura.*

Alloimmune neonatal thrombocytopenia is an uncommon but important disorder analogous to *hemolytic disease of the newborn* (ABO or Rh incompatibility). In most cases maternal anti-Pl^{A1} antibody in women who lack the Pl^{A1} platelet antigen is directed against fetal Pl^{A1}. Anti-Pl^{A1} is a naturally occurring antibody in Pl^{A1}-negative persons that occasionally causes thrombocytopenia in the first born as well as subsequent children, much like anti-A in ABO incompatibility. The maternal antibody develops in response to environmental antigens but crosses the placental barrier to attack fetal platelets.

If alloimmune neonatal thrombocytopenia is suspected from the mother's delivery history, cesarean delivery is recommended to avoid intracranial hemorrhage. Washed maternal platelet concentrate is used to treat hemorrhage, since the mother's platelets lack the specific antigen and are not attacked by the antibody. If the fetus is known to be at risk, platelet concentrate may be prepared in advance. Thrombocytopenia lasts for up to 8 weeks, but risk of dangerous hemorrhage is diminished after delivery.

Pl^{A2} and Bak are other antigens implicated in alloimmune neonatal thrombocytopenia. Besides anti-Pl^{A1}, other antibodies directed toward platelet-specific antigens have been described. Patients with Glanzmann's thrombasthenia lack the Pl^{A1} antigen as well as Pl^{A2} and Bak. It appears that these antigens are associated with the GP IIb–IIIa receptor. Pl^{A1} resides on the plasma membrane and is closely associated with GP IIIa.

Posttransfusion purpura (PTP) is a rare syndrome of unknown incidence, characterized by severe thrombocytopenia 7 to 10 days after a blood transfusion. The thrombocytopenia lasts 2 to 5 weeks and disappears without treatment.

PTP appears to result from increased platelet destruction caused by platelet alloantibodies. The majority of PTP cases occur in patients who lack the Pl^{A1} antigen on their platelets.[21] Only a small number of the fewer than 2% of the population who are Pl^{A1} negative who receive transfusions develop PTP. Other platelet-specific antigens such as Pl^{A2}, Duzo, and Bak are implicated in PTP, but the number of cases involving these antigens is far less than those involving Pl^{A1}. The majority of cases reported to date have been females, most of whom were previously pregnant or transfused. Sensitization may have been induced by fetal or donor platelets positive for Pl^{A1} reaching the patient's circulation.

The mechanism of the thrombocytopenia in PTP is not well understood. Even though the timing is typical of an anamnestic alloantibody response, it is difficult to explain the destruction of the patient's own platelets by an anti-Pl^{A1} antibody when the patient's platelets lack the antigen. A modification of the "innocent bystander" theory has been suggested, in which the donor platelet antigen becomes eluted from the transfused platelets, forming immune complexes with the anti-Pl^{A1} in the circulation. These immune complexes then destroy the patient's Pl^{A1}-negative platelets.[16] Another study postulates the adsorption of soluble Pl^{A1} substance from Pl^{A1}-positive donor plasma by patient platelets that causes them to become passively Pl^{A1} positive. This theory is supported by the realization that platelets have a strong tendency to adsorb plasma materials. In this case the patient's own anti-Pl^{A1} antibody attacks the passively positive platelets until the adsorbed Pl^{A1} substance has been eradicated.[8]

Clinically, patients with PTP usually present with platelet counts less than 20×10^3 cells per microliter. Purpura and mucocutaneous bleeding may be significant. Anti-Pl^{A1} antibodies are usually detectable in the patient's serum by reaction with Pl^{A1}-positive platelets. In most cases examination of the bone marrow demonstrates an increase in the number of megakaryocytes.

Corticosteroids have been used with limited success in the treatment of PTP. Exchange transfusions and plasmapheresis are the most commonly accepted therapies. Platelet transfusions are avoided because serious reactions may occur following infusion of Pl^{A1}-positive platelets.

THROMBOCYTOSIS AND THROMBOCYTHEMIA

Thrombocytosis means a PLC over 400×10^3 cells per microliter of peripheral whole blood.[18] In most cases thrombocytosis is secondary to inflammation or trauma (see Classification of Thrombocytosis) and is termed *reactive thrombocytosis*, in which case the PLC is elevated for a limited period and rarely exceeds 800×10^3. Thrombocytosis may exceed 1000×10^3 cells per microliter when it is a primary symptom of a myeloproliferative disorder such as *polycythemia vera, chronic myelocytic leukemia,* or *myelofibrosis with myeloid metaplasia*. Thrombocythemia is the name given to another myeloproliferative disorder, *essential thrombocythemia*, characterized by PLCs between 1000 and $2000 \times 10^3/\mu$l. Sometimes the term *thrombocythemia* is used as a synonym for *thrombocytosis*.

Reactive Thrombocytosis

PLCs between 440 and $800 \times 10^3/\mu$l with no change in platelet function are common in acute blood loss, after major surgery (particularly splenectomy) or childbirth, tissue necrosis, inflammatory disease, exercise, iron-deficiency anemia, and administration of epinephrine.[18] The MPV is normal or slightly decreased, and peripheral blood smear platelets appear normal in size and structure, in contrast to the platelets of essential thrombocythemia, which present with variation. Bone marrow aspiration is not required, but in those cases in which it has been performed, megakaryocytes are normal. Reactive thrombocytosis is associated with neither thrombosis nor hemorrhage. Thrombocytosis is not related to thrombopoietin levels. Studies were performed in which thrombocytotic animals were given thrombopoietin. A response that included marrow megakaryocyte regeneration and release of large (young) platelets occurred.

CLASSIFICATION OF THROMBOCYTOSIS

PRIMARY OR AUTONOMOUS

Essential thrombocythemia
Polycythemia vera
Chronic myelogenous leukemia
Myelofibrosis with myeloid metaplasia

SECONDARY OR REACTIVE

Exercise
Postsplenectomy
Acute or chronic blood loss
Inflammatory diseases
Iron deficiency
Redistribution
Epinephrine — endogenous and exogenous
Postpartum
Ovulation
Oral contraceptives

Reactive Thrombocytosis Associated With Blood Loss and Surgery

Acute hemorrhage without transfusion therapy is first followed by thrombocytopenia for 2 to 6 days, then thrombocytosis that lasts for several days. Major surgery that causes blood loss is followed by a similar pattern of thrombocytopenia and thrombocytosis. The PLC returns to normal 10 to 16 days after surgery.

POSTSPLENECTOMY THROMBOCYTOSIS. Severe or chronic hemorrhage may require multiple transfusions. Because stored bank blood platelets are not viable, they are rapidly cleared from the circulation. In these patients the PLC is monitored regularly. If it drops below $100 \times 10^3/\mu l$, one unit of platelet concentrate is administered for each new unit of cells.

Postsplenectomy thrombocytosis is a special case. The PLC typically reaches $1000 \times 10^3/\mu l$ after surgery regardless of the clinical reason for splenectomy. Thrombocytosis is expected intuitively, since the spleen normally sequesters one third of the circulating platelet mass; however, the actual elevation in PLC is several times greater than is predicted by simple mathematic computation. This suggests a possible role for the spleen in modulation of platelet production. In contrast to blood loss or other surgery, the PLC reaches a maximum 1 to 3 weeks postsplenectomy and remains elevated for 1 to 3 months. In some persons the PLC remains elevated for several years, especially if the splenectomy was therapeutic for hemolytic anemia. In these persons the risk of thrombosis is increased over that of other patients with splenectomy. The risk of thrombosis does not correlate with PLC results but rather with fibrin formation due to mild DIC. Anticoagulant therapy is used to lessen the risk of thrombosis in these patients.

IRON-DEFICIENCY ANEMIA. Mild iron-deficiency anemia secondary to chronic blood loss is associated with thrombocytosis in about 50% of cases. It is likely that the thrombocytosis is present only during periods of actual blood loss. The PLC has a wide range, but may go as high as $2000 \times 10^3/\mu l$. The PLC returns to normal soon after iron therapy is initiated. In severe iron-deficiency anemia, thrombocytopenia is more common than thrombocytosis, particularly in children. This suggests a role for iron in platelet production.

Reactive Thrombocytosis Associated With Inflammation

Like elevated plasma α- and β-globulin acute-phase reactants, thrombocytosis is an indicator of inflammation. Rheumatoid arthritis, rheumatic fever, osteomyelitis, ulcerative colitis, acute infections, and malignancy are all associated with thrombocytosis. An unexplained thrombocytosis may be an early indicator of malignancy. Administration of epinephrine and conditions associated with elevated plasma epinephrine levels such as chronic stress, pain, childbirth, and exercise are accompanied by thrombocytosis.

Reactive Thrombocytosis Associated With Exercise

Strenuous exercise causes relative thrombocytosis, a PLC increase that is caused by transfer of plasma water to the extravascular compartment, causing hemoconcentration. The change in PLC is reflected in changes in red and white cell components. All measures return to normal 30 minutes after completion of exercise. Aggregometry studies with ADP have shown increased platelet reactivity following exercise, but these were not confirmed by platelet factor 4 (PF_4) studies, nor do they indicate any clinical significance.

Rebound Thrombocytosis

Thrombocytosis follows the thrombocytopenia caused by marrow-suppressive therapy, reflecting an increase in thrombocytopoiesis.

Thrombocythemia

Essential thrombocythemia is a myeloproliferative disorder characterized by proliferation of marrow megakaryocytes and PLC values between 1000 and $2000 \times 10^3/\mu l$. Like most myeloproliferative disorders, it is prevalent in middle-aged and older patients, with an equal male–female distribution. Thrombocythemia is often accompanied by elevated erythrocyte and leukocyte counts. Tests of platelet function are inconclusive. BT values are usually normal, while aggregometry indicates hypoaggregation to ADP and epinephrine in some cases, normal responses in some, and hyperaggregation in others. Some studies reveal intravascular platelet aggregation and resistance to inhibitors of platelet function such as prostaglandin D_2.

In the majority of cases of essential thrombocythemia, patients experience no clotting disorders. Sometimes, however, there is increased risk of either thrombosis or hemorrhage. The pathophysiology in either case is unclear. Thrombosis is often a result of increased blood viscosity or release of procoagulant from granulocytes, but it may also be part of an infarctive process caused by the overwhelming platelet burden or by platelet hyperaggregability. Hemorrhage is most likely related to platelet hypoaggregability unmitigated by the huge excess. Paradoxically, bleeding occurs when platelets are present in counts above $1000 \times 10^3/\mu l$, yet is corrected when the PLC is lowered by chemotherapy.

Many clinicians choose to withhold treatment when patients are asymptomatic, reasoning that the risks of exposure to mutagenic alkylating chemicals are greater than the risk of thrombosis or hemorrhage. Melphalan, busulfan, or radioactive phosphorus is used if clotting symptoms or splenomegaly is experienced. If thrombosis is the main symptom, antiplatelet agents such as the NSAIAs are used in conjunction with heparin.

Primary or autonomous thrombocytosis is a typical finding in three other myeloproliferative disorders: polycythemia vera, chronic myelocytic leukemia, and myelofibrosis with (agnogenic) myeloid metaplasia. In these cases the PLC seldom reaches the extreme values achieved in essential thrombocythemia, and clotting disorders are uncommon. If thrombosis or hemorrhage occurs, treatment patterns for these disorders are similar to those for essential thrombocythemia.

QUALITATIVE PLATELET DISORDERS (THROMBOCYTOPATHIES)

All of the platelet disorders described to this point in this chapter are disorders affecting the PLC. In a few cases, like Bernard-Soulier syndrome and essential thrombocythemia, the change in count is accompanied by suppressed platelet function. Except for Bernard-Soulier syndrome, which is associated with thrombocytopenia, the disorders discussed in the remainder of the chapter are characterized by abnormal platelet function associated with a normal PLC.

To form a competent hemostatic platelet plug, platelets must be present in adequate numbers and have normal function. If the PLC is normal, a prolonged BT or the appearance of petechiae near the site of a tourniquet indicates a potential qualitative platelet abnormality. The BT (see Chap. 9) is the laboratory screen employed most commonly to detect abnormal platelet function. If the BT result exceeds 8 minutes and the patient has no evidence of vascular abnormalities, a qualitative platelet defect may exist.

The clinical manifestations of the thrombocytopathies mimic those of the quantitative platelet disorders: petechiae, purpura, ecchymosis, menorrhagia, epistaxis, and gastrointestinal, mucosal, and postoperative bleeding. Bleeding into joints or body cavities is rare.

Thrombocytopathies, like PLC disorders, are inherited or acquired. Bernard-Soulier syndrome, Glanzmann's thrombasthenia, aspirinlike syndrome, and storage pool disorder are hereditary thrombocytopathies. Storage pool disorders are common; the others are rare. Most acquired qualitative platelet disorders result from administration of drugs. Some thrombocytopathies result from intrinsic pathologic lesions of the platelets, some from extrinsic conditions. The classification of the congenital thrombocytopathies is given under Congenital Platelet Function Defects, earlier in this chapter. Defects are related to platelet adhesion, aggregation, or release. Von Willebrand disease is a deficiency of the high-molecular-weight multimers of Factor VIII R:Ag and is discussed in this chapter only as it relates to platelet function. (see chap. 5).

Disorders of Platelet Adhesion

The process whereby platelets cling to negatively charged foreign surfaces is called adhesion. The process of adhesion is distinct from aggregation and agglutination. Aggregation is energy-dependent coherence that is associated with platelet activation and secretion. Agglutination is energy-independent coherence that resembles the clumping of indicator cells in a serologic reaction. *In vivo* adhesion begins when disruption of the endothelial cell lining exposes subendothelial collagen associated with the basement membrane and *tunica media* (see Chap. 1). When platelets come into contact with the subendothelium, they change shape and cling to the exposed foreign surface. After new endothelium has grown to cover the exposed site, the platelet releases its hold on the subendothelium and returns to the circulation.

Adhesion characteristics change with the "shear rate" of blood flow, a measure of the lateral fluid force of blood as it passes the vessel wall. The shear rate of large arteries and veins is lower than the shear rate of small vessels and capillaries. In large vessels, platelets adhere directly to human fibrillar collagen types I or III, but in smaller vessels adhesion is mediated by the presence of vWF. vWF simultaneously binds a specific platelet surface surface glycoprotein, GP Ib and fibrillar collagen to promote adhesion (see Chap. 7). Diminished or abnormal vWF (von Willebrand disease), and absent GP Ib (Bernard-Soulier syndrome) both result in impaired adhesion and a hemorrhagic disorder typical of abnormal platelet function.[14]

Bernard-Soulier Syndrome

Bernard and Soulier first described the rare, autosomal-recessive Bernard-Soulier syndrome (BSS) in 1948, and to date only a few additional cases have been reported.[24] BSS is an inherited intrinsic platelet adhesion defect, often associated with consanguinity. The main laboratory characteristics of BSS are prolonged BT, inadequate prothrombin consumption, giant platelets seen on the stained peripheral blood smear, and absence of ristocetin-induced aggregation. Hemorrhagic symptoms are first observed during infancy or early childhood and tend to decrease with age. The prognosis is variable: some patients require platelet concentrate following superficial cuts or dental extractions or during menstruation. Others experience mild symptoms.

Mild to moderate thrombocytopenia is a frequent but inconsistent finding. Peripheral blood platelets in stained smears vary in size from normal (approximately 2 μm in diameter) to giant (as large as a lymphocyte). *In vivo* BSS platelets circulate in a spherical rather than normal discoid shape. This spherical shape is seen in heterozygous BSS carriers as well as patients. The internal structure of BSS platelets on the stained smear is usually normal, but occasionally there is a central clustering of granules called a *pseudonucleus* (see Fig. 10-6,*B*). BSS platelets contain higher than normal levels of granule contents, including vWF.

A BT in excess of 20 minutes is a common finding, but clot retraction is normal. Platelet factor 3 (PF_3, or platelet phospholipid) availability, as determined by the prothrombin consumption test with patient serum, is decreased (see Chap. 9), resulting in a shortened prothrombin consumption time result. A special method is employed in which BSS patient platelet-rich plasma is incubated with a suspension of kaolin. When this mixture is added to normal platelet-poor plasma, PF_3 availability is normal. Platelet retention tests using glass-bead columns yield prolonged results in BSS (Chap. 9). Plasma and platelet-derived Factor VIII – related antigen levels are normal to increased.

Aggregometry study results are diagnostic of BSS (Fig. 10-9). BSS platelets respond normally to addition of the agonists ADP, epinephrine, and arachidonic acid. The normal ristocetin-induced agglutination response is absent. The addition of fresh plasma that contains normal vWF activity fails to correct the abnormal response. Uncorrected failure to agglutinate in the presence of ristocetin is the key to the laboratory identification of BSS. In von Willebrand disease the missing response is corrected by addition of normal plasma; therefore, the ristocetin agglutination test is used to distinguish between BSS and von Willebrand disease.

The inability of BSS platelets to agglutinate in the presence of ristocetin and vWF is

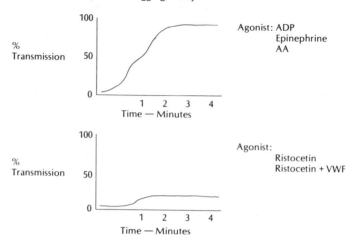

Bernard-Soulier Aggregometry

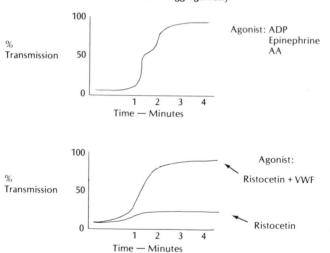

Von Willebrand's Disease Aggregometry

FIG. 10-9. Typical results of platelet aggregometry studies in Bernard-Soulier syndrome and von Willebrand disease. Note the normal response to ADP, epinephrine, and arachidonic acid (AA) but the lack of response to ristocetin. Addition of vWF does not correct the missing aggregation response to ristocetin in BSS but does correct in von Willebrand disease.

traced to the absence of the normal surface membrane glycoprotein termed GP Ib.[17] GP Ib is a receptor that binds vWF in the ristocetin agglutination reaction (see Chaps. 7 and 8) and is essential to platelet adhesion to subendothelial collagen through vWF in small vessels. BSS platelets also lack glycoprotein fractions V and IX (GP V, GP IX) and have reduced levels of sialic acid with reduced surface charge. The absence of GP Ib and the lack of capillary adhesion account for the hemorrhagic symptoms of BSS. Carriers have decreased levels of GP Ib and GP IX and increased platelet size, but no bleeding symptoms.

The aggregation response to thrombin is impaired in BSS platelets. Collagen-induced aggregation is sometimes absent as well. Nieuwenhuis and colleagues have described a separate glycoprotein deficiency, GP Ia deficiency, in a bleeding disorder associated with absent collagen-induced aggregation.[14]

Platelet aggregometry studies on BSS patient plasma are difficult to perform because it is hard to isolate the large platelets from erythrocytes and lymphocytes when using routine centrifugation methods for obtaining platelet-rich plasma. When the platelets are properly isolated, their increased size affects aggregometer light scattering, so aggregometry curves are altered. These problems affect the proper laboratory interpretation of ADP-, epinephrine-, arachidonic acid–, thrombin-, and collagen-induced aggregation.

In summary, the findings of prolonged BT, normal clot retraction, normal ADP and epinephrine aggregation, decreased platelet retention results, and absence of ristocetin agglutination in the presence of vWF permit distinction of BSS from von Willebrand disease, Glanzmann's thrombasthenia, and other disorders associated with giant platelets.

BSS patients are treated with platelet transfusions to manage bleeding episodes. The repeated use of platelet transfusions sometimes results in formation of plasma antibodies specific for the missing factor. Bone marrow transplantation may be a more long-lasting solution in severe cases.

Von Willebrand Disease

Von Willebrand disease (vWD) is a name given to a collection of at least three autosomal-recessive or autosomal-dominant plasma clotting factor deficiencies of variable genetic penetrance first described by von Willebrand in 1927.[19] Because vWD is a plasma factor deficiency producing extrinsic suppression of platelet adhesion, it is discussed in detail in Chapter 5. The discussion in this chapter is confined to the measurable platelet effects.

The clinical symptoms of vWD resemble those of other platelet disorders, as described earlier in this section, although severe vWD may also result in joint and internal hemorrhage similar to those seen in the hemophilias, described in Chapter 5. The platelet-mediated symptoms of vWD most resemble the symptoms of BSS and range from mild to severe. Results of laboratory tests of platelet activity and count are normal except for a prolonged BT and absence of ristocetin-induced aggregation that is corrected by the addition of vWF. Platelet morphology on stained peripheral blood smears is normal.

vWF is a multimeric plasma glycoprotein that is altered or diminished in vWD. vWF is produced by endothelial cells and megakaryocytes and circulates in the plasma in a noncovalent complex with Factor VIII procoagulant protein (antihemophilic factor). Type I and type III vWD are characterized by decreased levels of vWF in plasma. In type I vWD the vWF level is variable from case to case and from time to time within the individual patient. In type III vWD, vWF is absent, and symptoms are the most severe. Type II vWD is a family of at least four disorders characterized by structural abnormalities of the vWF molecule. Symptoms of type II vWD vary from mild to severe, depending on the molecular defect. In all cases the abnormality results in decreased adhesion of platelets to subendothelial collagen in small vessels. There is no abnormality of platelet structure except that platelet-stored vWF may exhibit the same structural abnormalities as plasma vWF in type II vWD. This fact is not fully established by experimental data.

vWF binds to GP Ib on the platelet surface.[22] It may also bind to GP Ia and the GPIIb–IIIa complex, although these reactions are still being debated, and their importance in vWD is unknown. A separate site on the vWF molecule binds to subendothelial fibrillar collagen, so the physiologic effect of the vWF molecule is to bridge the gap between platelets and subendothelium to promote adhesion (Fig. 10-10). Absence or structural deformation of the vWF molecule results in diminished adhesion and accounts for the hemorrhagic symptoms of vWD. In the case of types I or III vWD, adhesion abnormalities are related to the diminished concentration of vWF. In type II vWD, structural changes affect the affinity of binding sites on the vWF molecule for either GP Ib on platelets or binding sites on collagen. The presence of noncovalently bound Factor VIII procoagulant does not affect adhesion; even in hemophilia A, in which Factor VIII activity is absent, platelet–subendothelial adhesion is normal. The converse is not necessarily true. Diminished levels of vWF mean diminished levels of circulating Factor VIII procoagulant activity, so in type III vWD (complete absence of vWF), Factor VIII activity is nearly absent, and the patient exhibits not only the symptoms of a platelet disorder but also symptoms resembling those of hemophilia A. In other types of vWD the activity of Factor VIII is also diminished, but not enough to cause a bleeding problem by itself.

Laboratory findings in vWD resemble those of BSS. The BT is prolonged relative to diminished vWF concentration or function, but clot retraction is normal. The glass-bead platelet retention test reveals decreased retention, but preexposure of the beads to normal plasma corrects the percentage retention to normal. Immunologic testing by radioimmunodiffusion or electroimmunodiffusion (rocket assay) uses immunoglobu-

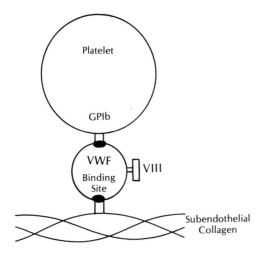

FIG. 10-10. Diagram demonstrating the position of vWF between the GP Ib platelet receptor and subendothelial collagen. The multimeric vWF molecule presents two binding sites, one specific for platelet GP Ib, the other specific for sites on the fibrillar collagen.

lin specific for an antigenic site on the vWF molecule termed *Factor VIIIR:Ag (Factor VIII–related antigen).* In vWD types I and III the plasma concentration of vWF by immunoassay is diminished or absent, respectively. In type II, VIIIR:Ag levels may be normal or decreased, depending on whether the molecular aberration affects the structure of the antigenic site.

Platelet aggregometry in vWD is normal with all agonists except ristocetin (see Chap. 9). Ristocetin agglutination is absent but corrected upon addition of plasma containing normal vWF (see Fig. 10-10). Ristocetin is able to promote agglutination because it bridges the charge-induced gap between neighboring vWF molecules bound to platelets. Live platelets are unnecessary for the demonstration of ristocetin agglutination, since agglutination is energy independent. Consequently, formalin-fixed reagent platelets from normal donors are often used in the ristocetin test for vWD. When reagent platelets are used, vWF is termed *ristocetin cofactor* and designated Factor VIIIR:RCo (Factor VIII–related ristocetin cofactor). Ristocetin cofactor activity ranges from 0% to 50% in all forms of vWD. Reagent platelets are, of course, not effective in the diagnosis of BSS, since in BSS ristocetin agglutination is affected by an intrinsic platelet defect. Table 10-5 gives the immunologic and ristocetin reactions in both vWD and BSS. In summary, the component that accounts for the absence of ristocetin agglutination in BSS is lack of GP Ib, while in vWD the deficient factor is vWF.

Assays for Factor VIII coagulant activity usually give diminished results in vWD, although Factor VIII activity is decreased to the level seen in hemophiliacs only in type III vWD. Since Factor VIII activity is normally present at tenfold excess, in vWD the Factor VIII coagulant activity is rarely low enough to promote hemorrhage as a separate mechanism from platelet-associated bleeding.

Treatment of vWD involves replacement of the missing plasma factor with fresh-frozen plasma or cryoprecipitate. Administration of 1-desamino-8-D-arginine vasopressin (DDAVP) induces release of Factor VIII/vWF from endothelial cells and provides temporary relief of symptoms.

TABLE 10-5
Laboratory Reactions in von Willebrand Disease and Bernard-Soulier Syndrome

Parameter	Type I vWD	Type II vWD	Type III vWD	BSS	Hemophilia A
VIII:C activity	Decreased	Normal or decreased	Absent	Normal	Decreased or absent
VIIIR:Ag	Decreased	Normal or decreased	Absent	Normal	Normal
VIIIR:RCo	Decreased	Decreased	Absent	Normal	Normal
BT	Prolonged	Prolonged	Prolonged	Prolonged	Normal
Ristocetin-induced aggregation	Decreased	Decreased	Decreased	Decreased	Normal
Correction with vWF	Yes	Yes	Yes	No	

BSS, Bernard-Soulier syndrome

Pseudo-von Willebrand Disease

Pseudo–von Willebrand disease (PvWD) is a name that Weiss and co-workers used to describe an autosomal-dominant trait they observed in one family.[26] This disease has been described by other investigators, who called it platelet-type von Willebrand disease.[11] The mild bleeding syndrome in these patients is associated with a deficiency of the high-molecular-weight vWF multimers (HMW VIIIR:Ag) in plasma, similar to types IIA and IIB vWD (see Chap. 5). In types IIA and IIB vWD the decreased plasma levels of HMW multimers is due to abnormalities of production, but in PvWD, production of these multimers is normal. In PvWD, platelets demonstrate increased avidity for HMW multimers; consequently, the rate of removal of HMW multimers from plasma is increased. The reason for increased avidity is unknown, but PvWD platelets may have a membrane abnormality.

In PvWD, platelets agglutinate in the presence of as little as 0.3 mg to 0.5 mg/ml of ristocetin, compared to normal agglutination, which requires at least 1 mg/ml. Furthermore, addition of vWF causes platelet aggregation in the absence of ADP or other agonists. These are the cardinal laboratory signs for PvWD. There is also a variable thrombocytopenia.

Symptoms of PvWD are similar to those of type IIB vWD. Low-dose cryoprecipitate is effective in treatment but should be used with caution.

Platelet Defects of Primary Aggregation

In platelet aggregometry, certain rare disorders result in failure to aggregate in response to ADP, epinephrine, collagen, or thrombin. These include *Glanzmann's* Thrombasthenia *(GT)* and *congenital afibrinogenemia.*

Glanzmann's Thrombasthenia

GT was first described in 1918 and termed *hereditary hemorrhagic thrombasthenia.*[17] GT is an autosomal-recessive hemorrhagic disorder with typical symptoms of platelet malfunction. Bleeding is frequent at birth and childhood and decreases with age. Laboratory findings in GT include a prolonged BT, impaired or absent clot retraction, and failure to aggregate to ADP or epinephrine. PLC is normal.

GT platelets are normal in size and appearance when examined in stained peripheral blood smears. They undergo shape change and form pseudopods normally when exposed to collagen. GT platelets degranulate and secrete PF_4, serotonin, and ADP normally upon exposure to thrombin, but do not aggregate. Exposure to thrombin and arachidonic acid yields normal thromboxane production. Platelets agglutinate normally in response to ristocetin. Glass-bead retention test results are markedly reduced, but *in vivo* adhesion to subendothelial collagen is normal. Prothrombin consumption test results are shortened, indicating impaired availability of PF_3 (platelet phospholipid) and diminished prothrombin activation.

Aggregometry results are used to identify GT. There is no primary wave of aggregation in the presence of ADP, epinephrine, collagen, or thrombin (Fig. 10-11). Ristocetin agglutination is normal.

The pathophysiology of GT is clear.[15] GT platelets lack surface glycoprotein fractions IIb and IIIa (GP IIb, GP IIIa). When ADP binds to normal platelets, GP IIb and GP IIIa combine to form a receptor complex that is exposed and binds fibrinogen. Fibrinogen is a necessary cofactor for the aggregation of normal human platelets, bridging the surface charge–induced gap between platelets in plasma. Lack of the GP IIb–IIIa

Glanzmann's Thrombasthenia — Aggregometry

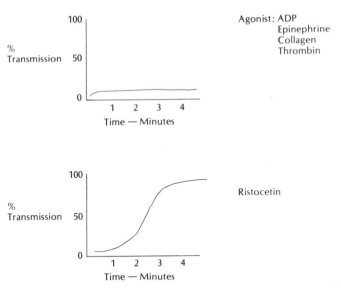

FIG. 10-11. Results of platelet aggregometry in GT. Note the lack of response to ADP, epinephrine, collagen, and thrombin, but normal ristocetin agglutination.

fibrinogen receptor prevents aggregation. In addition, alpha granules of GT platelets contain abnormally small levels of stored fibrinogen, suggesting that the GP IIb–IIIa complex not only binds but internalizes fibrinogen for storage. Other alpha granule proteins such as vWF, fibronectin, and thrombospondin are present at normal levels. Heterozygotes exhibit no bleeding disorder, although their platelets carry about half the normal levels of GP IIb–IIIa. *In vivo* secretion and adhesion are not impaired by the absence of the fibrinogen receptor, although in aggregometry, platelets incubated with ADP or epinephrine do not secrete their contents, since secretion does not occur without aggregation under these conditions.

GT exists in two forms, type I and type II. In type I the GP IIb–IIIa receptor and intracellular fibrinogen are absent, the bleeding disorder is severe, and there is no clot retraction. In type II GT, the GP IIb–IIIa is present at about 15% of normal concentrations, and intraplatelet fibrinogen levels are below normal. Type II clot retraction is observable but incomplete. Results of aggregometry studies are abnormal in both types.

The platelet-specific alloantigen Pl[A1] appears to be associated with GP IIIa and is absent in type I GT. Three other platelet surface antigens, Pl[A2], Bak[a], and Lek[a], are also associated with the complex. These antigens are present in normal amounts in BSS, demonstrating that they are not associated with GP Ib. GT patients who have received repeated platelet concentrate transfusions may develop an IgG alloantibody specific for the missing antigen, usually P1[A1], rendering future P1[A1]-positive platelet transfusions ineffective. Since 98% of the normal population is P1[A1] positive, platelet transfusion therapy for P1[A1]-negative patients must be approached with restraint. The addition of anti-P1^{A1} antibody to normal platelets inhibits their ability to bind fibrinogen and to aggregate with ADP.

Congenital Afibrinogenemia

Congenital afibrinogenemia is an autosomal-recessive absence or severe decrease of the plasma fibrinogen. Patients experience the symptoms of both impaired platelet function and clot formation. Prothrombin time, activated partial thromboplastin time, and thrombin time test results are greatly prolonged. The BT is prolonged, and ADP-induced aggregation of platelets is absent. Thrombin-induced aggregation is independent of fibrinogen and is normal.

Disorders of Platelet Secretion

Storage Pool Disorders

Disorders of platelet secretion are usually associated with an abnormal secondary wave of platelet aggregation. In secretion disorders, in vitro ADP-induced aggregation is impaired so that a primary wave of aggregation is followed by disaggregation instead of a secondary wave (Fig. 10-12). The aggregometer pen deflects upward for several seconds but then returns to the baseline. This tracing illustrates the fact that internal platelet ADP from dense bodies is not released during primary aggregation. In a normal tracing, reagent ADP causes the initial reorganization of platelets, contraction of their organelles, and expression of contents, including stored ADP from dense bodies. The released ADP then induces secondary aggregation. In disorders of secretion, internal ADP is not expressed; consequently, the reorganized platelets disperse and revert to their original shape, causing the tracing to return to the baseline value.

Disorders of secretion arise from two mechanisms. The first is the existence of diminished levels of granule and dense body content, known as *storage pool deficiency.* Platelets become activated normally, but the quantity of organelle contents is inadequate to support further aggregation.[25] The second mechanism occurs when normal storage pools of platelet contents are not fully expressed because there is a defect in the cell's activation mechanisms such as impaired prostaglandin production or inadequate biochemical response to thromboxane or calcium mobilization. Such impairment is often caused by drugs, such as the NSAIAs, that suppress or inactivate cyclooxygenase or some other enzyme essential to prostaglandin and thromboxane synthesis (see Chap.

Primary aggregation followed by disaggregation

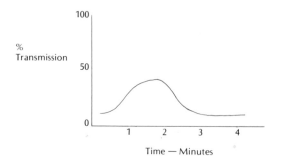

FIG. 10-12. Typical aggregometry tracing demonstrating a platelet secretion defect. Upon addition of the standard concentration of ADP, aggregation begins, reaches a plateau, then reverts to the baseline.

8). This explains why the platelets of patients who have taken aspirin undergo primary aggregation followed by disaggregation. There are rare congenital or acquired abnormalities of platelet activation that give results similar to the effects of NSAIAs; these are often called *aspirinlike disorders*. In most cases they are caused by deficiencies in cyclooxygenase or thromboxane synthetase activity.

DENSE BODY STORAGE POOL DEFICIENCY. The most common form of storage pool deficiency is caused by a decrease in dense body granules. Platelets from patients with storage pool deficiency have a marked decrease in dense bodies when viewed by transmission electron microscopy.[25] Quantitative measures reveal that the levels of ADP, calcium, and serotonin are diminished. The BT is increased in inverse relation to the level of ADP. Patients with storage pool deficiency experience a mild bleeding disorder most evident as prolonged bleeding after trauma or surgery and occasional epistaxis or menorrhagia. The BT may be normal or slightly prolonged but becomes increasingly prolonged upon ingestion of NSAIAs.

The cause of general storage pool deficiency is unknown. Some cases demonstrate defects in synthesis of platelet prostaglandins, thromboxane A_2, and malondialdehyde (see Chap. 8), but in others the functional pathways are intact. Impaired aggregation responses to arachidonic acid are seen in some cases, while platelets from others give a normal response. There are several inherited syndromes that include storage pool deficiency as part of their pathophysiology, including the *Hermansky-Pudlak syndrome (oculocutaneous albinism)*, *Chédiak-Higashi syndrome*, *Wiskott-Aldrich syndrome*, and *TAR*. Wiskott-Aldrich syndrome and TAR are described near the beginning of this chapter with other disorders of PLC.

Chédiak-Higashi syndrome (CHS) is a rare autosomal-recessive disease characterized by partial *oculocutaneous albinism* (inadequate skin and eye pigmentation), susceptibility to bacterial infections, and hemorrhage. Absence of intracellular skin pigmentation granules, myelocytic lysosomes, and the dense bodies of platelets may be traced to a common genetic lesion and account for the symptoms of this disorder. The abnormal bacteriolytic function of neutrophilic and monocytic lysosomes, reflected in the presence of large, dark-staining granules on peripheral blood smears, makes these patients chronically susceptible to infections.

The bleeding disorder in CHS is caused by defective platelet function. Platelets lack normal dense bodies and have diminished levels of ADP and serotonin. CHS platelets are able to take up radioactive serotonin at normal initial rates, but absorption ceases before normal serotonin levels are reached.[1] The ratio of ATP to ADP is higher than normal (6.3 compared to 1.5), indicating a dense body deficiency. The aggregation response of CHS platelets to the agonists ADP and epinephrine is variable but generally takes the pattern of primary aggregation followed by disaggregation.

Hermansky-Pudlak syndrome shares the diagnostic features of CHS, and the platelet abnormality is identical.[4] Mononuclear phagocytes in bone marrow and tissues contain an insoluble polyunsaturated lipid called *ceroid* in phagosomes, indicating a lipid metabolism disorder.

ALPHA GRANULE DEFICIENCY (GRAY PLATELET SYNDROME). Four cases of alpha granule deficiency in the presence of normal dense bodies have been reported.[17] Alpha granule deficiency is called gray platelet syndrome because on a Wright-stained peripheral blood smear platelets are larger than normal, with pale gray or blue-gray staining characteristics. Under the transmission electron microscope it is apparent that the alpha granules are missing.[25] Constituents of alpha granules, including PF_4, β-thromboglobulin, and fibrinogen, are decreased, while serotonin and ADP levels are normal.

Patients experience mild bleeding episodes, moderate thrombocytopenia, prolonged BT, and impaired aggregometry responses to collagen and thrombin. Plasma levels of PF_4 and β-thromboglobulin are increased, implying that the defect in this disorder is related to lysosomal packaging and not protein synthesis.

In summary, patients with storage pool deficiencies exhibit heterogeneity in granular abnormalities. The levels of dense body and alpha granule contents vary by the individual. In some cases there are diminished levels of lysosomal enzymes as well. Clinical bleeding manifestations vary from silent to severe and may be amplified by the presence of drugs that influence the release reaction. This group of syndromes emphasizes the importance of platelet granule contents in normal platelet function and normal plasma coagulation.

Abnormalities of the Arachidonic Acid Pathway

Secretion requires activity from several platelet enzymes. A series of phospholipases catalyze the release of arachidonic acid from membrane phospholipids. Arachidonic acid is converted to prostaglandin by cyclooxygenase and to thromboxane A_2 by thromboxane synthase. Thromboxane A_2 binds to adenylate cyclase to modulate production of cyclic adenosine monophosphate. The arachidonic acid pathway is described in detail in Chapter 8 with reference to each of the important enzymes.

Several acquired or congenital disorders of platelet secretion are traced to structural and functional modifications of arachidonic acid pathway enzymes. Acquired suppression of cyclooxygenase occurs upon ingestion of NSAIAs such as aspirin and ibuprofen. Hereditary absence or modification of the same enzymes is usually termed an *aspirin-like syndrome* because the clinical and laboratory manifestations resemble those following NSAIA ingestion. In either acquired or hereditary conditions the aggregometry response to ADP and epinephrine is the same as in the storage pool disorders: primary aggregation followed by disaggregation. Unlike storage pool disorders, ultrastructure and granular contents are normal.

DRUG-INDUCED ABNORMALITIES. Acetylsalicylic acid (aspirin) irreversibly acetylates the active site of the prostaglandin-producing enzyme cyclooxygenase and completely inhibits its activity. Because platelets are anucleate, they do not synthesize new enzymes, so the inhibitory effect is permanent. For this reason, ingestion of aspirin affects the secretory function of platelets for several days after the drug is discontinued. Aspirin suppression of platelet function disappears in relation to platelet life span. Eighty-five percent to 90% of normal persons demonstrate an increased BT of 2 to 9 minutes 2 hours after ingestion of 650 mg of aspirin. The degree of increase in BT is idiosyncratic and does not correlate with the pre-aspirin BT. Aggregometry on platelet-rich plasma from a person who has recently taken a routine dose of aspirin reveals the typical pattern of primary aggregation followed by disaggregation. BT and aggregometry results return to normal a few days after aspirin ingestion.

Persons with mild or silent bleeding disorders such as mild storage pool deficiency, thrombocytopenia, vascular disorder, vWD, or circulating anticoagulant experience a marked increase in their BT upon aspirin ingestion. Aspirin may be used for the so-called challenge test if a mild disorder is suspected. A BT is performed before and after administration of aspirin and the times compared. The BT is prolonged in inverse proportion to the level of ADP released from dense bodies.

There are other NSAIAs, including phenylbutazone, ibuprofen, indomethacin, and pyrazolone derivatives. These all inhibit cyclooxygenase, with results similar to those of aspirin except that the other NSAIAs bind reversibly to the enzyme. Consequently, their inhibitory effect is more short-lived.

ASPIRINLIKE SYNDROMES. Many individual cases of defects in one of the enzymes of the arachidonic acid metabolic pathway have been described. Liberation of arachidonic acid from membrane-bound phospholipids is the first step in thromboxane synthesis. A defect in one of the phospholipase enzymes responsible for release of the fatty acid, or, alternatively, a defect in calcium mobilization, may account for the diminished platelet activation. Platelets defective in arachidonic acid release have only primary aggregation to the agonists ADP, epinephrine, collagen, and platelet activating factor; they respond normally to arachidonic acid.

Defects of cyclooxygenase cause impaired aggregation results with ADP, epinephrine, collagen, and arachidonic acid but a normal response to the addition of prostaglandin G_2 (PGG_2). PGG_2 bypasses the cyclooxygenase-catalyzed point in the arachidonic acid pathway and serves as a substrate for thromboxane synthase. Immunoassay for the cyclooxygenase molecule has revealed normal concentrations in most patients. The assumption is made that the enzymatic defect in these cases is structural and not quantitative.

Defects in the thromboxane A_2 receptor, presumed to be located on the adenylate cyclase molecule, result in inadequate platelet stimulus in spite of normal production of thromboxane A_2. In this case, normal levels of thromboxane B_2 are produced by the platelet, yet aggregometry reveals abnormal responses to all agonists.

In all cases of aspirinlike syndromes the bleeding disorder is mild and need be treated only at times of clinical stress such as surgery or trauma. The BT is mildly prolonged, but prolongation is exaggerated upon administration of aspirin.

Although the abnormalities of secretion are poorly defined and, in the case of most persons; undetected, they are probably the single most common group of platelet disorders. Studies examining persons who "bleed a little longer than usual" may reveal more of these disorders.

REFERENCES

1. Apitz-Castro R, Cruz MR, Ledezma E et al: The storage pool deficiency in platelets from humans with the Chédiak-Higashi syndrome: Study of six patients. Br J Haematol 59:471–483, 1985
2. Brace LD, Fareed J, Tomeo J, Issleib S: Biochemical and pharmacological studies on the interaction of PL 10169 and its subfractions with human platelets. Haemostasis 16:93–105, 1986
3. Gewirtz AM: Human megakaryocytopoiesis. Semin Hematol 23:27–42, 1986
4. Hermansky F, Pudlak P: Albinism associated with hemorrhagic diathesis and unusual pigmented reticular cells in the bone marrow: Report of two cases with histochemical studies. Blood 14:162–174, 1959
5. Jordan SW, Larsen WE: Ultrastructure studies on the May-Hegglin anomaly. Blood 25:921–925, 1965
6. Karpatkin S: Autoimmune thrombocytopenic purpura. Semin Hematol 22:260–288, 1985
7. Kelton JG: Heparin-induced thrombocytopenia and thrombotic thrombocytopenic purpura: Destructive thrombocytopenic disorders characterized by acute arterial thrombosis. In International Hemostasis Symposium, Wayne State University, Detroit, 1986
8. Kickler TS, Ness PM, Herman JH, Bell WR: Studies on the pathophysiology of posttransfusion purpura. Blood 68:347–350, 1986

9. Kumar R, Ansell JE, Canoso RT, Deykin D: Clinical trial of a new bleeding time device. Am J Clin Pathol 70:640–645, 1978

10. McMillan R: Chronic idiopathic thrombocytopenic purpura. N Engl J Med 304:1135, 1981

11. Miller JL, Castella A: Platelet-type von Willebrand's disease: Characterization of a new bleeding disorder. Blood 60:790–794, 1982

12. Moschcowitz E: An acute febrile pleiochromic anemia with hyaline thrombosis of terminal arterioles and capillaries: An undescribed disease. Arch Intern Med 36:89, 1915

13. Murphy S: Platelets. In Spivak JL (ed): Fundamentals of Clinical Hematology, 2nd ed. Philadelphia, Harper & Row, 1984

14. Nieuwenhuis HK, Sakariassen KS, Houdijk WPM et al: Defiency of platelet membrane glycoprotein Ia associated with a decreased platelet adhesion to subendothelium: A defect in platelet spreading. Blood 68:692–695, 1986

15. Nurden AT, Caen JP: An abnormal platelet glycoprotein pattern in three cases of Glanzmann's thrombasthenia. Br J Haematol 28:253–260, 1974

16. Pegels JG, Bruynes ECE, Engelfreit CP, van dem Borne AEG: PTP: A serological and immunochemical study. Br J Haematol 49:521, 1981

17. Rao AK, Holmsen H: Congenital disorders of platelet function. Semin Hematol 23:102–118, 1986

18. Robbins G, Barnard DL: Thrombocytosis and microthrombocytosis: A clinical evaluation of 372 cases. Acta Haemat 70:175–182, 1983

19. Ruggeri ZM, Zimmerman TS: Platelets and von Willebrand disease. Semin Hematol 22:203–218, 1985

20. Schulman I, Abildgaard CF, Cornet J et al: Studies on thrombopoiesis II: Assay of human plasma thrombopoietic activity. J Pediatr 66:604–608, 1985

21. Shulman NR, Aster RH, Lerner A, Hiller MC: Immunoreactions involving platelets. V. Post transfusion purpura due to a complement-fixing antibody against a genetically controlled platelet antigen. J Clin Invest 40:1597, 1961

22. Stel HV, Sakariassen KS, de Groot PG et al: von Willebrand factor in the vessel wall mediates platelet adherence. Blood 65:85–90, 1985

23. Thompson AR, Harker LA: Manual of Hemostasis and Thrombosis, 3rd ed. Philadelphia, FA Davis, 1983

24. Weiss HJ: Congenital disorders of platelet function. Semin Hematol 17:228–241, 1980

25. Weiss HJ, Ames RP: Ultrastructural findings in storage-pool disease and aspirin-like defects of platelets. Am J Pathol 71:447–466, 1973

26. Weiss HJ, Meyer D, Rabinowitz R et al: Pseudo von Willebrand's disease: An intrinsic platelet defect with aggregation by unmodified human factor VIII/von Willebrand factor in subtypes of classic (type I) and variant (type II) von Willebrand's disease. J Lab Clin Med 101:411–425, 1983

Hypercoagulation and Thromboembolic Disorders

11

Barrett W. Dick

CASE STUDY A 52-year-old woman on hemodialysis for chronic renal failure first came to the attention of the hematology laboratory in the fall of 1985 when abnormal lymphoid forms (ALFs) were noted in her peripheral blood. At that time her white count was 13,000/mm³, with the abnormal forms making up less than 1% of the total; there was no enlargement of lymph nodes. No evidence of lymphoma was found on bone marrow examination.

In April of 1986 a breast mass was noted, which was excised and characterized as a T-cell lymphoma. Peripheral blood involvement was more apparent, with a white count of 55,000/mm³, and there were 46% ALFs with bone marrow involvement. The white count continued to rise rapidly, necessitating chemotherapy, but without evidence of a response.

In August of 1986 the patient was readmitted with signs and symptoms of an upper respiratory infection and some evidence of mental confusion. She was thought to have acute sinusitis and pneumonia. The white count on admission was 324,000/mm³, with 92% ALFs. Antibiotic therapy resulted in symptomatic improvement of her respiratory symptoms. Leukapheresis was performed several times, followed by initiation of chemotherapy. The white count fell to 34,000/mm³, with clearing of the confusion and further improvement in the patient's respiratory problem. On the 25th hospital day, the patient suffered a cardiac arrest and could not be resuscitated. The family refused to give permission for an autopsy.

This case illustrates hyperleukostasis syndrome, one potential cause of thrombosis. The patient's confusion was probably due to insufficient oxygen getting to the brain secondary to poor vascular perfusion due to a high white count. The symptoms improved after the white count was lowered by leukapheresis and chemotherapy, thus averting potential thrombus formation.

The hypercoagulable state is a group of hereditary or acquired conditions in which there is increased risk of venous or arterial thrombosis. Occlusion of arteriolar or capillary blood supply also occurs in a number of disorders in which the materials that block the blood vessels may not involve components of the hemostatic system. These are also included in the category of vaso-occlusive disorders.

Acquired hypercoagulable states, those secondary to underlying conditions (e.g., the thrombotic tendency in cancer patients and acute disseminated intravascular coagulation [DIC] associated with sepsis, are far more common than hereditary forms. The manifestations of hypercoagulability are frequently significant diagnostic or management problems, contributing to morbidity and mortality in these patients. Many clinical tests are available for diagnosing the presence of a thrombotic process, such as arteriography and venography. These tests establish that a thrombotic event has taken place so that appropriate treatment may be instituted; however, with the exception of tests used to establish the diagnosis of DIC, laboratory testing is yet to be accepted as a useful diagnostic modality in most of these acquired conditions.

Atherosclerotic cardiovascular disease is one of the two major contributors to death and disability in our society today. Hemostatic factors are postulated to play a role in its development. Although hereditary factors clearly play a role in the development of atherosclerotic vascular disease, its etiology at the molecular level is still poorly understood. Environmental factors such as diet and exercise also play a role. Therefore, this disease consists of both hereditary and acquired features.

Hereditary hypercoagulable states, excluding atherosclerosis, are relatively uncommon. The study of these disorders has led to a marked expansion of our knowledge of the control mechanisms in coagulation and fibrinolysis. Most of the disorders that have been identified are abnormalities of proteins that function to limit the extent of thrombus formation, acting as either inhibitors of the coagulation proteins or stimulators of the fibrinolytic mechanism. Examples of hereditary disorders are antithrombin III deficiency and protein C deficiency. Another class of these disorders, the dysfibrinogenemias, is characterized by increased resistance of fibrin to fibrinolysis.

In those few patients in whom a hereditary abnormality predisposing to thrombosis is suspected, laboratory tests are of diagnostic value. There are a growing number of laboratory tests that can be used to monitor an ongoing, acquired coagulation/thrombotic process. However, the clinical utility of these tests is not yet generally accepted, and in most instances they have not been sufficiently evaluated in prospective, controlled, clinical trials.

This chapter first describes the physiological processes that lead to acquired or hereditary hypercoagulable states, then discusses the currently available tests for diagnosis and the available treatments.

CHARACTERISTICS OF THROMBI

Thrombi are masses formed within the vascular system of the living person. They are composed of varying combinations of the formed elements of blood held together with fibrin; platelets frequently play an important pathogenetic role in thrombosis. In contrast, the term *clots* means an extravascular event, postmortem or in the test tube, involving activation of the coagulation sequence.

For a rational approach to the diagnosis and treatment of thrombi, an understanding of their characteristics is helpful if not essential. The composition of a thrombus varies depending on whether it forms in the arterial system or in the venous system. Each reflects a somewhat different pathogenetic mechanism. Arterial thrombi tend to be composed of platelet–fibrin complexes (Fig. 11-1, *B*). Venous thrombi are more likely to contain all of the formed elements of the blood (Fig. 11-1, *A*). Vascular damage

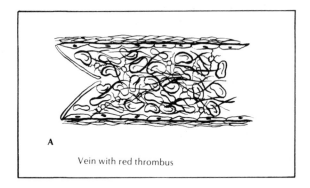

A

Vein with red thrombus

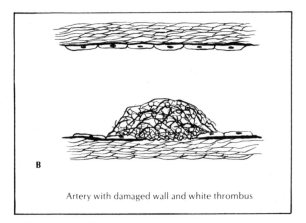

B

Artery with damaged wall and white thrombus

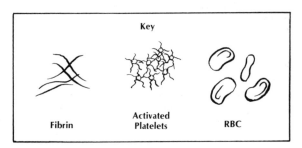

Key

Fibrin

Activated Platelets

RBC

FIG. 11-1. Characteristics of thrombi.

appears to be the critical factor in initiation of arterial thrombus formation, while stasis is usually the most important factor in venous thrombus formation.

Conditions that cause hypercoagulability enhance the tendency to form thrombi, but thrombi may also occur in the absence of an obvious predisposing cause in persons who have hereditary abnormalities causing hypercoagulability.

Venous Thrombi

The venous system is a relatively low-pressure system compared to the arterial system. When a person is upright, venous return from the legs is assisted by regular muscular contraction and relaxation, "pushing" blood back toward the heart. A system of valves in the deep veins of the legs prevents backflow. Stasis in the veins of the legs predisposes to venous thrombosis. Conditions in which this occurs include confinement to bed, immobilization or paralysis, compression of the veins by enlarged lymph nodes, or damage to the valves. Although stasis is clearly a contributing factor to venous thrombosis, the exact initiating factor is unclear. Most postulates suggest an activation of the coagulation process in venous valvular pockets, which are areas of possible turbulence and relative stasis. Activated coagulation factors or small platelet clumps have the potential for initiating the thrombotic process in these areas. In contrast, in areas of normal flow, activated coagulation factors and clumped platelets are diluted or carried away prior to initiating thrombus formation. Once begun, the thrombi could propagate either "downstream," with layering of additional elements, or retrograde if complete occlusion of the vein occurs.

Venous thrombi contain all of the formed elements of blood, appearing red, similar to a clot that forms in a test tube. This thrombus is called a "red thrombus." Irregularities of distribution of cellular elements and fibrin do occur. Layers of fibrin and platelets are found in some regions, presumably having occurred prior to complete occlusion of the vein while active blood flow continued.

Damage to a relatively thin-walled vein from surgical trauma or inflammation can also be a major factor in venous thrombus formation. This process is initiated by adherence of platelets to a damaged vascular wall, an example being deep vein thrombosis in patients who have had hip surgery. The incidence of this problem is quite high, with surgical trauma to the veins during the procedure thought to be a major contributing factor.

Arterial Thrombi

The arterial circulation is a fast-flowing, high-pressure system compared to the venous system. In the absence of stenosis, injury to the vessel wall is the major contributing factor to the generation of thrombi in the arterial system. Platelets adhere to an area of injury, and, depending on the strength of the stimulus, fibrin forms, resulting in a pale platelet–fibrin thrombus that adheres to the wall. If blood flow continues, fresh supplies of platelets and coagulation factors arrive at the site, contributing to the continued growth of the thrombus on the wall of the blood vessel, creating a so-called *mural thrombus*. This is the typical "white thrombus" that is characteristic of arterial thrombi. The major example of this type of thrombus is what forms in a region of atherosclerotic damage to the arterial wall. If there is ballooning or outpouching of the wall (aneurysm) or stenotic (narrowed) areas, blood flow in the region may be reduced, resulting in local stasis. In these situations red cells may also be found in the thrombus.

If there is stenosis, an occlusive thrombus with an appearance similar to that of a venous thrombus may occur.

ACQUIRED HYPERCOAGULABLE STATES

Hypercoagulability secondary to an underlying disease state or clinical condition is the most common cause of deep vein thrombosis and pulmonary embolism. The following groupings of vaso-occlusive problems are somewhat arbitrary, based on the primary components responsible.

Vaso-occlusive problems can be related to abnormalities in the formed elements of blood (*i.e.,* platelets, red cells, or white cells).

Platelet Abnormalities Associated With Vaso-occlusion

The platelet count is frequently increased as a nonspecific response to many kinds of stress (*e.g.,* blood loss, surgery, trauma, and underlying malignancy [see Chap. 10]). Very high elevations are sometimes seen for a period of time after splenectomy. Much concern has been expressed over the years that these increases, particularly when the count gets to a million or more per cubic millimeter, are associated with an increased risk of thrombosis. However, the reports appear to be largely anecdotal, with only a slightly increased risk at most.

In myeloproliferative disorders with high platelet counts, there is a poor correlation between the height of the platelet count and thrombotic risk.[6,84] Patients with comparable degrees of reactive thrombocytosis do not appear to be at increased risk of thrombotic events.[84,104] Paradoxically, there may be a bleeding tendency in myeloproliferative disorders, even with normal or elevated platelet counts. The tendency to bleed is generally attributed to acquired platelet function defects. Yet some patients with high platelet counts are clearly symptomatic, with microvascular ischemia. Burning and pain in the digits or symptoms of cerebral ischemia may be prominent complaints and may be relieved with aspirin therapy.[27,80,104] In the myeloproliferative disorder idiopathic (essential) thrombocythemia, young patients with the disorder, with some exceptions, are frequently asymptomatic, in contrast to elderly patients, who are more likely to have thrombotic episodes.[27] It is postulated that the major difference is underlying vascular disease in the latter group in combination with the high platelet count causing a thrombotic tendency.

In polycythemia vera, a myeloproliferative disorder characterized by a high hematocrit and platelet count and frequently associated with a thrombotic tendency, there is a poor correlation between the increased platelet count and thrombosis.

Increased sensitivity of platelets to agonists *in vitro* ("hyperaggregability") has been reported in association with a number of conditions such as smoking, diabetes mellitus, hyperlipidemia, and atherosclerotic vascular disease (see Chap. 10). In addition, circulating platelet aggregates as defined by *in vitro* testing have been found in a number of disorders associated with thromboembolic phenomena including microvascular thrombosis. Current questions relative to the interpretation of these tests revolve around whether these *in vitro* results reflect an *in vivo* phenomenon and, if they do, whether they represent cause or effect. The primary underlying factor may be the formation of the aggregates on the walls of damaged blood vessels with subsequent embolization.

Platelets may play an important pathogenetic role in thrombotic thrombocytopenic purpura (TTP) and related disorders, a poorly understood group of disorders in which platelet–fibrin thrombi are found in small blood vessels. Recent evidence suggests that abnormally high molecular weight multimers of von Willebrand factor causing platelet aggregation may be etiologically related to thrombosis in some cases of TTP,[53,71] but not all.[58] Why these thrombi have a predilection for certain target organs is still unexplained. In the hemolytic–uremic syndrome, a disorder very similar to TTP but occurring primarily in children, kidney involvement associated with renal failure is the more prominent feature. In TTP central nervous system involvement is more prominent.

Thrombocytopenia has frequently been reported in patients on heparin therapy (see Chap. 10).[2,8,17,52] It is manifested in a number of different ways: (1) acute onset, reversible thrombocytopenia occurring after an intravenous injection; (2) delayed onset, transient thrombocytopenia with the platelet count returning to normal even though heparin therapy is continued; (3) delayed onset, persistent thrombocytopenia with the platelet count remaining low until the heparin is discontinued; and (4) delayed onset, thrombocytopenia associated with recurrent venous thrombosis or arterial thrombosis. The exact cause of heparin-related thrombocytopenia is unknown. Some investigators have reported a factor in the IgG or IgM fraction of plasma that appears to be associated with the phenomenon.[2,17,82] In addition, the platelet agglutinating activity is more associated with the high-molecular-weight heparin fractions.[81] It has sometimes been associated with particular lots of heparin.[94] Regardless of the mechanism, it is clear that heparin causes thrombotic problems (usually arterial) in some patients. The exact incidence of this complication is unknown, most reports being anecdotal. No such events were reported in a prospective study of 1500 patients.[52]

Red Cell Abnormalities Associated With Vaso-occlusion

Increases in the red cell mass are seen in conditions associated with hypoxia, such as cyanotic cogenital heart disease and chronic lung diseases, and also as part of the myeloproliferative disorder polycythemia vera.

In polycythemia vera, thrombotic episodes are a significant management problem in some patients. Although controlling the disease with treatment decreases the thrombotic tendency, there is a poor correlation of the thrombotic tendency with the hematocrit and platelet count at the time of initial diagnosis. There is a better correlation with advanced age at diagnosis or with a history of previous thrombotic events. Other risk factors for thrombosis in these patients may be equally important.[84]

In most patients with cyanotic congenital heart disease, the risk of thrombosis is not significantly increased under most circumstances; however, these patients can be particularly susceptible if they become dehydrated.

White Cell Abnormalities Associated With Vaso-occlusion

White cells, aside from their role in inflammatory processes involving blood vessels, have been shown to participate in vaso-occlusive/ischemic problems through two mechanisms. In leukemia patients with very high white counts (greater than 100,000), leukocytes can apparently aggregate or become enclosed in a fibrin mesh, obstructing the microvasculature in vital organs such as the brain. This appears to be more common in myeloid leukemias, particularly myeloblastic, and has been partly attributed to the relative rigidity of myeloid precursors compared to other cells.

A somewhat unique group of patients that may or may not be related to myeloproliferative disorders is those with the Budd-Chiari syndrome, which is hepatic vein thrombosis. A high percentage of cases occur in patients with polycythemia vera, but the majority are idiopathic. In one group of young women with this syndrome, *in vitro* erythroid colony growth characteristics were those of a myeloproliferative disorder, even though peripheral blood changes were not characteristic.[97]

Another mechanism that may play a role in some diseases is granulocyte aggregation mediated by complement via complement receptors on the granulocyte membrane.[47] Complement can become activated on artificial surfaces such as in renal dialysis and cardiopulmonary bypass machines. Granulocyte aggregation then occurs, with the aggregates becoming lodged in the microcirculation. In the case of renal dialysis, the aggregates become lodged in the pulmonary circulation and are associated with a marked fall in the neutrophil count. Fortunately, this does not appear to cause any permanent pulmonary difficulty in these patients.

There is some evidence that complement-mediated leukostasis in the vascular bed of the lung may play a role in the adult respiratory distress syndrome, a form of pulmonary failure associated with shock from many different causes, such as trauma.

An additional relationship between leukocytes and thrombotic problems is the DIC syndrome associated with some acute leukemias, particularly acute promyelocytic leukemia. In most leukemias this is attributed to cell breakdown products activating the coagulation mechanism. The high incidence associated with acute promyelocytic leukemia has been attributed to procoagulant activity in the unique cytoplasmic granules that are characteristic of this type of leukemia.

Other Proteins and Thrombosis – Hyperviscosity

Hyperviscosity due to abnormal plasma proteins can lead to ischemic symptoms or thrombosis in small blood vessels. These proteins are usually immunoglobulins that may be present in abnormal amounts or have cryoprotein properties. Cryoproteins that cause clinical problems are those that tend to precipitate at temperatures lower than 37°C. This occurs in certain regions of the body, such as the fingers, toes, and earlobes and the tip of the nose. Examples are the monoclonal immunoglobulins (single idiotype) that can occur with Waldenström's macroglobulenemia (IgM) and other malignant lymphoproliferative disorders (IgA and certain IgG subclasses). Monoclonal proteins may or may not have cryoproperties. In addition, there is a group of disorders characterized by polyclonal increases of immunoglobulins with cryoproperties. When found, these disorders are frequently associated wth underlying disease, but some are idiopathic. Cryofibrinogens also occur and can be the cause of vaso-occlusive problems.

Hypercoagulability Secondary to Underlying Diseases

Underlying diseases or altered physiological states are by far the most common causes of a thrombotic tendency. Some examples are

Malignancy
Postoperative state
Nephrotic syndrome
Pregnancy
Hormonal therapy (birth control pills)?

Lupus anticoagulant
DIC
Atherosclerotic cardiovascular disease
Prosthetic heart valves and vascular grafts
Myeloproliferative disorders
Inhibitors of hemostatic factors
Hyperviscosity syndromes
Obesity
Homocystinuria
Paroxysmal nocturnal hemoglobinuria
Diabetes mellitus
Congestive heart failure

There is no one underlying pathophysiologic mechanism that is responsible. With the exception of the tests for the lupus anticoagulant, there is no single test or battery of tests that is currently accepted as being predictive. Thrombotic episodes in these disorders may be the initial presenting manifestation. In the absence of an obvious predisposing cause, when a patient presents with a thrombotic problem, the possibility of these disorders should be considered; diagnosis depends primarily on a careful history and physical examination followed by appropriate clinical and laboratory testing. A discussion of several of these conditions, illustrating the pathophysiology of thrombosis, follows.

Malignancy

The major example of hypercoagulability secondary to underlying disease is the patient with underlying cancer presenting with deep vein thrombosis. Cell breakdown with the "release" of tissue thromboplastin stimulating the coagulation system results in thrombosis and is one end of the spectrum of hypercoagulability, with DIC at the other end. Another mechanism that may contribute to thrombotic problems in cancer patients is physical impingement of the tumor masses on venous drainage or direct invasion of blood vessels.

Postoperative State

In certain surgical patients, actual physical damage to veins with resultant inflammation or thrombosis is a factor in thrombus formation. Postoperative bedrest and decreased mobility of the patient due to the procedure are additional contributory factors. A major example, orthopaedic surgery of the hip region, in which deep vein thrombosis is a significant, well-recognized complication, has already been discussed.

Nephrotic Syndrome

Diseases affecting the control mechanisms of coagulation are an additional mechanism by which thrombosis occurs. One example is the nephrotic syndrome. This is a group of diseases characterized by marked protein loss in the urine associated with an increased risk of thrombosis, particularly of the renal vein. Some of these patients have been demonstrated by loss of the protein in the urine to have an acquired antithrombin III deficiency.[51] A recent study reports a decrease in protein S levels in the patient with nephrotic syndrome.[23] A study of protein C in patients with the nephrotic syndrome demonstrated normal plasma activity even though the protein was being lost in the urine.[92]

Pregnancy and Hormonal Therapy

There are many changes that take place in the coagulation and fibrinolytic proteins in pregnancy in addition to the actual physical effects of pregnancy itself. As pregnancy progresses, most coagulation factors increase, accompanied by a decrease in fibrinolytic activity. These changes appear to be hormonally related. The physical mass of the uterus is also thought to interfere with venous return from the lower part of the body. In spite of these factors, the increased incidence of thromboembolic phenomena associated with pregnancy is largely in the postpartum period and may be related to the physical trauma of delivery. Recently, protein S levels have been reported to be significantly reduced during pregnancy and the postpartum period.[22] What role this may play in the thrombotic tendency is yet to be determined.

Likewise, the data relating to an increased risk of venous and arterial thromboembolic phenomena in women using hormonal birth control agents are to some degree conflicting. Increases in a number of coagulation factors and decreases in antithrombin III have been described in women on birth control pills and have been ascribed to the estrogen content of the pills. Some studies have found that the increased risk of thrombosis is primarily in smokers. Risk of cerebral arterial thrombosis and stroke has been reported to occur primarily in women with migraine. Overall, there appears to be some increased risk of thrombosis in women on birth control pills, but the magnitude of the risk and its interaction with other independent variables is uncertain. Most birth control pills currently in use have a lower estrogen content than did the earlier agents.

Lupus Anticoagulant

The lupus anticoagulant is primarily an *in vitro* phenomenon. It is usually discovered as an unexplained prolongation of the activated partial thromboplastin time in a patient without bleeding symptoms (see Chap. 4). A slight prolongation of the prothrombin time may be associated with it. It occurs in patients with systemic lupus erythematosus and in drug-induced lupus syndromes.[11,87] It also occurs in other so-called *collagen vascular diseases* ("autoimmune") and in persons with no apparent disease. Following are some of the disorders with which it has been associated:

Systemic lupus erythematosus (SLE)
Drug-induced lupus syndromes
   Chlorpromazine
   Hydralazine
   Procainamide
   Quinidine
Unspecified autoimmune diseases
Neoplasia, including myeloproliferative disorders

Lupus inhibitors have been characterized as being either IgM or IgG with specificity for a cardiolipinlike phospholipid. In the usual test systems they appear to react with the phospholipid used as a platelet substitute. Not all products are equally sensitive to the effects of the lupus inhibitor. Some appear to be relatively insensitive, depending on the character of the individual phospholipid substitutes.[87] The laboratory characteristics are described in Chapter 4.

Clinical bleeding is usually not associated with the presence of the lupus anticoagulant. However, some patients with prothrombin deficiency in conjunction with the inhibitor have a prolonged prothrombin time and a bleeding tendency.

Another potential cause of bleeding in patients with lupus erythematosus is autoimmune thrombocytopenia. Therefore, when bleeding does occur in these patients with the lupus anticoagulant, other abnormalities of hemostasis should be considered.

Paradoxically, the presence of the lupus anticoagulant has been associated with a thrombotic tendency.[10,30,34,72,83] This appears to be particularly true in those patients who also have biologically false-positive VDRL results. The VDRL (Venereal Disease Research Laboratories) is one of the classic serologic tests for syphilis (STSs) based on a reagent extracted from beef heart (cardiolipin). Biologically false-positive results can occur, meaning a positive VDRL result in the absence of syphilis. The most widely used STS, the RPR (rapid plasma reagin), is said to be less sensitive than the VDRL in detecting those at risk for thrombosis. Testing for the presence of a specific anticardiolipin antibody is now available and, according to some studies, is highly predictive for the subgroup at risk for a thrombotic tendency.[41]

An additional problem that has been identified in women with the lupus anticoagulant is repeated spontaneous abortions.[12,16,31,32,59] The cause of fetal death has generally been assumed to be placental infarction.

Several mechanisms for the thrombotic tendencies in lupus patients have been postulated:

- Inhibition of prostacyclin (PGI_2) production by vascular endothelial cells[16]
- Inhibition of vascular plasminogen activator release, either directly or indirectly[31]
- Associated inhibition of contact factors, causing decreased fibrinolytic activity[83]

Recent reports suggest that anticoagulation can prevent thrombosis in symptomatic patients.[30,72] Therapy with corticosteroids and aspirin has helped some women with the lupus anticoagulant carry their pregnancies to term.[12]

Inhibitors of Hemostatic Factors

A thrombotic tendency has been reported in association with an inhibitor of contact factors in a patient with discoid lupus erythematosus.[1] This report was made prior to the characterization of the lupus anticoagulant and recognition of its association with thrombosis and is therefore difficult to evaluate. In one report, an inhibitor of Factors XI and XII in a patient with SLE was associated with in vitro spontaneous platelet aggregation.[24] However, this patient did not have clinical problems with thrombosis.

There are rare reports of thrombosis secondary to inhibitors of fibrinolysis.[43,73,75] These reports are also relatively old and difficult to evaluate in light of current knowledge. There is a recent report of increased levels of a plasma inhibitor of tissue plasminogen activator in young persons who have survived myocardial infarctions.[38] The pathophysiologic significance of this is not clear.

Disseminated Intravascular Coagulation

DIC has already been discussed in Chapter 6 and under the topic of thrombosis secondary to malignancy. Although commonly thought of as a bleeding problem, stimulation of the coagulation system is generally considered to be the underlying pathophysiologic mechanism, and thrombosis is sometimes the major clinical manifestation. Thrombosis in DIC may be manifested in a number of different ways: deep vein thrombosis, thrombosis of the microcirculation of a vital organ, such as the kidney with renal failure, or as the purpura fulminans syndrome, in which there is hemorrhagic necrosis of areas of the skin and ischemic necrosis of the extremities due to vaso-occlusive phenomena.

Atherosclerosis

Atherosclerotic vascular disease and its complications is the most common contributor to morbidity and mortality in the United States. The role of hemostatic components in the genesis of atherosclerotic lesions is not yet clear and is currently the object of much study. One theory of the pathogenesis implicates platelet factors, in particular platelet-derived growth factor (PDGF), in the development of atherosclerosis by means of stimulation of smooth muscle proliferation in damaged vessel walls to which platelets have become adherent. A discussion of the relationship of hemostatic components to the etiology of atherosclerosis is beyond the scope of this text. The interested reader is referred to recent reviews of the subject, listed under Suggested Reading.

Regardless of the relationship of the hemostatic components to the etiology of atherosclerosis, thrombotic narrowing or occlusion superimposed on atherosclerotic vascular lesions clearly contributes to the complications. One of the major therapeutic thrusts in medicine today is the prevention of arterial thrombosis in high-risk patients, primarily through the use of platelet-inhibiting drugs, and lysis of thrombi with fibrinolytic agents once they have formed. Most studies have been in the area of coronary artery thrombosis and atherosclerotic cerebrovascular disease. The role of thrombosis in myocardial infarction had been a source of disagreement for many years. One of the old euphemisms for myocardial infarction was "coronary thrombosis." Yet, in some autopsy studies of patients dying after myocardial infarction, most were found to have severe coronary atherosclerosis, but many did not have a thrombosis. Some authors have postulated that in those who did have thrombi, the thrombi occurred after the infarction. Ultimately, when coronary arteriography became available and was used to study patients with acute myocardial infarction, it was discovered that 80% or more of patients with acute transmural myocardial infarctions had an occlusion if they were studied within 6 hours after the onset of symptoms. The percentage with occlusions decreased with an increasing interval between the onset of symptoms and the time of study. This was presumed to be due to spontaneous lysis of thrombi that had been present or relief of coronary artery spasm. It is now generally accepted that thrombosis is etiologically related to transmural myocardial infarction.[28,61,74]

Prosthetic Heart Valves and Vascular Grafts

Prosthetic devices made of artificial materials are used in the treatment of vascular disease when the natural tissues fail. Examples would be artificial heart valves and replacement grafts for major blood vessels with severe atherosclerotic disease. Although, relatively nonthrombogenic materials have been developed for these prostheses, the potential for forming thrombi is still present. In the case of heart valves, there is a particular potential for thrombi to be catastrophic; once formed, they can embolize to vital organs such as the brain and kidneys. These thrombi usually have the characteristics of arterial thrombi. When they form on artificial valve components, they usually have the appearance of pale, friable, fibrinous excrescences that are referred to as "vegetations."

HEREDITARY DISORDERS ASSOCIATED WITH THROMBOSIS

Hereditary disorders known to be associated with an increased tendency for thrombosis are disorders of

Protein S
Protein C
Antithrombin III
Plasminogen
Fibrinogen
Tissue plasminogen activator
Contact factors

In one recent study it was estimated that abnormalities of these proteins are causally related to thrombosis in approximately 20% of patients under the age of 45 who have repeated thromboses or have a family history suggesting a thrombotic tendency.[33] The defects are usually in proteins related to the control mechanisms of coagulation and fibrinolysis. The defect may be either a deficiency of one of these proteins or a structurally abnormal protein (dysprotein). If it is a dysprotein, it may not function properly even though it is present in a normal amount.

It is apparent that only a portion of the currently known factors that play a role in control mechanisms is listed above. It is likely that abnormalities of the other known factors or of control mechanisms not yet discovered will contribute to this list in years to come.

Protein C

Protein C is a vitamin K–dependent protein that has two known functions: inactivation of activated Factor V and activated Factor VIII and inactivation of a plasma inhibitor of tissue plasminogen activator (tPA), thus enhancing tPA release and activity.

In general, patients who have been symptomatic are heterozygotes with approximately half of normal amounts of protein C. Dysprotein C has also been described.[13,26,51] The deficiency is usually manifested as venous thrombosis, with half or more of the carriers being symptomatic.[13,36,37] Homozygous forms of the deficiency have been reported, usually presenting as catastrophic thrombotic problems in the newborn period, including neonatal *purpura fulminans*.[36,62,86,90] The fatality rate in these infants has been high. For reasons that are not clear, relatives of these unfortunate babies who are heterozygous for the deficiency have usually been asymptomatic, in contrast to the previous group of heterozygotes for protein C deficiency. Studies of protein C in normal newborns have demonstrated that it is low compared to adult values, as are other vitamin K–dependent factors.[49]

A rare syndrome that has been recognized for years but not understood until recently is the *purpura fulminans* syndrome, occurring in persons receiving coumarin anticoagulant therapy. In these persons, skin necrosis is the major manifestation, with a predilection for breast involvement in women. Many of these persons have now been demonstrated to be heterozygotes for protein C deficiency.[14,36,67] When they are anticoagulated, protein C, with a relatively short half-life, falls to even lower levels before the vitamin K–dependent coagulation factors reach therapeutic levels; thus, there is the apparent paradox of someone on anticoagulant therapy suffering from thrombotic problems.

Protein S

Protein S, also a vitamin K–dependent factor, is a cofactor for activated protein C (pC_a). Its function appears to be the binding of protein C to lipid membranes.[101] In the absence of protein S, pC_a is relatively ineffective as an inactivator of V_a and VIII_a. After its characterization, it was predicted that a deficiency of this protein would cause thrombotic problems. Shortly thereafter, the families with this disorder were described. The trait was autosomal in inheritance, with reportedly half or more of the heterozygotes having symptomatic thrombotic problems.[9,19-21,56,84] Of the known hereditary disorders causing thromboembolic phenomena, it is currently estimated that protein S abnormalities are among the most frequent, along with protein C abnormalities.[33]

Over half of the protein S circulates in a complex with C4b-binding protein and is not readily available to act as a cofactor for protein C. Therefore, patients who have symptomatic deficiencies of protein S may appear to have only slightly reduced amounts if total protein S is measured by immunologic methods. However, in these patients there may be little free protein S available.[9,19] Methods for testing for protein S deficiency have recently been developed. Of the immunologic methods, crossed immunoelectrophoresis is most helpful, allowing distinction between the free and bound fractions.[19]

Recent studies have shown that protein S has a relatively long half-life.[25] Therefore, it is predicted that the *purpura fulminans* syndrome is not likely to occur when these patients are anticoagulated, in contrast to protein C–deficient patients.

Antithrombin III

Antithrombin III (ATIII) was the first inherited plasma protein deficiency described that was associated with a thromboembolic tendency. It is an autosomal trait, in which the heterozygotes have approximately half the normal amount of protein and are at risk of thromboembolism. Although most of the cases reported have had deficiencies of the protein, some families with dysproteins have been described.

Plasminogen

Plasminogen is normally found in two forms: (1) free in the circulation and (2) incorporated in thrombi bound to fibrin. Under physiologic conditions, when circulating plasminogen is activated, it becomes rapidly inactivated by a circulating inhibitor, α-2-antiplasmin, thus preventing fibrinogenolysis. Bound plasminogen is protected from this inhibitor (see Chap. 2 for more detail), thereby allowing relatively specific fibrinolysis in regions of thrombus formation and limiting the extent of the process. Vessel wall tPA appears to be the major activator of fibrin-bound plasminogen. tPA also binds to fibrin through relatively specific binding sites.

Some families with a hereditary deficiency of plasminogen associated with a thrombotic tendency have been described.[60] It appears to be inherited as an autosomal trait. Additional families with dysplasminogens have been reported.[3,4,103]

Abnormal Fibrinogens

Most reported persons with dysfibrinogens have had a bleeding tendency or have been asymptomatic. A few in whom the dysfibrinogen is associated with a thrombotic tendency have been described. In these patients the fibrin multimers have been reported to be resistant to fibrinolysis.[7] The presence of a dysfibrinogen is frequently suspected in the presence of a prolonged thrombin time with no other identifiable causes. The confirmation of a dysprotein can be inferred by a discrepancy between functional assays and amounts measured by immunologic or protein precipitation methods.

Tissue Plasminogen Activator

A number of reports have described decreased release of tPA from the vessel wall associated with thromboembolic phenomena.[3,5,43,93] The physiology of tPA has been mentioned under the discussions of protein C and plasminogen. To review, tPA has a high specificity for activation of fibrin-bound plasminogen. Its release from the vascular wall is enhanced by pC_a, the latter inhibiting a plasma inactivator of tPA. Whether these deficiencies represent decreased production or decreased release is not always clear, but both mechanisms have been reported.

Factor XII and Other Contact Factors

Mr. Hageman, who was the index case of Factor XII deficiency, died in his early fifties of a massive pulmonary embolus. At the time of autopsy, he was reported to have atherosclerotic coronary artery disease but very mild aortic atherosclerosis.[78] Other patients with deficiencies of Factor XII who have had thromboembolic phenomena have been described.[35,45,68] This has led to speculation that persons who are heterozygous or homozygous for deficiencies of the contact factors may be at increased risk for thromboembolic events related to decreased activation of the fibrinolytic system. This is yet to be proven.

Platelets

At present there are no known thrombotic problems related to inherited disorders of platelets.

TESTING FOR HYPERCOAGULABILITY

To reiterate, the most common causes of "hypercoagulability" and thromboembolic phenomena are underlying diseases. A careful history and physical examination followed by appropriate clinical and laboratory testing are still the first line of approach. In a young patient with multiple episodes of thromboembolic phenomena or with a positive family history of these problems, testing for a deficiency is probably indicated. The best time to test for a deficiency is when the patient is at a baseline state; testing during an active thrombotic episode when factors are being consumed or while on anticoagulant therapy is clearly not optimal. For protein C determinations, a method has been devised for testing while the patient is on anticoagulant therapy by relating the levels to the other vitamin K–dependent factors and calculating the ratio.[26] In most situations testing first-degree relatives is probably the best first step if the patient is having an active thrombotic process or is on anticoagulant therapy. However, one has to realize that with the current level of technology, testing is time consuming, expensive, and frequently unrewarding.

Specific tests for the various proteins are discussed in detail in Chapter 12. In general, if one is going to perform one test, a functional assay is preferable so that dysproteins as well as decreased protein amounts can be detected. Ideally, both a protein quantitation test and a functional assay should be performed.

Testing for acquired hypercoagulable states is an area of active research. Molecular markers indicating that an active "clotting" process is taking place fall into two categories: (1) peptides released from coagulation proteins, discussed in Chapter 12, and (2) markers of the platelet release reaction, discussed in Chapters 9 and 12. The role that they may play in patient management decisions is still evolving. Currently, they have not replaced clinical and routine laboratory tests in the diagnosis and management of acquired thrombotic problems.

Platelet Tests in Arterial Thrombosis

Tests of platelet function that have been used in the study of arterial thrombosis are described in detail in Chapter 9. In general, there are two categories of testing: tests of intact platelets in *in vitro* systems and assays of molecular markers of the platelet release reaction performed on venous specimens or as a supplement to *in vitro* testing.

Platelet Aggregometry and Platelet Retention

Platelet aggregometry, originally used to define disorders of decreased platelet function, has been used with various modifications to test for hyperreactivity of platelets. Spontaneous aggregation of platelet-rich plasma (PRP) in the absence of aggregating agents is one type of test. Another approach is to use lower concentrations of the agonists than are normally used, testing for the threshold response compared to normal (*i.e.*, to see whether the test platelets will react at a lower concentration of agonists than normal platelets). A hypothetical example is shown in Figure 11-2. Details of these methods are described in Chapter 9.

These tests have generally not been accepted for routine patient testing, and they

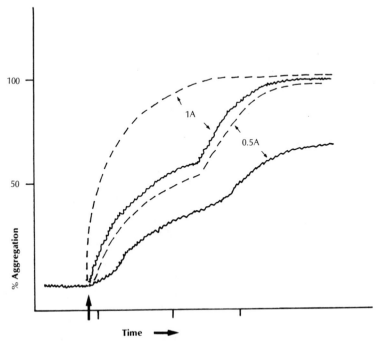

FIG. 11-2. Platelet aggregation curves of normal versus hyperaggregation states.

are currently being used primarily for research. The major unanswered questions, aside from disagreements over technical factors, are whether these measures of "hypercoagulability" reflect an *in vivo* phenomenon, and, if they do, is the phenomenon a cause or an effect of the underlying disease? Regardless of whether these tests are measuring a primary or secondary phenomenon, it is hoped that they will help to identify subgroups that may benefit from various types of therapeutic intervention.

Molecular Markers of the Platelet Release Reaction

As discussed in Chapter 8, many chemical mediators (*e.g.*, platelet factor 4 and β-thromboglobulin) are either involved in the platelet release reaction or are discharged during the reaction. These can be measured on carefully drawn venous specimens or on supernatant from *in vitro* testing. The details of these tests are discussed in Chapters 9 and 12.

Assays of these factors have been used for the study of both arterial and venous thrombosis. The use of these tests is still somewhat in its infancy, and they are being used primarily for research at present. As in the study of platelet hyperaggregability, the question of whether the abnormalities found are a cause or an effect of the underlying disease is still unresolved. The hope still remains, as with other tests of platelet function, that they will help identify high-risk subgroups of patients who would benefit from therapeutic intervention to prevent thrombotic problems.

TREATMENT

Several aspects must be considered when treating thrombotic problems:

- Treatment of thrombi that have already formed, be they arterial or venous
- Prevention and treatment of pulmonary embolism
- Prevention of thrombosis in patients who are identified as being at high risk

Medical Treatment of Deep Vein Thrombosis and Pulmonary Embolism

There are two basic approaches to the medical treatment of deep vein thrombosis and pulmonary embolism:

- Anticoagulation therapy, which prevents the extension or embolism of thrombi that have already formed or the formation of new thrombi
- Fibrinolytic therapy for purposes of lysing thrombi already formed

Anticoagulation has been the historic mainstay of treating deep vein thrombosis and pulmonary embolism. Therapy is initiated with heparin to obtain an immediate anticoagulant effect. Coumarin drug therapy is subsequently begun, with some overlap to allow the vitamin K–dependent coagulation factors to reach therapeutic levels before the heparin is stopped. In clinical studies the major effect of anticoagulation therapy in patients with deep vein thrombosis has been prevention of the potentially lethal complication of pulmonary embolism. Therapy with coumarin is usually continued for 3 to 6 months in patients in whom there are no hereditary deficiencies predisposing to thromboembolism. With our current state of knowledge, patients who have had one of the hereditary deficiencies identified, such as protein C deficiency, and who have had thromboembolic episodes may need to be anticoagulated for the remainder of their lives. However, long-term anticoagulation therapy also has its risks.

The goal of fibrinolytic therapy is lysis of thrombi or emboli. Several different substances have been used, some of which are endogenous to the body and one other that is exogenous. Some agents are intrinsically fibrinolytic, whereas other agents activate endogenous fibrinolytic activity.

Streptokinase, derived from streptococcal organisms, activates plasminogen in a two-step reaction: first, it complexes with circulating plasminogen, then the streptokinase–plasminogen complex "activates" plasminogen, forming plasmin, the active enzyme. Both fibrin and fibrinogen are subsequently cleaved indiscriminately. Therefore, not only are thrombi dissolved, but there is significant systemic fibrinogenolysis. An additional complication of fibrinolytic therapy, regardless of the agent used, is that the ensuing fibrinolysis does not discriminate between pathologic thrombi (*e.g.*, a pulmonary embolus) and those formed as part of normal hemostasis, such as in a recent surgical wound or needle puncture. One of the disadvantages of streptokinase is that it is a foreign protein to which some people may already be sensitized. For such people it is potentially ineffective and may cause an allergic reaction.

Urokinase is an enzyme of human origin normally found in urine. Preparations available for therapy are extracted from urine or from fetal kidney cell cultures. It is a direct activator of plasminogen to plasmin. Because of its human source, immunity or sensitivity to a foreign protein is not a problem, but it is much more expensive than streptokinase.

A new agent, tPA, manufactured by recombinant DNA techniques is now in the phase of clinical trials.[76] The gene for synthesis of tPA has been isolated from a human melanoma cell line and fused with a bacterium, allowing for synthesis of relatively large amounts of tPA. The theoretical advantage of tPA is that it should specifically activate plasminogen associated with fibrin thrombi, with little effect on fibrinogen. However, in initial trials in patients with myocardial infarction, there has been some systemic fibrinogenolysis, although less than is seen with streptokinase. tPA and other agents are discussed later in this chapter.

In patients with deep vein thrombosis and/or pulmonary embolism, fibrinolytic therapy is most effective if instituted within 48 hours of the onset of symptoms but can be used after longer intervals. Current simplified protocols recommend a loading dose followed by a fixed rate of infusion. It is usually monitored with any of the usual coagulation tests (prothrombin time, activated partial thromboplastin time, or thrombin time) to be certain that a fibrinolytic state has been attained. No particular therapeutic range has been recommended with the simplified protocols. After cessation of fibrinolytic therapy, heparin therapy is begun after results of the selected test return to less than two times the mean normal range.

Fibrinolytic therapy has also been used for lysis of venous thrombi in areas of the body other than the deep veins of the legs.[40,79,89]

Surgical Treatment of Deep Vein Thrombosis and Pulmonary Embolism

In selected patients in whom anticoagulation has either failed or is contraindicated because of clinical bleeding, surgery can be the preferred mode of therapy. Surgical techniques can prevent emboli through the use of procedures that impede venous return from areas with thrombi or can be used to remove large thromboemboli from the pulmonary arterial circulation. However, the availability of fibrinolytic therapy in recent years may obviate the surgical approach in some patients.[70]

Medical Treatment of Arterial Thrombosis

Antiplatelet Drugs

Aspirin and dipyridamole are the two currently most widely used antiplatelet drugs for prevention of thrombosis in patients with cardiovascular disease, although other drugs have been tried. Aspirin blocks the synthesis of thromboxane A_2 (TxA_2) at the cyclooxygenase step (see Chap. 8). It does so by irreversibly acetylating the active site, rendering the platelet incapable of synthesizing TxA_2 for the remainder of its life span. Many of the nonsteroidal anti-inflammatory drugs also block this enzyme but do so in a reversible fashion. When treatment with these drugs is stopped, they are cleared, and TxA_2 is again synthesized. Dipyridamole is thought to affect the metabolism of cyclic AMP, potentiating the effect of PGI_2.

Prospective studies on the clinical efficacy of these drugs are still underway, with encouraging results reported in some groups of patients.[15,39,42,57] The principle behind the use of these drugs in the therapy of arterial disease is based on the perceived role of platelets both in the genesis of atherosclerosis and in the thrombotic complications of atherosclerotic vascular disease. In addition, vasoactive chemical mediators released from platelets might play a role in myocardial ischemia and infarction by causing vasospasm.

Unfortunately, many of the studies have been criticized for various design flaws.[29] Because of the nature of the problem, it will probably take many years for the prospective studies to be completed. At the current time, aspirin has been shown to reduce the occurrence of strokes in male patients with transient ischemic attacks and to reduce myocardial infarction and death in patients with unstable angina or with previous myocardial infarction. Other groups of patients may benefit, but the evidence is not conclusive. The addition of other drugs to the regimen is currently of unproven benefit.

One of the unsettled questions has been the appropriate dose of aspirin. Low doses of aspirin will inhibit the production of TxA_2 without permanently affecting the endothelial cell's ability to synthesize PGI_2. Higher doses of aspirin affect endothelial synthesis of PGI_2, raising the criticism that they may be counterproductive.[44,65,69,77,102] Clinical studies have not borne out this latter hypothesis, but there is a tendency to prefer lower-dose therapy.

Aspirin therapy also appears to be effective in the prevention of thrombosis in coronary artery bypass grafts. Aspirin and/or other antiplatelet drugs in combination with anticoagulation have been shown to be effective in preventing thromboembolic complications in patients with artificial replacement valves in the heart and preventing occlusion in vascular grafts or synthetic cannulas.[39,42] Some of the combinations of aspirin with other drugs are as yet unproven to be of any additional benefit over aspirin alone. In some groups of patients the combination of aspirin with anticoagulation has had an unacceptable risk of bleeding complications.

Fibrinolytic Therapy

The principles of fibrinolytic therapy have previously been discussed. Most of the reported work in fibrinolytic therapy of arterial disease has been in the treatment of acute myocardial infarction. The role of thrombosis in the etiology of transmural myocardial infarction is now generally accepted.[43] If patients with electrocardiographic findings of transmural myocardial infarction have streptokinase infused directly into the occluded coronary artery within 4 to 6 hours after the onset of symptoms, there appears to be benefit to the patient. This benefit is manifested as a decreased mortality rate and a suggestion in some studies of better myocardial function.[54,55] There is improved benefit when the interval between onset of symptoms and perfusion is shorter. The major disadvantage of this method is that it requires a relatively sophisticated medical facility with angiography facilities and a cardiac angiography team on call for immediate availability at all times. Not only is this method expensive, in more remote areas it is frequently not available. Another approach is the use of intravenous streptokinase, a procedure that has been studied in many medical centers. Some groups have had reported results comparable to those with intracoronary streptokinase infusion; others have found the results to be less satisfactory. However, because of different study designs, the findings are not always comparable.

The disadvantages of systemic fibrinogenolysis with streptokinase have already been discussed. Newer agents currently being evaluated have specificity for activation of fibrin-associated plasminogen. These include tPA, prourokinase, and acylated streptokinase–plasminogen complex.[18,48,50,63,64,66,88,91,95,96,98–100] tPA has already been discussed. Prourokinase, also known as single-chain urokinase, becomes activated in the presence of fibrin. Acylated streptokinase–plasminogen complex is inert but still capable of binding to fibrin. Deacylation then occurs spontaneously with subsequent plasminogen activation. Initial studies with these substances are being reported and evaluated. Although some degree of systemic fibrinogenolysis has occurred with these agents, it is generally less severe than with streptokinase. Of course, as with streptokinase, these activators do not distinguish between pathologic thrombi (*i.e.,* those causing obstruction of critical blood vessels) and normal hemostatic thrombi such as those at a site of a recent injury or invasive procedure. Therefore, these agents do not appear likely to have fewer associated bleeding problems. This has been borne out so far by most studies performed.

CONCLUSIONS

The concept of hypercoagulability is far from new. The study of abnormalities of the control mechanisms related to coagulation and fibrinolysis that may lead to hypercoagulability is an active area of investigation in which our knowledge is rapidly expanding. It is probable that many more hereditary abnormalities will be discovered in the known and yet-unknown factors that regulate these processes. Molecular markers of hemostasis and thrombosis show promise of allowing more intelligent diagnosis and management of both hereditary and acquired hypercoagulability in the near future.

REFERENCES

1. Aberg H, Nilsson IM: Recurrent thrombosis in a young woman with a circulating anticoagulant directed against factors XI and XII. Acta Med Scand 192:419, 1972
2. Ansell J, Deykin D: Heparin-induced thrombocytopenia and recurrent thromboembolism. Am J Hematol 8:325, 1980
3. Aoki N: Genetic abnormalities of the fibrinolytic system. Semin Thromb Hemost 10:42, 1984
4. Aoki N, Moroi M, Sakata Y et al: Abnormal plasminogen: A hereditary molecular abnormality found in a patient with recurrent thrombosis. J Clin Invest 61:1186, 1978

5. Bachmann F, Kruithof IEKO: Tissue plasminogen activator: Chemical and physiologic aspects. Semin Thromb Hemost 10:6, 1984
6. Barbui T, Cortelazzo S, Viero P et al: Thrombohaemorrhagic complications in 101 cases of myeloproliferative disorders: Relationship to platelet number and function. Eur J Cancer Clin Oncol 19:1593, 1983
7. Beck EA, Charache P, Jackson DP: A new inherited coagulation disorder caused by an abnormal fibrinogen ("fibrinogen Baltimore"). Nature 208:143, 1965
8. Bell WR, Tomasulo PA, Alving BM et al: Thrombocytopenia occurring during the administration of heparin. Ann Intern Med 85:155, 1976
9. Bertina RM: Hereditary protein S deficiency. Hemostasis 15:241, 1985
10. Bowie EJW, Thompson JH, Pascuzzi et al: Thrombosis in systemic lupus erythematosus despite circulating anticoagulants. J Lab Clin Med 62:416, 1963
11. Boxer M, Ellman L, Carvalho A: The lupus anticoagulant. Arthritis Rheum 19:1244, 1976
12. Branch DW, Scott JR, Kochenour NK et al: Obstetric complications associated with the lupus anticoagulant. N Engl J Med 313:1322, 1985
13. Broekman AW: Hereditary protein C deficiency. Hemostasis 15:233, 1985
14. Broekman AW, Bertman RM, Loeliger EA et al: Protein C and the development of skin necrosis during anticoagulant therapy. Thromb Haemost 49:251, 1983
15. Cairns JA, Gent M, Singer J et al: Aspirin, sulfinpyrazone, or both in unstable angina: Results of a Canadian multicenter trial. N Engl J Med 313:1369, 1985
16. Carreras LO, Machin SJ, Deman R et al: Arterial thrombosis, intrauterine death and "lupus" anticoagulant: Detection of immunoglobulin interfering with prostacyclin formation. Lancet 1:244, 1981
17. Cimo PL, Moake JL, Wenger RS et al: Heparin-induced thrombocytopenia: Association with a platelet aggregating factor and arterial thromboses. Am J Hematol 6:125, 1979
18. Collen D, Topal EJ, Tieffenbrunn AJ et al: Coronary thrombolysis with recombinant human tissue-type plasminogen activator: A prospective, randomized, placebo-controlled trial. Circulation 70:1012, 1984
19. Comp PC, Doray D, Patton D et al: An abnormal plasma distribution of protein S occurs in functional protein S deficiency. Blood 67:504, 1986
20. Comp PC, Esmon CT: Recurrent venous thromboembolism in patients with a partial deficiency of protein S. N Engl J Med 311:1525, 1984
21. Comp PC, Nixon RR, Cooper MR et al: Familial protein S deficiency is associated with recurrent thrombosis. J Clin Invest 74:2082, 1984
22. Comp PC, Thurnau GR, Welsh J et al: Functional and immunologic protein S levels are decreased during pregnancy. Blood 68:881, 1986
23. Comp PC, Vigino S, D'Angelo AD et al: Acquired protein S deficiency occurs in pregnancy, the nephrotic syndrome, and acute systemic lupus erythematosus (abstr). Blood 66(Supp 1):348a, 1985
24. Cronberg S, Nilsson IM: Circulating anticoagulant against Factor XI and XII together with massive spontaneous platelet aggregation. Scand J Haematol 10:309, 1973
25. D'Angelo A, Esman CT, Comp PC et al: The half-life of protein S is much longer than protein C (abstr). Blood 66(Suppl 1):349a, 1985
26. D'Angelo SV, Comp PC, Esmon CT et al: Relationship between protein C antigen and anticoagulant activity during oral anticoagulation and in selected disease states. J Clin Invest 77:416, 1986
27. Davis RB: Acute thrombotic complications of myeloproliferative disorders in young adults. Am J Clin Pathol 84:180, 1985
28. Dewood MA, Spores J, Hensley GR et al: Coronary arteriographic findings in acute transmural myocardial infarction. Circulation 68(Suppl 1):I-39, 1983
29. Eichner ER: Platelets, carotids and coronaries: Critique on antithrombotic role of antiplatelet agents, exercise and certain diets. Am J Med 77:513, 1984
30. Elias M, Eldor A: Thromboembolism in patients with the "lupus"-type circulating anticoagulant. Arch Intern Med 144:510, 1984

31. Feinstein D: Lupus anticoagulant, thrombosis and fetal loss. N Engl J Med 313:1348, 1985

32. Firkin BG, Howard MA, Radford N: Possible relationship between lupus inhibitor and recurrent abortion in young women. Lancet 2:366, 1980

33. Gladson CL, Griffin JH, Hach V et al: The incidence of protein C and protein S deficiency in 139 young thrombotic patients (abstr). Blood 66(Suppl 1):350a, 1985

34. Glueck HI, Kant KS, Weiss MA et al: Thrombosis in systemic lupus erythematosus: Relationship to the presence of circulating anticoagulants. Arch Intern Med 145:1389, 1985

35. Glueck HI, Roehill W Jr: Myocardial infarction in a patient with Hageman (factor XII) defect. Ann Intern Med 64:390, 1966

36. Griffin JH: Clinical studies of protein C. Semin Thromb Hemost 10:162, 1984

37. Griffin JH, Evatt B, Zimmerman S et al: Deficiency of protein C in congenital thrombotic disease. J Clin Invest 68:1370, 1981

38. Hamsten A, Wiman B, de Faire U, et al: Increased plasma levels of a rapid inhibitor of tissue plasminogen activator in young survivors of myocardial infarction. N Engl J Med 313:1557, 1985

39. Harker LA: Clinical trials evaluating platelet-modifying drugs in patients with atherosclerotic cardiovascular disease and thrombosis. Circulation 73:206, 1986

40. Harrington JT: Thrombolytic therapy in renal vein thrombosis. Arch Intern Med 144:33, 1984

41. Harris EN, Boey ML, Mackworth-Young CG, et al: Anticardiolipin antibodies: Detection by radioimmunoassay and association with thrombosis in systemic lupus erythematosus. Lancet 2:1211, 1983

42. Harter HR, Burch JW, Majerus PW et al: Prevention of thrombosis in patients on hemodialysis by low-dose aspirin. N Engl J Med 301:577, 1979

43. Health and Public Policy Committee, American College of Physicians: Thrombolysis for evolving myocardial infarction. Ann Intern Med 103:463, 1985

44. Hirsh J: The optimal dose of aspirin. Arch Intern Med 145:1582, 1985

45. Hoak JC, Swanson LW, Warner ED et al: Myocardial infarction associated with severe factor XII deficiency. Lancet 2:884, 1966

46. Isacson S, Nilsson IM: Defective fibrinolysis in blood and vein walls in recurrent "idiopathic" venous thrombosis. Acta Chir Scand 138:313, 1972

47. Jacob HS, Craddock PR, Hammerschmidt DE et al: Complement-induced granulocyte aggregation: An unsuspected mechanism of disease. N Engl J Med 302:789, 1980

48. Jaffe AS, Sobel BE: Thrombolysis with tissue-plasminogen activator in acute myocardial infarction: Potentials and pitfalls. JAMA 255:237, 1986

49. Karpatkin M, Mannucci PM, Bhogal M et al: Low protein C in the neonatal period. Br J Haematol 62:137, 1986

50. Kasper W, Erbel R, Meinertz T et al: Intracoronary thrombolysis with an acylated streptokinase–plasminogen activator (BRL 26921), in patients with acute myocardial infarction. J Am Coll Cardiol 4:357, 1984

51. Kauffman RH, Veltkamp JJ, Van Tilburg NH: Acquired antithrombin III deficiency and thrombosis in the nephrotic syndrome. Am J Med 65:607, 1978

52. Kelton JG, Levine MN: Heparin-induced thrombocytopenia. Semin Thromb Hemost 12:59, 1986

53. Kelton JG, Moore J, Santos A et al: Detection of a platelet-agglutinating factor in thrombotic thrombocytopenic purpura. Ann Intern Med 101:509, 1984

54. Kennedy JW, Ritchie JL, Davis KB et al: Western Washington randomized trial of intracoronary streptokinase in acute myocardial infarction. N Engl J Med 309:1477, 1983

55. Kennedy JW, Ritchie JL, Davis KB et al: The Western Washington randomized trial of intracoronary streptokinase in acute myocardial infarction: A 12-month followup report. N Engl J Med 312:1073, 1985

56. Komiya T, Sugihara T, Ogata K et al: Inherited deficiency of protein S in a Japanese family with recurrent venous thrombosis: A study of three generations. Blood 67:406, 1986

57. Lewis HD Jr, Veterans Administration Cooperative Study Group: Unstable angina: Status of aspirin and other forms of therapy. Circulation 73(Suppl V):V-155, 1985

58. Lian EC-Y, Siddiqui FA: Investigation of the role of von Willebrand factor in thrombotic thrombocytopenic purpura. Blood 66:1219, 1985
59. Lockshin MD, Druzin ML, Goei S et al: Antibody to cardiolipin as a predictor of fetal distress or death in pregnant patients with systemic lupus erythematosus. N Engl J Med 313:152, 1985
50. Lottenberg R, Dolly FR, Kitchens CS: Recurring thromboembolic disease and pulmonary hypertension associated with severe hypoplasminogenemia. Am J Hematol 19:181, 1985
61. Luchi RL, Chakine RA: Coronary artery spasm, coronary artery thrombosis and myocardial infarction. Ann Intern Med 95:502, 1981
62. Marciniak E, Wilson HD, Marlar RA: Neonatal purpura fulminans: A genetic disorder related to the absence of protein C in the blood. Blood 65:15, 1985
63. Marder VJ: Pharmacology of thrombolytic agents: Implications for therapy of coronary artery thrombosis. Circulation 68(Suppl I):I-2, 1983
64. Marder VJ, Rothbard RL, Fitzpatrick PG et al: Rapid lysis of coronary artery thrombi with anisoylated plasminogen:streptokinase activator complex: Treatment by bolus intravenous injection. Ann Intern Med 104:304, 1986
65. Masotti G, Doggesi L, Galante G: Differential inhibition of prostacylin production and platelet aggregation by aspirin. Lancet 2:1213, 1979
66. Matsuo O, Collen D, Verstrete M: On the fibrinolytic and thrombolytic properties of active-site p-anisoylated streptokinase–plasminogen complex (BRL 26921). Thromb Res 24:347, 1981
67. McGehee WG, Klotz TA, Epstein DJ et al: Coumarin necrosis associated with hereditary protein C deficiency. Ann Intern Med 101(1):59, 1984
68. McPherson RA: Thromboembolism in Hageman trait. Am J Clin Pathol 68:420, 1977
69. Mehta J: Platelets and prostaglandins in coronary artery disease: Rationale for use of platelet-suppressive drugs. JAMA 249:2818, 1983
70. Miller GAH, Hall RCH, Paneth M: Pulmonary embolectomy, heparin and streptokinase: Their place in the treatment of acute massive pulmonary embolism. Am Heart J 93:568, 1977
71. Moake JL, Rudy CK, Troll JH et al: Unusually large plasma factor VIII:von Willebrand factor multimers in chronic relapsing thrombotic thrombocytopenic purpura. N Engl J Med 307:1432, 1982
72. Mueh JR, Herbst KD, Rappaport SI: Thrombosis in patients with the lupus anticoagulant. Ann Intern Med 92:156, 1980
73. Nilsson IM, Krook H, Sternby N et al: Severe thrombotic disease in a young man with bone marrow and skeletal changes and with a high content of an inhibitor in the fibrinolytic system. Acta Med Scand 169:323, 1961
74. Oliva PB: Pathophysiology of acute myocardial infarction, 1981. Ann Intern Med 94:236, 1981
75. Pandolfi M, Hedner U, Nilsson IM: Bilateral occlusion of the retinal veins in a patient with inhibition of fibrinolysis. Ann Ophthalmol 2:481, 1970
76. Pennica D, Holmes WE, Kohr WH et al: Cloning and expression of human tissue-type plasminogen activator cDNA in E. coli. Nature 301:214, 1983
77. Pitt B, Shea MJ, Romson JL et al: Prostaglandins and prostaglandin inhibitors in ischemic heart disease. Ann Intern Med 99:83, 1983
78. Ratnoff OD, Busse RJ Jr, Sheon RP: The demise of John Hageman. N Engl J Med 279:760, 1968
79. Rowe JM, Rasmussen RL, Mader SL: Successful thrombolytic therapy in two patients with renal vein thrombosis. Am J Med 77:1111, 1984
80. Salem HH, Van Der Weyden MB, Koutts J et al: Leg pain and platelet aggregates in thrombocythemic myeloproliferative disease. JAMA 244:1122, 1980
81. Salzman EW, Rosenberg RD, Smith MH et al: Effect of heparin and heparin fractions on platelet aggregation. J Clin Invest 65:64, 1980
82. Sandler RM, Seifer DB, Morgan K et al: Heparin-induced thrombocytopenia and thrombosis: Detection and specificity of a platelet-aggregating IgG. Am J Clin Pathol 83:760, 1985
83. Sanfelippo MJ, Drayna CJ: Prekallikrein inhibitor associated with lupus anticoagulant: A mechanism of thrombosis. Am J Clin Pathol 77:275, 1982
84. Schafer AI: Bleeding and thrombosis in the myeloproliferative disorders. Blood 64:1, 1984

85. Schwarz HP, Fischer M, Hopmeier P et al: Plasma protein S deficiency in familial thrombotic disease. Blood 64:1297, 1984
86. Seligsohn U, Berger A, Abend M et al: Homozygous protein C deficiency manifested by massive venous thrombosis in the newborn. N Engl J Med 310:559, 1984
87. Shapiro SS, Thiagarajan P: Lupus anticoagulants. Prog Hemost Thromb 6:263, 1982
88. Sherry S: Tissue plasminogen activator (t-PA): Will it fulfill its promise? N Engl J Med 313:1014, 1985
89. Sholar PW, Bell WR: Thrombolytic therapy for inferior vena cava thrombosis in paroxysmal nocturnal hemoglobinuria. Ann Intern Med 103:539, 1985
90. Sills RH, Marler RA, Montgomery RR et al: Severe homozygous protein C deficiency. J Pediatr 105:409, 1984
91. Smith RAG, Dupe RJ, English PD et al: Fibrinolysis with acyl-enzymes: A new approach to thrombolytic therapy. Nature 290:505, 1981
92. Soff GA, Sica DA, Marlar RA et al: Protein C levels in nephrotic syndrome: Use of a new enzyme-linked immunoadsorbent assay for protein C antigen. Am J Hematol 22:43, 1986
93. Stead NW, Bauer KA, Kinney TR et al: Venous thrombosis in a family with defective release of vascular plasminogen activator and elevated plasma factor VIII/von Willebrand's factor. Am J Med 74:33, 1983
94. Stead RB, Schafer AI, Rosenberg RD et al: Heterogeneity of heparin lots associated with thrombocytopenia and thromboembolism. Am J Med 77:185, 1984
95. TIMI Study Group: The thrombolysis infarction (TIMI) trial. N Engl J Med 312:932, 1985
96. Topal EJ, Bell WR, Weisfeldt ML: Coronary thrombolysis with recombinant tissue-type plasminogen activator: A hematologic and pharmacologic study. Ann Intern Med 103:837, 1985
97. Valla D, Casadevall N, Lacombe C et al: Primary myeloproliferative disorder and hepatic vein thrombosis. A prospective study of erythroid colony formation in vitro in 20 patients with Budd-Chiari syndrome. Ann Intern Med 103:329, 1985
98. Van de Werf F, Ludbrook PA, Bergmann SR et al: Coronary thrombolysis with tissue-type plasminogen activator in patients with evolving myocardial infarction. N Engl J Med 310:609, 1984
99. Van de Werf F, Nobuhara M, Collen D: Coronary thrombolysis with human single-chain, urokinase-type plasminogen activator (pro-urokinase) in patients with acute myocardial infarction. Ann Intern Med 104:345, 1986
100. Verstraete M, Borg M, Collen D et al: Randomised trial of intravenous recombinant tissue-type plasminogen activator versus intravenous streptokinase in acute myocardial infarction: Report from the European Cooperative Study Group for Recombinant Tissue-type Plasminogen Activator. Lancet 1:842, 1985
101. Walker FJ: Protein S and the regulation of activated protein C. Semin Thromb Hemost 10:131, 1984
102. Weksler BB, Pet SB, Alonso D et al: Differential inhibition by aspirin of vascular and platelet prostaglandin synthesis in atherosclerotic patients. N Engl J Med 308:800, 1983
103. Wohl RC, Summaria L, Robbins KC: Physiologic activation of the human fibrinolytic system: Isolation and characterization of human plasminogen variants, Chicago I and Chicago II. J Biol Chem 254:9063, 1979
104. Wu KK-Y: Platelet hyperaggregability and thrombosis in patients with thrombocythemia. Ann Intern Med 88:7, 1978

SUGGESTED READING

Colman RW, Hirsh J, Marder VJ, Salzman EW (eds): Hemostasis and Thrombosis: Basic Principles and Practice, 2nd ed. Philadelphia, JB Lippincott, 1987
Del Zoppo GJ, Harker LA: Blood/vessel interaction in coronary disease. Hosp Pract, p 163, May 1984

Duckert F: Thrombolytic therapy. Semin Thromb Hemost 10:87, 1984

Fareed J: Molecular Markers of Hemostatic Disorders. Semin Thromb Hemost 10(4), October 1984

Kitchens CS: Concept of hypercoagulability: A review of its development, clinical application, and recent progress. Semin Thromb Hemost 11:293, 1985

Robbins SL, Cotran RS, Kumar V: Pathologic Basis of Disease, 3rd ed, pp 91–112. Philadelphia, WB Saunders, 1984

Rosenberg RD, Bauer KA: New insights into hypercoagulable states. Hosp Pract, p 131, March 1986

Ross R: The pathogenesis of atherosclerosis—an update. N Engl J Med 314:488, 1986

Schafer AI: The hypercoagulable states. Ann Intern Med 102:814, 1985

Thrombolytic Therapy in Thrombosis: A National Institute of Health Consensus Development Conference. Ann Intern Med 93:141, 1980

Molecular and Automated Assessments of Coagulation

12

Jeanine M. Walenga

CASE STUDY

The impacts of newer tests on the laboratory evaluation of the hemostatic system are numerous; however, the diagnostic efficacy of these methods can be exemplified in the following case study.

Antithrombin III is also known as heparin cofactor and is required for the therapeutic action of heparin. Functional measurement of this important inhibitor in the identification of thrombotic disorders and heparinization responses is valuable.

A patient with deep vein thrombosis (DVT) was encountered at a midwestern medical center. He was given a routine dose of heparin for therapeutic anticoagulation. The patient did not respond to this dose, and his activated partial thromboplastin time (APTT) remained unaffected. He was given another dose of heparin and responded slightly. During the course of hospitalization the patient suffered pulmonary embolism on the first and third day.

The patient was treated with fresh-frozen plasma and after the fourth day of hospitalization was treated with Coumadin. The patient was eventually stabilized and was discharged on Coumadin. It was thought that the patient had a deficiency of antithrombin III (ATIII). Through the course of hospitalization, plasma samples were collected from this patient, and immunologic and functional ATIII levels were quantitated. The results are shown in Figure 12-1.

On the first day of hospitalization, both his functional and his immuno-

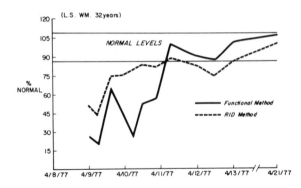

FIG. 12-1. Daily antithrombin III levels in a patient who suffered from pulmonary embolism as measured by both functional and immunologic (RID) assays.

logic levels of ATIII were low. However, the functional ATIII was much lower than the immunologic level. This is the day he suffered pulmonary embolism and resisted heparinization. After plasma infusion, his ATIII levels were increased; on the third day, however, he suffered another attack of pulmonary embolism. Although the immunologic ATIII levels were approximately 75%, his functional ATIII level was about 20%. The patient was given frozen plasma and twice the usual dose of heparin. This patient responded to therapy and was stabilized. On the subsequent days his ATIII levels were about normal in both the immunologic and the functional assays.

This patient suffered from a severe hypercoagulable crisis due to ATIII deficiency and subsequent consumption coagulopathy. A clear dichotomy in the functional and immunologic levels suggests that ATIII, when complexed with thrombin and X_a, retains its immunoreactivity yet loses its functionality. Therefore, in clinical states it is best to measure the functional ATIII level. Many methods based on chromogenic substrates are currently available for the measurement of ATIII. Immunologic ATIII levels are useful for correlating the consumptive index. A ratio between the functional activities and the immunologic levels can be calculated to determine the consumptive index.

Various scientific disciplines have contributed to a clearer understanding of hemostatic mechanisms at a molecular level. Routine coagulation tests cannot be used to thoroughly evaluate *hemostasis,* nor are they specific enough to identify the locale and nature of clotting or bleeding abnormalities. The prothrombin time (PT) and APTT are valid screening assays; however, a new molecular approach now provides more specific and sensitive biochemical analyses leading to differential diagnosis and more effective therapeutic intervention. Current developments combine biochemical, immunologic, and physical techniques with colorimetric, radiochemical, and physical end point detection. Adaptation of the newer methods to automated instrumentation is feasible.[46,165]

Although important to the evaluation of coagulation, early assay developments, as discussed in Chapter 1, focused only on clotting, with no direct evaluation of fibrinolysis or the full role of platelets. Emphasis was placed on bleeding disorders, with no concern for hypercoagulability. The period between 1970 and the early 1980s was explosive in the area of biochemical and molecular evaluation of blood fluidity—a process now referred to as *hemostasis*, which encompasses coagulation, fibrinolysis, platelets, endothelium, and interacting substances. In fact, hemostasis is no longer regarded merely as an independent system of clotting but rather as a general host response that, when uncontrolled, may contribute to the pathophysiology of inflammatory reactions, heart disease, and cancer.[97]

Individual activation and inhibition enzymes of both coagulation and fibrinolysis are quantitated with functional assays that rely not on the coagulation cascade but on a colorimetric end point detection.[44,74] Immunologic techniques are used to identify and quantitate proteins. Low-molecular-weight peptides and other substances such as prostaglandins that specifically define the initial stages of coagulant, fibrinolytic, or platelet activation well before changes can be detected by traditional coagulant assays can be quantitated by isotopic and nonisotopic immunoassay.[47] In addition, antithrombotic, fibrinolytic, and antiplatelet therapies are effectively monitored by newer techniques.

Hemostatic substances, their physical properties, and their most significant functions are indicated in Tables 12-1 to 12-4. Table 12-1 lists coagulant enzymes, proteins, and activation products (early peptide residues following enzymatic cleavage). Table 12-2 lists the circulating enzymes, activation products, and enzyme–inhibitor complexes associated with fibrinolysis. Table 12-3 lists substances and activation products related to platelets. Table 12-4 lists various substances related to hemostatic pathways, the interacting roles of which are yet to be clarified. Many enzymes have more than one direct function and can, for example, activate several major pro-enzymes and/or neutralize various active enzymes. Thus a categorical classification should be taken somewhat loosely.

TABLE 12-1
Newly Recognized Coagulant Proteins and Activation Products

Parameter	Molecular Weight (daltons)	Site of Origin	Plasma Level
COAGULANT ACTIVATORS AND ACTIVATION PRODUCTS			
Kinins	1,100	Liver	0–10 ng/ml
High-molecular-weight kininogen (HMWK)	108,000	Liver	7–18 mg/dl
Prekallikrein (PK)	32,000	Liver	5–10 mg/dl
Fibrinopeptide A (FPA)	1,600	Fibrinogen (coagulation)	0.5–3 ng/ml
Fibrinopeptide B (FPB)	1,600	Fibrinogen (coagulation)	0.5–3 ng/ml
D-Dimer	1,000,000	Fibrin	40–100 ng/ml
COAGULANT INHIBITORS			
Antithrombin III (ATIII)	65,000	Liver	18–30 mg/dl
Heparin cofactor II	66,000	Liver	90–100 μg/ml
C1 inhibitor (C1-INH)	105,000	Liver	18–22 mg/dl
α_1-Antitrypsin (α_1-AT)	54,000	Liver	200–400 mg/dl
Protein C (PrC)	62,000	Liver	2–4 μg/ml
Protein S (PrS)	69,000	Liver	1–2 μg/ml

TABLE 12-2
Newly Recognized Fibrinolytic Proteins and Activation Products

Parameter	Molecular Weight (daltons)	Site of Origin	Plasma Level
FIBRINOLYTIC ACTIVATORS AND ACTIVATION PRODUCTS			
Tissue plasminogen activator (tPA)	63,000	Endothelium, heart, uterus	2–5 ng/ml
Plasminogen (Plg)	90,000	Liver	10–20 mg/dl
Plasma plasminogen activator (pPA)	34,000		
Bβ 15–42 and related peptides	6,000–15,000	Fibrinogen	15–30 ng/ml
FIBRINOLYTIC INHIBITORS			
α_2-Antiplasmin (α_2-AP)	67,000	Liver	5–7 mg/dl
α_2-Macroglobulin (α_2-M)	725,000	Liver	150–400 mg/dl
Plasminogen activator inhibitor	75,000	Various	
SERINE PROTEASE–INHIBITOR COMPLEXES			
Xa–ATIII	122,000		0
Thrombin–ATIII	135,000		0
Plasmin–α_2-AP	155,000		0
Plasmin–α_2-M	810,000		0
Kallikrein–C1-INH	135,000		0
Complement–C1-INH	290,000		0

TABLE 12-3
Newly Recognized Platelet Substances and Activation Products

Parameter	Molecular Weight (daltons)	Site of Origin	Plasma Level
Platelet factor 4 (PF_4)	7780	Platelets (alpha granule storage)	4–8 ng/ml
β-Thromboglobulin (βTG)	8800	Platelets (alpha granule storage)	20–40 ng/ml
PROSTAGLANDINS			
Thromboxanes A_2 and B_2	350	Platelets, endothelium (arachidonic acid)	0–150 pg/ml
6-Keto prostaglandin ($PGF_{1\alpha}$)	350	Endothelium (arachidonic acid)	0–150 pg/ml
PGE_2, $PGF_{2\alpha}$, others	350	Various	

TABLE 12-4
Miscellaneous Hemostasis-Related Substances

Parameter	Site of Origin	Plasma Level
C5a, C4a, C3a (anaphylatoxins)		80–200 mg/dl
Histamine	Blood, mast cells	3–9 μg/dl
Lymphokines	Lymphocytes	
Monokines	Monocytes	
Angiotensins	Kidney	
Catecholamines	Various sites	0–10 ng/ml
Purines and pyrimidine	Various sites	0–10 μg/ml
Endorphins/enkephalins	Nervous system	
Glycosaminoglycans	Various sites	

Many newer tests are commercially available as manual kits adaptable to clinical chemistry instrumentation. A basic spectrophotometer is required for the enzymatic assays, and a basic gamma or beta counter or microtiter plate system is required for the immunologic assays. Centrifugal, solid-phase, flow, and kinetic analyzers and immunoanalytic instruments have hemostatic applications (Table 12-5).

Thrombotic disorders, whether directly acquired or associated with another disease, are a major health hazard. In 1985 the National Institutes of Health estimated that venous thromboembolism accounted for 300,000 hospitilizations and 50,000 deaths. An in-depth assessment of the individual parameters of coagulation, fibrinolysis, platelets, and endothelium through means described in this chapter may help alleviate many of these complications. Technologies are now available for biochemical analysis of individual activators, inhibitors, and early physiological markers of activation in hemostatic systems.[162] Application of these concepts will provide the clinical laboratory with the ability to clinically diagnose and therapeutically monitor thrombosis at a more effective level.

DEVELOPMENT OF ADVANCED HEMOSTATIC TECHNIQUES

Coagulant Techniques

The basic coagulation assays (see Chap. 4) are clot-based methods that employ the coagulant enzyme cascade and a fibrin end point. In 1935 Dr. Armand Quick introduced the one-stage PT.[123] The APTT assay evolved from original works of Quick, Biggs, and Douglas (1953).[19] The PT and APTT are global methods that do not provide precise quantitation of specific enzymes. Despite this generalized approach, these assays provide basic clinical information on the overall function of the coagulant system. The utility of these assays is proven by their long years of continued use in both research and clinical laboratories.

Clotting assays were originally performed in glass by a "tilt-tube" technique and visual clot end point detection. Although inherently error-prone and highly subjective,

TABLE 12-5

Instrumentation Available for Adaption of the Newer Hemostatic Parameters

Instrument Class	Detector	Representative Commercial Product	Adaptable Hemostatic Technique
Automated chemistry analyzers	Visible light, turbidimetric	Gilford 3500, Technicon RA-1000, Abbott ABA-100, DuPont aca, Boehringer Mannheim Hitachi	Synthetic substrate, coagulant
Centrifugal analyzers	Visible light, nephelometric, fluorescent light	Roche Cobas Bio, Instrumentation Laboratory Multistat, Electronucleonics Gemini/Gemsaec, J. T. Baker Centrifichem	Synthetic substrate, immunologic, coagulant
Kinetic analyzers	Visible light	Beckman, Gilford	Synthetic substrate
Solid-phase chemistry analyzers	Enzymatic, chemical, fluorescent light	Kodak Ektachem, Dade Stratus, IDT Fiax	Synthetic substrate, immunologic
Laser nephelometers	Immunoprecipitation	Hyland PDQ, Calbiochem, Baker	Immunologic
Rate nephelometers	Immunoprecipitation	Beckman ICS	Immunologic
Microtiter plate readers and wash systems	Visible light	Dynatech, Biotek, Behring, Cetus, Abbott	Enzyme immunoassay
Gamma or beta counters	Radioactivity	Beckman, Tracor, Packard, LKB	Radioimmunoassay
Dedicated hemostatic instruments	Visible light	Labsystems FP-910, Instrumentation Laboratory ACL	Synthetic substrate, immunologic, coagulant

the tilt-tube technique could be consistently performed by trained technicians. One of the first instruments developed to replace the tilt-tube technique in the late 1950s was the BBL Fibrometer (Becton Dickinson and Co., Rutherford, NJ 21030). This semiautomated clot timer employs an electromechanical detector of clot formation which, because of its versatility and reproducibility, has become the mainstay of many coagulation laboratories. In the 1970s, semiautomated and fully automated optical clot detectors were introduced. These instruments detect a change in light transmission upon fibrin polymerization and have been satisfactorily dedicated for PT and APTT analyses. Organon Teknika Corp. (Parsippany, NJ 07054); Lancer, a division of Sherwood Medical Industries (St. Louis, MO 63103); Medical Laboratory Automation, Inc.

(Mt. Vernon, NY 10570); and Ortho Diagnostic Systems, Inc. (Raritan, NJ 08869), are established manufacturers of these instruments.

Other clot-based instruments employ the concept of viscoelastic changes in whole blood or plasma as coagulation/fibrinolysis occurs. The Thromboelastograph (Hellige GmbH, Freiburg im Briesgau, W. Germany) and the Sonoclot (Sienco, Inc., Morrison, CO 80465) kinetically measure clot formation. The Hemachron (International Technidyne Corp., Metuchen, NJ 08840) and the Hepcon (HemoTec, Inc., Englewood, CO 80112) are used for monitoring heparin by viscomagnetic detector and optical detector, respectively.

The current trend in coagulation instrumentation is to combine multiple probes within one instrument for detection of coagulant, chromogenic (color), and immunologic assay end points. Several of these instruments will be discussed later in this chapter.

A recently developed assay based on coagulation end point detection is for the quantitation of protein C, an inhibitor of Factors V_a and VIII_a. Kits for use on the Fibrometer are commercially available from American Diagnostica, Inc. (Greenwich, CT 06830), and American Bioproducts Co. (Parsippany, NJ 07054). The assay is performed in a fashion similar to that for the factor assay for coagulant factors, in which diluted test sample is quantitated from a calibration curve of normal plasma diluted to various concentrations. Heptest from Haemachem, Inc. (St. Louis, MO 63144), is a recently developed clotting heparin assay that primarily measures inhibition of Factor X_a. It is performed like the APTT.

Synthetic Substrate Techniques

Since clot-based assays rely on an intact coagulation system and fibrin formation, techniques are complicated and often require multiple assay steps to ensure an accurate measure of individual proteins (see Chap. 4). For example, the original assay for ATIII was clot-based.[1,18] This procedure required an intact coagulation system and normal fibrinogen levels for accurate quantitation of ATIII. The assay suffered from nonlinearity. The presence of fibrin degradation products (FDPs) caused false elevations of results.

Synthetic substrate techniques make it possible to measure the activity of individual procoagulants and regulatory proteins. In the example of ATIII, quantitative interaction between the ATIII protein and the substrate is unaffected by FDPs, fibrinogen concentration, or the activity of other procoagulants. In general, synthetic substrate assays provide results with the sensitivity and specificity of a clinical chemistry technique. Synthetic substrate methods include fewer variables, fewer sources of error, and less speculation as to the identification of the analyte.

History of the Development of Synthetic Substrates

The use of synthetic substrates in enzyme analysis began with the observation of Sherry, Troll, and Wachman (1954) that coagulant and fibrinolytic proteins were able to hydrolyze arginine esters.[156] These proteins are termed *serine proteases*, since, like trypsin, they are able to cleave peptide bonds. Peptide substrates sensitive to specific enzymatic cleavage were subsequently synthesized, alleviating the difficulties of isolating physiological substrates in a natural and pure state. First-generation synthetic substrates were composed of simple amino acid-esters (*e.g.,* tosyl-arginine-methyl ester or benzoyl-arginine-ethyl ester) that possessed limited specificity. Colman was one of the first to report on the practical applications of this new principle to clinical problems.[30] He stated that synthetic substrate assays for the human kallikrein system, based on a simple biochemical design, are valuable for investigating alterations in these components in carcinoma, pancreatitis, bacteremia, liver disease, estrogen therapy, and allergic states.

Molecular Structure of Synthetic Substrates

The work of Blomback and co-workers gave an increased understanding of the molecular structure of serine proteases and their substrates, activators, and inhibitors.[20] Amino acids at positions 1, 2, and 9 of Fibrinopeptide A (FPA) (Phe-Val-Arg) were homologous across several species. Subsequent synthesis and evaluation of this oligopeptide revealed that it possesses anticoagulant activity and an affinity for thrombin. This observation led to the assumption that this sequence represented the active site for thrombin on the fibrinogen molecule.

Subsequently, Svendsen and co-workers introduced the first second-generation synthetic substrate in 1972.[44] It contained the tripeptide amino acid sequence Phe-Val-Arg coupled to the chromophore paranitroaniline (pNA); Bz-Phe-Val-Arg-pNa, Pentapharm, Basel, Switzerland). This chromogenic substrate provided a simple and direct means of assessing enzyme activity. Subsequent investigators used cleavage site sequencing of other natural substrates to produce synthetic equivalents. Substrates were also developed through the use of fluorophore tags. Available chromogenic substrates are shown in Table 12-6, and the currently available fluorogenic substrates are shown in Table 12-7.

Although in theory synthetic substrates appear to be highly applicable to hemostatic testing, one must be cautioned to several disadvantages. First, a synthetic substrate is less specific for an enzyme than its natural substrate. Most natural substrates are polypeptides of approximately 60,000 daltons molecular weight with specific secondary and tertiary structures. Synthetic substrates are simple straight-chain tripeptides. Thus, assays employing synthetic material are quantitative but not qualitative for enzyme activity, since nonspecific reactions may occur. Assay specificity can be increased, however, by addition of inhibitors to eliminate nonspecific reactions or by running specific controls. Second, synthetic substrates do not recognize the same degree of enzyme functionality as do the fibrin-forming natural substrates. For example, decarboxylated Factors II, VII, IX, and X (proteins induced by vitamin K antagonists [PIVKAs]) are produced during oral anticoagulant (Coumadin) treatment. These factors are not functionally active in clotting, but they are measured by synthetic substrates.[51] Although numerous reports on the clinical use of synthetic substrates for monitoring oral anticoagulant therapy have been published, certain irregularities do exist, indicating that further studies are needed to establish clinical relevance.[41,96,155]

Principle of Action of Synthetic Substrates

The principle of action of synthetic substrates is illustrated in Figure 12-2, in which a synthetic amino acid sequence is recognized as the active site of a specific enzyme. For example, the natural substrate of thrombin, fibrinogen, has the following amino acid sequence at its cleavage site: Phe-X_7-Val-Arg-Gly-Pro-Arg. An appropriate synthetic chromogenic substrate has the sequence CBz-Gly-Pro-Arg-pNA (Chromozym TH, Pentapharm, Basel, Switzerland). The tripeptide sequence is coupled at the carboxyl end to the optically active (405-nm), chemically stable, chromophore (pNA). An enzyme effectively cleaves the bond between the amino acid and the pNA, releasing the pNA tag. The optical characteristics of the free tag are significantly different from those of the

TABLE 12-6

Chromogenic Peptide Substrates for Serine Proteases and Their Applications in Hemostatic Testing

Substrate	Chemical Structure	Diagnostic Applications
FIRST-GENERATION SYNTHETIC SUBSTRATES		
AAMe	α-acetyl-L-arginine methyl ester	Measurement of trypsin-like
BAMe	α-benzoyl-L-arginine methyl ester	enzymes: Factor XII$_a$, kallikrein,
BA	α-benzoyl-L-arginine	thrombin, Factor X$_a$, plasmin,
TAMe	α-tosyl-L-arginine methyl ester	protein C$_a$, etc.
TA	α-tosyl-L-arginine	
LMe	L-lysine methyl ester	
ALMe	α-acetyl-L-lysine methyl ester	
AGLMe	α-acetyl-glycine-L-lysine methyl ester	
BLMe	α-benzoyl-L-lysine methyl ester	
TLMe	α-tosyl-L-lysine methyl ester	
SECOND-GENERATION SYNTHETIC SUBSTRATES		
Chromozym TH	Tos-or-CBZ-Gly-Pro-Arg-pNA	ATIII, heparin cofactor II, PT,
S-2160	Bz-Phe-Val-Arg-pNA	APTT; Factors II(a), V, and VIII;
S-2238	H-D-Phe-Pip*-Arg-pNA	PF$_3$, PF$_4$
Abbott	CH$_3$-Gly-Pro-Arg-pNA	
S-2222	Bz-Ile-Glu-(O-R†)-Gly-Arg-pNA	ATIII, heparin, Factors VII, VIII,
S-2337	Bz-Ile-Glu-(O-R†)-Glu-Arg-pNA	IX, and X
CBS 31.39	CH$_3$-SO$_2$-D-Leu-Gly-Arg-pNA	
S-2251	H-D-Val-Leu-Lys-pNA	Plasminogen, α$_2$-AP, plasmin,
Chromozym PL	CBZ-Gly-Pro-Arg-pNA	plasminogen activator
S-2288	H-D-Ile-Pro-Arg-pNA	Plasminogen activator or inhibitor
S-2390	H-D-Val-Phe-Lys-pNA	
S-2302	H-D-Pro-Phe-Arg-pNA	(Pre)kallikrein, Factor XII,
Chromozym PK	Bz-Pro-Phe-Arg-pNA	antikallikrein
CBS 33.27	H-D-Phe-Gly-Phe-Arg-pNA	
S-2266	H-D-Val-Leu-Arg-pNA	Glandular kallikrein
Chromozym UK	Bz-Val-Gly-Arg-pNA	Urokinase, antiurokinase titer,
S-2444	Pyro-Glu-Gly-Arg-pNA	C1-esterase inhibitor
Spectrozyme UK	Cbo-L-(γ)Glu(α-t-Buo)-Gly-Arg-pNA	
Chromozym Try	H-D-Val-Gly-Arg-pNA	α$_1$-AT, trypsin, α$_2$-M
Chromozym Try	Cbo-Val-Gly-Arg-pNA	
Chromozym Try	Z-Val-Gly-Arg-pNA	
CBS 40.17	Bz-D-Ala-Ala-Arg-pNA	
S-2423	CH$_3$-CO-Ile-Glu-Gly-Arg-pNA	
Spectrozyme TRY	Cbo-Gly-D-Ala-Arg-pNA	Trypsin activity
S-2422	Bz-Phe-Glu-Gly-Arg-pNA	Limulus procoagulant enzyme,
S-2421	Ace-Phe-Glu-Gly-Arg-pNA	endotoxin
C1-I	C$_2$H$_5$CO-Lys-(ξ-Cbo)-Gly-Arg-pNA	C1-esterase
Spectrozyme C$_1$E	Me-CO-Lys(γ-Cbo)-Gly-Arg-pNA	
	H-D-or Boc-Leu-Ser-Thr-Arg-pNA	Activated protein C, antiprotein C

(Continued)

TABLE 12-6
Chromogenic Peptide Substrates for Serine Proteases and Their Applications in Hemostatic Testing *(Continued)*

Substrate	Chemical Structure	Diagnostic Applications
SECOND-GENERATION SYNTHETIC SUBSTRATES *(Continued)*		
Spectrozyme PC$_a$	H-D-Lys(γ-Cbo)-Pro-Arg-pNA	
S-2484	Glu-Pro-Val-pNA	Granulocyte elastase
THIRD-GENERATION SYNTHETIC SUBSTRATES		
CBS 34.47	H-D-CHG-But-Arg-pNA	ATIII, (pro)thrombin, heparin,
Spectrozyme TH	H-D-HHT-Ala-Arg-pNA	PT, APTT
Th-1	H-D-CHG-Ala-Arg-pNA	
Spectrozyme Fx$_a$	MeO-CO-D-CHG-Gly-Arg-pNA	ATIII, heparin, Factors VIII, IX, X
Xa-1	CH$_3$-OCO-D-CHA-Gly-Arg-pNA	
CBS 30.41	H-D-But-CHA-Lys-pNA	Plasminogen, plasminogen
CBS 33.08	H-D-Nleu-CHA-Arg-pNA	activator, α_2-AP
Spectrozyme PL	H-D-Nleu-HHT-Lys-pNA	
PL-1	N-D-Nleu-CHA-Lys-Arg-pNA	
Spectrozyme t-PA	CH$_3$SO$_2$-D-CHT-Gly-Arg-pNA	Tissue plasminogen activator
Spectrozyme P.kal	H-D-Pro-HHT-Arg-pNA	(Pre)kallikrein, Factor XII,
PK-1	H-D-But-CHA-Arg-pNA	antikallikrein
Chromozym GK	H-D-Val-CHA-Arg-pNA	Glandular kallikrein
CBS 23.41	H-D-Val-CHA-Arg-pNA	
Spectrozyme G.Kal	H-D-Val-CHA-Arg-pNA	Glandular and urinary kallikrein
Spectrozyme Pro	H-D-CHG-Pro-Arg-pNA	α_1-AT, α_2-M
Spectrozyme LAL	CH$_3$O-CO-D-HHT-Gly-Arg-pNA	Endotoxin, limulus enzyme

Note:

Substrates of the S series are available from KabiVitrum, Stockholm, Sweden; or Helena Laboratories, Beaumont, TX.

Substrates of the Chromozym series are available from Boehringer-Mannheim, Indianapolis, IN; or Pentapharm, Basel, Switzerland.

Substrates of the CBS series are available from Diagnostica Stago, Asnieres, France; or American Bioproducts Company, Parsippany, NJ.

Substrates of the Spectrozyme series are available from American Diagnostica, Greenwich, CT.

Substrates of the X-1 series are available from Immuno Diagnostics, Vienna, Austria.

* Piperidyl

† CH$_3$ or H

native substrate (Fig. 12-3). Thus, it is feasible to quantify enzymatic activity based on changes in optical density. These assays are measured kinetically during the initial phases of the reaction or by an end point technique in which acetic acid is used to quench or stop the reaction after a specified time prior to measuring the reaction. The scheme below represents a general sequence of the biochemical reaction.

$$\text{Bz-CO-Phe-Val-Arg-pNA} \xrightarrow{\text{Serine protease}} \text{Bz-CO-Phe-Val-Arg-OH} + \text{pNA}$$

   (Achromogenic)   (Chromogenic)

TABLE 12-7
Fluorogenic Peptide Substrates for Serine Proteases in Hemostatic Testing

Enzyme	Chemical Structure
Thrombin	Boc-Val-Pro-Arg-MCA*
	CBZ-Gly-Pro-Arg-βNA
	H-D-Phe-Pro-Arg-AIE
Factor X_a	Boc-Ile-Glu-Gly-Arg-MCA*
Urokinase	Glut-Gly-Arg-MCA
Plasmin	H-D-Val-Leu-Lys-AIE*
	Boc-Gly-Lys-MCA
	Boc-Val-Leu-Lys-MCA
	Boc-Glu-Lys-Lys-MCA
Urinary kallikrein	Pro-Phe-Arg-MCA
Pancreatic kallikrein	Pro-Phe-Arg-MCA
Plasma kallikrein	Z-Phe-Arg-MCA
Trypsin	Bz-Arg-MCA
	Boc-Phe-Ser-Arg-MCA
	Leu-Thr-Arg-MCA
Limulus clotting enzyme	Boc-Leu-Gly-Arg-MCA
XI_a, XII_a	Boc-Phe-Ser-Arg-MCA
	Boc-Leu-Thr-Arg-MCA
Protein C (activated)	Boc-Leu-Ser-Thr-Arg-MCA
Cathepsin H	Arg-MCA

* Substrate available in the Protopath kits (American Dade, Division of American Hospital Supply Corp., Miami, FL). All other substrates are available from Protein Research Institute, Minoh Osaka, Japan.

Fluorescent tags may be preferred for their higher level of sensitivity compared with chromophores, particularly when enzyme concentrations are excessively low. Fluorescent groups include 5-aminoisophthalic acid dimethyl ester, with emission at 430 nm and excitation at 335 nm; trifluoromethyl coumarin amide, with excitation at 400 nm and emission at 505 nm; 7-amino-7 methylcoumarin, with excitation at 380 nm and emission at 460 nm; and 4-methoxy-2-naphthylamine, with excitation at

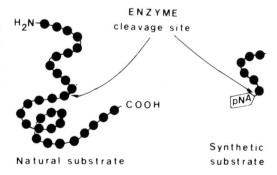

FIG. 12-2. The synthetic substrate mimics the enzymatic active site of the natural physiologic substrate, thereby providing a readily accessible reagent for sensitive and specific enzymatic analysis. The release of a chromophore, paranitroaniline *(pNA)*, due to enzymatic cleavage, produces a color that is easily quantitated. (Courtesy of Goran Cleason, KabiVitrum, Stockholm, Sweden)

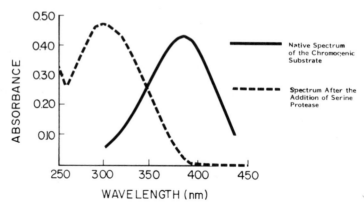

FIG. 12-3. Absorbance spectra of 0.25mM native substrate and free pNA. Because of the action of a serine protease on the substrate, the liberated pNA produces a shift in the peak absorbance compared to that of the native (coupled) substrate-pNA. Quantification of free pNA is easily performed at 405 nm, where no interference from the native substrate occurs.

340 nm and emission at 425 nm. The structure of each of these detector groups is illustrated in Figure 12-4.

Inclusion of a pseudoamino acid may increase the solubility, specificity, and kinetic characteristics of synthetic substrates. A pseudoamino acid is a synthetically modified naturally occurring amino acid (see Spectrozyme UK in Table 12-6). Some examples of pseudoamino acids are cyclohexylglycine (CHG), cyclohexyltyrosine (CHT), cyclohexylalanine (CHA), and norleucine (Nleu). The synthetic substrates that include pseudoamino acids are referred to as third-generation substrates.

Although simple substrate esters coupled to a color-enhancing agent continue to be used for reasons of feasibility and cost-effectiveness, the reaction is nonspecific and must be used only where the biochemical reaction is well defined. Several of the coagulation assays for the aca (E. I. Du Pont de Nemours & Co., Wilmington, DE 19803) use a thiobenzyl ester substrate coupled to Ellman's reagent (5,5'-dithio-bis-2-nitro benzoic acid). The benzyl mercaptan released from the substrate reacts with Ellman's reagent to give a thioperoxide that can be monitored at 412 nm.

The generalized schemes below illustrate various enzymatic reactions with synthetic substrates employed in the quantification of hemostatic parameters.

> **Proenzyme (indirect) assay:** measures either proenzyme or activator activity level by measuring the generated enzyme
>
> 1. Proenzyme $\xrightarrow{\text{Activator}}$ Enzyme
>
> 2. R-pNA $\xrightarrow{\text{Enzyme}}$ R-COOH + pNA
>
> **Enzyme (direct) assay:** directly quantitates the activity of an enzyme
>
> 1. R-pNA $\xrightarrow{\text{Enzyme}}$ R-COOH + pNA
>
> **Inhibitor assay:** quantitates the activity level of an endogenous inhibitor against exogenously added purified enzyme

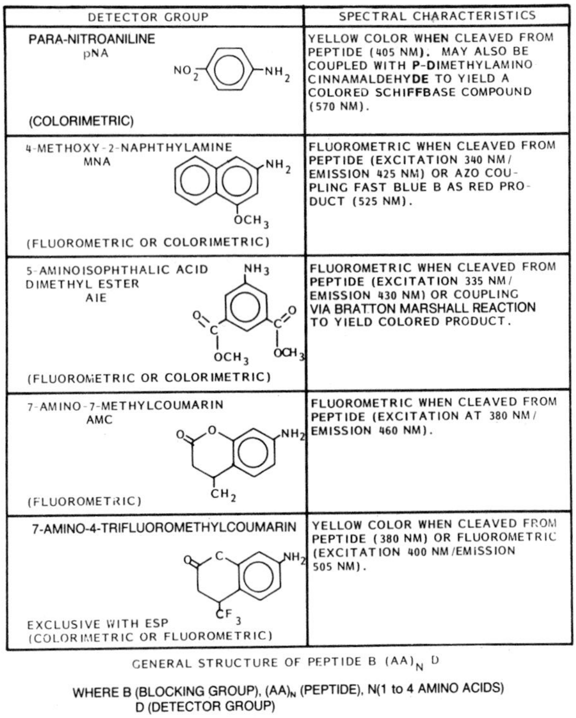

DETECTOR GROUP	SPECTRAL CHARACTERISTICS
PARA-NITROANILINE pNA (COLORIMETRIC)	YELLOW COLOR WHEN CLEAVED FROM PEPTIDE (405 NM). MAY ALSO BE COUPLED WITH P-DIMETHYLAMINO CINNAMALDEHYDE TO YIELD A COLORED SCHIFFBASE COMPOUND (570 NM).
4-METHOXY-2-NAPHTHYLAMINE MNA (FLUOROMETRIC OR COLORIMETRIC)	FLUOROMETRIC WHEN CLEAVED FROM PEPTIDE (EXCITATION 340 NM/ EMISSION 425 NM) OR AZO COUPLING FAST BLUE B AS RED PRODUCT (525 NM).
5-AMINOISOPHTHALIC ACID DIMETHYL ESTER AIE (FLUOROMETRIC OR COLORIMETRIC)	FLUOROMETRIC WHEN CLEAVED FROM PEPTIDE (EXCITATION 335 NM/ EMISSION 430 NM) OR COUPLING VIA BRATTON MARSHALL REACTION TO YIELD COLORED PRODUCT.
7-AMINO-7-METHYLCOUMARIN AMC (FLUOROMETRIC)	FLUOROMETRIC WHEN CLEAVED FROM PEPTIDE (EXCITATION AT 380 NM/ EMISSION 460 NM).
7-AMINO-4-TRIFLUOROMETHYLCOUMARIN EXCLUSIVE WITH ESP (COLORIMETRIC OR FLUOROMETRIC)	YELLOW COLOR WHEN CLEAVED FROM PEPTIDE (380 NM) OR FLUOROMETRIC (EXCITATION 400 NM/EMISSION 505 NM).

FIG. 12-4. Various fluorogenic detector groups and their spectral characteristics.

GENERAL STRUCTURE OF PEPTIDE B (AA)$_N$ D

WHERE B (BLOCKING GROUP), (AA)$_n$ (PEPTIDE), N(1 to 4 AMINO ACIDS) D (DETECTOR GROUP)

1. Pure enzyme + inhibitor $\longrightarrow$ Enzyme – inhibitor complex + residual enzyme

2. R-pNA $\xrightarrow{\text{Residual enzyme}}$ R-COOH + pNA

Cofactor assay: quantitates the activity level of a cofactor normally present to enhance the rate of an enzymatic reaction

1. Proenzyme $\xrightarrow{\text{Cofactor and activator}}$ enzyme

2. R-pNA $\xrightarrow{\text{Enzyme}}$ R-COOH + pNA

Synthetic Substrates and Automated Instrumentation

Certain automated instruments may be used to measure hemostatic parameters.[49,101] Table 12-5 lists various classes of instruments, with commercial examples in which hemostatic parameters are quantitated through the use of synthetic substrate, clot formation, or immunologic reactions. The instruments are designed for batch processing of single tests on multiple samples or multiple test panels on a single sample. Versatility ranges from instruments that only measure the final reaction solution, by end point or kinetic analysis, to instruments that automatically pipet reagents and sample, incubate, and analyze the reaction.

One automated system for hemostatic testing is the aca (E. I. du Pont de Nemours & Co., Inc., Wilmington, DE 19803; Fig. 12-5). Plasminogen, ATIII, fibrinogen, FDP, and heparin determinations are available through the use of individually assembled test packs for discrete sample analysis.[61,119,164] The packs contain reagents in tablet form and are marked with a binary code that signals a microprocessor control. Under the direction of the microprocessor, the test pack is automatically filled with designated quantities of sample and diluent; the reaction proceeds according to design, and the results are determined photometrically.

The FP-910 Coagulation Analyzer (Labsystems, Inc., Morton Grove, IL 60053; Fig. 12-6) is a unique, semiautomated, microprocessor-controlled system compatible with spectrophotometric, enzyme-linked immunosorbent assay (ELISA), and coagulant technologies. It simultaneously pipets and measures nine test samples in a cuvette block and measures them by vertical photometry. It is flexible, easy to use, economical, and compatible with commercial reagents, and allows high throughput (150–200 tests/hr).

The concept of centrifugal analysis was formulated by Anderson (1967) in an effort to design an automated instrument not based on continuous flow, in which analyses could be performed in parallel and computer interfaced.[165] The basic concept is of a radial block of cuvettes rotating through a stationary light beam, in which absorbance readings are taken. A typical rotor contains twenty cuvettes and rotates at approximately 500 rpm, taking a reading every 100 ms. The major advantage to this system is the apparent simultaneous analysis of blank and test samples, allowing minimal electronic noise or signal shift between samples (Fig. 12-7).

Individual cuvettes consist of at least two separate compartments divided by a dam (Fig. 12-8) separating reagents and test samples until centrifugal force causes them to mix. Mixing is completed in seconds, and data acquisition can begin just seconds after initiation of the reaction. The results may be photometric, fluorimetric, or turbidimetric and may be measured kinetically or by end point analysis.

The centrifugal analyzer has become the most popular instrument for automated synthetic substrate assays.[6,40,65,67,73,77,84,92] The most recent development in centrifugal analysis has been the ACL (Instrumentation Laboratory, Inc., Lexington, MA 02173).

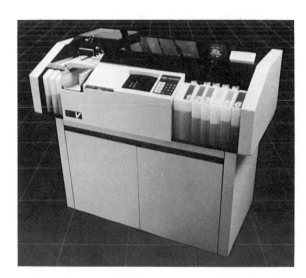

FIG. 12-5. The aca V (E.I. Du Pont de Nemours & Co., Inc., Wilmington, DE 19803) offers hemostasis assays for ATIII, plasminogen, fibrinogen, FDPs, and heparin.

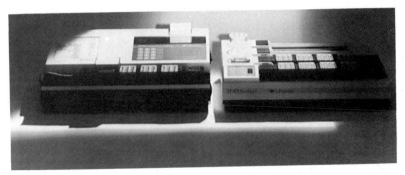

FIG. 12-6. The FP-910 (Labsystems, Inc., Morton Grove, IL 60053) is a dedicated hemostasis instrument capable of measuring coagulant, synthetic substrate, and immunologic assays.

This instrument automatically performs both traditional clotting assays and synthetic substrate assays. Calibration and quality control programs are also automated and can be stored in the instrument memory. The ACL is currently programmed for PT, APTT, and fibrinogen (individual or simultaneous testing), as well as factor assays (individual or simultaneous profiling), heparin, ATIII, plasminogen, and α_2-AP (Fig. 12-9).

The Ektachem device (Eastman Kodak Co., Rochester, NY 14650) was introduced in 1978 for miniaturized, simplified dry chemistry analysis. Dry reagents are positioned in multiple layers sandwiched between two plastic covers. Ten microliters of patient sample are transferred to a porous spreading layer. The uniform sample then filters to the first reagent layer, where an initial reaction occurs. As the solution passes

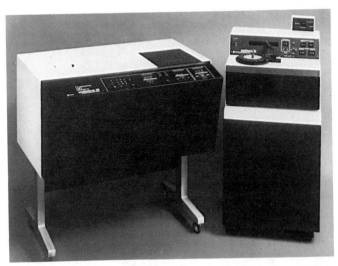

FIG. 12-7. The Multistat III centrifugal analyzer (Instrumentation Laboratory, Inc., Lexington, MA 02173). The loader is on the right and the analyzer on the left. This instrument is capable of measuring coagulant, synthetic substrate, fluorescent, and immunologic assays.

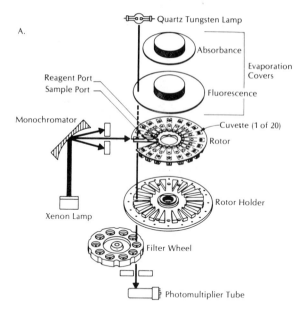

A.

Quartz Tungsten Lamp

Absorbance

Evaporation
Covers

Reagent Port
Sample Port

Fluorescence

Monochromator

Cuvette (1 of 20)

Rotor

Xenon Lamp

Rotor Holder

Filter Wheel

Photomultiplier Tube

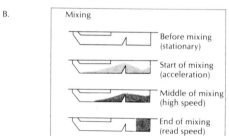

B.

Mixing

Before mixing
(stationary)

Start of mixing
(acceleration)

Middle of mixing
(high speed)

End of mixing
(read speed)

FIG. 12-8. (*A*) Optics schematic for the Multistat III (Instrumentation Laboratory, Inc., Lexington, MA 02173), showing the cuvette rotor, its housing in the analyzer, and the light source. (*B*) Diagrammatic representation of an individual cuvette during analysis in the centrifugal analyzer. (*A*, Hills LP: Semin Thromb Hemost 9[3]:219, 1983; *B*, courtesy of Electronucleonics, Inc., Fairfield, NJ 07006)

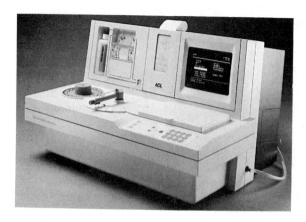

FIG. 12-9. The ACL (Instrumentation Laboratory, Inc., Lexington, MA 02173) is a dedicated hemostasis instrument capable of performing coagulant and synthetic substrate assays. It is currently programmed for PT, APTT, factor assays, ATIII, plasminogen, α_2-AP, and heparin.

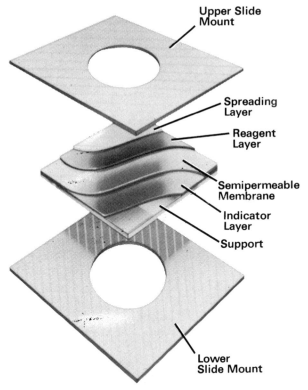

Upper Slide Mount

Spreading Layer

Reagent Layer

Semipermeable Membrane

Indicator Layer

Support

Lower Slide Mount

FIG. 12-10. Diagrammatic illustration of a dry chemistry slide from the Ektachem system, showing the various reaction layers. (Courtesy of Eastman Kodak Co., Rochester, NY 14650)

to the second layer, enzymatic reactions result in color development. The color is proportional to analyte activity and is measured by reflectance photometry (Fig. 12-10).

The dry reagents may be stored at room temperature. Accuracy is high because of the elimination of pipetting, mixing, reconstitution, and dilution. Coagulation assays are feasible and currently under development in this and similar systems.

Immunologic Techniques and Instrumentation

Immunologic assays measure antigenically characterized protein without regard to the utility of the protein. These assays (immunoassays) are designed to measure the concentration of proteins in nanogram-per-milliliter and picogram-per-milliliter ranges (Table 12-8). The sensitivity of immunoassay exceeds the sensitivity of synthetic substrate and coagulant techniques, which measure in the milligram- and microgram-per-milliliter ranges. All immunoassays are based on antigen–antibody reactions, in which the antigen is the substance to be analyzed (analyte) and the reactant is an antibody or immunoglobulin. Recent developments have encouraged the development of immunoassays in hemostasis.

TABLE 12-8
Relative Sensitivity of Various Techniques Used to
Evaluate Hemostatic Parameters

Technique	Detection Limit
Coagulant techniques	10^{-6} g/ml
Synthetic substrate techniques	10^{-6} g/ml
Immunologic techniques	
Latex agglutination	10^{-6} g/ml
Nephelometry	10^{-6} g/ml
Radial immunodiffusion	10^{-6} g/ml
Electroimmunodiffusion	10^{-6} g/ml
Radioimmunoassay	10^{-12} g/ml
Enzyme immunoassay	10^{-12} g/ml
Fluoroimmunoassay	10^{-12} g/ml

Antibodies to all the hemostatic proteins are now produced either as polyclonal antibodies raised against human proteins in laboratory animals or as monoclonal antibodies raised in hybridoma culture. Monoclonal antibodies are more specific than polyclonal antibodies. A marker, or *ligand,* is covalently bound to the reagent antibody to provide a means of detection. Most antibodies are marked with radioactive ligands such as ^{125}I or enzymes such as peroxidase or alkaline phosphatase. Enzymes will react with reagent substrates to produce measurable color or fluorescence.

Some inherited hemostatic disorders result in the production of proteins in normal concentration that carry molecular aberrations. Such qualitative changes have been described for ATIII, fibrinogen, prothrombin, plasminogen, α_2-AP, and Factors VII, VIII, IX, and X.[50,82,133,134,145] Immunoassays are rarely sensitive to qualitative changes; thus, normal concentrations of dysfunctional proteins would be detected. For example, in dysfibrinogenemia, clot-based assays like the APTT are prolonged, but the immunoassay result may be normal. On the other hand, some aberrant proteins carry modifications that affect immunoassay reactions, particularly if the specific determinant of molecular structure that accounts for the antigen–antibody reaction is modified or if the molecular charge is affected. For example, when the charge is affected, electrophoretic mobility is modified.

A recently advanced concept for the diagnosis of hemostatic disorders is measurement of *molecular markers.*[47] Because these markers are protein fragments (oligopeptides) of hemostatic proteins or other low-molecular-weight substances, immunologic techniques are the only means of measuring their blood levels. Coagulant and synthetic substrate methods, although adequate for the larger proteins such as ATIII and plasminogen, do not provide the sensitivity level required for molecular markers.

The normal state of blood fluidity is maintained through integration of diverse enzymatic and cellular systems that act as continual checks and balances on one another (see Chap. 2). This complex network consists of coagulation and fibrinolytic enzymes, platelets and vascular endothelium, and the less readily associated but clearly involved systems of *complement,* prostaglandins, *leukotrienes,* immunologic proteins, and inorganic ions. Activation of or imbalance in any of these systems generates certain well-defined peptide cleavage products or cellular release products that have been termed molecular markers. These markers are of low molecular weight ($<$ 10,000 daltons) and are found at nanogram-per-milliliter or picogram-per-milliliter levels in blood. Based on their origin, they identify a specific pathway of activation. Because of the nature of their formation and their naturally low plasma concentrations, elevated levels of molecular markers indicate the initial stages of activity. Thus their measurement provides a reliable tool for identifying early underlying events leading to hemorrhagic or hypercoagulable disorders. Furthermore, with an early diagnosis, specifically targeted therapeutic intervention can be started prior to the establishment of a major pathologic state.

The assay for molecular markers quantitates the native substance and does not involve *in vitro* activation, generation, or other manipulations prior to measurement, as was required in earlier methods such as the PT and APTT. This eliminates sources of error and possible nonphysiological interfering reactions.

Latex Agglutination

Latex agglutination assays for fibrin(ogen) degradation products (FDPs) X, Y, D, and E in serum and urine were developed in the early 1970s. Latex particles coated with specific antibody crosslink with soluble antigenic particles and create a visible precipitate. Elevated levels of FDP have been found in pulmonary embolism, myocardial infarction, and disseminated intravascular coagulation (DIC). Results are usually expressed semiquantitatively, but FDPs may be quantitated by titration. The limitations of this technique allow for identification of particles no smaller than the relatively large D and E fragments (90,000 and 50,000 daltons, respectively) at greater than 2 μg/ml. Since these fragments are derived from both fibrinogen and fibrin, elevated levels cannot be directly correlated to active coagulation. False-positive findings result from the presence of rheumatoid factor in plasma or blood in urine. Although plasma is considered a more physiologic sample, serum must be used as a sample to eliminate the cross-reactivity of fibrinogen. Assay kits are available from Burroughs-Wellcome Co. (Research Triangle Park, NC 27709) and American Dade (Miami, FL 33152).

D-dimer, a digestion product of fibrin, is a definitive indicator of active coagulation. A semiquantitative latex agglutination assay has been developed and is commercially available from AGEN U.S.A., Inc. (Mountain View, CA 94941). Sensitivity of the assay is 20 ng/ml, normal values being less than 200 ng/ml. The assay does not detect fibrinogen or its degradation products (X, Y, D, E). Positive results can be indicative of DIC, postoperative thrombosis, and pulmonary embolism.

Nephelometry

Nephelometric techniques, first reported by Schultze and Schwick in 1959, employed a change in light scatter to quantitate the level of antigen–antibody complex formation.[137] Original nephelometers measured the intensity of light scatter at a 90° angle to the incident light. To increase sensitivity, modifications were made, including the measurement of only forward light scatter and incorporation of electronic devices to minimize background noise due to dust and other contaminants (Fig. 12-11). The use of a polymeric buffer intensified light scatter by enhancing the insolubility of antigen–antibody complexes. The laser was a major development that created a more sensitive system with high-intensity monochromatic light sharply focused into one beam (Fig. 12-12).

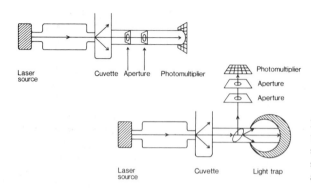

FIG. 12-11. Optics diagram for the measurement of forward light scatter *(top left)* and for the measurement of light scatter at a 90° angle *(bottom right)*.

Nephelometric immunoassay is performed either by end point analysis (1 – 2-hour incubation required) or by a kinetic rate analysis (immediate measure). Assays are available for Factor VIIIR:Ag, protein C, prothrombin, ATIII, α_1-AT, α_2-M, C1-INH, plasminogen, fibrinogen, fibronectin, FDPs, and anaphylatoxins (C3a, C4a, C5a). Applications can be found for the PDQ Laser Nephelometer (Hyland Diagnostics, Division of Travenol Laboratories, Costa Mesa, CA 92626), the Laser Nephelometer System (Behring Diagnostics, Division of American Hoechst Corp., La Jolla, CA 92112), the Beckman Immunochemistry System (Beckman Instruments, Inc., Brea, CA 92621), the J. T. Baker Immunology Series 420 (J. T. Baker Instruments Corp., Allentown, PA 18001), and the Multistat III centrifugal analyzer (Instrumentation Laboratory, Inc., Lexington, MA 02173). Several advantages of nephelometry, such as nonisotopic reagents and ease of automation, may lead to an expansion of this technique in clinical areas.

Radial Immunodiffusion

Immunodiffusion, originally described in 1948 by Ouchterlony, holds that the concentration of an antigen is directly proportional to the rate of precipitate produced as a result of its diffusion in an antiserum-containing agarose preparation.[116] Current radial immunodiffusion (RID) methodology is based on the technique of Mancini, in which a test sample, placed in a well cut into the agarose, diffuses radially from the well.[93] The precipitate area is allowed to reach a maximal size; the square of the diameter of the ring is linearly proportional to the antigen concentration (Fig. 12-13). This simple tech-

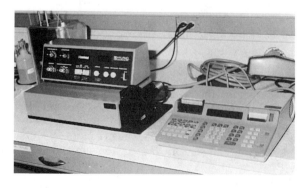

FIG. 12-12. The PDQ laser nephelometer (Hyland Diagnostics, Costa Mesa, CA 92626).

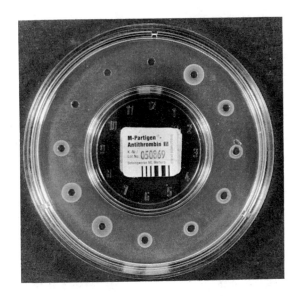

FIG. 12-13. A radial immunodiffusion plate (Calbiochem-Behring, LaJolla, CA 92112), showing a calibration curve for ATIII and several patient samples.

nique is reproducible but time consuming. Forty eight hours are required to obtain results. Assays are commercially available for ATIII, plasminogen, α_1-AT, α_2-M, α_2-AP, and fibrinogen.

Electroimmunodiffusion

First described by Grabar and Williams in 1953, the technique of electroimmunodiffusion (EID or EIP) has remained a powerful analytical tool.[52] In the Laurell rocket technique, antigen migrates under an electric current through an antibody-containing medium, forming precipitate patterns in the shape of a rocket. Quantitation of antigen,

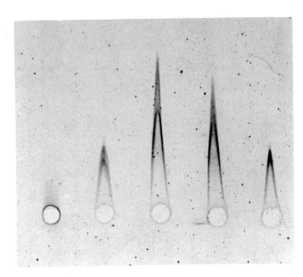

FIG. 12-14. Rocket (Laurell) electroimmunodiffusion showing a calibration of Factor XII antigen and a patient sample of low concentration.

which is proportional to the length of the rocket, can be achieved within 1 to 2 hours (Fig. 12-14).[88]

Two-dimensional electroimmunodiffusion, first described by Ressler in 1960[126] provides more specific identification and characterization of antigens. In practice, one performs the first electrophoretic step as in the rocket assay, then rotates the agar containing antigen–antibody complexes 90° and performs a second electrophoretic step (second dimension) on the pre–electrophoretically separated antigens (Fig. 12-15). Any antigen–antibody combination can be measured with this technique.

Radioimmunoassay

Yalow and Berson[172] were the first reported users of radioimmunoassay (RIA) based on competitive binding of radiolabeled and unlabeled (test sample) antigen to monospecific antibody. The concentration of remaining free, unbound, radiolabeled antigen is quantitated and related to the concentration of unlabeled test antigen through the use of standards. The amount of labeled protein bound to the antibody is inversely proportional to the concentration of bound unlabeled test protein (Fig. 12-16). Radioimmunoassay is the most sensitive technique available for hemostatic testing, although it requires special equipment (semiautomated and fully automated systems are available) and handling of isotopic material. Assays include FPA, $B\beta$ $15-42$–related peptides, PF_4, βTG, prostaglandins, leukotrienes, anaphylatoxins, Factor VIIIR:Ag, ATIII, and plasminogen.

Enzyme Immunoassay

The technique of enzyme immunoassays (EIA) is similar to RIA except that the radionuclide marker is replaced by an enzyme. The final immunologic step is therefore followed by an indicator reaction to allow enzyme activity within the antigen–antibody complex to be photometrically determined. Enzyme markers bound to antibody can be any of the following: peroxidase, alkaline phosphatase, glucose galactosidase, malate dehydrogenase, or glucose-6-phosphate dehydrogenase. Advantages of EIA over RIA are that reagents have a longer shelf-life, there are no strict regulations governing the handling of isotopes, and there is less expense.

Two distinct EIA methods are homogeneous and heterogeneous assays. The homo-

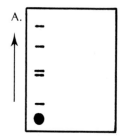 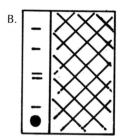 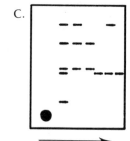

FIG. 12-15. Diagram of the crossed-immunoelectrophoresis technique. (A) First-dimension separation of proteins from sample well origin in an antibody-containing agar. (B) Removal of agar and replacement with new antibody containing agar. (C) Second-dimension separation of proteins at 90° to the first dimension.

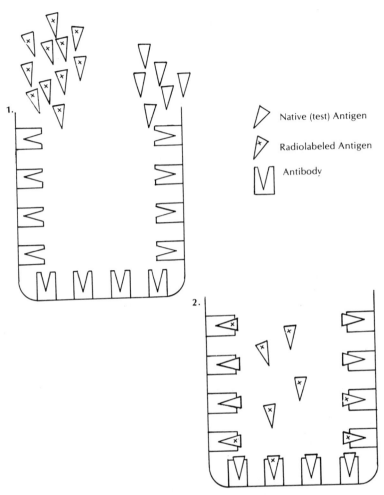

FIG. 12-16. Diagram of the competitive binding principle of radioimmunoassay. *(1)* Antibody is bound to a solid surface. Added test unlabeled and labeled antigen compete for a limited number of antibody binding sites. *(2)* Bound, labeled (*) antigen is then quantitated, and the concentration of the bound, unlabeled test antigen is mathematically determined from the proportion of the total labeled antigen that was able to bind to the antibody in the presence of test antigen.

geneous test involves competitive binding between enzyme-labeled antigen and unlabeled test antigen for a fixed number of antibody binding sites. The principle of quantitation is based on inhibition of the catalytic activity of the enzyme by the antigen–antibody complex. Because a separation step of reagents is not required, this system is referred to as a homogeneous test. This allows for ease of automation, yet it also allows for interference from plasma components (Fig. 12-17).

The heterogeneous test principle, known by the term ELISA (enzyme-linked immunosorbent assay), requires that the free reactant be separated from the solid-phase bound reactant after each reaction. The separation technique is usually a simple aspira-

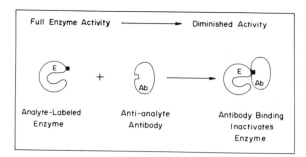

FIG. 12-17. Diagram of a homogeneous enzyme immunoassay. The antigen–(analyte–enzyme) antibody (antianalyte) complex reduces the activity of the enzyme. By competitive binding of the enzyme-labeled analyte and unlabeled (test) analyte for the antibody, quantitation of the test analyte is possible.

tion. However, some procedures may require centrifugation, sedimentation, double-antibody, or glass-bead separation. The ELISA principle involves either a competitive or noncompetitive binding system using an enzyme-linked antigen or an enzyme-linked antibody.

The competitive ELISA principle involves several steps. In a first incubation step, there is competition between plasma antigen and enzyme-labeled antigen for a limited number of antibody molecules previously coated on the inside surface of a plastic container. In a second incubation step, substrate specific for the enzyme label is added. A colored product is released by enzymatic cleavage. The absorbance of the product is inversely proportional to the enzyme–antigen complex bound to the wall. Thus, increasing plasma antigen concentrations result in less color intensity (Fig. 12-18). The ratio between the amount of antibody-bound plasma antigen and antibody-bound enzyme-labeled antigen is used to calculate the relative concentration of the plasma antigen.

The noncompetitive or "sandwich" ELISA principle is often employed in the measurement of relatively large antigens possessing several antigenic determinants. The

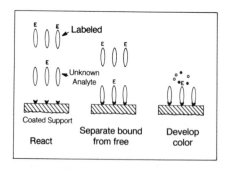

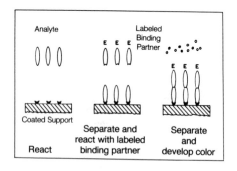

FIG. 12-18. Comparison of the competitive heterogeneous-phase and sandwich enzyme immunoassays. Heterogeneous assays use competitive binding to labeled and unlabeled (test) antigen for solid-phase fixed antibody. Sandwich assays use a second enzyme-labeled antibody to bind to free antigenic sites of the bound antigen–antibody complex. Both use an enzymatic reaction with the labeled antibody in a second step for quantitation.

first step requires antibody to be coated to the inside surface of a plastic support medium. Second, the plasma antigen is added. This antigen binds to the previously coated antibodies. Third, specific enzyme-labeled antibodies are added, producing a "sandwich" complex of antigen bound on two sides by antibody. Next, substrate and chromogen are added to photometrically determine the amount of enzyme-linked antibody bound to the support. Hence, the color intensity is directly proportional to the concentration of antigen (see Fig. 12-17).

Several semiautomated and fully automated ELISA systems for microtiter plates are available with one or more of the following components: a wash/aspiration module, a pipettor/dilutor, and a reader (Fig. 12-19). The microtiter plate allows up to 96 tests per run. Microsampling and low reagent consumption are positive features. Assays currently available by the ELISA technique include PF_4, βTG, FPA, D-dimer, Factors VIIIR:Ag, X, IX, and VII, platelet-bound (direct and indirect) antibodies, and $B\beta$ 15–42–related peptides.

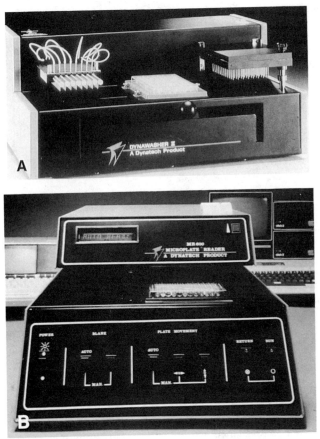

FIG. 12-19. The Dynatech microELISA system (Dynatech, Laboratories, Inc., Alexandria, VA 22314). *(A)* Wash/aspirate instrument. *(B)* Reader.

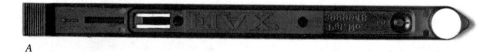

A

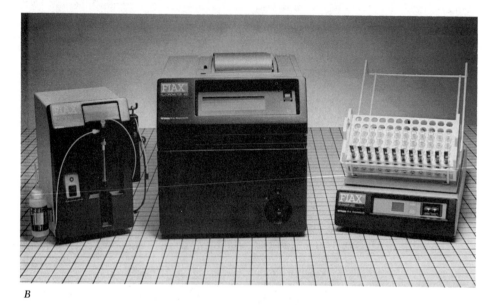

B

FIG. 12-20. The solid-phase dipsticksystem StiQ (International Diagnostic Technology, Inc., Santa Clara, CA 95051). (A) StiQ reaction strip. (B) Strip reader.

Fluoroimmunoassay

Fluoroimmunoassay (FIA) employs the same principle as ELISA, with the exception that a fluorophore is used in place of a chromophore–enzyme conjugate. This may enhance the sensitivity of the reaction. Applications to microbeads and solid-phase dipsticks have been developed.

The FIAX Test System (International Diagnostic Technology, Inc., Santa Clara, CA 95051) offers a dipstick technique. Reagents are contained on a StiQ sampler, upon which the reaction takes place and is read in a specially designed fluorometer. Currently applied coagulation parameters include α_1-AT, α_2-M, and the anaphylatoxins C3, C4, and C5 (Fig. 12-20).

The automated Stratus system (American Dade, Division of American Hospital Supply Corp., Miami, FL 33152) provides fluorometric enzyme immunoassay capability in a dry test tab. The test tab contains immobilized antibody to which sample antigen binds. Added next is enzyme-labeled antigen, which binds to the remaining antibody sites not bound by patient sample. Substrate, which reacts with the enzyme-labeled antigen to produce fluorescence, is then added. This system is capable of performing both sequential (described above) and competitive methodologies in which sample and enzyme-labeled antigen are simultaneously added (Fig. 12-21).

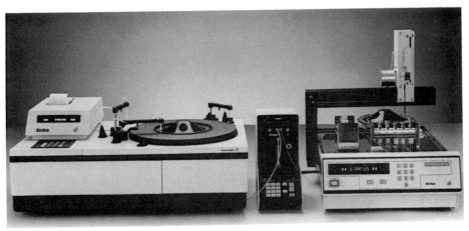

FIG. 12-21. The Stratus system (American Dade, Division of American Hospital Supply Corp., Miami, FL 33152), capable of performing dry chemistry enzyme immunoassays.

SYNTHETIC SUBSTRATE ASSAYS

Synthetic substrate technology may be used to measure procoagulants, activated coagulants, coagulant cofactors, and protease inhibitor activities. This technology has been most successfully applied to protease inhibitors because the prior techniques were tedious, nonspecific, and qualitative. Of all the new hemostatic technologies, synthetic substrates may provide the most significant contribution to the revolution in laboratory testing. Following is a description of the applications currently in use. Commercially available kits for some of the assays are available from American Bioproducts Co. (Parsippany, NJ 07054); Boehringer Mannheim, Diagnostics Division (Indianapolis, IN 46250); and Helena Laboratories (Beaumont, TX 77704).

Antithrombin III

ATIII plays a central role in the regulation of the coagulation system, strongly inhibiting thrombin and Factor X_a.[32,63,138] It also inhibits Factors XII_a, XI_a, and V_a, kallikrein, C1-INH, and plasmin. It is naturally a slow, progressive inhibitor; however, in the presence of heparin, ATIII is potentiated 1000-fold to become a fast-acting inhibitor.[128] The therapeutic efficacy of heparin depends on the presence of ATIII, such that persons lacking this inhibitor fail to respond to heparin therapy. Qualitative abnormalities and quantitative deficiencies of ATIII are associated with an increased risk of thromboembolism, as observed in resistance to heparin therapy, use of oral contraceptives, liver disease, DIC, nephrotic syndrome, and L-asparaginase therapy.[29,48,83,94,163,176] Recently, several commercial therapeutic ATIII preparations have become available.

    Functional assays for ATIII are based on its mechanism of action with heparin.[13,43,53,136] Plasma ATIII, complexed with reagent heparin, inhibits a known amount of thrombin. The residual thrombin (not inhibited) hydrolyzes a thrombin-specific synthetic chromogenic substrate. The measured amidolytic activity ($\Delta A_{405}/\text{min}$) is inversely proportional to the amount of ATIII in the sample, which can be quantitated by comparison to a standard.[3] The principle of this assay is illustrated as follows:

1. Heparin + ATIII $\longrightarrow$ Heparin – ATIII complex
2. Heparin – ATIII + thrombin $\longrightarrow$ Heparin – ATIII – thrombin + residual thrombin
3. R-pNA $\xrightarrow{\text{Residual thrombin}}$ R-COOH + pNA

R-pNA can be any thrombin-specific substrate (see Table 12-6).

Similarly, ATIII can be quantitated by measuring Factor X_a inhibition with the same principle as for thrombin inhibition.

1. Heparin + ATIII $\longrightarrow$ Heparin – ATIII complex
2. Heparin – ATIII + X_a $\longrightarrow$ Heparin – ATIII – X_a + residual X_a
3. R-pNA $\xrightarrow{\text{Residual } X_a}$ R-COOH + pNA

This assay requires a Factor X_a – specific synthetic substrate (see Table 12-6).

Heparin Cofactor II

Heparin also interacts with heparin cofactor II (HCII), a plasma inhibitor distinguishable from ATIII, to inhibit thrombin.[153] This reaction proceeds in a 1 : 1 molar ratio and is similar to the ATIII – heparin reaction except that HCII is a weak inhibitor of Factor X_a. Dermatan sulfate (DS), a glycosaminoglycan similar to heparin, specifically activates HCII but not ATIII. This reaction was used to develop a clinical assay for HCII based on the inhibition of thrombin. Recent clinical evidence has associated a low circulatory level of HCII with thrombosis.[29,39,142] The method of Abildgaard for HCII assay is described below.[2,115]

1. HCII + thrombin + DS $\longrightarrow$ HCII – thrombin – DS + residual thrombin
2. R-pNA $\xrightarrow{\text{Residual thrombin}}$ R-COOH + pNA

Synthetic substrates specific for thrombin are suitable (see Table 12-6).

Indirect assays for the quantitation of HCII have been proposed based on the fact that HCII has minimal interactions with Factor X_a. Assays for ATIII can be performed by both the thrombin and the X_a inhibition techniques, and the difference in activity (thrombin inhibition greater than X_a inhibition) would be attributed to HCII.[56]

α_2-Antiplasmin

Several plasma components inhibit plasmin (see Chap. 2). α_2-AP, also termed α_2-plasmin inhibitor, is the most rapid and specific of the plasmin inhibitors. α_2-AP binds to the light (β) chain of plasmin to form an inactive complex in a reaction that exceeds the speed of the ATIII – heparin – thrombin reaction 100-fold.[108,169] The inhibitory activity of α_2-AP is directed against both fluid-phase and fibrin-bound plasmin. α_2-AP has also been shown to directly bind to fibrin, causing interference in the plasmin – fibrin reaction. α_2-AP inhibits serine proteases other than plasmin such as Hageman factor fragment, kallikrein, Factor XI_a, thrombin, Factor X_a, and urokinase.

In certain disorders of fibrinolysis the level of α_2-AP may be significantly decreased, leading to enhanced or uncontrolled fibrinolysis and excessive bleeding. α_2-AP concentration is decreased in hepatic cirrhosis and DIC and during the course of thrombolytic therapy.[7,8]

The assay for α_2-AP is as follows: a known amount of plasmin is inhibited by test α_2-AP; residual (noninhibited) plasmin is then assayed by a plasmin specific synthetic substrate.[57,75,76]

1. Plasmin $+ \alpha_2$-AP $\longrightarrow$ Plasmin $- \alpha_2$-AP $+$ residual plasmin

2. R-pNA $\xrightarrow{\text{Residual plasmin}}$ R-COOH $+$ pNA

R-pNA can be any plasmin-specific substrate (see Table 12-6).

α_2-Macroglobulin

α_2-M is a dimeric protein with pairs of subunit chains held together by disulfide bridges. Plasma levels of α_2-M drop from 625 mg/dl in infancy to 250 mg/dl in adults. Increases are observed during pregnancy and oral contraceptive use, whereas decreases are observed during thrombolytic therapy.[68,157]

α_2-M has the widest spectrum of protease inhibiting activity, forming complexes with thrombin, plasmin, and kallikrein. Complexes can also be formed with neutral proteases, elastase, collagenase, and cathepsin D. Thus α_2-M may play a regulatory role at cell surfaces or on endothelium. The mechanism of action of α_2-M remains unsolved. In comparison to α_2-AP α_2-M is a slow-acting inhibitor of plasmin.

α_2-M can be quantified in the following manner: α_2-M forms a complex with excess reagent trypsin, and the complex is directly measured by synthetic substrate. Prior to adding the substrate, aprotinin (Trasylol, a basic polypeptide of 6500 daltons that inhibits kallikrein and trypsin) is added to the mixture to inhibit the noncomplexed (residual) trypsin to prevent free trypsin from being measured by the substrate.

1. Trypsin $+ \alpha_2$-M $\longrightarrow \alpha_2$-M$-$trypsin $+$ residual trypsin
2. Residual trypsin $+$ aprotinin $\longrightarrow$ Trypsin $-$ aprotinin

3. R-pNA $\xrightarrow{\alpha_2\text{-M}-\text{trypsin}}$ R-COOH $+$ pNA

Substrates for trypsin can be used (see Table 12-6).

C1-Esterase Inhibitor

C1-INH is a plasma protease inhibitor of C1-esterase (C1-E, the activated first component of complement), kallikrein, plasmin and Factors XI_a, XII_a, and XII_f.[124,135] No hemostatic abnormalities have been reported in persons with C1-INH deficiency, perhaps because of the overlapping inhibitory activity of the other plasma proteases, ATIII and plasminogen activator inhibitor. However, observation of decreased levels has been valuable in the diagnosis of angioneurotic edema, a major life-threatening disease.[38]

C1-INH activity is assayed by various methods through the use of synthetic substrates. In the most direct method, C1-E is mixed with premeasured C1-INH to form a complex. The residual (noncomplexed) C1-E is then measured chromogenically. The concentration of the inhibitor is inversely related to the intensity of the chromophore.

1. C1-E $+$ C1-INH $\longrightarrow$ C1-E$-$C1-INH $+$ residual C1-E

2. R-pNA $\xrightarrow{\text{Residual C1-E}}$ R-COOH $+$ pNA

Synthetic substrates for C1-E are suitable (see Table 12-6).

Protein C

Protein C (PrC) inhibits Factors V_a and VIII_a and stimulates fibrinolysis. PrC is activated by thrombin, the cofactor protein S (PrS), and thrombomodulin, an endothelial cell surface cofactor. It is inhibited by vitamin K antagonists but not by heparin or ATIII.[31,81] Numerous congenital deficiencies of PrC that are directly related to thrombotic complications have been reported.[16,42,55,95,139] Additionally, PrC contained in prothrombin-complex concentrates may be responsible for the undesired anticoagulant activity associated with these treatments.

At present, a reliable functional assay for activated PrC (PrC_a) based on synthetic substrates is not available. However, a model reaction in which PrC_a is measured is presented here.

$$1.\ PrC + thrombomodulin + PrS \longrightarrow PrC_a$$

$$2.\ R\text{-}pNA \xrightarrow{PrC_a} R\text{-}COOH + pNA$$

Synthetic substrates for PrC are suitable but currently do not possess complete specificity. Substrates for thrombin are used, but they are even less specific for PrC. Clotting assays based on the same reaction are presently more reliable.

Protein S

PrS is a vitamin K–dependent serine protease that acts as a cofactor in the activation of PrC. It is quantitated by immunoelectrophoresis.

Plasminogen Activator Inhibitor

Plasminogen activator inhibitor (PAI), a plasma protein of approximately 75,000 daltons, inhibits Factor XII_a and urokinase- or streptokinase-induced activation of plasminogen. However, PAI fails to inhibit plasmin, kallikrein, or Factors XI, X, and IX. The concentrations of this inhibitor and Factor XII are both decreased following cholecystectomy, suggesting that PAI has physiological importance in the control of the Hageman system.[62] The synthetic substrate assay is performed as follows, using premeasured tPA-specific substrates. The inhibition of tPA due to PAI is inversely proportional to the intensity of the chromphore.

$$1.\ tPA + PAI \longrightarrow tPA\text{-}PAI + residual\ tPA$$

$$2.\ R\text{-}pNA \xrightarrow{Residual\ tPA} R\text{-}COOH + pNA$$

α_1-Antitrypsin

The role of α_1-AT as a protease inhibitor is minor even though its plasma concentration is highest of all protease inhibitors. α_1-AT slowly inhibits thrombin; the rate depends on the molar ratio of α_1-AT to thrombin. As the concentration of α_1-AT increases relative to the thrombin concentration, the rate of thrombin inhibition progressively increases. α_1-AT also inhibits plasmin, Factor XI_a, and possibly Factor X_a. There is evidence that α_1-AT regulates the actions of white blood cell enzymes.

Congenital deficiencies of α_1-AT are not associated with major thrombotic or bleeding tendencies.[90,107] α_1-AT is an acute-phase reactant showing increased levels in inflammatory and necrotic diseases (especially hepatocellular diseases), oral contraceptive use, and pregnancy. Proteolytic destruction of pulmonary tissue in congenital α_1-AT deficiency is a direct cause of lung disease.

The test principle for the assay of α_1-AT employs a premeasured trypsin reagent and a trypsin-specific substrate (see Table 12-6).

1. Trypsin $+ \alpha_1$-AT $\longrightarrow \alpha_1$-AT–trypsin complex $+$ residual trypsin

2. R-pNA $\xrightarrow{\text{Residual trypsin}}$ R-COOH $+$ pNA

Heparin

Heparin is a naturally occurring anticoagulant widely used as a therapeutic agent. It is a heterogeneous mixture of straight-chain anionic glycosaminoglycans of variable molecular weight (3,000–30,000 daltons), sulfation, and saccharidic sequencing.

As described previously, heparin potentiates the activity of ATIII and HCII, thereby inhibiting numerous proteases (in particular Factors II_a and X_a but also Factors XII_a, XI_a, and IX_a and kallikrein). Heparin is also suspected in modulating platelet and endothelial cellular activities. The antithrombin action of heparin appears to be highly important for clot inhibition, and it seems to be closely associated with a bleeding tendency.[25] Clinical studies indicate that conventional heparin therapy regulation is best monitored with a clot-based assay such as the APTT (see Chap. 4). Alternate routes of administration of heparin and newer antithrombotic agents produce blood levels of heparin and antithrombotic effects that differ from those of conventional heparin therapy. Thus, a more sensitive assay than the coagulant APTT is required to monitor these therapeutic regimens.

Synthetic substrate assays of individual enzymatic reactions provide useful information not obtainable by clot-based assays. Regulation of heparin therapy through measurement of absolute — not functional — heparin levels or measurement of one isolated heparin effect may, however, be inadequate. Nevertheless, these are the only current means of measuring the activities of heparin derivatives. Several chromogenic assays are available based on either thrombin or Factor X_a inhibition.[12,77,103,166]

ANTITHROMBIN HEPARIN ASSAY

1. Heparin $+$ ATIII $\longrightarrow$ Heparin–ATIII complex
2. Heparin–ATIII $+$ thrombin $\longrightarrow$ Heparin–ATIII–thrombin $+$ residual thrombin

3. R-pNA $\xrightarrow{\text{Residual thrombin}}$ R-COOH $+$ pNA

This assay is a modification of the original amidolytic assay of Odegard.[115] Synthetic substrates for thrombin are suitable (see Table 12-6).

ANTI–FACTOR X_a HEPARIN ASSAY

1. Heparin $+$ ATIII $\longrightarrow$ Heparin–ATIII complex
2. Heparin–ATIII $+ X_a \longrightarrow$ Heparin–ATIII–$X_a +$ residual X_a

3. R-pNA $\xrightarrow{\text{Residual } X_a}$ R-COOH $+$ pNA

This assay is a modification of the original amidolytic assay of Teien.[152] Synthetic substrates for Factor X_a are suitable (see Table 12-6).

Chromogenic assays of heparin depend on the presence of ATIII. The ATIII may be from the patient plasma only or may be supplemented to the assay by addition of excess exogenous ATIII. When endogenous ATIII alone is used, assay results reflect the native response of patient plasma components. When exogenous ATIII is added, the native response is lost, but the measure of absolute heparin concentration is more accurate. Therapeutic levels of heparin are 0.2 to 0.4 USP U/ml. Patient plasma levels are determined by comparison to heparin standards.

Plasminogen

Plasminogen is the precursor of plasmin, the most significant activator of fibrinolysis. Immunologically abnormal plasminogen has been described in persons with thromboembolic disease.[134] Plasminogen deficiencies have been correlated with hyaline membrane disease in premature infants, with DIC, and with promyelocytic leukemia.[4,7,170] Plasminogen measurement is useful in differentiating primary and secondary fibrinolysis. It is essential to have adequate plasminogen levels during thrombolytic therapy for effective treatment.

Plasminogen can be quantitated either in its active form (plasmin) or in the form of an enzymatically active complex that is not affected by endogenous plasma antiplasmins. Streptokinase, a bacterially derived enzyme, is used to activate plasminogen by forming a complex with it. The amidolytic activity of the plasminogen–streptokinase complex (SK-PL) is directly proportional to the plasminogen concentration of the test sample.[120,143,146]

$$1.\ \text{Plasminogen} + \text{streptokinase} \longrightarrow \text{SK-PL}$$

$$2.\ \text{R-pNA} \xrightarrow{\text{SK-PL}} \text{R-COOH} + \text{pNA}$$

Synthetic substrates specific for plasmin are suitable (see Table 12-6).

Plasminogen Activator

Plasminogen activators are a heterogeneous group of serine proteases that convert plasminogen to plasmin. They have been isolated from vascular tissue, plasma, and other body fluids and tissues. Plasminogen activators exist in both zymogenic and active forms. As enzymes they show varying degrees of amidolytic and protease activities. All plasminogen activators cleave the Arg_{560}–Val peptide bond of Glu–plasminogen to create plasmin. The most commonly used activators of plasminogen are urokinase (from urine and kidney tissue culture) and streptokinase (from bacterial cell culture). Urokinase has been isolated in two molecular forms: 55,000 daltons (high molecular weight) and 32,000 daltons (low molecular weight), with specific activities of 100,000 IU/mg protein and 220,000 IU/mg protein, respectively. Streptokinase, isolated from β-hemolytic streptococci, has a molecular weight of 48,000 daltons and a specific activity of 100,000 IU/mg protein. In contrast to urokinase, it is not a serine protease. Rather, streptokinase activates plasminogen by forming a 1:1 molar complex. Human tPA has a molecular weight of 70,000 daltons and a specific activity of 40,000 IU/mg protein. It appears to be a serine protease.

Plasminogen activator levels are known to increase in certain pathologic bleeding states, particularly in the presence of malignant tumors. Decreased levels of tPA are correlated with thromboembolic disease.[62]

tPAs are assayed by synthetic substrate or by an indirect method in which exogenously added plasminogen is transformed into plasmin upon activation by plasminogen activator. The generated plasmin is then measured with plasmin-specific substrates (see Table 12-6). The reaction schemes are given in the following.

DIRECT ASSAY

$$\text{R-pNA} \xrightarrow{\text{Plasminogen activator}} \text{R-COOH} + \text{pNA}$$

INDIRECT ASSAY

1. $\text{Plasminogen} \xrightarrow{\text{Plasminogen activator}} \text{Plasmin}$

2. $\text{R-pNA} \xrightarrow{\text{Plasmin}} \text{R-COOH} + \text{pNA}$

Specificity of these assays remains to be validated. Other, more specific immunologically based (ELISA) assays are available for tPA.

Urokinase and streptokinase used as activators in the above assays are also thrombolytic agents used in the treatment of thromboembolic diseases. Specific chromogenic substrates are employed for direct quantitation of these agents to determine agent potency or circulating levels.[71,150] Activity is expressed in terms of caseinolytic units (CU) or Council on Thrombolytic Agent (CTA) units based on standard agent preparations.

1. $\text{Streptokinase} + \text{plasminogen} \longrightarrow \text{SK-PL}$

2. $\text{R-pNA} \xrightarrow{\text{SK-PL}} \text{R-COOH} + \text{pNA}$

or

$$\text{R-pNA} \xrightarrow{\text{Urokinase-PL}} \text{R-COOH} + \text{pNA}$$

Synthetic substrates for plasmin are suitable for the streptokinase assay, and substrates for urokinase are suitable for the urokinase assay (see Table 12-6).

Factor II$_{(a)}$

Factor II (prothrombin) is quantitated after activation with *Echis carinatus* venom, staphylocoagulase (a secretion product of *Staphylococcus aureus*), or a Factor X_a-V_a- phospholipid$-Ca^{2+}$ mixture. The venom and staphylocoagulase activate both PIVKAs and normal prothrombin, leading to a falsely high level of activity for orally anticoagulated patients. Only prothrombin activated by X_a-V_a-phospholipid$-Ca^{2+}$ is physiologically relevant to a functional defect or coumarin therapy, since this activator most closely simulates the natural coagulation system.[17,80,85] Thrombin generation by Factor X_a is inhibited by synthetic substrates for thrombin; therefore, a two-stage assay is necessary for accurate quantitation.

1. $\text{Prothrombin} \xrightarrow{\text{Activator}} \text{Thrombin}$

2. $\text{R-pNA} \xrightarrow{\text{Thrombin}} \text{R-COOH} + \text{pNA}$

Reagent thrombin can be standardized with a similar assay in which thrombin is directly measured by adding sample to substrate.

Factor V$_{(a)}$

Factor V$_a$ is a cofactor for the enzymatic conversion of prothrombin to thrombin by Factor X$_a$. Platelet phospholipid and free calcium are also required for this reaction. In a proposed amidolytic assay, excess prothrombin, X$_a$, Ca^{2+}, and phospholipid are added to test plasma, wherein Factor V$_a$ is the limiting factor.[58,75,112] Thrombin-specific substrates are used (see Table 12-6).

1. Prothrombin $\xrightarrow{\text{X}_a - \text{Ca}^{2+} - \text{V}_a - \text{phospholipid}}$ Thrombin

2. R-pNA $\xrightarrow{\text{Thrombin}}$ R-COOH + pNA

Factor VII$_{(a)}$

There is no synthetic peptide substrate specific for the direct measurement of Factor VII$_a$. However, several reactions are coupled together to form a measurable product. First, Factor VII is activated by tissue thromboplastin. Second, Factor VII$_a$ activates Factor X. Third, factor X$_a$ is measured by a X$_a$-specific substrate (see Table 12-6).[10,96,121,140]

1. Factor VII $\xrightarrow{\text{Tissue thromboplastin}}$ Factor VII$_a$

2. Factor X $\xrightarrow{\text{Factor VII}_a + \text{Ca}^{2+}}$ Factor X$_a$

3. R-pNA $\xrightarrow{\text{Factor X}_a}$ R-COOH + pNA

One problem exists with this reaction. Since Factor X$_a$ activates additional Factor VII through a feedback loop (see Chap. 2), there is competition by Factor X$_a$ for both Factor VII and synthetic substrate, creating a less than ideal biochemical reaction for measuring Factor X$_a$.

Factor VIII$_{(a)}$

Native Factor VIII acts as a cofactor in the coagulation cascade; it has no protease activity. To measure Factor VIII, it is first modified by thrombin to VIII$_a$, which in turn helps catalyze the activation of Factor X by Factor IX$_a$. Phospholipid and Ca^{2+} must also be present for this reaction. The activated Factor X then cleaves the synthetic substrate. The intensity of the released chromophore is proportional to X$_a$ activity, which is in turn proportional to VIII$_a$ activity.[127]

1. Factor VIII $\xrightarrow{\text{Thrombin}}$ Factor VIII$_a$

2. Factor X $\xrightarrow[\text{VIII}_a]{\text{Ca}^{2+}, \text{ phospholipid, Factor IX}_a}$ Factor X$_a$

3. R-pNA $\xrightarrow{\text{Factor X}_a}$ R-COOH + pNA

Circulating inhibitor of Factor VIII is measured by the same system (see Chap. 4). Plasma containing inhibitor is mixed with pooled normal plasma. Factor VIII from the mixture is measured as above and compared to the Factor VIII level of normal plasma without inhibitor. The difference represents the extent of Factor VIII inhibition. The inhibitor titer is determined by serial dilution of the test plasma.

Factor IX$_{(a)}$

Factor IX activity is measured in a coupled assayed. Factor IX is activated by contact activation reagents such as kaolin or by addition of purified Factor XI$_a$. In the presence of exogenous VIII$_a$, Ca^{2+}, and phospholipid, the generated Factor IX$_a$ then catalyzes activation of Factor X, and X$_a$ in turn is measured. Factor X$_a$ activity is proportional to Factor IX$_a$ activity, which is proportional to the level of Factor IX zymogen in the test plasma. The assay is designed so that Factor IX$_a$ limits the rate of Factor X$_a$ formation.[24,28,102]

1. Factor IX $\xrightarrow{\text{Factor XI}_a,\ \text{Ca}^{2+}}$ Factor IX$_a$

2. Factor X $\xrightarrow[\text{Ca}^{2+},\ \text{phospholipid}]{\text{Factor VIII}_a,\ \text{Factor IX}_a}$ Factor X$_a$

3. R-pNA $\xrightarrow{\text{Factor X}_a}$ R-COOH + pNA

Factor X$_{(a)}$

Factor X is quantified after activation with Russell's viper venom (RVV), and Ca^{2+} is quantified through the use of Factor X$_a$–specific substrates (see Table 12-6).[9,159]

1. Factor X $\xrightarrow{\text{RVV}-\text{Ca}^{2+}}$ Factor X$_a$

2. R-pNA $\xrightarrow{\text{Factor X}_a}$ R-COOH + pNA

Since Factor X activity is decreased during anticoagulant therapy, its quantitation by chromogenic substrates may prove useful in monitoring the therapeutic action of these drugs.[41,72,86,100] However, one must be aware that synthetic substrates are capable of measuring both normal and PIVKA forms of Factor X$_a$.

The trace amount of Factor X$_a$ that is ordinarily formed in blood is instantaneously inhibited by the plasma inhibitors. However, during certain activated states (hypercoagulable states) in which inhibitors are consumed, increased levels of circulating Factor X$_a$ are detected. Freely circulating Factor X$_a$ can be directly quantitated by synthetic substrates by the following method.

R-pNA $\xrightarrow{\text{Factor X}_a}$ R-COOH + pNA

Factor XI$_{(a)}$

No synthetic substrate assay currently exists for the quantitation of plasma Factor XI$_a$. Purified Factor XI or XI$_a$ can, however, be measured directly by the fluorogenic substrate Boc-Phe-Ser-Arg-MCA. (Peptide Research Institute, Minoh, Osaka, Japan).

Factor XII$_{(a)}$

Factor XII is measured indirectly through the use of a substrate for plasma kallikrein. Plasma Factor XII is activated to XII$_a$ via contact activation with kaolin or similar substances. Since plasma prekallikrein is also activated, the sample is incubated at 37°C for 60 minutes to inactivate the formed kallikrein. This does not inactivate Factor XII_a. Factor XII_a is now added to a known amount of prekallikrein, which is thereby converted to kallikrein. Kallikrein is then measured chromogenically.[36,161]

$$1. \text{ Factor XII} \xrightarrow{\text{Kaolin}} \text{Factor XII}_a$$

$$2. \text{ Prekallikrein} \xrightarrow{\text{Factor XII}_a} \text{Kallikrein}$$

$$3. \text{ R-pNA} \xrightarrow{\text{Kallikrein}} \text{R-COOH} + \text{pNA}$$

Note that the apparent simultaneous activation of Factor XII and prekallikrein is a complicated biochemical mechanism of which the kinetics are largely unknown. Therefore, the precise conditions for an accurate quantitation are yet to be determined.

Prekallikrein

Prekallikrein (Fletcher factor) is quantified by converting the proenzyme to the active enzyme, kallikrein, and directly measuring kallikrein activity.[5,78,147-149] Activators that can be used to activate prekallikrein include dextran, ellagic acid, micronized silica, and kaolin. Substrates specific for kallikrein are suitable (see Table 12-6).

$$1. \text{ Prekallikrein} \xrightarrow{\text{Activator}} \text{Kallikrein}$$

$$2. \text{ R-pNA} \xrightarrow{\text{Kallikrein}} \text{R-COOH} + \text{pNA}$$

Platelet Factor 3 (Platelet Phospholipid)

A chromogenic substrate method to determine platelet factor 3 (PF_3) has been described by Sandberg and coworkers.[132] Platelet-rich plasma (PRP) is prepared from patient whole blood. The PRP contains both factors, Factors V and X, required for the reaction. Factor X is activated by addition of Russell's viper venom. The amount of PF_3 is the rate-limiting factor in the reaction mixture containing Factors X_a and V_a and Ca^{2+}. This complex converts reagent prothrombin to thrombin, which in turn is measured by synthetic substrate. Cleavage of substrate releases chromophore, the intensity of which is proportional to the concentration of PF_3. This method is relatively new, and normal values have not yet been established.

$$1. \text{ Prothrombin} \xrightarrow{X_a, V_a, Ca^{2+}, PF_3} \text{Thrombin}$$

$$2. \text{ R-pNA} \xrightarrow{\text{Thrombin}} \text{R-COOH} + \text{pNA}$$

Platelet Factor 4

Vinazzer and colleagues[160] described a chromogenic substrate method for measurement of platelet factor 4 (PF_4). Patient PRP is either treated with epinephrine or collagen to activate platelets or homogenized to release all PF_4 from the platelet granules. The ability of PF_4 to inactivate heparin is used to measure PF_4. The PRP supernate or homogenate is added to a mixture of heparin, ATIII, and Factor X_a. Heparin ordinarily inhibits the activity of Factor X_a but is rendered unable to do so in the presence of PF_4. Therefore, increased PF_4 in the patient plasma results in suppression of reagent heparin. More X_a is then available to cleave chromophore from the substrate. The intensity of chromophore is directly proportional to the original concentration of PF_4.

1. Heparin $+ PF_4 \longrightarrow$ Heparin $- PF_4 +$ residual heparin
2. Residual heparin $+ ATIII \longrightarrow$ Heparin $- ATIII$ complex
3. Heparin $- ATIII +$ Factor $X_a \longrightarrow$ Heparin $- ATIII -$ Factor $X_a +$ residual Factor X_a
4. R-pNA $\xrightarrow{\text{Residual Factor } X_a}$ R-COOH $+$ pNA

Similarly, a thrombin-based heparin assay can be employed for the measurement of PF_4. S-2222 (KabiVitrum, Stockholm, Sweden) was the substrate used in this reaction.

Synthetic Substrate – Based Prothrombin Time

In the clot-based PT, citrated plasma is activated with tissue thromboplastin and calcium chloride (see Chap. 4). The thrombin that is generated catalyzes the formation of detectable fibrin from fibrinogen. A chromogenic substrate may be substituted for fibrinogen to detect thrombin formation.[14,45]

1. Plasma $\xrightarrow[\text{Ca}^{2+}]{\text{Tissue thromboplastin}}$ Thrombin

2. R-pNA $\xrightarrow{\text{Thrombin}}$ R-COOH $+$ pNA

Thrombin-specific substrates inhibit the Factor X_a generated during coagulation. Numerous attempts have been made to develop substrates devoid of this undesirable effect, but none have been successful to date.

Synthetic Substrate – Based Activated Partial Thromboplastin Time

In the clot-based APTT, partial thromboplastin and calcium chloride are used to initiate clot formation. A chromogenic substrate may be substituted for fibrinogen, as in the PT.[45,173]

1. Plasma $\xrightarrow[\text{Ca}^{2+}]{\substack{\text{Partial thromboplastin and} \\ \text{contact activation}}}$ Thrombin

2. R-pNA $\xrightarrow{\text{Thrombin}}$ R-COOH $+$ pNA

As in the PT, thrombin-specific synthetic substrates devoid of Factor X_a inhibition have not been produced to date. Synthetic substrate – based techniques are currently available for routine PT or APTT assay; however, their reliability in clinical laboratory use is under investigation.

Total Serine Protease Activity Screen

In certain diseases, plasma, serum, ascitic fluid, amniotic fluid, and pleural fluid contain free serine protease activity, such as measurable levels of trypsin, thrombin, or kallikrein. These enzymes, in activated forms, are usually not present in body fluids. To assay for activity, test fluid is added to a pH-specific buffer and an enzyme-specific synthetic substrate such as S-2302. The reaction rate of the activity is monitored, and test serine protease activity is directly quantitated by comparison to specific enzyme standards. Activities are confirmed by blocking the protease activity with a suitable inhibitor; for example, kallikrein activity is blocked by the addition of aprotinin. Serine proteases are unstable, so test samples are tested immediately or frozen. Centrifugation may be necessary to remove fibrin and cellular debris.

IMMUNOASSAYS

Low-molecular-weight ($<$10,000 daltons) products of hemostatic activation are excellent markers for the physiologic or pathologic processes responsible for their formation. Immunoassay is the only practical way to measure these molecular markers because they circulate in nanogram or picogram levels and are very small in structure.

The following section describes various immunologic assays used in the quantitation of these markers and makes reference to clinical applications. Older methods for immunologic determination of the larger hemostatic proteins have been described in this chapter and will not be discussed further.

Because of the nature of molecular markers, special collection and handling procedures are required to maintain a physiologic sample for accurate quantitation:

1. Only a nontraumatic, double-syringe venipuncture is acceptable (see Chap. 3). Second-syringe blood is used for analysis.
2. Special anticoagulants containing specific inhibitors must be used to avoid either degradation or generation of the molecular markers ex vivo. EDTA anticoagulant for PF_4 studies or a mixture of EDTA, aprotinin, thrombin inhibitor, and indomethacin to inhibit all coagulation, platelet, and fibrinolytic activities can be used.
3. Collection tubes must be prechilled.
4. Collected blood must be placed immediately on ice and be centrifuged at high speed (4°C) within 30 minutes of the draw. Only the middle third of plasma is separated from cells and either assayed immediately or frozen at −70°C.
5. The general status of the patient should be noted to account for possible elevated levels of certain markers due to exercise, stress, or medication.
6. Other body fluids, such as urine and spinal fluid, are also suitable samples.

Fibrinopeptides A and B

Thrombin hydrolysis of fibrinogen yields two small soluble peptides: fibrinopeptide A and fibrinopeptide B (FPA and FPB).[113] As FPA and FPB are released, polymerization sites on the central "D" and "E" domains of the remaining fibrinogen molecule are exposed (see Chap. 2). The cleaved fibrinogen molecules assemble side to side and end to end, joining at the exposed sites. This reaction is facilitated by Factor XIII_a and Ca^{2+}. The resulting polymer is crosslinked fibrin.

$$\text{Fibrinogen} \xrightarrow{\text{Thrombin}} \text{Fibrin} + 2\text{FPA} + 2\text{FPB}$$

Immunoassay of FPA provides an early, specific indication of thrombin activation. The plasma FPA reference range is 0.5 to 3 ng/ml. Increased plasma FPA levels are found in DIC, neoplasia, burns, and various leukemias and following hip surgery.[33,104,110,117,158,175] Decreased levels are seen in antithrombotic therapy.[118,153,174]

FPB is not measured, because of its 30-second half-life. Commercial ELISA kits are available from American Bioproducts Co. (Parsippany, NJ 07054).

Bβ-Related Peptides

Plasmin progressively degrades fibrin or fibrinogen to first release a series of peptides from the B chain. These are Bβ-related peptides that include Bβ 1–118, Bβ 1–42, and the most common, Bβ 15–42. Numbers indicate the amino acid region cleaved from the fibrin molecule.[151] Subsequent cleavage yields larger Fragments X, Y, D, and E from the D and E domains. These larger fragments are released in complexes from normally crosslinked fibrin or as singular fragments from noncrosslinked fibrin, as is seen in Factor XIII deficiency. Immunoassay of Bβ-related peptides yields elevated results in DIC, primary fibrinolysis, and burns.[87,114] Bβ-related peptides are normally present in plasma at a concentration range of 0.5 ng to 30 ng/ml.

Both FPA and Bβ fibrinopeptides are associated with hypercoagulable conditions. Furthermore, the specific origins of both substances allow differentiation between primary and secondary fibrinolysis. Primary fibrinolysis associated with plasmin activity will show an increased level of Bβ peptides but a normal level of FPA, PF_4, and βTG. Conversely, in secondary fibrinolysis or DIC, the coagulant, fibrinolytic, and platelet pathways are activated, producing increased levels of FPA, Bβ peptides, and platelet release products.

Kits are commercially supplied by IMCO Corp. (Stockholm, Sweden) for RIA analysis and by the New York Blood Center (New York, NY 10021) and American Bioproducts Co. (Parsippany, NJ 07054) for ELISA-based analysis.

Platelet Factor 4

PF_4 is a specific platelet release protein secreted in complex with a proteoglycan carrier. It is stored in the alpha granules and released upon platelet activation.[11,106] Physiologically, PF_4 functions as an antiheparin substance binding to heparin at a site different from the binding site of ATIII.[111] PF_4 has also been shown to inhibit collagenase and to potentiate granulocyte elastase, thus regulating cell growth.[66,91] Normal plasma PF_4 levels are 4 ng to 8 ng/ml. Elevated levels have been observed during myocardial infarction, venous thrombosis, myeloproliferative syndrome, diabetes, and inflammatory states.[59,110,114,171]

PF_4 is quantitated by RIA or ELISA techniques available from Abbott Laboratories (Diagnostic Division, North Chicago, IL 60064) and American Bioproducts Co. (Parsippany, NJ 07054), respectively.

β-Thromboglobulin

βTG is a specific platelet release protein stored in the alpha granules.[105] Its physiologic function is considered to be antiheparin. Normal plasma levels are 20 ng to 40 ng/ml. Elevated levels have been associated with similar conditions associated with increased PF_4 levels.[35,110,114,144]

βTG is quantitated by an RIA technique available from Amersham, Inc. (Arlington Hts., IL 60005).

Prostaglandins

Prostaglandins are unsaturated hydroxylated fatty acids derived from phosphatidylino-sitol and phosphatidylcholine by the enzymatic action of phospholipases C and A_2, respectively. These substances produce profound effects at very low concentrations, interacting with specific receptors at a cellular level. Prostaglandins are associated with the reproductive, cardiovascular, renal, pulmonary, immunologic, nervous, and gastro-intestinal systems, and only those assays relevant to hemostasis will be described here. Leukotrienes are substances of a similar nature that can also be quantitated with immu-nologic assays.[21,23,131]

Because of the extremely short half-lives (about 8 minutes) of prostaglandins, they are measured by their biologically inactive stable metabolites. Thromboxane B_2 is a stable metabolite of thromboxane A_2 (TxA_2) derived from arachidonic acid through the cyclooxygenase pathway. TxA_2 is a very potent vasodilator and a potent platelet aggre-gating agent. Conversely, prostacyclin (PGI_2 or $PGF_{1\alpha}$), also derived from arachidonic acid through the cyclooxygenase pathway, is a potent vasoconstrictor and inhibitor of platelet aggregation. A homeostatic balance exists between thromboxane production in the platelet and prostacyclin production in the endothelium.

Nonsteroidal anti-inflammatory agents (NSAIAs) like aspirin and indomethacin are used in antiplatelet therapy. NSAIAs react with cyclooxygenase, so their effects may be monitored through measurement of prostaglandin end products like TXB_2 and $PGF_{1\alpha}$ (see Chap. 8). Other prostaglandins produced by platelets, such as PGE_2, PGF_2, and PGD_2, are also measurable, although their physiologic roles are less clear. Normal plasma levels of all prostaglandins are 0 pg to 5 pg/ml. Preliminary studies have shown possible involvement of prostaglandins in uremia, hypertension, endotoxic shock, ischemic heart disease, diabetes, cerebrovascular disease, and artheroscler-osis.[26,69,89,98,99,125,130,167,174] RIA kits are commercially available through New England Nuclear (Boston, MA 02118) and Seragen, Inc. (Boston, MA 02122).

Platelet-Associated Immunoglobulins

An ELISA platelet antibody assay has been developed by Organon Teknika Corp. (Par-sippany, NJ 07054) to investigate drug-induced thrombocytopenia. This assay mea-sures either platelet-bound (direct) or circulating plasma (indirect) IgG or IgM antibod-ies to platelets. Platelet immunoglobulins may consist of true antiplatelet antibodies binding to platelet Fc receptors or endogenous IgG bound to normal platelets.[79] The increased amount of bound immunoglobulin is responsible for rapid clearance of plate-lets by the mononuclear phagocytic system, resulting in the clinical manifestations of thrombocytopenia.[141,142] Platelet-associated IgG is elevated in isoimmune neonatal thrombocytopenia, alloimmune thrombocytopenia, idiopathic or autoimmune throm-bocytopenic purpura, and drug-induced thrombocytopenia.[60]

Coagulant Factors

ELISA-based kits have been introduced for Factors VII, VIII, IX, and X and PrC from American Bioproducts Co. (Parsippany, NJ 07054). These allow rapid screening and quantitation of the antigenically reactive factors.

Serine Protease–Inhibitor Complexes

Activated serine proteases form complexes with their respective inhibitors, for example, X_a–ATIII, II_a–ATIII, plasmin–α_2-AP, plasmin–α_2-M, kallikrein–C1-INH, complement–C1-INH, and PrC_a–C_a inhibitor. The presence of formed complexes in circulation indicates hemostatic activation.[28] Activated systems can be identified by the specific complexes. Monoclonal antibodies to these complexes are being developed to be used in RIA or ELISA techniques.

Complement

Circulating complement system zymogens are activated by antibodies, endotoxin, plasmin, or trypsin (classic pathway) or by bacterial lipopolysaccharides and parasitic antigens (alternative pathway). Complement activation leads to cellular lysis, chemotaxis, and phagocytosis, effecting removal of foreign particles from the host. These same factors cause tissue damage when overactivated. The hemostatic system has been linked with the complement system in DIC; for example, thrombin cleaves C3 and C5, and several platelet–complement and coagulation factor–complement factor interactions have been observed (see Chap. 8).[22,54,64,70,122,148]

Individual components of the complement system are assayed by chromogenic substrate and nephelometric techniques, by solid-phase chemistry through the use of the FIAX systems from International Diagnostic Technology (Santa Clara, CA 95051), and by RIA through the use of the Upjohn Co. (Kalamazoo, MI 49001) assay.

MISCELLANEOUS

Circulating biologically active substances of a chemically heterogeneous nature interact with the various biochemical pathways of hemostasis. Serotonin, a platelet release product, is measured by RIA and high-pressure liquid chromatography. Other platelet-related products include platelet activating Factor (PAF) a β-lysin, and substances that increase vascular permeability, proliferation of smooth muscle cells, and chemotaxis.[15,27,34,37,109,129,168] Lymphokines and monokines are currently under investigation for their effects in thrombotic disorders, demonstrating certain interactions with platelets, fibrinogen, and vessel walls. Current indications are that the leukocyte may be an important component of the hemostatic mechanism. Angiotensin is closely associated with the contact phase of coagulation via bradykinin. Several neurotransmitters— catecholamines, purines, pyrimidines, endorphins, and enkephalins—may act as messengers to regulate the activation or inhibition of clotting. Glycosaminoglycans, including heparins, heparans, dermatans, and chondroitins, are endogenous regulators of thrombotic activity.[111]

The current status of these substances is not as clearly demarcated as that of the coagulation and fibrinolytic proteins or molecular marker peptides. However, taking into account the integrated nature of physiology and the complexity of hemostasis, the future may reveal a direct relevance of these substances to the regulation of hemostasis.

CLINICAL RELEVANCE

It is often difficult to identify and differentiate hemostatic disorders on the basis of global screening tests such as the PT and APTT and tests of fibrinogen and fibrin(ogen) split products, which are designed only for hemorrhagic disorders and not thrombotic disorders. As a result, relatively high rates of morbidity and mortality associated with thrombotic complications have occurred. Due to an increased understanding of the biochemistry and molecular biology of hemostasis, recent developments in clinical methodology with application to automated instrumentation have been made.

Hemostasis is a balance between complex interactions of directly opposing systems (coagulation and fibrinolysis) with seemingly unrelated systems on both the enzymatic (complement) and cellular (platelets, endothelium, leukocytes) levels. It should not be surprising that coagulation disorders often accompany many different disease states. Individual enzymes, inhibitors, cellular release products, and low-molecular-weight products of activation reactions (molecular markers) are now measured in sensitive, specific assays that go far beyond the limits of the global PT and APTT. With this new perspective in assessing pathologic hemostatic conditions, not only can therapeutic intervention begin during early stages of disease (*i.e.,* at subclinical stages before major pathologic complications are established), but it can also be more specifically targeted to the particular abnormality. Advanced therapeutic approaches recently introduced are plasma fractions for procoagulant therapy, antiplatelet agents, depolymerized heparins, subcutaneous heparin, and fibrinolytic agents. Furthermore, prophylactic therapy can be administered to those considered at risk to develop thrombosis.

It is interesting to note that many of the newer therapeutic and prophylactic regimens, while effective in the patient, demonstrate no effect on the PT and APTT. However, certain molecular markers or synthetic substrate assays are capable of monitoring the effects of these therapies. Through the use of these newer assays, it has become apparent that many therapeutic and nontherapeutic invasive techniques such as plasmapheresis and administration of contrast media cause an activation of the hemostatic system. Widespread use of the more sensitive assays may identify other such unforeseen stresses so that possible medical complications can be avoided.

Technological advances in methodology and instrumentation have changed the scope of all clinical laboratories, but in particular the coagulation laboratory. An overall development has been the result of influences from clinical chemistry, clinical immunology, pharmacology, biochemistry, and biotechnology. Analytical instruments for use in hemostatic testing go beyond the clot-based readers and platelet aggregometers to a range of automated discrete chemistry analyzers, batch processors, microtiter systems, and the newest multiprobe instruments designed to measure two or three different physical end points. Moreover, automation has the distinct advantages of operational simplicity, microsampling, low reagent consumption, cost-effectiveness, and computer compatibility for fast and accurate data reduction.

The capabilities of these newer technologies in evaluating hemostasis provide a means for standardization and quality control of therapeutic agents, assay reagents, and methodology. The global PT and APTT assays were not capable of these types of assessments.

At present, the clinical relevance of the newly identified parameters described in this chapter must be established in many clinical instances. However, a future in which the potential of monitoring these parameters will be a reality can be visualized.

REFERENCES

1. Abildgaard U, Gravem K, Godal HC: Assay of progressive antithrombin in plasma. Thromb Diath Haemorrh 24:224, 1970
2. Abildgaard U, Larsen ML: Assay of dermatan sulfate cofactor (heparin cofactor II) activity in human plasma. Thromb Res 35:257, 1984
3. Abildgaard U, Lie M, Odegard OR: Antithrombin (heparin co-factor) assay with "new" chromogenic substrates (S-2238 and Chromozym TH). Thromb Res 11:549, 1977
4. Ambrus CM, Weintraub DH, Dunphy D et al: Studies on hyaline membrane disease. I. The fibrinolytic system in pathogenesis and therapy. Pediatrics 32:10, 1963
5. Amundsen E, Svendsen L: A new assay for plasma kallikrein activity utilizing a synthetic chromogenic substrate. In Witt I (ed): New Methods for the Analysis of Coagulation Using Chromogenic Substrates, pp 211–219. New York, Walter de Gruyter, 1977
6. Andreasen T: Automated two-stage assay for determination of antithrombin III with a centrifugal analyzer. Haemostasis 9:65, 1980
7. Aoki N, Saito H, Kamiya T et al: Congenital deficiency of α_2-plasmin inhibitor associated with severe hemorrhagic tendency. J Clin Invest 63:877, 1979
8. Aoki N, Yamanaka T: The α_2-plasmin inhibitor levels in liver diseases. Clin Chim Acta 84:99, 1978
9. Aurell L, Friberger P, Lenne C et al: Method for the determination of factor X in plasma using the chromogenic substrate S-2337. In Fareed J (ed): Perspectives in Hemostasis, pp. 382–388. New York, Pergamon Press, 1981
10. Avvisati G, ten Cate JW, Van Wijk EM et al: Evaluation of a new chromogenic assay for factor VII and its application in patients on oral anticoagulant treatment. Br J Haematol 45(2):343, 1980
11. Barber AG, Kaser-Glanzmann R, Jakabova M, Luscher EF: Characterization of chrondroitin sulfate proteoglycan carrier for heparin neutralizing activity-(PF₄) released from human blood platelets. Biochim Biophys Acta 286:316, 1972
12. Bartl K, Dorsch E, Lill H, Ziegenhorn J: Determination of the biological activity of heparin by use of a chromogenic substrate. Thromb Haemost 42:1446, 1979
13. Bartl K, Lill H: A versatile essay method of antithrombin III using thrombin and Tos-Gly-Pro-Arg-PNA. Thromb Res 18(1–2):267, 1980
14. Baughman DJ, Lytwyn A: Thrombin activation rate constant: One stage chromogenic assay for the extrinsic system. Thromb Res 26(1):1, 1982
15. Beneviste J, Le Couedic JP, Polonsky J, Tence M: Structural analysis of purified platelet-activating factor by lipases. Nature 269:170, 1977
16. Bertina RM, Broekmans AW, van der Linden IK, Mertens K: Protein C deficiency in a Dutch family with thrombotic disease. Thromb Haemost 48:1, 1982
17. Bertina RM, Marel VD, Nieuwkoop W, Loeliger EA: Spectrophotometric assays of prothrombin in plasma of patients using oral anticoagulants. Thromb Haemost 42:1296, 1979
18. Bick RL, Kovacs I, Fekete LF: A new two-stage functional assay for antithrombin III (heparin cofactor): Clinical and laboratory evaluation. Thromb Res 8:745, 1976
19. Biggs R, Douglas AS: The measurement of prothrombin in plasma. J Clin Pathol 6:15, 1953
20. Blomback B: Synthetic substrates and synthetic inhibitors: The use of chromogenic substrates in studies of the hemostatic mechanism. Haemostasis 7:183, 1978
21. Borgeat P, Sirois P: Leukotrienes: A major step in the understanding of immediate hypersensitivity reactions. J Med Chem 24:121, 1981
22. Branson HE, Wyatt DO, Schmer G: Complement consumption in acute disseminated intravascular coagulation without antecedent immunopathology. Am J Clin Pathol 66:967, 1976
23. Bray MA: Leukotriene D4: An inflammatory mediator with vascular actions in vivo. Agents Actions 11:51, 1982
24. Byrne R, Link RP, Castellino JF: A kinetic evaluation of activated bovine blood coagulation factor IX toward synthetic substrates. J Biol Chem 225(11):5336, 1980

25. Carter CJ, Kelton JG, Hirsh J et al: The relationship between the hemorrhagic and antithrombotic properties of low molecular weight heparin in rabbits. Blood 59:1239, 1982
26. Chen LS, Itu T, Ogawa K, Staka T: Changes of plasma 6-keto-PGF_1 alpha and thromboxane B_2 levels and platelet aggregation after tourniquet on the upper limb in normal subjects in patients with ischemic heart disease. Jpn Circ J 46:651, 1982
27. Chignard M, Le Couedic JP, Vargaftug BB, Benveniste J: Platelet-activating factor (PAF-acether) secretion from platelets: Effect of aggregating agents. Br J Haematol 46:455, 1980
28. Collen D, de Cock F: Thrombin antithrombin-III and plasma α_2-antiplasmin complexes as indicators of in vivo activation of coagulation and/or fibrinolytic systems. Thromb Haemost 38:173, 1975
29. Collen D, Schertz J, de Cock F, Holmer E, Verstraete M: Metabolism of antithrombin-III (heparin cofactor) in man: Effects of venous thrombosis and heparin administration. Eur J Clin Invest 7:27, 1977
30. Colman RW, Mason JW, Sherry S: The kallikreinogen–kallikrein enzyme system of human plasma: Assay of components and observations in disease state. Ann Intern Med 71:763, 1969
31. Comp PC, Jacocks RM, Ferrell GL, Esmon CT: Activation of protein C in vivo. J Clin Invest 70:127, 1982
32. Conard J, Samama M: L'antithrombine III. Rev Med 19:2343, 1978
33. Cronlund M, Hardin J, Burton J et al: Fibrinopeptide A in plasma of normal subjects and patients with disseminated intravascular coagulation and systemic lupus erythematosus. J Clin Invest 58:142, 1976
34. Demopoulos CA, Pinkard RN, Hanahan DJ: Platelet activating factor: evidence for 1-O-alkyl-2-acetyl-sn-glyceryl-3-phosphorylcholine as the active component (a new class of lipic chemical mediators). J Biol Chem 254:9355, 1979
35. Denham MJ, Fisher M, James G, Hassan M: Plasma concentration of β-thromboglobulin in venous and arterial thrombosis. Lancet i:1154, 1977
36. Dick W, Cullmann W, Muller N, Adler K: Factor XII assay with the chromogenic substrate chromozyme PK. J Clin Chem Clin Biochem 19(6):357, 1981
37. Donaldson DM, Tew JG: Beta-lysin of platelet origin. Bacteriol Rev 41:501, 1977
38. Donaldson WH, Evans RR: A biochemical abnormality in hereditary angioneurotic edema: Absence of serum inhibitor of C'1-esterase. Am J Med 35:37, 1963
39. Duckert F, Tran TH, Marbet GA: Association of hereditary heparin cofactor II deficiency with thrombosis. Lancet 2:413, 1985
40. Dunikowski LK, Myrmel KH, Derzack MT: Automated chromogenic antithrombin III assay with a centrifugal analyzer. Clin Chem 25:1076, 1979
41. Erskine JG, Walker ID, Davidson JF: Maintenance control of oral anticoagulant therapy by a chromogenic substrate assay for factor X. J Clin Pathol 33(5):445, 1980
42. Esmon CT: Protein C: Biochemistry, physiology and clinical implications. Blood 62:1155, 1983
43. Fareed J, Messmore HL, Bermes EW Jr, Bick RL: Laboratory evaluation of antithrombin III: A critical overview of currently available methods for antithrombin III measurements. Semin Thromb Hemost 8(4):288, 1982
44. Fareed J, Messmore HL, Walenga JM, Bermes EW Jr: Synthetic peptide substrates in hemostatic testing. CRC 19(2):71, 1983
45. Fareed J, Messmore HL, Walenga JM et al: Synthetic peptide substrates in the monitoring of anticoagulant and procoagulant therapy J Clin Chem biochem 19(8):663, 1981
46. Fareed J, Walenga J (guest eds): Automation in Coagulation Testing, Parts 1 and 2. Semin Thromb Hemost 9(3/4), 1983
47. Fareed J, Walenga JM, Bick RL et al: Impact of automation on the quantitation of low molecular weight markers of hemostatic defects. Semin Thromb Hemost 9(4):349, 1983
48. Filip DJ, Eckstein JD, Veltkamp JJ: Hereditary antithrombin III deficiency and thromboembolic disease. Am J Hematol 2:343, 1976

49. Friberger P: Synthetic peptide substrate assays in coagulation and fibrinolysis and their application on automates. Semin Thromb Hemost 9(4):275, 1983

50. Girolami A, Bareggi G, Brunetti A, Sticchi A: Prothrombin Padua: A "new" congenital dysprothrombinemia. J Lab Clin Med 84:654, 666, 1974

51. Girolami A, Patrassi G, Toffanin F, Saggin L: Chromogenic substrate (S-2238) prothrombin assay in prothrombin deficiencies and abnormalities: Lack of identity with clotting assays in congenital dysprothrombinemias. Am J Clin Pathol 74(1):83, 1980

52. Grabar P, Williams CT: Methode permettant l'etude conjugee des proteines: Application au serum sanguim. Biochim Biophys Acta 10:193, 1953

53. Gray AJ, Uhlmeyer KA, Fedor EJ: Quantichrom AT-III: Diagnostic kit for the quantification of total antithrombin-III in plasma (abstr). Thromb Haemost 42:225, 1979

54. Graybill JR, Hawiger J, Des Prez RM: Complement and coagulation in Rocky Mountain spotted fever. South Med J 66:410, 1973

55. Griffin JH: Clinical studies on protein C. Semin Thromb Hemost 10:162, 1984

56. Griffith M, Carraway T, White G, Dombrose F: Heparin cofactor activities in a family with hereditary antithrombin III deficiency: Evidence for a second heparin cofactor in human plasma. Blood 61:111, 1983

57. Gyzander E, Friberger P, Myrwold H et al: Antiplasmin determination by means of the plasmin specific substrate S-2251 — methodological studies and some clinical applications. In Witt I (ed): New Methods for the Analysis of Coagulation Using Chromogenic Substrates, pp 229–245. Berlin, Walter de Gruyter, 1977

58. Hagglund N, Blomback M: Amidolytic assay of factor V in plasma. Proc World Fed Hemophilia Congr, 27 June–1 July, 1983, Stockholm, p 61, abstr #243

59. Handin RI, McDonough M, Leach M: Elevation of platelet factor 4 in acute myocardial infarction: Measurement by radioimmunoassay. J Lab Clin Med 91:340, 1978

60. Harmon JA, Miller WV: Platelet antibodies: Their detection and significance. Am J Med Technol 47(10):797, 1981

61. Harris AL, Calvert KM, Collins RE, Fan PE: Evaluation of the DuPont "aca" methods for the assay of FBG, PLG, and AT III. Clin Chem 28:1585, 1982

62. Hedner U: Inhibitor(s) of plasminogen activation distinct from the other plasma protease inhibitors—a review. In Collen D, Wiman B, Verstraete M (eds): The Physiological Inhibitors of Coagulation and Fibrinolysis, p 189. Amsterdam, Elsevier/North-Holland Press, 1979

63. Hensen A, Loeliger EA: Antithrombin-III: Its metabolism and its function in blood coagulation. Thromb Diath Haemorrh 9(Suppl 1):1, 1963

64. Hensikveld RS, Leddy JP, Klemperer MR, Breckenridge RT: Hereditary deficiency of the sixty components of complement in man. II. Studies of hemostasis. J Clin Invest 53:554, 1974

65. Hills LP, Lorenzi-Anderson M, Huey E, Tiffany T: Use of a centrifugal analyzer in coagulation testing. Semin Thromb Hemost 9(3):217, 1983

66. Hiti-Harper J, Wohl H, Harper E: Platelet factor 4: An inhibitor of collagenase. Science 199:991, 1978

67. Holmes EW, Fareed J, Bermes EW: Automated antithrombin III determination using two assay systems. Clin Chem 26:1073, 1980

68. Horne CHW, Howie PW, Wier RJ, Goudie RB: Effect of combined oestrogen–protestogen oral contraceptives on serum levels of α_2-macroglobulin, transferrin, albumin, and IgG. Lancet i:49, 1970

69. Hornych A, Safar M, Bariety J et al: Urinary thromboxane B_2 in hypertensive patients. Arch Mal Coeur 75:109, 1982

70. Hugli TE: Complement factors and inflammation: effects of α-thrombin on components C3 and C5. In Lundblad RL, Fenton JW, Mann KG (eds): The Chemistry and Biology of Thrombin, pp 345–360. Ann Arbor, Ann Arbor Press, 1977

71. Huseby R, Clavin S, Smith R et al: Studies on tissue culture plasminogen activator. II. The detection and assay of urokinase and plasminogen activator from LLLC-PK cultures (porcine) by the synthetic substrate N α-benzyloxycarbonyl-glycyl-glycyl-arginyl-4-methoxy-2-naphthylamide. Thromb Res 10:679, 1977

72. Italian Cismel: Multicenter evaluation of a new chromogenic factor X assay in plasma of patients on oral anticoagulants. Thromb Res 19(4/5):493, 1980
73. Ito R, Statland BE: Centrifugal analysis for plasma kallikrein activity, with use of the chromogenic substrate S-2302. Clin Chem 27:586, 1981
74. Ito RK, Statland B: Hemostasis testing with synthetic substrates. Diagnostic Medicine, January 1984
75. Kahle LH: A simple two stage amidolytic assay for factor V (abstr #0833). Thromb Haemost 50(1):226, 1983
76. Kahle LH, Lamping RJ, ten Cate JW: Evaluation of an automated amidolytic antiplasmin assay. Thromb Haemost 42:49, 1979
77. Kapke GF, Johnson GF, Witte DL, Feld RD: Automated fluorometric heparin assay on the Multistat III. Clin Chem 27:1107, 1981
78. Kato H, Adachi N, Iwanasa S et al: A new fluorogenic substrate method for the estimation of kallikrein in urine. J Biochem (Tokyo) 87(4):1127, 1980
79. Kelton JG, Gibbons S: Autoimmune platelet destruction: Idiopathic thrombocytopenia purpura. Semin Thromb Hemost 8(2):83, 1982
80. Kirchhof BRJ, Vermeer C, Hemker HC: The determination of prothrombin using synthetic chromogenic substrates: Choice of a suitable activator. Thromb Res 13(2):219, 1978
81. Kisiel W, Canfield WM, Ericsson LH, Davie EW: Anticoagulant properties of bovine plasma protein C following activation by thrombin. Biochemistry 16:5824, 1977
82. Kluft C, Los N: Demonstration of two forms of α_2-antiplasmin by modified crossed immunoelectrophoresis. Thromb Res 21:65, 1981
83. Kobayaski N, Takeda Y: Studies of the effect of estradiol, progesterone, cortisone, thrombophlebitis, and typhoid vaccine on synthesis and catabolism of antithrombin-III in the dog. Thromb Haemost 37:111, 1977
84. Konings CH: Measurement of antitryptic activity of serum with a centrifugal analyzer. Clin Chem 23:1760, 1977
85. Korsan-Bengtsen I, Axelsson G, Waldenstrom J: Determination of plasma prothrombin with the chromogenic peptide substrate H-D-phe-pip-arg-pNA (S-2238). In Witt I (ed): New Methods for the Analysis of Coagulation Using Chromogenic Substrates, pp 145–154. Berlin, Walter de Gruyter, 1977
86. Lammle B, Bounameaux H, Marbet GA et al: Monitoring of oral anticoagulation by an amidolytic factor X assay: A long term study in 42 patients. Thromb Haemost 44(3):150, 1980
87. Lane DA, Ireland H, Wolff S et al: Plasma concentrations of fibrinopeptide A, fibrinogen fragment B beta 1–42 and beta-thromboglobulin following total hip replacement. Thromb Res 26:111, 1982
88. Laurell CB: Antigen–antibody crossed electrophoresis. Anal Biochem 10:358, 1965
89. Leach CM, Thorburn GC: A comparative study of collagen induced thromboxane release from platelets of different species: Implications for human atherosclerosis models. Prostaglandins 24:47, 1982
90. Lewis JH, Iammarino RM, Spero JA, Hasiba U: Antithrombin Pittsburgh: An alpha-l-antitrypsin variant causing hemorrhagic disease. Blood 51:129, 1978
91. Lonky SA, Marsh J, Wohl H: Stimulation of human granulocyte elastase by platelet factor 4 and heparin. Biochem Biophys Res Commun 85:1113, 1978
92. Madaras F, Chew MY, Parkin JD: Automated estimation of factor Xa using the chromogenic substrate S-2222. Haemostasis 10:271, 1981
93. Mancini G, Carbonara AO, Heremans JF: Immunochemical quantitation of antigens by single radial immunodiffusion. Immunochemistry 2:235, 1965
94. Marciniak E, Farley CH, DeSimone PA: Familial thrombosis due to antithrombin III deficiency. Blood 43:219, 1974
95. Marlar RA, Endres-Brooks J: Recurrent thromboembolic disease due to heterozygous protein C deficiency (abstr). Thromb Haemost 50:351, 1983
96. Marsaritella P, Deutsch E: Clinical use of a method for the determination of factor VII by a chromogenic substrate. Thromb Res 21(6):585, 1981

97. Marx J: Coagulation as a common thread in disease. Science 218:145, 1982
98. Matsumoto M, Kusunoki M, Uyama O et al: Platelet aggregation induced by arachidonic acid and thromboxane generation in patients with hypertension or cerebrovascular disease. Prostaglandins 7:553, 1981
99. Mehta J, Mehta P: Significance of platelet function and thromboxane B2 levels across the human myocardial vascular bed. Acta Med Scand 651:111, 1981
100. Mibashan RS, Scully MF, Birch AJ et al: Automated control of coumarin therapy by chromogenic factor X assay. Thromb Haemost 42:291, 1979
101. Mitchell GA: Development and clinical use of automated synthetic substrate methods for the evaluation of coagulation and fibrinolysis. Semin Thromb Hemost 9(4):262, 1983
102. Mitchell GA, Abdullahad CM, Ruiz JA et al: Flurogenic substrate assays for factors VIII and IX: Introduction of a new solid phase fluorescent detection method. Thromb Res 21(6):573, 1981
103. Mitchell GA, Garguilo RJ, Huseby RM et al: Assay for plasma heparin using a synthetic peptide substrate for thrombin: Introduction of the fluorophore aminoisophthalic acid, dimethyl ester. Thromb Res 13(1):47, 1978
104. Mombelli G, Roux A, Haeberli A, Straub PW: Comparison of ^{125}I-fibrinogen kinetics and fibrinopeptide A in patients with disseminated neoplasia. Blood 60:381, 1982
105. Moore S, Pepper DS, Cash JD: The isolation and characterization of a platelet-specific β-globulin (β-thromboglobulin) and the detection of anti-urokinase and antiplasmin released from thrombin aggregated washed human platelets. Biochim Biophys Acta 379:360, 1975
106. Moore S, Pepper DS, Cash JD: Platelet antiheparin activity: The isolation and characterization of platelet factor 4 released from thrombin-aggregated washed human platelets and its dissociation into subunits and the isolation of membrane-bound antiheparin activity. Biochim Biophys Acta 379:370, 1975
107. Morse JO: Alpha 1-antitrypsin deficiency. N Engl J Med 299:1045, 1978
108. Mullertz S, Clemmensen I: The primary inhibitor of plasmin in human plasma. Biochem J 159:545, 1976
109. Nachman RL, Weksler B, Ferris B: Increased vascular permeability produced by human platelet granule cationic extract. J Clin Invest 49:274, 1970
110. Nichols AB, Owen J, Kaplan KL et al: Fibrinopeptide A, platelet factor 4, and beta-thromboglobulin levels in coronary heart disease. Blood 60:650, 1982
111. Niewiarowski S, Rucinski B, James P, Lindahl U: Platelet antiheparin proteins and antithrombin III interact with different binding sites on heparin molecule. FEBS Lett 102:75, 1979
112. Nishibe H: The assay of factor V in plasma using a synthetic chromogenic substrate. Clin Chem Acta 106(3):301, 1980
113. Nossel HL: Release of fibrinopeptides. N Engl J Med 295:428, 1976
114. Nossel HL, Wasser J, Kaplan KL et al: Sequence of fibrinogen proteolysis and platelet release after intrauterine infuson of hypertonic saline. J Clin Invest 64:1371, 1979
115. Odegard OR, Lie M, Abildgaard U: Heparin cofactor activity measured with an amidolytic method. Thromb Res 6:287, 1975
116. Ouchterlony O: Antigen–antibody reactions in gel. Ark Kem Min Geol 26B:1, 1948
117. Peuscher RW, Cleton FJ, Armstrong L et al: Significance of plasma fibrinopeptide A (FPA) in patients with malignancy. J Lab Clin Med 96:5, 1980
118. Peuscher RW, van Aken WG, Flier OT et al: Effect of anticoagulant treatment measured by fibrinopeptide A (FPA) in patients with venous thromboembolism. Thromb Res 13:33, 1980
119. Pierson-Perry JF, Wehrly JA, Siefring GE: Coagulation testing with the DuPont aca discrete clinical analyzer. Semin Thromb Hemost 9(4):315, 1983
120. Pochron SP, Mitchell GA, Sibareda I: A fluorescent substrate assay for plasminogen. Thromb Res 13:733, 1978
121. Poller L, Thomson JJ, Bodzenta A et al: An assessment of an amidolytic assay for factor VII in the laboratory control of oral anticoagulants. Br J Haematol 49(1):69, 1981

122. Polley MJ, Nachman R: The human complement system in thrombin-mediated platelet function. J Exp Med 147:1713, 1978

123. Quick AJ: Prothrombin in hemophilia and in obstructive jaundice. J Biol Chem 109: LXXIII–LXXIV, 1935

124. Ratnoff OD, Pensky J, Ofston D, Naff BF: The inhibition of plasmin, plasma kallikrein, plasma permeability factor, and the C1r subcomponent of the first component of complement by serum C'1 esterase inhibitor. J Exp Med 129:315, 1969

125. Remuzzi G, Cavenaghi AI, Mecca G: Bleeding in uremic patients: A possible role for prostacyclins (PGI$_2$). Blood 50(Suppl 1):280, 1977

126. Ressler RN: Electrophoresis of serum protein antigens in an antibody containing buffer. Clin Chim Acta 5:359, 1960

127. Rosen S, Friberger P, Anderson M, Vinazzer H: A new chromogenic assay for determination of human factor VIII:C activity. In Triplett DA (ed): Standardization of Coagulation Assays: An Overview, pp 255–260. Skokie, IL, College of American Pathologists, 1982

128. Rosenberg RD: Actions and interactions of antithrombin and heparin. N Engl J Med 292:146, 1975

129. Ross R, Glomset J, Kariya B, Harker L: A platelet-dependent serum factor that stimulates the proliferation of arterial smooth muscle cells in vitro. Proc Natl Acad Sci USA 71:1207, 1974

130. Ross R, Glomset JA: The pathogenesis of atherosclerosis. N Engl J Med 295:369, 1976

131. Samuelsson B, Hammarstrom S: Leukotrienes: A novel group of biologically active compounds. Vitam Horm 39:1, 1982

132. Sandberg H, Anderson LO: A high sensitive assay of platelet factor 3 using a chromogenic substrate. Thromb Res 14(1):113, 1979

133. Sas G, Blasko G, Banhegyi D et al: Abnormal antithrombin III (antithrombin III "Budapest") as a cause of a familial thrombophilia. Thromb Diath Haemorrh 32:105, 1974

134. Scharrer I, Robbins K, Wohl R et al: Investigations on two congenital abnormal plasminogens (Frankfort I and Frankfort II): Their relationship to thrombosis. Thromb Haemost 50(1):257, 1983

135. Schreiber AD, Kaplan AP, Austen KF: Inhibition by C1 INH of Hageman factor fragment activation of coagulation, fibrinolysis and kinin generation. J Clin Invest 52:1402, 1973

136. Scully MF, Kakkar VV: Methods for semi-micro or automated determination of thrombin, antithrombin and heparin cofactor using the substrate H-D-phe-pip-arg-P-nitroanilide-2HCl. Clin Chim Acta 79:595, 1977

137. Schultze HE, Schwick G: Quantitative immunologische Bestimmung von Plasmaprotenen. Clin Chim Acta 4:15, 1959

138. Seeger WH: Antithrombin III: Theory and clinical applications. Am J Clin Pathol 68:367, 1978

139. Seligsohn U, Berger A, Abend M et al: Homozygous protein C deficiency manifested by massive venous thrombosis in the newborn. N Engl J Med 310:559, 1984

140. Seligsohn U, Osterud B, Rapaport SI: Coupled amidolytic assay for factor VII: Its use with a clotting assay to determine the activity state of factor VII. Blood 52:978, 1978

141. Shulman NR, Weinrach RS, Libre EP, Andrews HL: The role of the reticuloendothelial system in the pathogenesis of idiopathic thrombocytopenic purpura. Trans Assoc Am Physicians 78:374, 1965

142. Sie P, Dupouy J, Pichon J, Boneu B: Constitutional heparin co-factor II deficiency associated with recurrent thrombosis. Lancet ii:414, 1985

143. Silverstein R: A rapid kinetic assay for determining plasminogen in plasma (abstr). Blood 44:935, 1974

144. Smith RC: β-Thromboglobulin and deep vein thrombosis. Thromb Hemost 39:338, 1978

145. Sorensen P, Sas G, Pezo I et al: Distinction of two pathologic antithrombin III molecules: Antithrombin III "Aaborg" and antithrombin III "Budapest." Thromb Res 26:211, 1982

146. Soria C, Soria J: A plasminogen assay using a chromogenic synthetic substrate: Results from clinical work and from studies of thrombolysis. Prog Chem Fib Thrombolysis 3:337, 1978

147. Soulier JP, Gozin D: Assay of Fletcher factor (plasma prekallikrein) using an artificial clotting reagent and a modified chromogenic assay. Thromb Haemost 42(2):538, 1979

148. Stichaikul T, Puwasatien P, Karnjanajetanee J, Bokisch V: Complement change and disseminated intravascular coagulation in *Plasmodium falciparum* malaria. Lancet i:770, 1975

149. Stormorken H, Baklund A, Gallimore M, Ritland S: Chromogenic substrate assay of plasma prekallikrein with a note on its site of biosynthesis. Haemostasis 7:69, 1978

150. Svendsen L: Estimation of urokinase activity by means of a highly susceptible synthetic chromogenic peptide substrate. In Witt I (ed): New Methods for the Analysis of Coagulation Using Chromogenic Substrates, pp 251–262. Berlin, Walter de Gruyter, 1977

151. Takagi T, Doolittle RF: Amino acid sequence studies on plasmin-derived fragments of human fibrinogen: Amino-terminal sequences of intermediate and terminal fragments. Biochemistry 14:940, 1975

152. Teien A, Lie M, Abildgaard U: Assay of heparin in plasma using a chromogenic substrate for activated factor X. Thromb Res 8:413, 1976

153. Tollefsen DM, Majerus DW, Blank MK: Heparin cofactor II: Purification and properties of a heparin-dependent inhibitor of thrombin in human plasma. J Biol Chem 257(5):2162, 1982

154. Torngren S, Noren I, Savidge G: The effect of low-dose heparin on fibrinopeptide A, platelets, fibrinogen degradation products and other haemostatic parameters measured in connection with intestinal surgery. Thromb Res 14:871, 1979

155. Tripodi A, DiSanto C, Mannucci PM: A chromogenic assay of prothrombin compared with coagulation tests during anticoagulant therapy and liver disease. Ric Clin Lab 11(3):215, 1981

156. Troll W, Sherry S, Wachman J: The activation of thrombin on synthetic substrates. J Biol Chem 308:85, 1954

157. Tunstall AM, Merriman JML, Milne I, James K: Normal and pathological serum levels of α_2-macroglobulins in men and mice. J Clin Pathol 28:133, 1975

158. Van Mourik JA: The significance of fibrinopeptide A (FPA) in the diagnosis of low-grade intravascular coagulation and venous thromboembolism. Haematologica (Pavia) 66:259, 1981

159. Van Wijk EM, Kahle LH, ten Cate JW: A rapid manual chromogenic factor X assay. Thromb Res 22(56):681, 1981

160. Vinazzer H: A simplified assay method for platelet factor 4 in plasma and in platelets with a chromogenic substrate. Haemost 7:352, 1978

161. Vinazzer H: Assay of total factor XII and of activated factor XII in plasma with a chromogenic substrate. Thromb Res 14(1):155, 1979

162. Vogel G, Sturzebecher J, Klessen C, Lauten G: Use of chromogenic substrates in the clarification of disorders in the early stages of blood coagulation. Folia Haematol (Leipz) 109(1):115, 1982

163. von Kaulla E, von Kaulla KN: Antithrombin-III diseases. Am J Clin Pathol 48:69, 1967

164. Walenga J, Kelly J, Fareed J et al: Performance characteristics of an automated antithrombin III, plasminogen and fibrinogen on the DuPont ACA system. Clin Chem 28:1585, 1982

165. Walenga JM, Fareed J, EW Bermes Jr: Automated instrumentation and the laboratory diagnosis of bleeding and thrombotic disorders. Semin Thromb Hemost 9:172, 1983

166. Walenga JM, Fareed J, Messmore HL: New avenues in the monitoring of antithrombotic therapy: The role of automation. Semin Thromb Hemost 9(4):340, 1983

167. Webb PJ, Westwick J, Scully MF et al: Do prostacyclin and thromboxane play a role in endotoxic shock? Br J Surg 68:720, 1981

168. Weksler BB, Coupal CE: Platelet-dependent generation of chemotactic activity in serum. J Exp Med 137:1419, 1973

169. Wilman B, Collen D: Purification and characterization of human antiplasmin, the fast-acting plasmin inhibitor in plasma. Eur J Biochem 78:19, 1977

170. Wohl RC, Summaria L, Robbins KC: Physiological activation of the human fibrinolytic system: Isolation and characterization of human plasminogen variants, Chicago I and Chicago II. J Biol Chem 254:9063, 1979

171. Workman EF, Clark DM, Fedor EJ: Platelet factor 4 levels in hypercoagulable states. Thromb Haemost 42:208, 1979
172. Yalow RS, Berson SA: Assay of plasma insulin in human subjects by immunological methods. Nature 184:1648, 1959
173. Yamada K, Meguro T: Novel method of APTT using the chromogenic substrates for thrombin and an autoanalyzer. Thromb Haemost 42:225, 1979
174. Ylikorkala O, Kaila J, Viinikka L: Prostacyclin and thromboxane in diabetes. Br Med J [Clin Res] 283:1148, 1981
175. Yudelman I, Greenberg J: Factors affecting fibrinopeptide A levels in patients with venous thromboembolism during anticoagulant therapy. Blood 59:787, 1982
176. Yue RH, Gertler MM, Starr R, Koutrouby R: Alteration of plasma antithrombin-III levels in ischemic heart disease. Thromb Haemost 35:598, 1976

SUGGESTED READING

Bick L: Disorders of Hemostasis and Thrombosis. New York, Thieme Stratton 1985

Colman RW, Hirsh J, Marder VJ, Salzman EW (eds): Hemostasis and Thrombosis: Basic Principles and Clinical Practice, 2nd ed. Philadelphia, JB Lippincott, 1987

Fareed J: Perspectives in Hemostasis. New York, Pergamon Press, 1981

Hemker HC: Handbook of Synthetic Substrates for the Coagulation and Fibrinolytic System. The Hague, Martinus Nijhoff, 1983

Murano G, Bick RL: Basic Concepts of Hemostasis and Thrombosis. Boca Raton, FL, CRC Press, 1980

Ogston D: The Physiology of Hemostasis. Cambridge, MA, Harvard University Press, 1983

Parvez Z: Immunoassays in Coagulation Testing. New York, Springer-Verlag, 1984

Ratnoff OD, Forbes CD: Disorders of Hemostasis. Orlando, Grune & Stratton, 1984

Thompson AR, Harker LA: Manual of Hemostasis and Thrombosis, 3rd ed. Philadelphia, FA Davis, 1983

Thomson JM: Blood Coagulation and Haemostasis. New York, Churchill Livingstone, 1980

Verstraete M, Vermylen J: Thrombosis. Elmsford, NY, Pergamon Press, 1984

Walenga JM: In vitro evaluation of heparin fractions: Old vs. new methods. CRC Press, Inc. 22(4):361, 1986

Glossary

Accuracy: The measure of how near a test result is to the theoretical "correct" result

Activated Partial Thromboplastins: Mixtures of contact activators (kaolin, ellagic acid, or Celite) with organically extracted brain and lung phospholipids used to initiate intrinsic clot formation

Examples:

BBL Platelet Factor Reagent (Celite)
Dade Cephaloplastin (ellagic acid)
Hyland P.T. Reagent (kaolin)
Organon Teknika Platelin (Celite)
Ortho Thrombofax (ellagic acid)

Actomyosin (Thrombosthenin): A contractile protein that forms the substance of muscle tissue and is found in many other motile cells. *Thrombosthenin* is a term used for actomyosin, which is found in the platelet, but there is no physical difference between platelet and other actomyosin.

Acute Lymphocytic Leukemia: A progressive malignant disease of the blood, resulting in abnormal proliferation of lymphoblasts in the bone marrow. It is primarily a malignancy of childhood although seen later in life. Severe thrombocytopenia and easy bruising may be the earliest diagnostic clues.

Acute Nonlymphocytic Leukemia: A progressive malignancy of the blood, resulting in abnormal proliferation of myeloblasts, monoblasts, or erythroblasts in the bone marrow. It is primarily a malignancy of adults. Severe thrombocytopenia and easy bruising may be the earliest diagnostic clues.

Adenosine Diphosphate (ADP): A purine nucleotide that induces platelet aggregation. The hydrolysis of ADP, forming cyclic adenosine monophosphate (cAMP), releases 36,000 J/mol of energy.

Adsorbed Plasma: Plasma from which the vitamin K–dependent factors have been removed. Adsorbed plasma contains Factors V, VIII, XI, XII, and XIII and fibrinogen. Common adsorbents are barium sulfate and aluminum hydroxide.

Afibrinogenemia: The absence of fibrinogen in the blood. This severe hemorrhagic disorder may be inherited as an autosomal-recessive trait or may occur in disseminated intravascular coagulation.

Aged Serum: A reagent made by incubating normal serum for 24 hours at 37°C. The serum contains Factors VII, IX, X, XI, and XII.

Agglutination: Formation of cell aggregates without the activation of the cells

Aggregometry: Quantitative measurement of platelet cohesion in a photometer, which measures changes in light transmission through a plasma suspension of platelets. The suspension is prepared from whole blood, then activated with a variety of agonists. The pattern of light transmission change is recorded and analyzed.

Agonist: A substance that attaches to a receptor and causes activation of a cell. In platelets, some agonists are ADP, epinephrine, collagen, arachidonic acid, and thrombin.

Alpha granule: The storage organelle in platelets that contains various hemostatic proteins

Alternative Pathway: A minor or feedback series of reactions that activate the intrinsic and extrinsic coagulation systems

Anaphylatoxins: Polypeptides cleaved from the complement components C3 and C5, termed *C3a* and *C5a*, that mediate mast cell degranulation with release of histamines These increase vascular permeability and cause a drop in blood pressure.

Antagonist: A substance that attaches to a receptor and opposes activation of a cell. In platelets some antagonists are prostaglandins I_2 and E_2.

Antecubital Fossa (Crease): The space opposite the elbow

Anticoagulant: A substance that inhibits the formation of clots. Those used in blood specimen collection include EDTA, citrate, and oxalate, all of which bind calcium to prevent coagulation. Heparin, an anticoagulant that occurs *in vivo*, and is used in collection, acts against thrombin to prevent coagulation.

α_2**-Antiplasmin:** A naturally occurring inhibitor of fibrinolysis

Antiplatelet Antibody: An immunoglobulin specific for platelet antigens, such as Pl^{A1}. The antibody may be responsible for an autoimmune or alloimmune disorder.

Antithrombin III (ATIII): An alpha globulin synthesized by the liver and found in many body fluids. ATIII is a naturally occurring inhibitor of coagulation.

Antithrombotic: The ability of a substance to inhibit the formation or generation of a thrombus (clot). Major endogenous inhibitors of coagulation are antithrombin III and protein C. Therapeutic products such as heparin are widely used as antithrombotic agents to prevent thrombosis.

Aplastic Anemia: A pancytopenia resulting from aplasia of the bone marrow, which is replaced by fat cells. There is severe depletion of marrow megakaryocytes, with resulting thrombocytopenia, which leads to bleeding and formation of purpura. Often the evidence of hemorrhage is the most visible clinical symptom.

Arachidonic Acid: A 20-carbon fatty acid with four unsaturations, abundant in the phospholipid bilayer that forms most membranes. It is the substrate for prostaglandin and thromboxanes and is used as an agonist in platelet aggregometry.

Aspirinlike Syndrome: A thrombocytopathia in which platelet secretion (release) is impaired, probably due to an enzymatic defect in the thromboxane synthesis pathway. Aggregometry results are similar to those seen in aspirin-treated platelets. There is primary aggregation followed by disaggregation with ADP and epinephrine but no aggregation with collagen.

Asymmetric Mitosis: Production of dissimilar daughter cells, one that is able to differentiate into a specific pathway, another that retains the capacity for subsequent asymmetric mitosis

Autoimmune Thrombocytopenic Purpura (AITP): A chronic or acute disorder caused by the presence of circulating antiplatelet autoantibodies, which results in severe depression of platelet count, formation of purpura, and anemia. It was formerly known as idiopathic thrombocytopenic purpura.

Bβ-Related Peptides: A group of peptides of amino acid sequences 1–15, 1–24, 1–118, and most commonly 15–42 released from the B chain of fibrin by the action of plasmin, in the initial stages

Bernard-Soulier Syndrome: A rare, severe congenital bleeding disorder, transmitted as an autosomal-recessive trait, in which platelets demonstrate abnormal adhesion and thrombocytopenia. The morphology is of large, gray platelets in Wright stain. There is a normal aggregation response to ADP, epinephrine, and collagen, but no response to ristocetin even when von Willebrand factor is added.

Biphasic Curve: A curve produced by the intersection of two arcs

Bleeding Diathesis: A predisposition or tendency to bleed

Bleeding Time: The time required for a standard wound to stop bleeding under controlled conditions of intracapillary pressure and skin thickness. The bleeding time test is the initial screen for assessment of platelet function in the clinical laboratory.

Borchgrevink Technique: An *in vivo* platelet retention technique. A capillary puncture is made and a platelet count is performed on the first blood that appears. After a specified period, a second count is done from the same puncture. The second count is expected to be lower than the first.

Brecher-Cronkite Platelet Count: A manual technique that has been regarded as the standard method for platelet counting, developed in 1950. Blood is diluted in ammonium oxalate and counted on a Neubauer grid by means of phase microscopy.

C1 inhibitor (C1-INH): A plasma inhibitor of C1-esterase, the first component of complement

Capillary Fragility: The unexpected escape of red cells through capillary walls as a result of capillary disorders such as vasculitis. Fragility results in the appearance of petechiae, ecchymoses, and purpura in the skin.

Capillary Fragility Test: A clinical test to measure the escape of blood from capillaries under stress. A suction device, called a petechiometer, is applied to the skin for a specified period. Then it is removed and the area underneath observed for formation of petechiae. The appearance of one petechiae or more may indicate abnormal fragility.

Chemiluminescence: The emission of light due to a chemical reaction

Clot: A gel-like mass formed in whole blood, composed of fibrin, platelets, and erythrocytes, or in plasma, composed of fibrin and platelets

Coagulation: The process by which several glycoproteins interact with platelets to form an insoluble blood clot to stop blood loss or flow; to change from a fluid state to a thickened mass

Coagulation Cascade: A hypothesis that bases the theory of coagulation on a series of enzymatic reactions that lead to the formation of a fibrin clot. The reactions are like a waterfall or cascade, in which a protein is activated to activate the next protein in the sequence.

Coefficient of Variation (CV): Standard deviation divided by the mean and expressed as a percentage

Collagen: A protein present in connective tissue that is formed by fibroblasts. It is found in the form of slender fibrils with a high tensile strength and high amounts of hydroxyproline.

Colony Forming Unit (CFU): Any of several hematopoietic stem cells that have been identified by their ability to give rise to monoclonal colonies in the spleen when transplanted into isogeneic, lethally radiated mice

Complete Thromboplastin: Acetone-dried extracts from animal brain or lung tissues

Consumption Coagulopathy: See *Disseminated Intravascular Coagulation.*

Contact Activation: The process by which coagulation is initiated in the intrinsic pathway by contact with a surface

Contact Activators: Substances added to coagulation reagents that maximize surface activation *in vitro*

Coumarin (Warfarin): An antagonist to the production of the vitamin K–dependent factors, used routinely as a therapeutic anticoagulant

Cryoprecipitate: A preparation used to restore coagulation in patients with hemophilia or von Willebrand disease. The cryoprecipitate is prepared by freezing and slowly thawing fresh plasma. Cryoprecipitate, a solution rich in Factor VIII, von Willebrand factor, and fibrinogen, is extracted by centrifugation.

Cytology: The study of cells: their origin, structure, function, and pathology

Cytoskeleton: The system of microtubules and microfilaments that serves as a framework for a cell, functioning to maintain cell shape and provide support

DDAVP: 1-Desamino-8-D-arginine-vasopressin, an analogue of antidiuretic hormone used as a vasoconstrictor. DDAVP stimulates release of Factor VIII and von Willebrand factor from endothelium.

D-Dimer: A peptide release product of the action of plasmin on fibrin, with a molecular weight of 10^6 daltons

Demarcation Membrane System: Proliferation of plasma membrane throughout the megakaryocyte during its cytoplasmic growth phase in the bone marrow. The demarcation system becomes the plasma membrane of individual platelets.

Dense Body: A platelet storage organelle containing ADP, serotonin, calcium, and pyrophosphate. These materials are released upon activation of the platelet to amplify the platelet thrombus-forming mechanism.

Dense Tubular System: A series of membranes, closely apposed to the open canalicular system, that contain several structures important to the activation of platelets, such as adenyl cyclase, cyclooxygenase, and bound calcium. The dense tubular system forms as a condensation of the smooth endoplasmic reticulum of the megakaryocyte.

Dimer: Two identical molecules that are joined by covalent bonds

Disseminated Intravascular Coagulation (DIC): A disturbance in the hemostatic balance, activated by a procoagulant stimulus, that produces the release of tissue factor into the circulation, or conditions that lead to endothelial cell injury and/or Factor XII activation. Both platelets and coagulation factors are consumed, fibrin is deposited in small vessels in many organs, and the fibrinolytic system is activated, with the subsequent accumulation of fibrinogen degradation products in the circulation, which may inhibit clot formation.

Dysfibrinogenemia: A qualitative abnormality in the fibrinogen molecule due to a possible amino acid substitution. The condition is usually an autosomal-dominant trait. More than 40 abnormal fibrinogens have been reported, with only a few of the actual defects known. Defects can result in abnormal aggregation of fibrin monomer, abnormal release of the fibrinopeptides, or abnormal crosslinking. The thrombin, prothrombin, and Reptilase times in these patients are prolonged.

Ecchymosis: Hemorrhage into the skin greater than 3 cm in diameter

EDTA: Ethylenediamine tetraacetic acid, edetic acid, molecular weight 292.24 daltons. A chelating agent that sequesters many divalent or trivalent metals, including calcium. Sodium and potassium salts of EDTA bind calcium and are used as anticoagulants in whole blood collection. Trade names include Sequestrene and Versene.

Elastin: The essential component of elastic fibers. It is a fibrous protein that allows certain tissues to expand and then return to normal shape. Elastin differs from collagen in that it contains little hydroxyproline, does not have a triple helical structure, and does not occur in a repeating peptide unit.

Endomitosis: The process of DNA replication and nuclear proliferation without formation of daughter cells

Endoplasmic Reticulum: A system of internal cellular membranes that controls the production of internal and secretory cell materials. Rough endoplasmic reticulum is lined with ribosomes and produces protein. Smooth endoplasmic reticulum has no ribosomes and produces lipids. Various specialized structures of cells, such as the dense tubular system in platelets, may be derived from endoplasmic reticulum.

Epinephrine: A hormone secreted by the adrenal medulla in response to fear, anger, stress, or hypoglycemia, which increases various metabolic activities. It is used as an agonist in platelet aggregometry.

Epsilon-Aminocaproic Acid (EACA or Amicar): An *in vitro* and *in vivo* inhibitor of fibrinolysis

Erythropoiesis: The production of red cells

Erythropoietin: A glycoprotein that induces formation of cells in the erythropoietic cell line

Essential Thrombocythemia: A myeloproliferative disorder characterized by proliferation of megakaryocytes, extreme thrombocytosis, and neutrophilic leukocytosis. Platelet counts regularly go above $1000 \times 10^3/\mu l$, and a frequent sign is gastrointestinal hemorrhage.

Euchromatin: Extended chromatin that is actively involved in translation

Extrinsic Pathway: That part of the cascade mechanism of coagulation that begins with activation from an extrinsic source: tissue factor released from damaged endothelium. Tissue factor, along with Factor VII, then activates Factor X in the common pathway, which leads to thrombin formation, which in turn acts on fibrinogen to convert it to fibrin.

Fenestration: A thin area or opening in the membrane of a cell, seen in the endothelial lining of sinusoids. Fenestrae allow for the passage of other cells or cellular elements.

Fibrin: The insoluble protein that is formed when thrombin acts on fibrinogen

Fibrin Clot: A thrombus composed of platelets and fibrin

Fibrin Degradation Products: The breakdown products of fibrinogen and fibrin that result from activation of fibrinolysis. There are four main fibrin degradation products (X, Y, D, E). All can act as strong anticoagulants and are seen in patients with disseminated intravascular coagulation, renal transplant patients, and patients with primary fibrinolysis.

Fibrin Monomer: The altered fibrinogen molecule that results from thrombin's action on fibrinogen, cleaving off fibrinopeptides A and B

Fibrinogen: A large glycoprotein that circulates in the plasma. It is composed of three pairs of nonidentical polypeptide chains, designated alpha, beta, and gamma.

Fibrinogenolysis: Pathologic dissolution of a clot, resulting from excess free plasmin destroying fibrinogen and other coagulation factors. Fibrinogenolysis is a component of disseminated intravascular coagulation.

Fibrinolysis: The process of breaking down or lysing fibrin through enzymatic dissolution

Fibrinopeptide: One of the two acidic polypeptide fragments, fibrinopeptide A and fibrinopeptide B, that account for 3% of the weight of fibrinogen. They are released from the terminal ends of the alpha and beta chains of the fibrinogen molecule in response to the action of thrombin.

Fibrinopeptide A (FPA): A cleavage peptide containing 16 amino acids released from the amino terminal of the A chain of fibrinogen in the initial stages of the action of thrombin. For every molecule of fibrinogen, two FPA molecules are released; the approximate half-life is 4 minutes.

Fibrinopeptide B (FPB): A 14-amino-acid peptide released from the B chain of fibrinogen in the initial stages of the action of thrombin. For every molecule of fibrinogen, two FPB molecules are released, but at a slower rate than the release of FPA. The approximate half-life is 30 seconds, though the molecule is too unstable for accurate measurement.

Fibroblast: A connective tissue cell derived from the mesenchyme that produces collagen, ground substance, and elastic fibrils

Fibronectin: A glycoprotein found on the fibroblast surface. It is involved in stabilization of the fibrin clot and is also called *cold-insoluble globulin*. Fibronectin helps bind the membranes of adjoining cell surfaces.

Firefly Extract: See *Luciferin*.

Friable: Easily broken down into smaller pieces

Giant Platelet: A morphologically abnormal platelet present in myeloproliferative disorders, acute leukemia, and certain platelet disorders. A giant platelet is greater than 6 μm in diameter on a peripheral blood smear and generally exceeds the diameter of surrounding erythrocytes.

Glanzmann's Thrombasthenia: A rare, severe congenital bleeding disorder, transmitted as an autosomal-recessive trait, in which platelets function abnormally although they are normal in number. There is usually no aggregation response to ADP, epinephrine, or collagen. The bleeding time is prolonged and clotting factors are normal.

Globular Protein: Proteins that are soluble, usually in the presence of salt. The molecules are usually spheroid or ellipsoid when in solution.

Glycocalyx: The thick surface coat of a platelet that contains several types of glycoproteins and absorbs and concentrates several of the plasma procoagulants

Glycoprotein: A substance containing proteins covalently linked to carbohydrates. Glycoproteins occur in extracellular fluids, the ground substance of cartilage, basement membrane, the surface coat of epithelial cells, and as antigens and receptors in and on membranes. All of the plasma proteins except albumin are glycoproteins.

Golgi Apparatus: A complex intracellular network of flattened membrane-bound sacs near the nucleus that processes proteins produced in the endoplasmic reticulum, adding side-chains and packaging them in granules or secretory vesicles. The Golgi apparatus stains poorly in Wright stain preparations.

Granulopoiesis: Production of granulocytes, including basophils, eosinophils, neutrophils, and monocytes

Gray Platelet Syndrome: A rare platelet release defect caused by a deficiency of alpha granules, resulting in platelets that appear gray when stained with Wright's stain

Hemacytometer: A counting chamber for blood cells. It is a rectangular glass block the central area of which is a measured depression and the floor of which is ruled into several adjacent squares such as a Neubauer grid. A suspension of blood is introduced into the chamber and the cells in designated squares counted with the aid of a microscope.

Hematoma: A swelling filled with clotted blood that has escaped from a blood vessel into the tissues or a cavity

Hemolytic–Uremic Syndrome (HUS): A disorder characterized by endothelial damage in glomerular capillaries and renal arterioles, resulting in platelet and fibrin being deposited in the vasculature. Clinically, it resembles thrombotic thrombocytopenic purpura except that hypertension and renal failure are more common in this disorder.

Hemophilia: A group of hereditary bleeding disorders of coagulation in which one of the coagulation proteins is missing or defective

Hemorrhage: Uncontrolled bleeding into the skin or surrounding environment

Hemorrhagic Diathesis: A bleeding problem caused by a pathophysiologic mechanism

Hemostasis: A physiologic system based on blood vessel integrity, platelet function, and a set of plasma proteins, which functions to preserve blood vessel integrity and prevent hemorrhage

Hemostatic Plug: The thrombus formed to arrest the flow of blood

Heparan Sulfate: A glycosaminoglycan found in connective tissue

Heparin: A complex heteropolysaccharide with a structure similar to that of heparan sulfate, but with more sulfate groups. Heparin is found *in vivo* in the metachromatic granules of mast cells. It is also manufactured synthetically and used to treat thrombosis. *In vitro*, heparin is used as an anticoagulant to prevent the tube of blood from clotting so that it can be tested.

Heparin Cofactor II: A heparin-dependent protein inhibitor of thrombin distinguishable from antithrombin III

Heparin Derivatives: The molecularly heterogeneous antithrombotic agent heparin can be fractionated into more homogenous components of low, medium, and high molecular weight or high and low antithrombin III affinity. Other fractions of the parent heparin material may possess more homogeneous sulfation or charge characteristics. By fractionating heparin into its various components, the individual activities characteristic of each component can also be isolated.

Hermansky-Pudlak Syndrome: An inherited disorder of platelet release characterized by reduced concentrations of ADP in the dense granules. It is a defect in secondary aggregation and is commonly associated with albinism.

Heterochromatin: Condensed, nonfunctional chromatin

Histogram: A bar or line graph that displays the frequency distribution of a statistical sample

Humoral: Pertaining to molecules in solution in body fluids, such as antibodies or complement

Hyaline: Glassy and transparent

Hydrodynamic Focusing: A physical phenomenon employed in the operation of several types of cell counters in which a stream of cells in a fluid column is concentrated toward the center of the column by a sheath of clear fluid. This approach enhances discrimination of cell volumes and increases counting sensitivity.

Hydrophilic: Soluble in water

Hydrophobic: Insoluble in water

Hypercoagulability: A tendency to thrombose

Hypofibrinogenemia: An abnormally low concentration of fibrinogen in the blood. This is usually inherited as an autosomal-recessive trait and may occur in disseminated intravascular coagulation.

Immune Thrombocytopenic Purpura (ITP): A chronic or acute acquired disorder caused by the presence of circulating antiplatelet autoantibodies or isoantibodies or deposition of immune complexes, resulting in severe depression of platelet count, formation of purpura, and anemia

Inosithin: A soybean phospholipid that is useful as a partial thromboplastin

Intrinsic Pathway: That part of the cascade mechanism of coagulation that begins with activation of Factor XII by a negatively charged surface. XII$_a$ then proceeds to activate Factor XI, which activates IX in the presence of calcium. Activated IX then feeds into the common pathway of Factor X activation.

Ion Pump: A membrane-bound molecule that functions metabolically to move charged ions into or out of a cell against an ionic gradient. Pumps expend energy in the process of moving ions.

Isoimmune Thrombocytopenic Purpura: An acute disorder caused by the presence of exogenous antiplatelet antibodies as a result of transfusion or transplacental introduction. There is severe depression of platelet count, formation of purpura, and anemia. The disorder is self-limited and disappears when the source of antibody is removed.

Juxtaglomerular Apparatus: An interrelated group of cells in the distal convoluted tubules and the glomerulus including the macula densa, juxtaglomerular cells, and the mesangial cells, which secrete several hormones in response to various blood measurements

Keloid: The accumulation of an abnormally large amount of collagen within a scar. Keloids occur more often in blacks or those with a deficiency of Factor XIII.

Labile: Unstable or easily changed by heat or chemical oxidation

Lacuna: A clear area surrounding the dense-staining material within the platelet dense body, thought to be an artifact of preparation caused by contraction of the material in the granule

Lentiform: Bean-shaped

Leukopoiesis: Bone marrow and lymphoid production of white cells

Ligand: A molecule bound to an antibody or antigen and used as an indicator in immunochemical reactions. Examples are isotopes, fluorescein, and various enzymes.

Log-Normal: A statistical probability distribution the logarithm of which has a normal distribution

Luciferin: A material extracted from firefly tails that emits light upon reaction with ATP

Lumen: The channel within a tubular organ such as blood vessel through which substances pass

Lumiaggregometry: A form of platelet aggregometry in which luminescence and light transmission are measured simultaneously

Lupus Erythematosus: An autoimmune inflammatory disease that is either discoid or systemic (SLE). The discoid variety is mainly a skin disorder, while the systemic type involves organs such as the kidneys, central nervous system, and joints. Antinuclear antibodies have been shown to be increased in this disorder.

Lupus Inhibitor: A circulating anticoagulant seen in 5% to 10% of patients with lupus erythematosus that causes a prolonged APTT. The lupus inhibitor is often associated with a thrombotic tendency.

Lysosome: An intracellular granule containing a variety of lytic enzymes, usually for the purpose of digestion of phagocytosed materials. Lysosomes are found in macrophages and granulocytes as well as platelets. Their function in platelets is unclear. In granulocytes the lysosomes are usually called granules.

Macrophage: The end stage of the monocyte–macrophage cell system, a large cell that circulates in the blood and populates most tissues. Macrophages are capable of phagocytosis, immunologic reactions, and inflammatory responses.

Marker: A property used to identify a structure. On cells, specific surface proteins may be used as markers and may be detected by specific antibodies.

May-Hegglin Anomaly: A disorder of autosomal-dominant inheritance characterized by the presence of Döhle bodies in leukocytes, increased platelet size, and occasional thrombocytopenia

Mean Platelet Volume (MPV): The average volume of a population of platelets expressed in femtoliters (fl) or cubic micrometers (μm^3). The MPV is computed by integrative analysis of the histogram of platelet size distribution. The reference range is given as 9 fl to 12 fl at a platelet count of $150 \times 10^3/\mu l$, but the MPV varies inversely with the platelet count.

Megakaryocyte: A bone marrow cell that is the precursor to the platelet. Megakaryocytes are uninucleate but multiploid and are the largest cells found in the bone marow. Platelets are formed from megakaryocytes by cytoplasmic fragmentation.

Megakaryocytic Hypoplasia: A thrombocytopenic condition due to a decrease in the production of megakaryocytes following bone marrow damage, replacement, or intrinsic abnormalities

Microfilament: The contractile fiber formed by actomyosin, about 5 nm to 7 nm in diameter

Micromegakaryocyte: A megakaryocyte similar in size and appearance to a small lymphocyte that passes through the peripheral blood. These cells are usually found in relation to a myeloproliferative disorder.

Microtubule: A cylindrical structure, 20 nm to 27 nm in diameter, found in many types of cells. It is composed of protein subunits about 4 nm in diameter called tubulin. Microtubules serve as part of the cytoskeleton.

Mitochondria: Intracellular organelles containing enzyme systems that generate ATP by means of oxidative phosphorylation. Mitochondria also contain binding sites. These organelles are abundant in cells that require high levels of energy to function.

Molecular Marker: A term used for defined chemical products, usually of low molecular weight, released or generated during early hemostatic activation processes. These markers not only detect thrombotic or fibrinolytic disorders at their onset, before a major clinical condition is established, but also identify the locale and exact nature of the disorder. Examples include fibrinopeptide A, Bβ peptides, platelet factor 4, β-thromboglobulin, prostaglandins, anaphylatoxins, platelet activating factor, and serotonin.

Mononuclear – Phagocyte System: A collection of phagocytic cells, which are numerous in the lymph nodes, the sinusoids of the spleen, liver, and bone marrow, and the peritoneum, pericardium, and pleural sac. The system includes monocytes and macrophages but does not include neutrophils.

Monophasic Curve: A curve that describes a single arc

Multiparametric Instrument: A hematologic instrument that is capable of reporting several whole blood measurements simultaneously. Many instruments provide red blood cell counts, white blood cell counts, hemoglobin, hematocrit, red blood cell indices, mean platelet volume, and erythrocyte, leukocyte, and platelet histograms.

Multipotential: Able to differentiate into one of many cell lines. The multipotential stem cell may give rise to several pluripotential stem cells.

Myeloid: Pertaining to, derived from, or resembling the bone marrow

Myeloproliferative Disorder: A blood neoplasm characterized by proliferation of bone marrow cells. Examples of myeloproliferative disorders include chronic myelocytic leukemia, myelofibrosis with myeloid metaplasia, essential thrombocythemia, and polycythemia vera.

National Committee for Clinical Laboratory Standards (NCCLS): A committee of representatives of the professions, government, and industry who develop standards and guidelines to improve the quality and efficiency of laboratory performance

Neonatal Isoimmune Thrombocytopenic Purpura: The form of isoimmune thrombocytopenic purpura in which maternal antibody is transported across the placental barrier and introduced into the fetal circulation, resulting in severely decreased platelet counts and bleeding at birth

Neubauer Grid: A particular configuration of contiguous squares etched into the floor of a hemacytomer. The overall grid covers nine square millimeters ruled in square-millimeter sections. Each square is ruled into 16 smaller squares, except for the center square, which is ruled into 25 smaller squares. This grid is most often used for red cell, white cell, and platelet counts.

Open Canalicular System: A membrane system that permeates the normal platelet and connects to the surface. The OCS absorbs large quantities of plasma proteins to form the glycocalyx.

Osmium Tetroxide (OsO$_4$): An oxide of osmium used as a histologic fixative for electron microscopy, used to demonstrate lipids and darken the benzidine reaction product

Osteoclast: A large multinucleate cell of the bone marrow responsible for breakdown of mineralized bony matrix and return of free calcium ion to the blood plasma. Osteoclasts resemble megakaryocytes in size but are derived from the monocyte–macrophage cell line.

Partial Thromboplastin: A lipid reagent used as a substitute for platelets in clotting tests

Patent: Clear, unobstructed

Petechia: A hemorrhage into the skin of less than 3 mm in diameter

Plasminogen Activator: A heterogeneous group of serine proteases capable of converting plasminogen to plasmin; for example, tissue plasminogen activator (endothelium, uterus, heart), circulating plasma plasminogen activator, urokinase, and kidney tissue cell cultures

Platelet (Thrombocyte): An anucleate cell produced by cytoplasmic fragmentation of a bone marrow cell known as the megakaryocyte. The platelet is responsible for ongoing repair of blood vessel intima and initiation of plasma coagulation in the case of vascular trauma.

Platelet Activating Factor: An ether–lipid release product from antigen-stimulated leukocytes of the composition acetyl glyceryl ether phosphorylcholine. It acts to induce platelet aggregation and is a mediator of hypersensitivity.

Platelet-Derived Growth Factor: A protein in the alpha granules of the platelet that stimulates growth of smooth muscle cells

Platelet Distribution Width (PDW): A measure of the shape and breadth of the frequency distribution histogram of platelet size. A high PDW indicates abnormal variation in platelet size.

Platelet Estimate: Approximation of the platelet count by examination of peripheral blood smear. The accuracy of the estimate depends on the quality of the smear, selection of the appropriate fields, and the erythrocyte count.

Platelet Factor 3: Fragments of plasma membrane phospholipid released from the platelet upon activation that serve as a point of assembly for certain of the plasma coagulation reaction complexes such as prothrombinase, also called platelet phospholipid

Platelet Factor 4: A protein contained in the alpha granules of platelets that is released upon activation and is capable of neutralizing heparin

Platelet Immune Complexes: Immune complexes attached to platelets. An immune complex is the reaction product of an antibody and soluble antigen. In most cases immune complexes circulate until they are cleared by the mononuclear–phagocyte system, but often they attach to the Fc receptors of platelets, triggering platelet phagocytosis by macrophages and resulting in an acute but limited thrombocytopenia. The source of circulating antigen may be drugs, viruses, or secretions of bacteria.

Platelet Phospholipid: See *Platelet Factor 3.*

Platelet-Poor Plasma (PPP): The plasma preparation used for most coagulation studies and for setting 100% transmission of light in platelet aggregometry. It is prepared by centrifugation of whole blood at 1600g to 2000g for 5 to 10 minutes.

Platelet Retention: A test designed to measure the adhesion of platelets to a foreign surface. A platelet count is performed before and after whole blood is exposed to glass or some like surface. The count is expected to drop at least 30%, but certain diseases, such as von Willebrand disease, result in diminished adhesion. Results of tests of platelet retention are influenced by platelet aggregation as well as adhesion.

Platelet-Rich Plasma (PRP): The supernatant of whole blood required for platelet aggregometry, having a high concentration of platelets. It is prepared by centrifugation of whole blood at 75g to 100g for 5 to 10 minutes.

Platelet Satellitism: The tendency for platelets to adhere closely to neutrophils when the blood is collected in EDTA. It is believed that platelet satellitism is immune-mediated, but there are no known clinical symptoms. The phenomenon is visible in the Wright-stained blood smear.

Pluripotential: Able to differentiate into one of several cell lines

Poietin: A humoral substance that induces a pluripotential stem cell to differentiate into a specific cell line

Posttransfusion Purpura (PTP): A condition characterized by delayed thrombocytopenia and bleeding following transfusion. Most patients who have this disorder lack the Pl^{A1} antigen, which is present in 98% of the donors.

Precision: The degree of agreement among individual measurements performed at a specific laboratory under prescribed conditions

Primary Hemostasis: The part of the hemostatic mechanism that is responsible for initiation. *Primary hemostasis* usually refers to the role of the platelet in triggering coagulation.

Procoagulant: Proteins or other material that when activated may provide the constituents necessary for coagulation

Proplatelet Process: An extension of megakaryocyte cytoplasm through endothelial fenestra into bone marrow sinusoids. The proplatelet process is the source of platelets, which form by fragmentation into the passing blood.

Prostacyclin: One of the metabolic oxidation products of arachidonic acid. Prostacyclin is a product of the prostacyclin synthetase reactions on prostaglandin (PGH_2) and is a smooth muscle relaxant that inhibits platelet aggregation.

Prostaglandin: Naturally occurring 20-carbon fatty acids that have numerous and diverse biologic actions such as constriction or dilation of blood vessels, enhancement or inhibition of platelet aggregation, and induction of labor or termination of pregnancy, depending on the specific prostaglandin and target tissue involved

Protein C: A vitamin K–dependent serine protease possessing anticoagulant properties characterized by inhibitory action against Factors V and VIII. It has the additional property of stimulating fibrinolysis. Protein C is converted to its enzymatic form (protein C_a) by a complex of thrombin and thrombomodulin, an endothelial cell thrombin receptor.

Protein S: A vitamin K–dependent factor that markedly enhances the activity of protein C

Prothrombinase: A complex composed of Factors X_a and V_a, phospholipid, and calcium that acts as an enzyme to convert prothrombin to thrombin

Pseudo–von Willebrand Disease: A platelet disorder characterized by increased binding of von Willebrand factor to the platelet, resulting in the depletion of the factor from the plasma

Purpura: A hemorrhage into the skin between 3 mm and 10 mm in diameter. Also, a group of hemorrhagic diseases characterized by hemorrhage into the skin, mucous membranes, and serosal surfaces

Receptor: A specific molecule on the surface of a cell, usually glycoprotein, which reacts to bond a humoral substance. In the case of the platelet, this binding often results in activation of the cell.

Rees-Ecker Platelet Count: A manual technique that was widely used before the introduction of the Brecher-Cronkite technique. Whole blood is diluted in a solution of brilliant crystal blue dye that stains the platelets light blue. Cells are counted on a Neubauer grid under transmitted light microscopy.

Reptilase: Trade name for a thrombin substitute derived from the venom of the pit viper *Bothrops atrox* that is used in a clot-based assay similar to the thrombin time

Ristocetin: An antibiotic that induces agglutination of platelets in the presence of von Willebrand factor. It is used as an agonist of platelet aggregation. Platelets will not agglutinate to ristocetin in von Willebrand disease or Bernard-Soulier syndrome.

Russell's Viper Venom (Stypven): A form of tissue thromboplastin derived from snake venom that activates the coagulation pathway at the level of Factor X. It is useful in detecting Factor X deficiency.

Salzman Technique: An *in vitro* platelet retention technique. Blood is passed through a glass-bead–filled column, and a platelet count is performed. This is compared to a count on untreated whole blood. The second count is expected to be lower than the first.

Sarcoplasmic Reticulum: A system of connecting tubes within a muscle fiber that serve to conduct calcium ions to the actomyosin molecules for activation

Schizocyte (Schistocyte): A split or broken erythrocyte, often present as a result of microangiopathic anemia with destruction of red cells. Schizocytes may be erroneously included in an automated platelet count.

Sensitivity: A value representing the lowest concentration of a substance that can be quantitated with confidence

Serine Protease: A classification of proteins the enzymatic action of which is like that of trypsin in that they selectively hydrolyze peptide bonds containing arginine or lysine. These enzymes circulate in a zymogenic form, and their activities are regulated by specific activators and inhibitors.

Serine Protease–Inhibitor Complexes: An endogenously formed complex between an enzyme (serine protease) and its specific inhibitor. These complexes are usually cleared rapidly from circulation but may show elevated levels in certain disease states.

Serotonin: An amine hormone, metabolite of L-tryptophane, that is secreted by the chromaffin cells of the gastrointestinal mucosa and is found in the dense bodies of platelets. It is a powerful vasoconstrictor and participates in the formation of the hemostatic platelet plug.

Simplastin A: Trade name for a lyophilized preparation of thromboplastin and calcium with additional amounts of Factors I and V

Simplate: Trade name for a spring-loaded, disposable lancet that produces a standard wound for performance of the bleeding time test (Organon Teknika, Parsipanny, NJ 07054)

Sinusoid: A distended capillary, the endothelium of which is fenestrated and supports the presence of macrophages on its surface. Sinusoids are found in the bone marrow, spleen, and liver.

Specificity: The ability to determine only the single component that is being assayed and not other substances that may be present

Spleen: A highly vascular hematopoietic organ located within the left upper quadrant of the peritoneum. The spleen consists of the red pulp, which is the main phagocytic constituent of the body and is full of branching sinusoids, and the white pulp, which is filled with small lymphocytes. The spleen is surrounded by a thick connective tissue capsule and supported throughout with branching connective tissue trabeculae.

Spurious Thrombocytopenia: A falsely diminished platelet count caused by platelet clumping, the presence of giant platelets, or platelet satellitism. Platelets pass through the orifice of the particle counter in clumps that are counted as single pulses.

Standard Deviation (SD): The measurement of the spread in individual laboratory results about the laboratory mean value

Stem Cell: A cell capable of asymmetric mitosis

Storage Pool Disorder: A thrombocytopathy in which platelet secretion (release) is impaired, probably because of diminished levels of ADP or serotonin in dense body granules. Aggregation patterns are usually diminished or may show primary aggregation followed by disaggregation, and no aggregation with collagen.

Streptokinase: A proteolytic enzyme of the hydrolase class that activates plasminogen. It is not found in the human, but rather is produced by group A streptococci and used therapeutically to dissolve thrombi.

Stromal Cells of the Bone Marrow: Cells such as osteoblasts that make the supporting mineralized bony matrix

Subendothelium: The layer of the blood vessel wall external and adjacent to the innermost endothelial layer. The subendothelium is rich in collagen fibrils, which induce adhesion and activation of platelets and the coagulation mechanism.

Syncytium: A multinucleate mass of protoplasm produced by the fusion of uninucleate cells

Systolic Pressure: The blood pressure in the artery during the period of contraction of the ventricles

TAR Syndrome: Congenital hypoplastic thrombocytopenia with absent radii inherited as an autosomal-recessive trait. Patients have reduced platelets as well as platelet functional abnormalities due most likely to a storage pool defect.

Thrombasthenia: A rare, severe congenital bleeding disorder, transmitted as an autosomal-recessive trait, in which platelets function abnormally although they are normal in number. There is usually no aggregation response to ADP, epinephrine, or collagen, a prolonged bleeding time, and normal clotting factors; also called Glanzmann's thrombasthenia.

Thrombocythemia: A fixed increase in circulating platelets associated with an increase in megakaryocyte number and volume. The term is usually used in reference to myeloproliferative disorders such as essential thrombocythemia in which the platelet count is frequently greater than $1,000,000/\mu l$.

Thrombocytopathy: The term at one time referred to abnormal platelet function seen in storage pool disorder or aspirinlike syndrome. Aggregometry often shows a pattern of primary aggregation followed by disaggregation when ADP or epinephrine is used as an agonist, or no aggregation to collagen.

Thrombocytopenia: A decrease in the number of circulating platelets; a platelet count below $1.5 \times 10^3/\mu l$

Thrombocytosis: An increase in the number of circulating platelets; platelet count above $4 \times 10^3/\mu l$

β-Thromboglobulin: A protein contained in the alpha granules of platelets that is released upon activation and that neutralizes heparin weakly. It is often used as a marker for platelet activation because it is unique to the platelet and because it is mildly vasoactive.

Thrombolytic Therapy: Exogenous administration of fibrinolytic agents, such as urokinase, streptokinase, or tissue plasminogen activator, to induce a lytic action or dissolution of a preformed clot

Thrombomodulin: A cofactor found on the endothelium that helps to inactivate thrombin

Thromboplastin: A substance having procoagulant properties that is found in most tissues

Thrombopoietin: The poietin that induces formation of the megakaryocytic cell line

Thrombosis: Formation of a clot in a blood vessel, a lung, or the heart. The clot is composed of platelets, fibrin, and usually erythrocytes.

Thrombospondin: A high-molecular-weight glycoprotein released from the platelet alpha granule of thrombin-stimulated platelets that may play a role in platelet aggregation

Thrombotic Thrombocytopenic Purpura: A clinical condition marked by increased platelet consumption and thrombi in the microcirculation

Thromboxane: A prostaglandin product of platelet activation formed from arachidonic acid through the cyclooxygenase pathway. This substance is one of the most potent aggregating agents and produces strong contraction of vascular muscles and platelet shape change.

Thrombus: A gel-like aggregation of blood elements, particularly platelets and fibrin, but also other elements like red blood cells; also referred to as a blood clot

Tissue Plasminogen Activator (tPA): A glycoprotein, produced and secreted by the vascular intima, that activates plasminogen within a fibrin clot

Tourniquet Test: A clinical test to measure the escape of blood from capillaries under stress. A pressure cuff is applied to the arm and inflated to between the systolic and diastolic pressures for a specified period. When it is released, the arm is observed for petechiae below the level of the tourniquet. The presence of more than five petechiae in a 3-cm circle is evidence of abnormal fragility.

Transaminase: That group of enzymes that catalyzes the transfer of amino groups in the interconversion of a-amino acids and a-oxoacids; also called aminotransferases

Trilaminar: Demonstrating three layers

Tubulin: Dimeric repeating subunits about 4 nm in diameter that combine to make up microtubules

Ultrastructure: Cell structure beyond the resolving power of the light microscope

Vasculature: The system of the body pertaining to blood vessels

Volar: Referring to the palm of the hand or the sole of the foot

Von Willebrand Disease: An autosomal-dominant bleeding disorder in which the bleeding is from the mucous membranes and skin. There are many variants, with mild to severe expression depending on the amount of decrease of the von Willebrand factor.

Von Willebrand Factor: That part of the Factor VIII molecule responsible for platelet adhesion and function. It is also referred to as Factor VIII/vWF, ristocetin cofactor, and VIIIR:Ag.

Wright Stain: A polychromatic Romanowsky-type stain, commonly used for blood smears

Index

The letter *f* following a page number indicates a figure; the letter *t* following a page number indicates a table.

Drugs Affecting Platelets

Platelet Agglutination
Ristocetin

Platelet Aggregation, Inhibition
Aspirin
Calcium channel blockers
Chlorpheniramine
Cyproheptadine
Diflunisal
Diltiazem
Diphenhydramine
Dipyridamole
Fenoprofen
Hydroxychloroquine
Ibuprofen
Indomethacin
Isoproterenol
Methapyrilene
Mezlocillin
Nifedipine
Persantin(e)
Piperacillin
Promethazine
Propranalol
Ticarcillin
Urokinase
Valproic acid

Platelet Survival, Increased
Dipyridamole

Purpura
Acetaminophen
Aminosalicylic acid
Amitriptyline
Amobarbital
Amphotericin B
Arsenicals
Aspirin
Butabarbital
Carbamazepine
Carbenicillin
Carbimazole
Cephalothin
Chloral hydrate
Chlorophenothane
Chloroquine
Chlorothiazide
Chlorpheniramine
Chlorpropamide
Cloxacillin
Cycloserine
Desipramine
Diazepam
Diazoxide
Diphenhydramine
Erythromycin
Ethambutol
Furosemide
Glutethimide
Gold
Griseofulvin
Hydralazine
Hydrochlorothiazide
Ibuprofen
Imipramine
Indomethacin
Iodides
Isoniazid
Levodopa
Measles vaccine
Mefenamic acid
Meprobamate
Methaqualone
Methylthiouracil
Nalidixic acid
Nitrofurantoin

Oxazepam
Oxyphenbutazone
Oxytetracycline
Penicillin
Pentobarbital
Perphenazine
Pertussis vaccine
Phenobarbital
Phenylbutazone
Practolol
Propylthiouracil
Protriptyline
Quinacrine
Quinidine
Quinine
Rifampin
Salicylazosulfapyridine
Streptomycin
Sulfadoxine
Sulfamerazine
Sulfamethazine
Sulfamethizole
Sulfamethoxypyridazine
Sulfanilamide
Sulfapyridine
Sulfathiazole
Sulfisoxazole
Tetanus vaccine
Tolbutamide
Trimethoprim-sulfamethoxazole

Purpura, Nonthrombocytopenic
Aminosalicylic acid
Antidepressants
Antihistamines
Arsenicals
Aspirin
Betamethasone
Carbamazepine
Carbenicillin
Carbimazole
Carbromal
Carphenazine
Chlorophenothane
Chloroquine
Chlorothiazide
Chlorpheniramine
Chlorpromazine
Chlorpropamide
Chlortetracycline
Colchicine
Corticotropin
Cortisone
Dexamethasone
Diatrizoate
Digoxin
Diphenyhydramine
Diphenylhydantoin
Dobutamine
Erythromycin
Glucocorticoids
Glyburide
Hydrocortisone
Indomethacin
Influenza vaccine
Isoniazid
Isoxicam
Lithium
Meclofenemate
Meprobamate
Methylprednisolone
Moxalactam
Naproxen
Oxytetracycline
Penicillamine
Penicillin

Pentazocine
Pertussis vaccine
Phentolamine
Phenylbutazone
Piperacillin
Prednisolone
Prednisone
Promethazine
Propranolol
Propylthiouracil
Quinidine
Quinine
Reserpine
Smallpox vaccine
Stibophen
Sulfapyridine
Sulfisoxazole
Sulfonamides
Sulindac
Theophylline
Tolbutamide
Triamcinolone
Trichlormethiazide
Trifluoperazine
Trimethadione

Thrombocytopenia
Acetaminophen
Acetazolamide
Acetohexamide
Allopurinol
Aminopyrine
Aminosalicylic acid
Amitriptyline
Amobarbital
Amodiaquine
Amphotericin B
Ampicillin
Amrinone
Antazoline
Antihistamines
Arsenicals
Arsine
Aspirin
Azathioprine
Bendroflumethiazide
Benzene
Butabarbital
Carbamazepine
Carbimazole
Carbon tetrachloride
Carbromal
Cefazolin
Cephalexin
Cephaloridine
Cephalothin
Chloramphenicol
Chlorate
Chlordiazepoxide
Chloroguanide
Chlorophenothane
Chloroquine
Chlorothiazide
Chlorpheniramine
Chlorpromazine
Chlorpropamide
Chlortetracycline
Chlorthalidone
Clindamycin
Clofibrate
Cloxacillin
Colchicine
Contraceptive agents, oral
Dantrolene sodium
Dapsone
Desipramine
Dexamethasone